KU-067-239

COLOR
ATLAS OF
CLINICAL
HEMATOLOGY

FOURTH EDITION

E141   WH 17 HOF

369 0160382

E141   WH 17 HOF

COLOR ATLAS OF
CLINICAL HEMATOLOGY

FOURTH EDITION

A. Victor Hoffbrand, MA, DM, DSc, FRCP, FRCPath, FRCP (Edin), FMedSci
Emeritus Professor of Hematology
The Royal Free and University College Medical School
Honorary Consultant Hematologist
Royal Free Hospital
London, United Kingdom

John E. Pettit, MD (Otago), FRCPA, FRCPath
Director and Hematologist, Medlab South Ltd
Christchurch, New Zealand
Formerly Associate Professor of Hematology
University of Otago Medical School
Dunedin, New Zealand

Paresh Vyas, BM, FRCP, FRCPath, DPhil
Department of Haematology and MRC Molecular Haematology Unit
John Radcliffe Hospital and Weatherall Institute of Molecular Medicine
Oxford, England

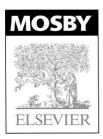

MOSBY

ELSEVIER

1600 John F. Kennedy Blvd.
Ste 1800
Philadelphia, PA 19103-2899

COLOR ATLAS OF CLINICAL HEMATOLOGY, FOURTH EDITION   ISBN: 978-0-323-04453-0

Copyright © 2010 by Mosby, LTD., an affiliate of Elsevier Ltd.
© 2002 Elsevier Science Limited 2002. All rights reserved.
© Harcourt Publishers Limited 2000.

All rights reserved. No part of this publication may be reproduced or transmitted in any form or by any means, electronic or mechanical, including photocopying, recording, or any information storage and retrieval system, without permission in writing from the publisher. Permissions may be sought directly from Elsevier's Rights Department: phone: (+1) 215 239 3804 (US) or (+44) 1865 843830 (UK); fax: (+44) 1865 853333; e-mail: healthpermissions@elsevier.com. You may also complete your request on-line via the Elsevier website at http://www.elsevier.com/permissions.

Notice

Knowledge and best practice in this field are constantly changing. As new research and experience broaden our knowledge, changes in practice, treatment and drug therapy may become necessary or appropriate. Readers are advised to check the most current information provided (i) on procedures featured or (ii) by the manufacturer of each product to be administered, to verify the recommended dose or formula, the method and duration of administration, and contraindications. It is the responsibility of the practitioner, relying on their own experience and knowledge of the patient, to make diagnoses, to determine dosages and the best treatment for each individual patient, and to take all appropriate safety precautions. To the fullest extent of the law, neither the Publisher nor the Authors assume any liability for any injury and/or damage to persons or property arising out of or related to any use of the material contained in this book.

The Publisher

Library of Congress Cataloging-in-Publication Data

Color atlas of clinical hematology / A. Victor Hoffbrand ... [et al.].
—4th ed.
 p. ; cm.
 Rev. ed. of: Color atlas of clinical hematology / A. Victor Hoffbrand,
John E. Pettit. 3rd ed. 2000.
 Includes bibliographical references and index.
 ISBN 978-0-323-04453-0
 1. Blood—Diseases—Diagnosis—Atlases. 2. Hematology—Atlases. 3. Hematology—Atlases.
I. Hoffbrand, A. Victor. II. Hoffbrand, A. Victor.
Color atlas of clinical hematology.
 [DNLM: 1. Hematologic Diseases—Atlases. WH 17 C7188 2009]
 RC636.H63 2010
 616.1'50758—dc22

                                        2008012157

Acquisitions Editor: Dolores Meloni
Developmental Editors: Elena Pushaw, Kimberly DePaul, John Ormiston
Design Direction: Lou Forgione
Business Controller: Patrick Corcoran

Printed in China

Last digit is the print number: 9 8 7 6 5 4 3 2 1

Working together to grow
libraries in developing countries

www.elsevier.com | www.bookaid.org | www.sabre.org

ELSEVIER   BOOK AID International   Sabre Foundation

PREFACE

Since the previous edition was published in 2000, major advances have occurred in the understanding of the molecular basis of hematological diseases. The World Health Organization (2008) Classification of Hematological Malignancies has incorporated this new knowledge to define many of these diseases and to add new entities. Molecular genetics are also now used more widely to classify benign disorders such as the thalassemias, inherited bone marrow failure syndromes, iron refractory iron deficiency anemia, hemochromatosis, and inherited coagulation disorders. We have attempted to fully illustrate this new knowledge in the fourth edition of the *Color Atlas of Clinical Hematology*. Scientific diagrams, images of cytogenetics, fluorescent in-situ hybridization (FISH), and gene arrays are included throughout. Fluorescent-activated cell sorting (FACS) and new imaging techniques, including FDG-PET, widely used in the diagnosis of Hodgkin and non-Hodgkin lymphoma, are also extensively included.

The two original authors have been joined for this edition by Dr. Paresh Vyas from the Weatherall Institute of Molecular Medicine; Dr. Vyas has taken responsibility for the first three chapters, which deal with the basic science of blood formation, including cell machinery, cellular aspects of hematopoiesis, and growth factors. We give only brief descriptions of therapy and have omitted the section from the previous edition on fine needle aspirate (FNA) appearances in nonhematological disease since FNA has now largely been replaced by tru-cut biopsy in hematological practice.

We thank the many colleagues throughout the world who have generously provided images. They are acknowledged on the individual figures. We particularly thank Dr. Elisabeth Nacheva and Dr. Wendy Erber for many cytogenetic, FISH, FACS, and hematopathology images, without which the book would have been incomplete. Professor Elias Campo came to our rescue when we needed many additional figures to comprehensively illustrate the new WHO 2008 classification of lymphomas, and we thank him and Professor Elaine Jaffe for giving us access to the provisional 2008 WHO classification prior to its publication. Professor Peter Isaacson and Dr. Alan Ramsay have also generously given many immunohistological images. We are sad that Professor David Mason, an outstanding hematopathologist and colleague, who was a major contributor to the Atlas in the third edition, died in 2008.

We are grateful to our Publishers and particularly Dolores Meloni, Michael Troy, Joan Sinclair, and John Ormiston for their unstinting help in assembling this vast amount of complex material into its final form. We are grateful to Jane Fallows for her expert scientific diagrams and the Department of Medical Illustration, Royal Free Hospital for expertise in assembling many electronic images into a publishable form. They have all been remarkably patient during our multiple additions and updating. We are also grateful to Avril van der Loo, who expertly typed and retyped the majority of the chapters.

We hope this book in its printed and electronic versions will be used as a comprehensive, up-to-date illustrated encyclopedia of blood diseases. We would be grateful to receive offers of new images for future editions and also advice if any errors or omissions have occurred in what has been an immense task.

A. Victor Hoffbrand
John E. Pettit
Paresh Vyas
2009

CONTENTS

CHAPTER

CELL MACHINERY

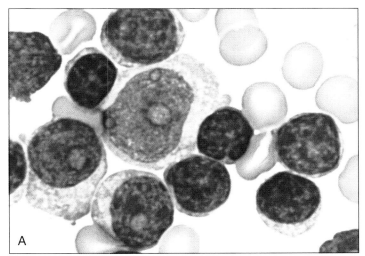

MOLECULAR AND CELLULAR BIOLOGY OF THE CELL

There have been and continue to be rapid advances in our understanding of the basic mechanisms that regulate the molecular and cellular processes within a cell. The aim of this chapter is to provide a primer of our understanding of these processes. This is relevant to clinical hematology because when these processes are deregulated, for example, by acquisition of genetic mutations, this can give rise to hematologic disorders.

COMPARTMENTALIZATION OF THE CELL

A central evolutionary advance was the compartmentalization of cells. Figure 1-1 shows the compartments in a cell. The cell is bounded by a complex cell membrane that allows regulation of molecules into and out of the cell. Within the cytoplasm a number of different organelles perform key functions. For example, as described later in this chapter, mitochondria are critical for adenosine triphosphate (ATP) generation and heme biosynthesis. Proteins are translated from amino acids and undergo posttranslational modification in the Golgi complex and rough endoplasmic reticulum. Depending on the cell type, there are specialized structures within the cytoplasm, such as granules, that allow the cell to perform its specialized role.

THE NUCLEUS

As we focus in on the nucleus, it is clear that it is also bounded by a specialized nuclear envelope and membrane (Fig. 1-2). Entry into and exit out of the nucleus is regulated by nuclear pores. Within the nucleus, deoxyribonucleic acid (DNA) is tightly packaged by proteins and the DNA-protein complex is known as chromatin. Chromatin has different appearances under the light and electron microscope. When DNA is tightly packaged (and the genes more likely to be not expressed) it is known as heterochromatin. Under the light/electron microscope it appears darker. When DNA is less tightly packaged it is described as euchromatin and is lighter in appearance. The other visible structure within the nucleus, in some cells, is the nucleolus, where ribosomal genes are transcribed and assembly of the ribosome takes place.

The DNA in the nucleus is distributed among 22 pairs of autosomal chromosomes (numbered 1 to 22, in order of size) and two sex chromosomes (Fig. 1-3, A). When cells are in the metaphase of the cell cycle (see Fig. 1-32), chromosomes condense and can be visualized by a technique called *karyotyping*. Chromosomes are divided into two arms, a short arm, p, and a longer arm, q. The region where the chromosomes join is termed the *centromere*. Chromosomes are further subdivided into numeric light and dark bands (depending on how they stain with the Giemsa dye). These structures can be visualized (Fig. 1-3, B). Furthermore, when cells are not in metaphase, chromosomes are more diffusely spread through the nucleus. Most current evidence suggests that the chromosomes

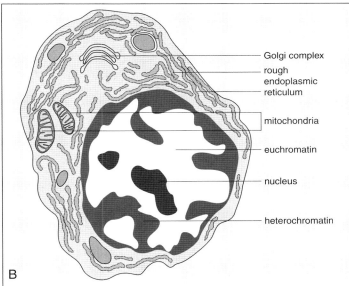

Fig. 1-1. A, Photomicrograph showing the morphology of many cells with prominent nucleoli, in this case, B cells. **B,** A schematic representation of the intracellular composition as visualized by electron microscopy. The nucleus is composed of euchromatin, which is less condensed, paler, and more transcriptionally active, and heterochromatin, which is more condensed, darker, and less transcriptionally active. In cytoplasm subcellular organelles including mitochondria, rough endoplasmic reticulum, and the Golgi complex are shown. The function of these organelles is discussed later. (A, Courtesy of Professor J.V. Melo.)

occupy discrete territories (chromosomal territories) within a nucleus (Fig. 1-3, C). These territories need not be contiguous and can be shared with other chromosomes. However, there are still many aspects of how chromosomes are organized that remain unclear. Just two questions include, first, what constrains chromosomes to territories and, second, how do territories affect gene regulation.

1

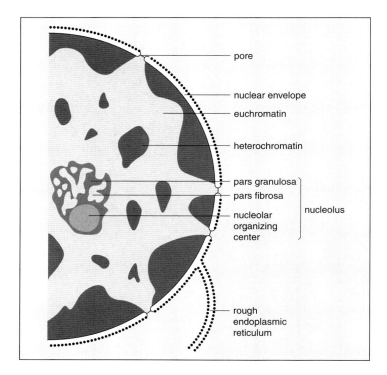

Fig. 1-2. A schematic representation of a portion of the nucleus. The nucleus is highly compartmentalized, containing specialized structures. The nucleolus is composed of a pars granulosa, a pars fibrosa, and a nucleolar organizing center and makes t-RNA. The nucleus is bounded by a nuclear envelope that is lined by rough endoplasmic reticulum. There is controlled entry and exit into the nucleus via nuclear pores.

More recent work over the last decade has suggested that within chromosomal territories chromatin exists in loops and that actively expressed genes along the chromosome and possibly even from different chromosomes may congregate in specialized structures called *transcription factories* (see later).

The sequencing of the human genome was a landmark in biology. It has enabled scientists to catalog all of the human genes arrayed along the chromosomes (Fig. 1-4). Genes are divided into protein coding genes (of which there are approximately 21,000), genes that encode different types of ribonucleic acid (RNA) (e.g., ribosomal RNA, micro-RNAs, small nuclear RNA), and genes that make an RNA moiety that is not translated into a functional protein or RNA (pseudogenes). This provides a primary description of our genetic makeup. The characterization of the human genome is still being refined as we understand more about how genes are organized.

Genes themselves are composed of deoxyribonucleic acid (DNA) (Fig. 1-5). DNA is composed of four nucleotides. Each nucleotide consists of a phosphate group linked by a phosphoester bond to a pentose sugar molecule (ribose) that lacks a hydroxyl group (thus is deoxyribose) that is then attached to one of four heterocyclic carbon- and nitrogen-containing organic rings: adenine (A), cytosine (C), guanine (G), and thymine (T). C and T are known as pyrimidines and A and G as purines. These are then linked together into polynucleotides via phosphoester bonds. As Watson and Crick correctly proposed, these are organized into two associated antiparallel polynucleotide strands that have a 5′ to 3′ direction and form a double helix. The strands are held in register by base-pairing between the two strands such that an A is paired with a T via two hydrogen bonds and a C with a G via three hydrogen bonds. Hydrophobic and van der Waals interactions combine with the thousands of hydrogen bonds to give the double

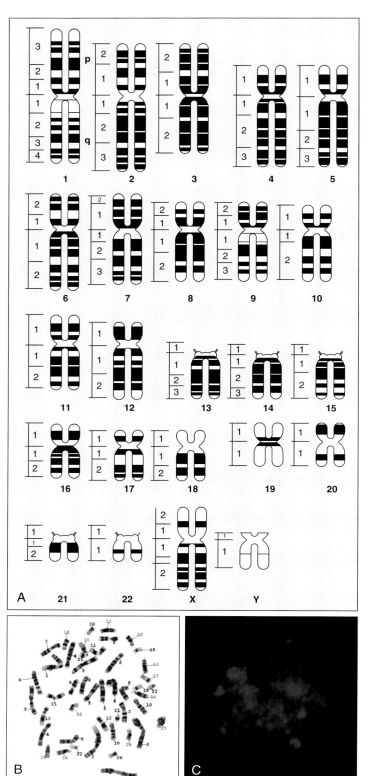

Fig. 1-3. A, DNA in the nucleus is organized into 46 chromosomes. There are two copies of chromosomes 1 to 22 with two sex chromosomes (XX or XY). Each chromosome is divided into a short arm (p) and a long arm (q) and then subdivided into major numeric subsections. For example, the short arm of chromosome 1 (1p) has three subsections and the long arm (1q) has four subsections. **B,** The gross subdivision of chromosome can be visualized by Giemsa staining of chromosomes that have been subject to brief proteolytic cleavage. **C,** Within an interphase nucleus chromosomes occupy discrete territories. The figure shows the territory occupied by chromosome 11 (red color) in a primary erythroblast. (*B,* Courtesy of Professor H. Lodish. *C,* Courtesy of Jo Green and Dr. Veronica Buckle.) (See also Chapter 12.)

Chromosome 1
Length: 247,249,719 bps
Known Protein coding Genes: 2,146
Novel Protein coding Genes: 54
Pseudogene Genes: 159
miRNA Genes: 43
rRNA Genes: 42
snRNA Genes: 178
snoRNA Genes: 60
Misc RNA Genes: 93
SNPs: 959,707

Chromosome 2
Length: 242,951,149 bps
Known Protein coding Genes: 1,375
Novel Protein coding Genes: 84
Pseudogene Genes: 40
miRNA Genes: 23
rRNA Genes: 24
snRNA Genes: 116
snoRNA Genes: 37
Misc RNA Genes: 74
SNPs: 897,485

Chromosome 3
Length: 199,501,827 bps
Known Protein coding Genes: 1,111
Novel Protein coding Genes: 47
Pseudogene Genes: 45
miRNA Genes: 24
rRNA Genes: 21
snRNA Genes: 89
snoRNA Genes: 30
Misc RNA Genes: 66
SNPs: 741,052

Chromosome 4
Length: 191,273,063 bps
Known Protein coding Genes: 828
Novel Protein coding Genes: 59
Pseudogene Genes: 32
miRNA Genes: 21
rRNA Genes: 13
snRNA Genes: 81
snoRNA Genes: 16
Misc RNA Genes: 58
SNPs: 775,836

Chromosome 5
Length: 180,857,866 bps
Known Protein coding Genes: 922
Novel Protein coding Genes: 63
Pseudogene Genes: 23
miRNA Genes: 19
rRNA Genes: 22
snRNA Genes: 74
snoRNA Genes: 18
Misc RNA Genes: 67
SNPs: 662,967

Chromosome 6
Length: 170,899,992 bps
Known Protein coding Genes: 1,103
Novel Protein coding Genes: 29
Pseudogene Genes: 81
miRNA Genes: 17
rRNA Genes: 16
snRNA Genes: 82
snoRNA Genes: 25
Misc RNA Genes: 56
SNPs: 724,817

Chromosome 7
Length: 158,821,424 bps
Known Protein coding Genes: 984
Novel Protein coding Genes: 68
Pseudogene Genes: 48
miRNA Genes: 31
rRNA Genes: 14
snRNA Genes: 64
snoRNA Genes: 27
Misc RNA Genes: 62
SNPs: 612,979

Chromosome 8
Length: 146,274,826 bps
Known Protein coding Genes: 736
Novel Protein coding Genes: 32
Pseudogene Genes: 19
miRNA Genes: 17
rRNA Genes: 14
snRNA Genes: 61
snoRNA Genes: 21
Misc RNA Genes: 39
SNPs: 579,334

Chromosome 9
Length: 140,273,252 bps
Known Protein coding Genes: 921
Novel Protein coding Genes: 38
Pseudogene Genes: 66
miRNA Genes: 26
rRNA Genes: 11
snRNA Genes: 43
snoRNA Genes: 15
Misc RNA Genes: 47
SNPs: 582,297

Chromosome 10
Length: 135,374,737 bps
Known Protein coding Genes: 819
Novel Protein coding Genes: 35
Pseudogene Genes: 52
miRNA Genes: 16
rRNA Genes: 17
snRNA Genes: 64
snoRNA Genes: 8
Misc RNA Genes: 42
SNPs: 584,001

Chromosome 11
Length: 134,452,384 bps
Known Protein coding Genes: 1,390
Novel Protein coding Genes: 52
Pseudogene Genes: 61
miRNA Genes: 19
rRNA Genes: 19
snRNA Genes: 51
snoRNA Genes: 40
Misc RNA Genes: 47
SNPs: 566,679

Chromosome 12
Length: 132,349,534 bps
Known Protein coding Genes: 1,088
Novel Protein coding Genes: 51
Pseudogene Genes: 38
miRNA Genes: 21
rRNA Genes: 15
snRNA Genes: 77
snoRNA Genes: 21
Misc RNA Genes: 65
SNPs: 532,785

Chromosome 13
Length: 114,142,980 bps
Known Protein coding Genes: 358
Novel Protein coding Genes: 10
Pseudogene Genes: 41
miRNA Genes: 14
rRNA Genes: 9
snRNA Genes: 29
snoRNA Genes: 12
Misc RNA Genes: 34
SNPs: 405,240

Chromosome 14
Length: 106,368,585 bps
Known Protein coding Genes: 661
Novel Protein coding Genes: 28
Pseudogene Genes: 25
miRNA Genes: 51
rRNA Genes: 14
snRNA Genes: 42
snoRNA Genes: 56
Misc RNA Genes: 38
SNPs: 351,504

Chromosome 15
Length: 100,338,915 bps
Known Protein coding Genes: 657
Novel Protein coding Genes: 65
Pseudogene Genes: 34
miRNA Genes: 15
rRNA Genes: 6
snRNA Genes: 43
snoRNA Genes: 95
Misc RNA Genes: 35
SNPs: 336,612

Chromosome 16
Length: 88,827,254 bps
Known Protein coding Genes: 915
Novel Protein coding Genes: 49
Pseudogene Genes: 25
miRNA Genes: 14
rRNA Genes: 13
snRNA Genes: 39
snoRNA Genes: 14
Misc RNA Genes: 31
SNPs: 372,250

Chromosome 17
Length: 78,774,742 bps
Known Protein coding Genes: 1,232
Novel Protein coding Genes: 60
Pseudogene Genes: 56
miRNA Genes: 32
rRNA Genes: 10
snRNA Genes: 47
snoRNA Genes: 29
Misc RNA Genes: 52
SNPs: 311,411

Chromosome 18
Length: 76,117,153 bps
Known Protein coding Genes: 293
Novel Protein coding Genes: 20
Pseudogene Genes: 8
miRNA Genes: 9
rRNA Genes: 5
snRNA Genes: 42
snoRNA Genes: 12
Misc RNA Genes: 21
SNPs: 314,228

A

Fig. 1-4. All the genes and open reading frames in the human genome have been provisionally characterized from the sequencing of the human genome. This figure shows the number of base pairs, known protein coding genes, novel protein coding genes, pseudogenes, genes encoding micro-RNAs (miRNAs), ribosomal genes (rRNAs), small nuclear RNAs (snRNAs), small nucleolar RNAs (snoRNAs), other RNAs (miscellaneous RNAs), and single-nucleotide polymorphisms (SNPs) encoded by each chromosome. MT, mitochondrion. (Data from NCBI database, Human genome, Build 36.3, www.ncbi.nlm.nih.gov.)

Continued

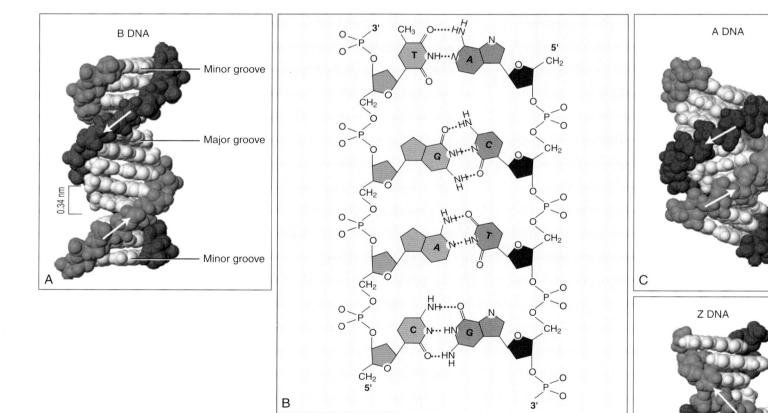

Chromosome 19
Length:	63,811,651 bps
Known Protein coding Genes:	1,428
Novel Protein coding Genes:	49
Pseudogene Genes:	45
miRNA Genes:	71
rRNA Genes:	6
snRNA Genes:	14
snoRNA Genes:	12
Misc RNA Genes:	18
SNPs:	243,927

Chromosome 20
Length:	62,435,964 bps
Known Protein coding Genes:	612
Novel Protein coding Genes:	15
Pseudogene Genes:	29
miRNA Genes:	16
rRNA Genes:	8
snRNA Genes:	32
snoRNA Genes:	16
Misc RNA Genes:	34
SNPs:	324,911

Chromosome 21
Length:	46,944,323 bps
Known Protein coding Genes:	271
Novel Protein coding Genes:	23
Pseudogene Genes:	9
miRNA Genes:	7
rRNA Genes:	3
snRNA Genes:	10
snoRNA Genes:	5
Misc RNA Genes:	6
SNPs:	169,215

Chromosome 22
Length:	49,691,432 bps
Known Protein coding Genes:	509
Novel Protein coding Genes:	26
Pseudogene Genes:	39
miRNA Genes:	15
rRNA Genes:	2
snRNA Genes:	18
snoRNA Genes:	11
Misc RNA Genes:	20
SNPs:	196,364

Chromosome X
Length:	154,913,754 bps
Known Protein coding Genes:	878
Novel Protein coding Genes:	37
Pseudogene Genes:	80
miRNA Genes:	58
rRNA Genes:	19
snRNA Genes:	64
snoRNA Genes:	25
Misc RNA Genes:	48
SNPs:	424,094

Chromosome Y
Length:	57,772,954 bps
Known Protein coding Genes:	86
Novel Protein coding Genes:	27
Pseudogene Genes:	2
miRNA Genes:	2
rRNA Genes:	6
snRNA Genes:	14
snoRNA Genes:	3
Misc RNA Genes:	2
SNPs:	60,414

Chromosome MT
Length:	16,571 bps
Known Protein coding Genes:	13

B

Fig. 1-4, cont'd.

B DNA

Minor groove

Major groove

0.34 nm

Minor groove

A

B

A DNA

C

Z DNA

D

Fig. 1-5. Models of various structures adopted by DNA. **A,** A space-filling model of the "B" form of DNA. This is the common form of DNA, with a helical turn every 10 base pairs. The major and minor grooves of DNA are visible. **B,** A stick model shows that DNA is composed of a sugar phosphate backbone with the bases ("A," "C," "G," and "T") pointing inward (blue and light brown). **C,** More compact "A" form of DNA with 11 bases pairs per helical turn. **D,** "Z" form of DNA is a left-handed helix. (Courtesy of Professor H. Lodish.)

helix great stability. In the common "B" form, the helix is right handed and makes a complete turn every 3.4 nm (about 10 base pairs) (Fig. 1-5). The space between the strands creates a major and minor groove. In low humidity, DNA can adopt a more compact form with 11 base pairs per helical turn ("A" form). Finally, short stretches of DNA composed of alternate purines and pyrimidines can form an alternate stacked Z structure.

GENE TRANSCRIPTION AND mRNA TRANSLATION: THE PRODUCTION AND JOURNEY OF mRNA

A copy of DNA of genes is transcribed into ribonucleic acid (RNA) in the nucleus by a process called transcription. RNA is processed and transported into the cytoplasm. RNA corresponding to protein genes is then translated in the cytoplasm in a process called translation. Not surprisingly, these processes are very complex, affording opportunities to the cell to exquisitely regulate the complement of proteins made, but also making it vulnerable to errors that lead to disease.

Genes are transcribed by one of three different RNA polymerases (RNA Pols). Most protein coding genes are transcribed by RNA Pol II. In addition to RNA Pol II–transcribed genes, genes encoding ribosomal RNAs, small nuclear RNAs, and some transfer RNAs (involved in protein translation) involved in RNA processing are transcribed by RNA Pol I and Pol III, but these genes will not be discussed further in this book. However, it is important to remember that in a typical rapidly growing mammalian cell, approximately 80% of total RNA is ribosomal RNA and approximately 15% is transfer RNA.

When RNA is transcribed, a gene is said to be *expressed*. Transcription of each gene begins at the 5′ end of the gene at its transcriptional start site (TSS) (Fig. 1-6). For any one gene the TSSs can either be single or multiple over several neighboring nucleotides. The DNA sequence 5′ of the gene helps regulate transcription and is known as the *promoter*. This sequence works with other sequences (called regulatory sequences or cis-elements; see later discussion) to provide finely tuned control over the amount of messenger RNA (mRNA)

produced. In Chapter 9, the regulatory sequences involved in globin gene expression are described.

The body of the gene is segmented into exons separated by intervening sequences (introns). Exonic sequence is divided into protein coding and noncoding sequence. RNA Pol II makes an RNA copy of the entire gene (primary transcript). This RNA species is then processed within the nucleus. As the nascent elongating primary transcript is being produced, a 5′ 7-methylguanine cap is added to the 5′ end to protect the RNA from enzymatic degradation. In addition, as nascent RNA transcript (heterogeneous RNA [hnRNA]) emerges from the RNA Pol II, it is sheathed in a large set of nuclear proteins in structures called heterogeneous ribonuclear particles (hnRNPs). hnRNP-associated proteins are important for transport of the RNA species and probably aid in the processing of RNA. Once the primary transcript is made, the 3′ end of the transcript is recognized by a protein complex that includes an enzyme called an endonuclease that cleaves the RNA transcript to produce a 3′ end of the RNA. This then allows the enzyme poly(A) polymerase to attach a homopolymeric string of A residues to the 3′ end called a poly-A tail. Increasing recent evidence suggests that the processes of transcription initiation, elongation by RNA Pol II, and 3′ end processing may be co-regulated.

The introns are then spliced out to form the mature messenger (m)RNA species (a simplified version of this process is presented in Fig. 1-7). Splicing is an elaborate process that involves a large number of steps, catalyzed by a splicing complex (or splicesome) that contains small nuclear RNAs (snRNAs) and proteins to form small nuclear ribonuclear particles (snRNPs). It is estimated that over 100 proteins are involved in splicing. At first approximation, this process is probably a complex as regulation of transcriptional initiation and translation. One reason why a cell invests this degree of effort into splicing is that it allows a cell to generate multiple different mRNA species from a single gene—contributing to the biologic complexity that an organism can achieve from a limited gene set. One important part of splicing is that the two nucleotides that lie in the intron and mark the boundary of an exon-intron are almost always invariant (see Fig. 1-7). Thus the 5′ end of the intron is usually marked by the dinucleotide "GU" whereas the 3′ end is marked by "AG."

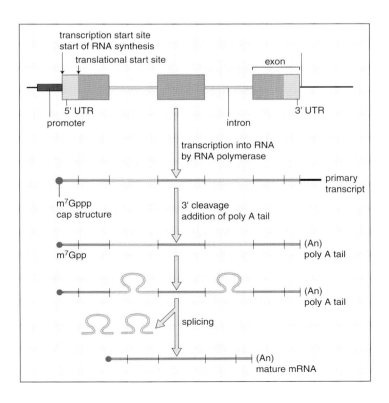

Fig. 1-6. Most genes encoding proteins are first transcribed into mature messenger RNA (mRNA) via multiple steps. *Top,* Genes are divided into exons (shown as boxes) separated by introns (shown as pink lines). Preceding the transcribed region is a promoter region (brown box) that helps regulate transcription timing and rate. A transcriptional initiation site marks the beginning of transcription. The beginning and end of the transcribed regions are usually not translated into protein and are known as the 5′ and 3′ untranslated regions (UTRs) (depicted as yellow boxes). Translated areas are shown as green boxes.

The whole gene from the transcriptional start site is transcribed by RNA polymerase to make a primary transcript. This has a specialized cap structure at its 5′ end to protect the transcript from degradation. The 3′ end of the transcript is then cleaved and a tail of "A" nucleotide residues (known as a poly-A tail—"An") is added at the 3′ end of the transcript (to protect the end from degradation). Then the introns loop out (see later for details) and are spliced out to create mRNA moiety.

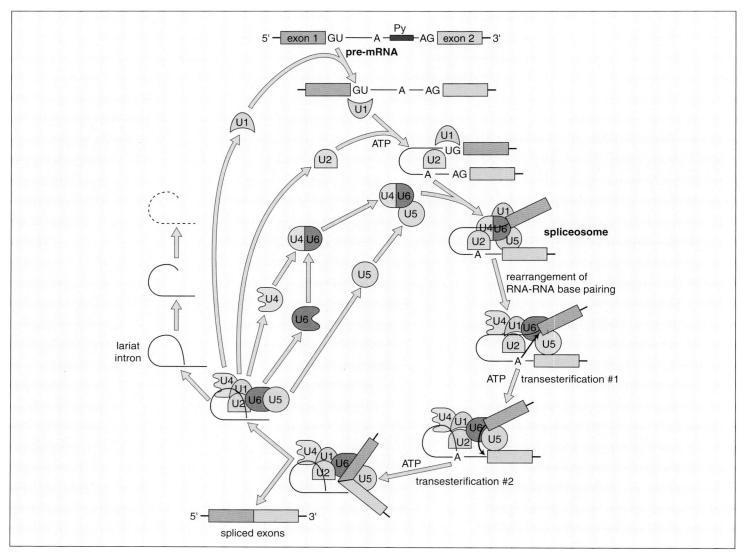

Fig. 1-7. Detail of splicing out of introns coordinated by splicing small nuclear ribonuclear protein particles (snRNPs) U1, U2, and U4 to U6. U1 and U2 snRNPs associate with unspliced transcript in an ordered sequence at specific nucleotides ("GU") at the 5' intron-exon boundary and a pyrimidine tract (Py) near an "A" nucleotide known as the branch point. U4 to U6 then assemble, catalyzing an ATP-dependent rearrangement of RNA base-pairing structure. The snRNPs then catalyze two transesterification reactions that allow the exons to join. The intervening intron forms a lariat structure that is degraded. The snRNPs are recycled.

Like hnRNA, mRNA is wrapped in chaperone proteins, to form messenger ribonuclear particles (mRNPs) that are exported from the nucleus through a water-impermeable phospholipid bilayer, the nuclear envelope, that is studded with proteins and pores (Figs. 1-8 and 1-9). The nuclear pore complex (NPC) is a large structure (approximately 125 million Daltons) about 30 times the size of the ribosome. It is made of multiple copies of a large number of proteins (approximately 100). It has a ring-basket structure. The ring points into the nucleus and filaments form a basket. The structure is embedded in the nuclear envelope. mRNPs are exported to the cytoplasm in a guanosine triphosphate- (GTP-) dependent process through the NPC. It is facilitated by a subset of RNP proteins that contain amino acid sequences that function as nuclear export signals (NESs). Similarly, proteins made in the cytosol have to be imported into the nucleus through NPCs. Such proteins often, but not always, have nuclear localization signal (NLS) sequences.

Once in the cytoplasm, mRNA is covered by cytosolic proteins. The stability of mRNAs is variable and can be regulated (see Chapter 5). This can help determine the amount of mRNA available for protein synthesis.

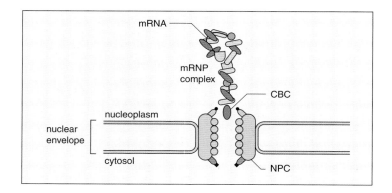

Fig. 1-8. Nascent primary transcripts and mRNAs are associated with nuclear proteins to form heterogeneous ribonuclear protein particles (hnRNPs). Some of these hnRNPs help transport mRNA out of the nucleus. The 5' end of the mRNA-hnRNP complex (mRNP) associates with a cap-biding complex (CBC) that is exported through a specialized nuclear pore complex (NPC). Some of the hnRNPs remain in the nucleus and are recycled. mRNA then interacts with cytosolic mRNP-binding proteins that escort the mRNP to ribosomes to be translated. mRNP export is an active, controlled, and coordinated process.

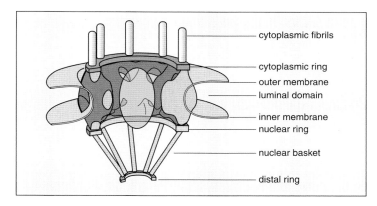

Fig. 1-9. A detailed schematic view of a eukaryotic nuclear pore complex. It is a highly ordered structure that is embedded in the nuclear and cytosolic membranes.

Just as large macromolecular machines are required to make DNA and mRNA, proteins are translated from mRNA in a large structure called a *ribosome*. The details of translation are set out in Fig. 1-10. The large and small ribosomal subunits, with the aid of specific translational initiation proteins (factors), locate the translational start site, which is usually the first codon (the three RNA nucleotides) for the amino acid methionine, in an ATP- and GTP-dependent process. As codons are composed of triplets of mRNA nucleotides, there are three different reading frames or ways in which mRNA triplets can be read by the ribosome. The frame that is selected is defined by the position of the start codon. Once engaged, the ribosome processes along the mRNA and sequentially adds amino acids to the growing peptide chain by recognizing sequential triplets of mRNA nucleotides (codons) (Fig. 1-10B).

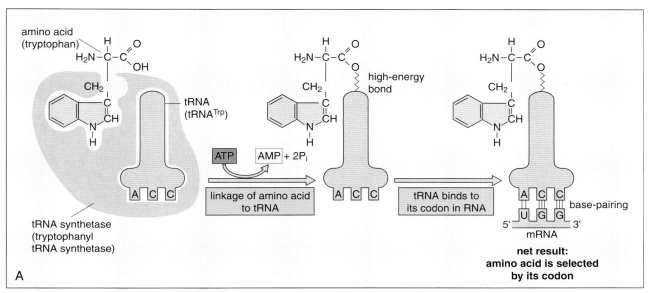

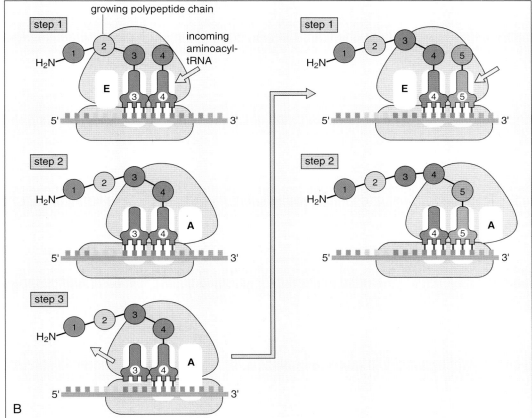

Fig. 1-10. mRNA is translated into proteins. **A,** mRNAs docked in the ribosome interact with transfer RNAs (tRNAs) that bind amino acids. Different amino acids bind specific tRNA molecules. Here, the amino acid tryptophan is coupled to a specific tRNA^{Trp} by an adapter aminoacyl-tRNA synthetase in an ATP-dependent reaction. The triple RNA nucleotide "ACC" sequence in the tRNA^{Trp} (anticodon sequence) then base pairs to a triple RNA sequence "UGG" (codon) in mRNA. Thus the amino acid is selected by specific codon-anticodon recognition. **B,** To form an elongating protein polypeptide in a ribosome from mRNA, amino acids are added sequentially as specific tRNAs are recruited by codon-anticodon base pairing. In this figure, in step 1 on the left-hand side, amino acids 1, 2, and 3 have already been added. Amino acid is docked (via the specific tRNA) next to amino acid 3. In step 2, amino acid 4 is bound to amino acid 3 and a new tRNA docking position ("A") is available for the next tRNA to dock. In step 3, mRNA moves along and is opposite position "A" and the tRNA that brought in amino acid 3 is ejected. These steps are then repeated on the right-hand side to allow docking of tRNA that brings in amino acid 5, which is added to growing polypeptide chain.

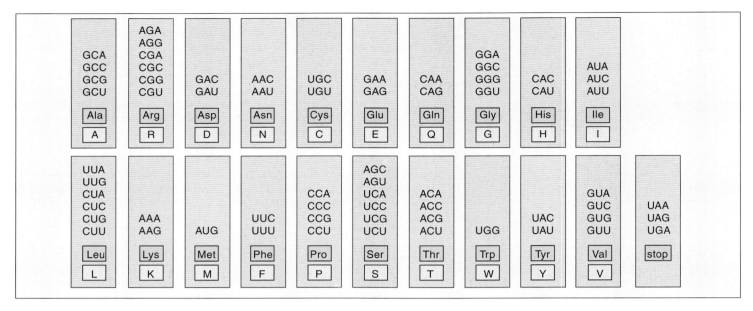

Fig. 1-11. This shows how different RNA codons are used to code for amino acids. Thus, on the top on the left, the amino-acid alanine (three-letter code is Ala, yellow box, and the one-letter code is A, blue box) is coded by the codons "GCA," "GCC," "GCG," and "GCU." The codons "UAA," "UAG," and "UGA" bring a halt to addition of amino acids and are thus a "stop" signal and are known as stop codons.

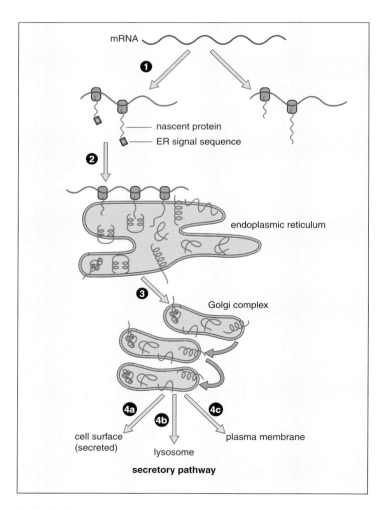

Fig.1-12. Newly synthesized proteins that are secreted are folded and posttranslationally modified in the rough endoplasmic reticulum and the Golgi apparatus. Step 1, Ribosomes (green rectangles) synthesize polypeptide chains (blue lines) from an mRNA template (red line). Proteins with a signal sequence (pink square) are taken up by the rough endoplasmic reticulum, where translation is completed. Proteins without a signal sequence complete translation in the cytosol on free ribosomes. Step 2, In the rough endoplasmic reticulum the proteins are folded and posttranslationally modified. Step 3, They are transferred to the Golgi via transport vesicles. Step 4, The folded protein is then sorted for onward transport.

The amino acid added to the peptide is defined by the RNA codon selected, and as shown in Fig. 1-11 there is a code for how the different RNA codons specify particular amino acids. Of note, specific RNA codons have specific "stop" signals (as well as a start signal; see previous discussion) that cause peptide chain termination. In eukaryotic cells (i.e., organisms with cells that have internal compartments, like mammalian cells) multiple ribosomes commonly engage and concurrently translate a single mRNA to form a circular polysome to increase the efficiency of protein translation. As ribosomes finish translation at the 3′ end, the subunits quickly reassemble to reinitiate synthesis at the 5′ end of the mRNA.

Nascent peptide chains have to be properly folded, and amino acids are modified and then sorted and either directed to the right cellular compartments or labeled for export. Proteins with a specific signal sequence direct the ribosome to the endoplasmic reticulum where protein synthesis is completed, and peptides are directed to the Golgi complex and sorted for different destinations (the secretory pathway) (Figs. 1-12 and 1-13). In other cases, proteins complete synthesis in cytosolic ribosomes and are directed to other compartments (the nucleus, mitochondria, or peroxisome). The transport of proteins depends on signal sequences (e.g., a nuclear localization signal) and interaction with specific receptor/transport proteins.

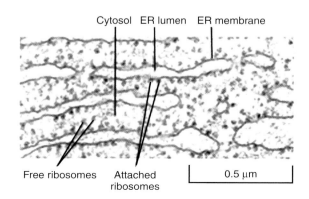

Fig. 1-13. Representation of an electron micrograph of ribosomes attached to the rough endoplasmic reticulum in a pancreatic cell.

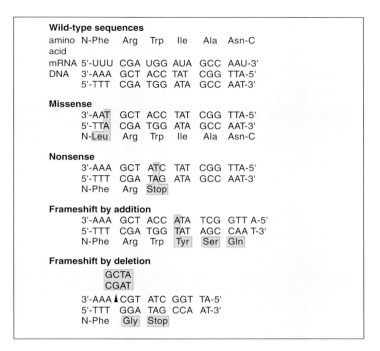

Fig. 1-14. Changes in coding parts of the DNA sequence of a gene can alter the protein produced. In this example, the wild-type (normal) protein and corresponding mRNA and DNA sequences are shown on top. Point mutations that change the amino acid encoded in the protein are known as missense mutations. Here a "T" to "A" change in the DNA (reading 5´ to 3´) alters protein sequence from phenylalanine (Phe) to leucine (Leu). On occasion the amino acid change can alter protein function. Below, the point change ("C" to "A") introduces a stop codon. This is a nonsense mutation. Below, if nucleotide/nucleotides is/are added (the nucleotide "T") or deleted ("CGAT"), this alters the reading frame (the order in which the triplets of nucleotides are read as codons) and alters protein sequence. This is a frameshift mutation. Nonsense and frameshift mutations usually have a more profound effect on protein sequence.

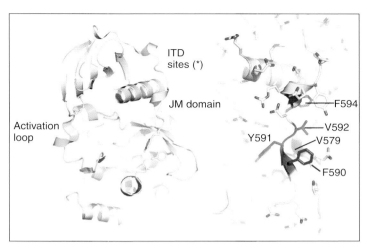

Fig. 1-16. A ribbon model of the crystal structure of the FLT3 kinase domain (with green activation loop and yellow juxtamembrane, JM domain) is shown. The positions of internal tandem duplications (ITDs) in JM domain, leading to FLT3 activation, are indicated. *Right,* Close view of the mutation sites in the JM domain (yellow). The structure is shown as a ribbon backbone, with side chains shown as colored sticks.

DNA MUTATIONS CAN ALTER PROTEIN SYNTHESIS BY A NUMBER OF MECHANISMS

DNA mutations at a variety of places in the gene locus can cause aberrant mRNA and protein production (Figs. 1-14 and 1-15). For example, point nucleotide substitutions in the coding sequence (see Fig. 1-14) can cause either an amino acid substitution (missense mutation) or introduce a stop codon (nonsense mutation). Deletions or additions of nucleotides (other than of multiples of

three nucleotides) can cause an alteration in the reading frame (frameshift mutation). In addition to mutations in the coding sequence, mutations can also occur in the promoter (or other distal cis-regulatory elements) to alter transcription; in the invariant splice acceptor donor sites in the intron at the intron-exon boundary to affect splicing; and in sequences that control 3´ end processing (poly A addition sites) and 5´ end processing (addition of the cap site) (see Figs. 1-15 and 9-6). The whole spectrum of these mutations is exemplified in the germline in the β-globin gene in β-thalassemia (see Chapter 9) or, to a lesser extent, in acquired mutations in the FMS-like tyrosine kinase 3 (FLT3) kinase in AML (Fig. 1-16) (see Chapter 12). In the case of FLT3 mutations the DNA mutations cause augmented abnormal proliferative signaling that promotes growth of the leukemia cells.

TRANSCRIPTIONAL CONTROL OF GENE EXPRESSION

One major level of control of protein production is by regulating mRNA transcription. For any gene, expression is regulated by regulatory DNA sequences (cis-elements), proteins (transcription

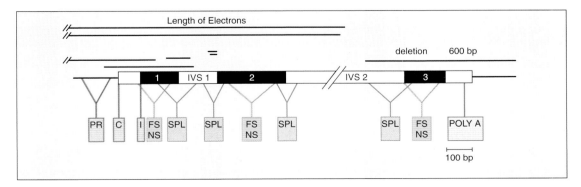

Fig.1-15. β-Thalassemia: the classes of mutations that underlie β-thalassemia. The 600 base pair deletion may also cause β-thalassemia. Other rare deletions may occur that affect the β-globin gene, the β and δ genes, or the γ, δ and β genes. PR, promoter; C, CAP site; I, initiation codon; FS, frameshift; NS, nonsense (premature chain termination) mutation; SPL, splicing mutation; POLY A, polyA addition site mutation. (Courtesy of Professor D. J. Weatherall.)

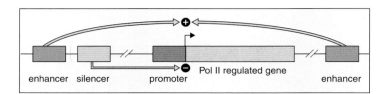

Fig. 1-17. Regulation of genes transcribed by RNA polymerase II is controlled by multiple DNA sequences (cis-elements). Here, the gene is regulated by proximal sequences—a promoter that abuts the transcriptional initiation site *(arrow)* and distal sequences that function to both enhance (enhancers) and repress (silencers) gene expression.

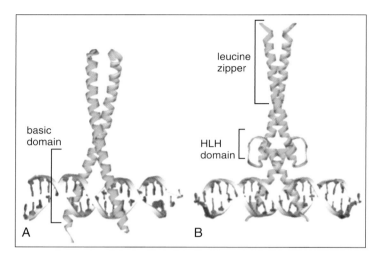

Fig. 1-18. A, Crystal structure of two TFs (green shades) shows the intimate contact between basic residues (basic domain) and specific sequences in the major groove of DNA (white double helix). The two TF then interact with each other via helical structures that are rich in leucine residues (so-called leucine zipper domain). Thus these TFs contain bzip domains. **B,** Here are crystal structure of two TFs (green shades) that bind the major groove of DNA (white shade) via basic residues (basic domain). Immediately following this domain are helix-loop-helix domains (HLH) followed by leucine zipper regions. Therefore these TFs have bHLH domains with leucine zippers.

factors and transcriptional cofactors) that regulate the transcription of the gene by binding either directly or indirectly to cis-elements and by access to the cis-elements regulated by packing of the DNA in chromatin (regulation at the level of chromatin structure).

CIS-ELEMENTS AND TRANSCRIPTION FACTORS

Figure 1-17 shows that cis-elements can be located near the gene. For example, the promoter defines the location of transcription start site(s) and the direction of transcription. Cis-elements located at a distance from the gene can either promote (enhancer) or repress (silencer) transcription. Cis-elements are composed of multiple binding sites for transcription factors (TFs). Thus the cis-element acts as a docking site for multiple DNA-binding TFs that in turn tether other TFs and cofactors that do not bind DNA.

Like many other proteins, TFs have a modular structure. For example, DNA-binding TFs such as MAX have a domain called the basic region (b) that binds DNA and an adjacent region, the helix-loop-helix (HLH) motif that interacts with other TFs and cofactors (Fig. 1-18). These domains allow TFs to be organized into families that share similar amino acid sequences and structural domains. Thus MAX is part of the bHLH TF family. TFs in a common family often bind approximately 6 to 10 similar DNA base pair sequences (binding sites) and physically interact with similar protein partners.

Once TFs and cofactors bind cis-elements proximal and distal to the gene most, but not all, evidence suggests that the cis-elements come together by looping out intervening DNA (Figs. 1-19 and 1-20). Either before or after looping, the complex of TFs and cofactors recruits RNA Pol II containing preinitiation complex. RNA Pol II is then phosphorylated on a specific domain (the C-terminal domain) that allows RNA Pol II to disengage from the preinitiation complex and elongate the RNA chain as it proceeds along the gene.

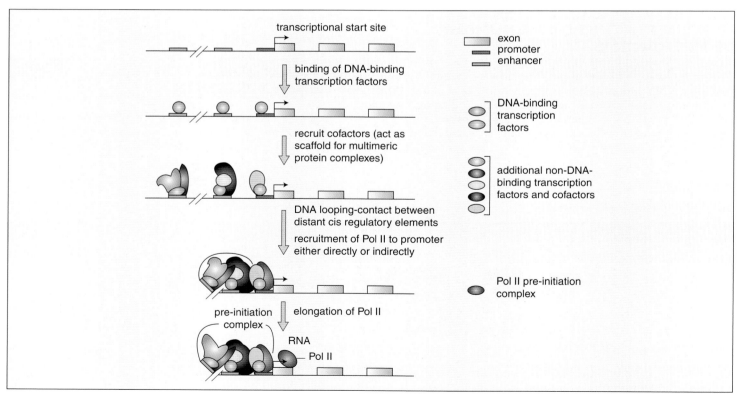

Fig. 1-19. Gene expression is controlled by transcription factors that bind cis-elements. DNA-binding transcription factors binding to cis-elements then recruit cofactors and other transcriptional regulators. It is also likely that DNA-binding TF and non-DNA-binding TF/cofactors may form pre-formed complexes that bind directly to DNA. Binding of RNA polymerase II, the preinitiation complex, and DNA looping between different cis-elements triggers transcription and elongation of polymerase II along the gene.

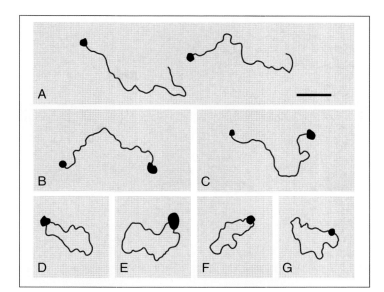

Fig. 1-20. Looping between cis-elements can be visualized. **A,** Schematic representation of an electron micrograph of the transcription factor Sp1 (shown as a black spot) bound to a cognate binding site at one end of DNA (irregular line). **B** and **C,** Two cognate DNA-binding sites were engineered at either end of the DNA fragment. **D–G,** Over time Sp1 bound to the ends of the DNA self-associated and looped the intervening DNA out.

Study of hematopoietic genes has contributed significantly to our understanding of eukaryotic gene expression. Examples include the α- and β-globin gene loci (Fig. 1-21). In the β-globin locus, multiple closely spaced distal cis-elements combine to form a specific type of enhancer, known as a locus control region (LCR). TFs and cofactors bound at the LCR and even more distal cis-elements are thought to bind together by looping out intervening DNA and promote transcription of different globin genes in a developmental-stage–specific manner.

CHROMATIN AND EPIGENETIC CONTROL OF GENE EXPRESSION

DNA is highly packaged in a nucleus. For a TF to gain access to a short DNA sequence in a particular cis-element of an individual gene, the chromatin associated with that sequence has to be specifically unpacked (Figs. 1-22 and 1-23). Metaphase chromosomes are progressively unpackaged via intermediate states that are poorly defined, to a 30 nm chromatin fiber, to DNA wrapped around

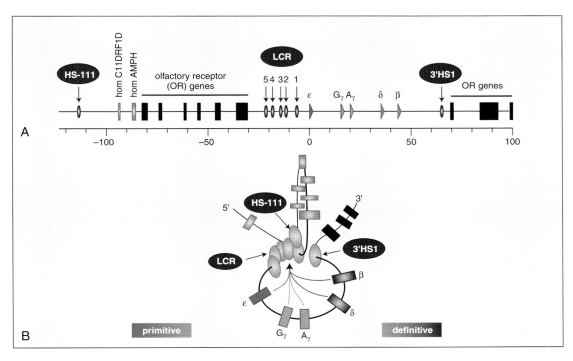

Fig. 1-21. Cis-elements that regulate gene expression can be distributed over a large area and can be complex. One of the best-studied gene loci is the human β-globin gene cluster on chromosome 11. **A,** There are five genes in the β-globin gene cluster (ε, Gγ, Aγ, δ, and β, depicted as arrowheads). At 5′ of the gene cluster there are five cis-elements (numbered 1 to 5, marked by arrows and collectively termed the locus control region, LCR). Two more cis-elements are located 111 kilobases 5′ (HS-111) and approximately 65 kilobases 3′ (3′ HS1). The whole β-globin domain (genes and cis-elements) is embedded in the midst of a bank of olfactory receptor (OR) genes (purple blocks) and two other genes (pink blocks). The scale below the locus is in kilobases. **B,** In a nucleus current evidence supports a model where all the β-globin cluster cis-elements physically interact (even though widely dispersed) with each other and with a β-like globin gene. Embryonic ε globin is expressed first (in primitive red cells), then the fetal γ genes, and finally the adult δ− and β-globin genes (both in definitive red cells).

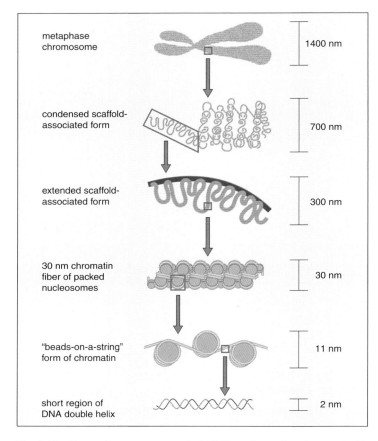

Fig. 1-22. Genes do not exist as naked DNA in the nucleus but are highly packaged. This figure shows that when metaphase chromosomes are unpackaged they are composed of fibrils of chromatin and may be associated with nuclear structures (one example that has been suggested is nuclear scaffolds that are often attached to nuclear membranes). When further unpacked, these chromatin fibrils are composed of 30 nm chromatin fibers, which in turn are composed of DNA wrapped around histone protein octamers called nucleosomes. When the 30 nm fiber is unwrapped the nucleosomes are linked by intervening DNA (like beads on a string). Nucleosomes can be temporarily shifted (remodeled) to expose naked DNA. The exact physical structure of higher-order chromatin structure (30 nm fiber and higher orders of packaging) is unclear. Regulating the wrapping and unwrapping of DNA also affords a layer of regulation on controlling which genes are expressed (unwrapped) and which are not (wrapped).

nucleosomes (composed of histone octamer—two units of H2A, H2B, H3, and H4) and finally to naked DNA. Regulation of the selective packing or unpacking of chromatin affords another level at which control on gene expression can be exerted. Control of expression of specific genes by regulation of the state of chromatin is not encoded in the DNA of the gene and thus is termed *epigenetic regulation of gene expression.* Huge advances have been made in our understanding of the epigenetic regulation and chromatin structure and its influence on gene expression both in normal cells and to a lesser extent in diseases such as some of the hematologic malignancies (Table 1-1). This is exemplified in Fig. 1-23, *A,* where the cis-elements that regulate expression of a key gene are shown either in an open chromatin conformation allowing access to TFs and expression of the gene or in a closed chromatin conformation (where gene expression is repressed). The normal chromatin state at key genes that control cell fate (e.g., growth, self-renewal, and differentiation) can be altered in a pathogenic manner in cancer.

This increased knowledge has led to the development of a new class of therapies for hematologic disease. To understand how these drugs may work in outline, it is helpful to consider epigenetic regulation of gene expression in more detail.

Control of packing is principally mediated by histones and methylation of DNA at the dinucleotide CpG (see Fig. 1-23). Histones can

be posttranslationally modified (acetylated, phosphorylated, methylated, or ubiquinated) at multiple residues by a large number of enzymes in a complex manner. Posttranslation modification of histones allows them to interact with a large number of different chromatin-associated proteins that either allow the chromatin to be packed or unpacked to different degrees. At its simplest, histones are acetylated by a family of histone acetyltransferases (HATs). Acetylation is broadly associated with activation of gene expression. By contrast, acetyl moieties can be removed by enzymes called histone deacetylases (HDACs). This is associated with repression of gene expression.

Similarly, CpG dinucleotides can be methylated by DNA methyltransferases and methylated CpG residues bind methyl CpG binding proteins (MeCPs). Methylation of DNA is associated with more

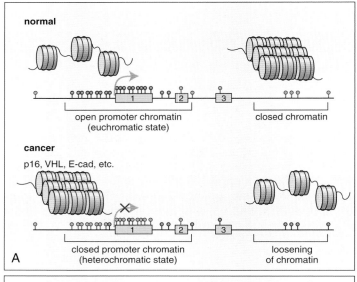

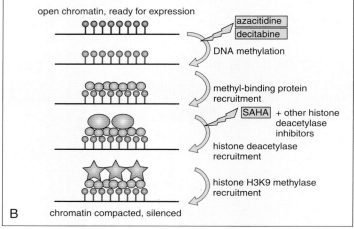

Fig. 1-23. A, Genes are in yellow boxes. Unwrapped genes (Gene 1) are in an open chromatin, euchromatic state. These genes have unmethylated CpG DNA residues (shown as pink lollipops) and are transcribed (green arrow). Genes that are not transcribed (genes 2 and 3) often have methylated CpG residues (blue lollipops). Closed chromatin is shown as closely packaged nucleosomes. In cancer gene expression is often inappropriate, and this is reflected in the changed chromatin structure. Thus genes such as p16, VHL, and E-cadherin (E-cad) are not transcribed. CpG residues are methylated and the chromatin is in a closed conformation. **B,** The transition from an open to a closed chromatin state occurs via multiple steps that can be targeted by drugs. Top, a gene locus is in an open chromatin conformation and the dinucleotide CpGs are not methylated (pink lollipops). DNA can then be methylated (blue lollipops). This can be inhibited by DNA methyltransferase inhibitors that are used in clinical practice (azacitidine and decitabine). Methyl CpG binding protein (brown circles) is recruited to methylated DNA and this is thought to facilitate binding of histone deacetylases and histone H3K9 and H3K27 methylases. Acetylated histones are associated with open chromatin and facilitate transcription whereas deacetylated histones and histone H3 methylated at residue lysine (K) 9 and K27 are associated with closed chromatin and transcriptional repression. A number of drugs in clinical use inhibit histone deacetylases. These include sodium valproate, SAHA, and MGCD0103.

TABLE 1-1. EXAMPLES OF HEMATOLOGIC DISEASES WHERE TRANSCRIPTIONAL EXPRESSION OF GENES THOUGHT TO BE IMPORTANT IN DISEASE CAUSATION IS MODIFIED BY EPIGENETIC PROCESSES

Disease	Gene silenced by epigenetic mechanism
Leukemia	
AML M2	p15 silencing AML1-ETO
AML M4 eo	p15 silencing by CBFβ-SMMHC
APML (AML M3)	RARAβ promoter silencing by PML/RARα
AML/MDS	p15, E-Cadherin promoter methylation
ALL	p15, p16, FHIT methylation
B-cell lymphoma	
Follicular lymphoma	SHP1 promoter methylation – increased proliferation
Mantle cell lymphoma	SHP1 and SOCS1 promoter methylation – activation of JAK-STAT pathway
High grade NHL	SHP1, p15 and p16 methylation – increased proliferation
MALT lymphoma	SHP1 promoter methylation
Hodgkins lymphoma	
Hodgkins lymphoma	CD19, CD20, CD79a, BLNK, Bob1, TSG, RASSF1A
T-cell lymphoma	
Cutaneous T-cell lymphoma	SHP1 promoter methylation – increased proliferation
Multiple myeloma	
Myeloma	SOCS-1, p16, E-Cadherin, DAP kinase, p73 promoter methylation

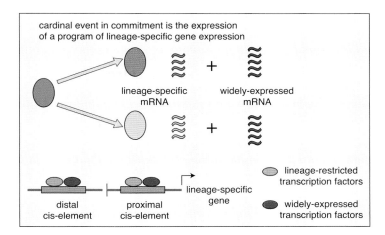

Fig. 1-24. A cardinal event in lineage specification is the expression of a program of lineage-specific gene expression. A multipotential cell (blue) differentiates into cells of two different lineages (pink and yellow). Though the phenotype of any cell, including cells of a specific lineage, is the sum of the lineage-specific and widely expressed RNAs, the specific phenotype of a lineage is a function of the lineage-specific RNAs. Below, expression of a lineage-specific gene is controlled by DNA sequences (cis-elements) and widely expressed and lineage-restricted transcription factors. Thus, ultimately, one important element in regulating lineage specification is the complement of lineage-restricted transcription factors that are expressed and the transcriptional networks they control.

hematopoietic TFs generate all blood cells by working in a combinatorial manner to direct lineage-specific programs of expression (Fig. 1-25). These TFs are not only crucial for normal blood cell program but the genes encoding them are often a target of acquired mutation that leads to hematologic malignancy (see Chapter 12).

highly packaged DNA and repression of gene expression. Methylation of CpG residues and the posttranslational modifications of histones are linked such that methylation of CpG residues and binding of MeCPs promotes binding of HDACs (and thus gene repression as histones become deacetylated). Novel classes of drugs that inhibit DNA methyltransferases (e.g., azacitidine and decitabine) and HDAC (e.g., vorinostat or SAHA) would potentially reverse the repression of genes, especially those that promote differentiation of malignant cells.

TRANSCRIPTION FACTORS, CONTROL OF GENE EXPRESSION, AND LINEAGE COMMITMENT

A cardinal event in differentiation of a lineage-specific cell is the elaboration of a lineage-specific program of gene expression (Fig. 1-24). Expression of lineage-specific genes, like that of all genes, is dependent on cis-elements and TFs (see previous discussion). These TFs themselves can either be widely expressed or have a restricted pattern of expression. For example, there is a small subset of TFs that are principally or exclusively expressed in blood cells. It is the action of these hematopoietic TFs that is critical in directing hematopoietic-specific gene expression. One such hematopoietic TF is GATA1, which is expressed in erythroid cells and megakaryocytes, as well as eosinophils and mast cells. In all of these cell types, but especially the former two lineages, it is critically required for expression of most of the genes associated with terminal maturation of red cells and megakaryocytes and platelets. Extrapolating this more broadly to hematopoiesis, accumulating evidence suggests that a small subset of critical

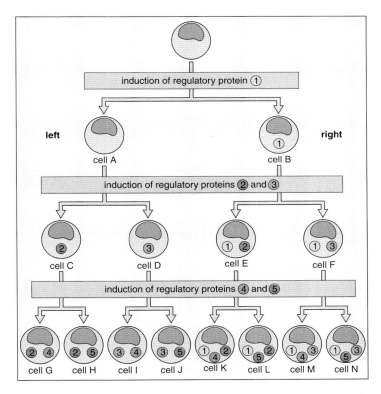

Fig. 1-25. This simplified diagram illustrates the principle that combinations of a limited number of critical regulatory proteins can generate different cell types (lineages) during development and adult life. Thus, in the embryonic life, the cell at the apex of the hierarchy and all its progeny divide asymmetrically such that the cell on the left always produces an even-numbered regulatory protein whereas the cell on the right produces an odd-numbered protein. The protein complement produced by a cell is then perpetuated by its progeny (cellular memory). In this simplistic scenario, five different regulatory proteins generate eight cell types (G to N). With continuation of this scheme, 10,000 cell types would be generated by only 25 different gene regulatory proteins.

MICRO-RNAS

Over the last decade or so a previously unrecognized class of RNAs, micro-RNAs (miRNAs), have been shown to play important biologic roles in controlling expression of proteins (Fig. 1-26) in normal cells. miRNAs may also play a role in disease (Table 1-2). The importance of the discovery of miRNAs led to the Nobel Prize being awarded to two investigators in 2006.

miRNAs are encoded by RNA Pol II–transcribed genes to produce pre-miRNAs. These are processed initially in the nucleus and then in the cytoplasm. Here, mature 22 base pair miRNAs bind principally to the untranslated regions of mRNA transcripts leading either to mRNA degradation or repression of translation of mRNAs.

TABLE 1-2. miRNAS THAT MAY BE FUNCTIONAL IN HEMATOPOIESIS

miRNA	Candidate target genes	Function
miR-181a	None identified	Lymphopoiesis
miR-223	NFI-A	Granulopoiesis
miR-221, miR-222	c-kit	Erythropoiesis
miR-130a	MafB	Megakaryopoiesis (assumed)
miR-10a	HoxA1	Megakaryopoiesis (assumed)

DNA REPLICATION AND TELOMERES

Every time a human cell divides, its 6 billion base pairs have to be faithfully replicated. This extraordinary task is accomplished daily in billions of cells, for the most part without deleterious consequence. When a cell enters the phase in the cell cycle (S, synthesis phase; see later discussion) where the genome is replicated, replication is initiated at multiple areas in the genome called *replication foci*. DNA replication then proceeds in a semiconservative manner, meaning that the two DNA strands in a double helix, separate, are individually replicated and the resulting two double helices segregate into daughter cells (Fig. 1-27, *A*). Thus each daughter cell has a strand of newly synthesized DNA and a strand from the parental cell. Given that DNA polymerase, the enzyme that replicates DNA, does so in a 5′ to 3′ manner, only one strand is replicated continuously (the leading strand) whereas the other strand has to be replicated in short fragments (Okazaki fragments) (Fig. 1-27, *B* and *C*). For the lagging strand a number of additional steps are required to ligate the discontinuous Okazaki fragments into a continuous DNA strand. DNA synthesized from multiple foci is then ligated together.

One special problem created by the semiconservative mode of DNA replication is the replication of the lagging DNA strand at the ends of chromosomes (Fig. 1-28). This is overcome by having repetitive sequences (called telomeres) at the ends of chromosomes that decrease with each round of replication. For cells that need to self-renew and maintain a high proliferative potential (e.g., germ and other stem cells), the enzyme telomerase can extend the repetitive sequences and compensate for loss at replication. Telomerase is a specialized ribonuclear protein complex composed of an RNA component called TERC that binds to the end of the leading strand, and this is replicated by a specialized reverse transcriptase that is also a component of telomerase, called TERT. This is discussed further in Chapter 17. Loss of telomerase function leads to progressive telomere shortening, and this can have catastrophic consequences for cell viability and can lead to transformation of the cell (Fig. 1-28). The degree of maintenance of telomeres determines the number of generations a cell can produce and is often increased above normal in malignant cells. The importance of telomeres in humans is elegantly demonstrated by acquired and germline mutations in patients with dyskeratosis congenita (DKC) and aplastic anemia (see Chapter 17).

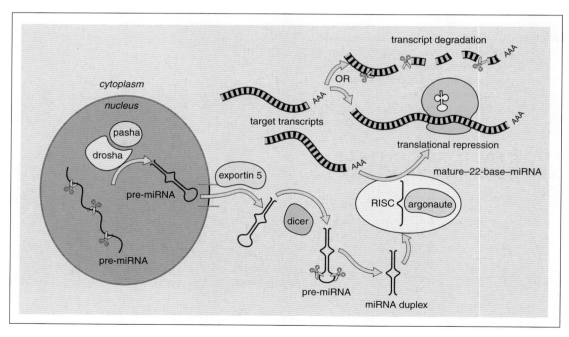

Fig. 1-26. An important class of molecules that regulates gene expression are micro-RNAs (miRNAS). A simplified diagram illustrates how miRNAs are produced and how they regulate miRNA and protein levels. Most miRNAs are expressed from RNA polymerase II regulated genes as pre-miRNAs. This is cleaved by a nuclear RNAse III Drosha and its partner protein DGCR8 Pasha into 50 to 80 base pair stem loop pre-miRNAs. These pre-miRNAs are actively exported with the help of exportin-5 into the cytoplasm where another nuclease, Dicer excises them into 20 to 24 base pair mature miRNA duplexes. One of the two miRNA strands is then bound by the multiprotein complex called RISC, which contains, among other proteins, the protein argonaute (RISC/Argonaute). This strand can then repress gene expression by binding to mRNAs by partial sequence complementarity. Binding of mature miRNAs can either inhibit translation of mRNAs or target the mRNA for degradation.

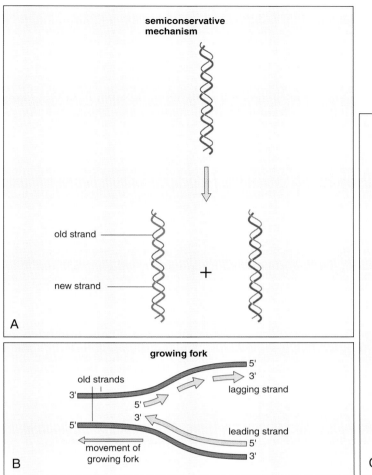

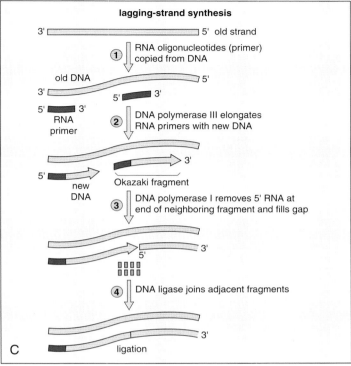

Fig. 1-27. DNA replication is semiconservative. **A,** This shows that the parental DNA is composed of two strands. During replication each of the parental strands acts as a template for replication, and thus progeny strands contain one new strand and one old strand. **B,** DNA replication is initiated at origins of replication, and as replication proceeds the parental strands are separated and a replication fork is formed. DNA is synthesized from a 5′ to a 3′ direction, and this creates two types of strands of newly replicated DNA. One strand, called a leading strand, is continuously synthesized by DNA polymerase III by sequential addition of deoxyribonucleotides in the same direction as the movement of the replication fork (the bottom strand in this figure). In contrast, the other newly synthesized strand is made discontinuously (top strand) and is known as the lagging strand. **C,** Synthesis of the lagging strand requires multiple steps. First, multiple RNA oligonucleotides (primers) are synthesized from parental DNA strand templates. These serve to prime synthesis of fragments (called Okazaki fragments) of the new (lagging) strand. DNA polymerase I then removes the RNA primers, fills in the gaps with DNA, and finally DNA ligase joins adjacent DNA fragments.

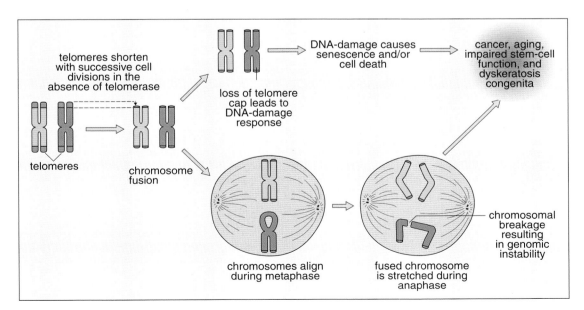

Fig. 1-28. The enzyme complex telomerase is essential for maintaining telomere length, and this is critical for chromosomal and cell viability. Lack of telomerase activity leads to telomere shortening with successive cell division. This can activate DNA damage responses and lead to cell senescence and cell death. Alternatively, telomere shortening can precipitate chromosomal fusion, and genomic instability. A specific condition associated with impaired telomerase activity is dyskeratosis congenita (see Chapter 17), in which children and young adults can have hematopoietic stem cell failure and leukemia. More generally impaired telomere function has been implicated in many cancers and ageing.

MUTATIONS AND HOW THEY RESULT IN DISEASE

During DNA replication errors in fidelity can lead to single base changes (Fig. 1-29, *A*) that will create allele-specific changes in DNA sequence composition that are known as single-nucleotide polymorphisms (SNPs).

When SNPs occur in nongenetic parts of the genome they can be without consequence. However, if they occur in a coding sequence they can result in mutation with a functional consequence (see Figs. 1-14 and 1-29, *B*). The single-nucleotide missense substitution of a T to G in the sixth codon of the β-globin gene that changes a valine to a glutamine to produce a βs-globin allele (a sickle β-globin allele) is an example of a pathogenic SNP. Because of selective pressure, multiple such functional missense mutations can be detected even in

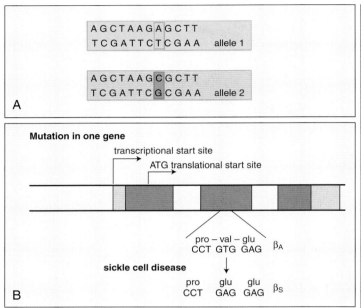

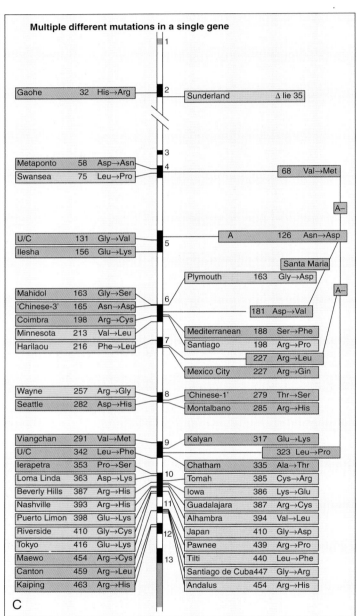

Fig. 1-29. Errors in DNA replication or the maintenance of the methylated state of CpG residues can change DNA sequence. **A,** When DNA sequence change occurs at single nucleotide it is known as single-nucleotide polymorphism (SNP). In this example, the "A" residue on allele 1 is changed to a "C" residue on allele 2. **B,** When SNP occurs in coding sequence it can alter protein sequence. In this example, a "T" residue at the sixth codon in exon 2 of the human β-globin gene is changed to an "A" residue. This changes a valine (val) to glutamic acid (glu). This results in a β-sickle allele. In the homozygous state this causes sickle cell disease (see Chapter 9). **C,** Mutations can occur at multiple positions in the gene. In the glucose-6-phosphate dehydrogenase (G6PD) gene, many different mutations cause G6PD deficiency. These may cause drug sensitivity (pink) or more rarely chronic non spherocytic hemolytic anemia (NSHA) (yellow). The exons are shown in black bands except exon 1, which is noncoding and shown in gray. **D,** SNPs can occur in the promoters of genes and alter gene expression. This can cause a phenotype. Here, a "G" to "A" change creates a binding site for the transcription factor OCT1 in the promoter of the TNF gene. This causes increased expression of the TNF gene. This mechanism has been implicated in the pathogenesis of cerebral malaria. (*C,* Adapted with permission from Vulliamy TJ, Mason PJ, Luzzatto L: Molecular basis of glucose-6-phosphate dehydrogenase deficiency, *Trends Genet* 8:138-143, 1992.)

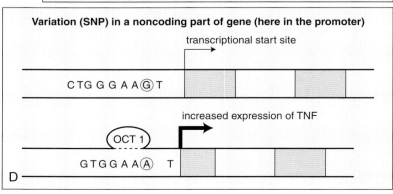

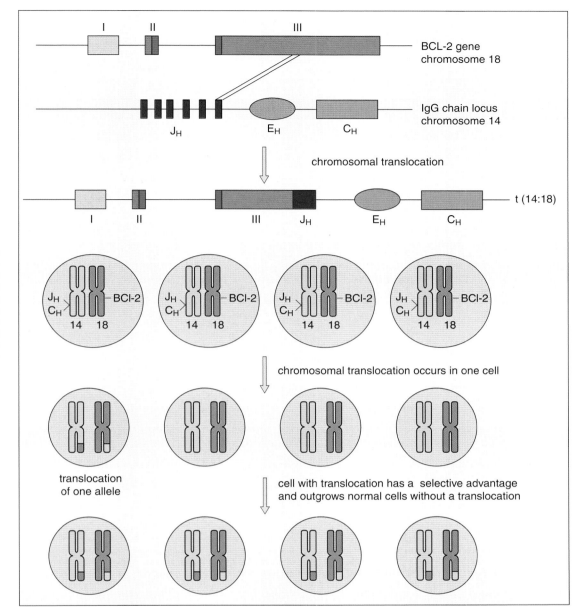

Fig. 1-30. This shows how chromosomal translocation leads to disease-causing mutation. In this example the BCL-2 gene on chromosome 18 is involved in a translocation with the Ig heavy chain locus on chromosome 14. In this case the translocation breakpoints are inside the genes and give rise to a fusion transcript. Acquisition of this translocation provides a selective advantage to cells.

a single gene such as β-globin or glucose-6-phosphate dehydrogenase (G6PD) (see Fig. 1-29, *C*, and Chapter 8), producing a large of number of alleles associated with disease. Finally, it is being increasingly appreciated that SNPs in cis-elements (promoters or enhancers) can alter expression of a gene from a single allele with the SNP by altering the binding, and thus activity of DNA-binding TFs (see Fig. 1-29, *D*). This has been shown to be the case for an SNP in the tumor necrosis factor α (TNFα) promoter where a "G" to "A" change creates a binding site for the TF OCT-1 leading to increased TNFα expression and increased susceptibility to cerebral malaria. More examples such as this are now coming to light from SNP association studies.

DNA replication errors can also lead to translocation of chromosomes (Fig. 1-30). This is one of the most common karyotypic abnormalities in hematologic malignancy, which affects the expression of the gene either quantitatively (especially frequent in acute lymphoblastic leukemia) or qualitatively. Pathologically important translocations often lead to production of fusion transcripts where the genes at the sites of translocation produce proteins of altered function, for example, BCR-ABL in chronic myeloid leukemia, PML-RARA in acute promyelocytic leukemia or AML M3, and PBX-EHA in pre–B-ALL (see Chapters 12 and 13). Translocation can also cause disease by altering gene expression (see Fig. 1-30) with pathologic consequences by altering the cell fate of hematopoietic stem/progenitor cells (Fig. 1-31). Control of cell fate is discussed more extensively in Chapters 2 and 3.

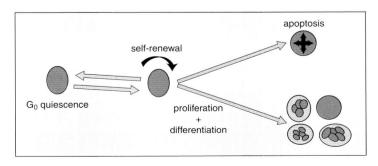

Fig. 1-31. This schematically shows the cell fate choices available to a hematopoietic stem/progenitor cell.

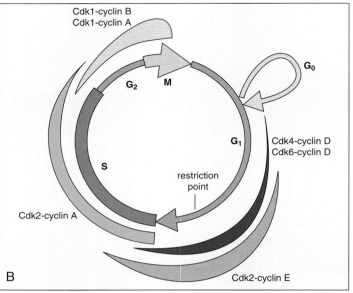

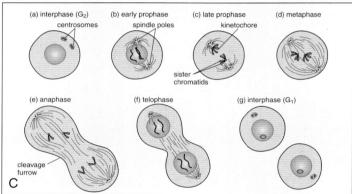

Fig. 1-32. A, A schematic representation of the cell cycle. Quiescent cells ("G$_0$") enter the cycle in "G$_1$" and progress to synthesize DNA in the "S" phase. In the G$_2$ phase cells have 4n DNA content and this leads to mitosis "M." The G$_1$, S, and G$_2$ phases collectively are known as interphase. Though chromosomes are condensed only in mitosis, they are shown in condensed form to emphasize that the number of chromosomes are different stages in the cell cycle. **B,** Passage through the cell cycle is, in part, regulated by proteins that themselves cycle. These include the cycle-dependent kinases (Cdk) that are physically associated (i.e., are a complex) with proteins that regulate them, called cyclins. Different combinations of Cdks and cyclins are required to progress through different stages of the cell cycle. Thus CDk2-cyclin E complex is important in G$_1$. Critical regulatory points in the cell cycle are called restriction points, and the location of the G$_1$ restriction point is shown. **C,** During the cell cycle a key facet is the proper separation of sister chromatids (generated in "S" phase). *a)* In late G$_2$, structures called centrioles are replicated. *b)* In early prophase, chromosomes and associated centrioles move to cell poles. Now the chromosomes start to condense and can be seen as threads. The nuclear membrane begins to disaggregate. *c)* Late prophase, chromosome condensation is complete. The chromosome centromeres are visible, and they progressively move to the pole and microtubular spindle fibers connect the centromeres to the poles of the cell. *d)* Metaphase; chromosomes move to the cell equatorial plane. *e)* Anaphase; the sister chromatids separate into independent chromosomes. Each centromere is connected to the pole by a spindle fiber and moves to the pole. Simultaneously, the cell elongates. Cytokinesis begins and cleavage furrows appear. *f)* Telophase; new nuclear membranes are seen and chromosomal decondensation starts. The cells now reenter G$_1$ and interphase.

CELL CYCLE

One critical determinant of cell fate is whether cells enter the cell cycle. Though much is known about the molecular controls and cell biology of the cell cycle, we are still unearthing the complexity of how cell cycle is linked with external cues, the cellular history of the cell, and the cell compartment a cell is located (i.e., stem cell or progenitor cell).

Cell cycle is divided into phases (Fig. 1-32, *A* and *C*). There is cyclic synthesis of DNA (S phase), a pause known as G2, followed by chromosome condensation, nuclear envelope breakdown and chromosome segregation followed by chromosome decondensation, nuclear envelope reformation, and cytokinesis leading to separation of two daughter cells (mitosis or M phase). A critical set of proteins that control passage through the cell cycle are the cyclins, the expression of which differs throughout the cell cycle by periodic changes in synthesis and degradation (Fig. 1-32, *B*). They activate a set of protein kinases (CDKs) (Fig. 1-33), which then phosphorylate various proteins. Phosphorylation of the retinoblastoma susceptibility gene product RB prevents RB from blocking the transcription factors (e.g., E2F) essential for transition from the G1 to the S phase of the cell cycle. The cyclin CDK complexes are regulated by inhibitors. Thus cyclin D–CDK4 and cyclin D–CDK6 complexes are inhibited by a 16 kDa protein encoded by the INK4a gene and a 15 kDa protein encoded by the INK4b gene, inhibiting progress from mid to late G1.

The p53 gene codes for a 53 kDa transcription control factor that mediates a block in the cell cycle at the G1–S phase boundary. This is mediated by a p21 cyclin CDK inhibitor, p21CIPI. Expression of p53 is induced by DNA damage that results from radiation or drugs (Fig. 1-34). The cell is therefore held up in G1 to allow the cell to repair the damage. If the damage is extensive, p53 induces apoptosis by increased expression of the pro-apoptotic gene BAX (Fig. 1-34). This is not the only example of how progression through the cell cycle and response to external cues (in this case DNA damage) is linked with another cell fate choice option, namely apoptosis.

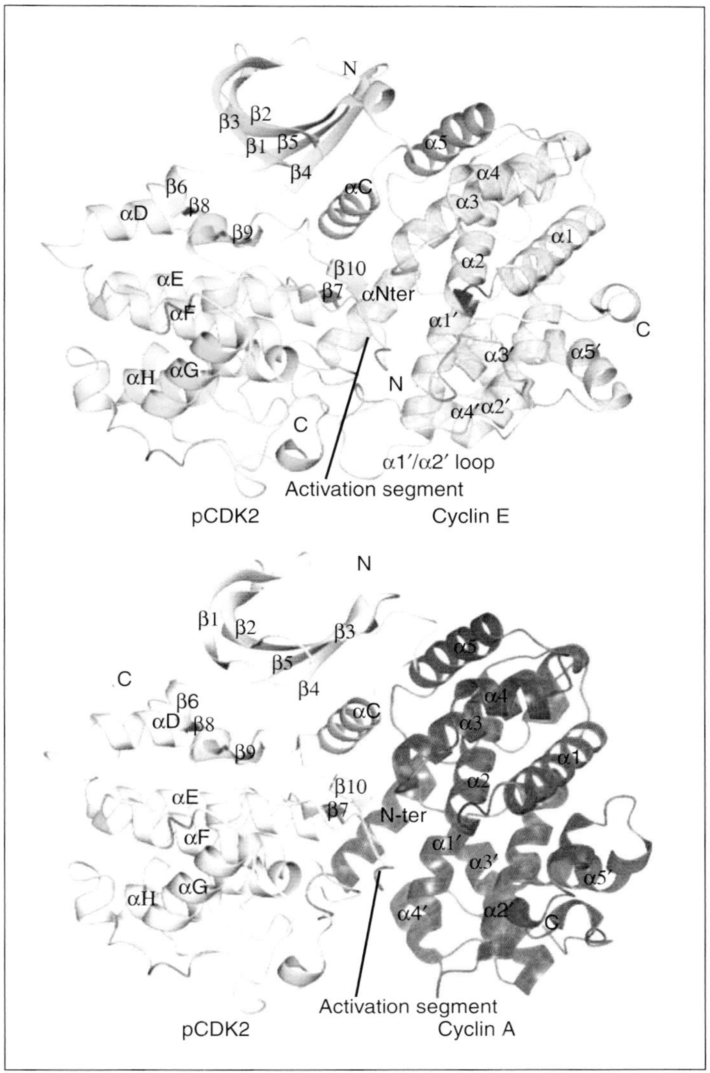

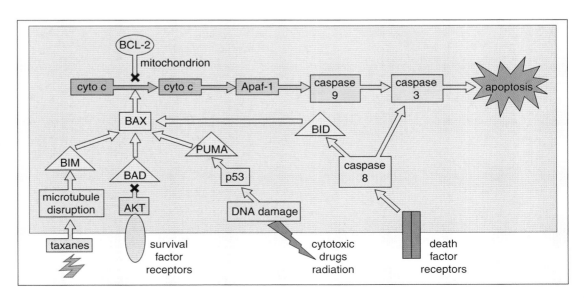

Fig. 1-33. The intimate contacts between Cdks and cyclins are shown by the crystal structures of the pCDK2 (green)/cyclin E (cyan) (top) and the pCDK2 (yellow)/cyclin A (magenta) complexes.

APOPTOSIS

Cell death can occur by necrosis or by a physiologically active mechanism (*apoptosis,* programmed cell death) (Fig. 1-34). Necrosis occurs in response to ischemia, chemical trauma, or hyperthermia. It affects many adjacent cells, and is characterized by cell swelling, with early loss of plasma membrane integrity and swelling of organelles and

nucleus. There is usually an inflammatory infiltrate of phagocytic cells in response to spillage of cell contents into the surrounding space.

Programmed cell death occurs by an active process that requires calcium ions. Nuclear condensation, nuclear fragmentation, and cytoplasmic vacuolation occur early, with later changes in the organelles and plasma membrane (Fig. 1-35). Apoptosis also involves

Fig. 1-34. This simplified diagram shows key elements of the pathways that lead to caspase 3 activation and apoptosis. A number of stimuli can activate the pathway. See text for details.

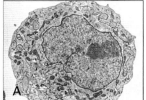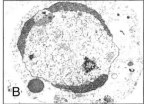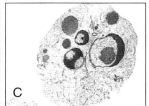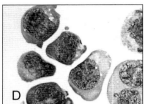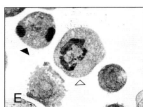

Fig. 1-35. Apoptosis: **(A–C)** electron microscopic and **(D, E)** light microscopic appearances. **A,** Normal K562 cell line. **B,** Early apoptotic cell showing chromatin condensation at the nuclear periphery. **C,** Later apoptotic cell showing both chromatin condensation and nuclear fragmentation. **D,** Normal K562 cell line. **E,** Early apoptotic cell (open arrowhead) with peripheral chromatin condensation and late apoptotic cell (solid arrowhead) with both chromatin condensation and nuclear fragmentation. (Reproduced with permission from Riordan FA, Bravery CA, Mengubas K, et al: Herbimycin A accelerates the induction of apoptosis following etoposide treatment or gamma-irradiation of bcr/abl-positive leukaemia cells, *Oncogene* 16:1533-1542, 1998.)

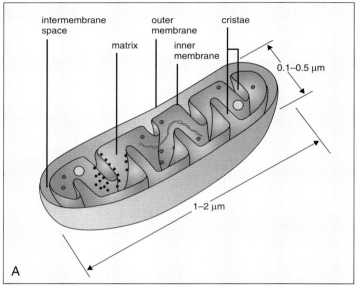

Fig. 1-36. A, A three-dimensional schematic diagram of a mitochondron cut longitudinally. The ATP-producing complexes (F_0F_1, red cell dots) are located on the inner membrane protruding inward. Mitochondrial DNA (blue), ribosomes (blue circles), and granules (yellow dots) are shown. **B,** Summary of aerobic oxidation of pyruvate illustrates some of the complexity of the biochemistry within the mitochondria.

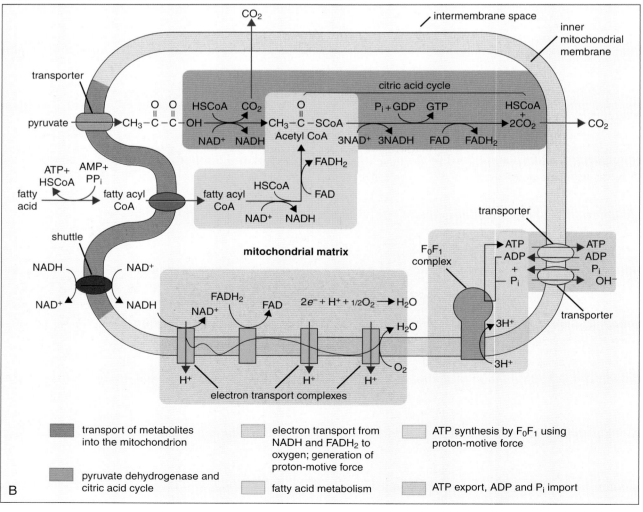

digestion of cell DNA by an endonuclease to produce on a gel, a ladder of regular bands 180 base pairs apart. Cleavage occurs by double-stranded breaks on linker regions between nucleosomes. The final part of the apoptosis pathway involves caspase enzymes. The executioner caspase 3 cleaves a restricted set of cellular proteins, including polyadenosine diphosphate–ribose polymerase, laminin, and gelsolin (see Fig. 1-34). Caspase 3 is activated by caspase 9. This in turn is activated by the apoptotic protease 1 (APAF-1), which itself is activated by cytochrome c. Cytochrome c is released from mitochondria when the pro-apoptotic protein BAX is in excess and forms homodimers. Cells are protected from apoptosis by BCL-2, which binds to BAX and thereby inhibits cytochrome c release and caspase activation. Apoptosis is promoted by BAD, which forms heterodimers with BCL-2. Apoptosis may also be stimulated by direct DNA damage (e.g., by radiation or drugs) or by withdrawal of a growth factor (e.g., interleukin-3) that promotes survival by stimulating phosphorylation of BAD by protein kinase B, thus preventing its association with BCL-2.

ORGANELLES IN CELLS

MITOCHONDRIA

Mitochondria are complex organelles that are the main sites of ATP production (Fig. 1-36) during aerobic metabolism, are important for heme biosynthesis (see Chapter 5), and play a role in apoptosis. They are among the largest organelles and can make up to 25% of the cellular volume. They are composed of two structurally and functionally distinct inner and outer membranes. The inner membrane has a large number of invaginations or cristae that protrude into the central space or matrix of the mitochondria. The complex biochemical pathways that produce ATP from aerobic metabolism of glucose (via pyruvate produced by the glycolytic pathway) can result in up to 34 molecules of ATP for every molecule of glucose. This involves phosphorylation and oxidation. Fatty acids can also be metabolized to CO_2 to generate ATP. Metabolism of pyruvate and fatty acids generates NADH and $FADH_2$ molecules that are oxidized to NAD^+ and FAD, and the resulting protons are pumped across the inner mitochondrial membrane. ATP generation is powered by the resulting proton-motive force. Thus it is easy to see why mitochondria are required to provide energy for a cell.

LYSOSOMES

Lysosomes are closed intracellular compartments composed of a single membrane that are responsible for degrading intracellular components that are no longer required for the cell's metabolism. Material is taken up by a lysosome by at least three routes (Fig. 1-37). Endocytosis is the process by which small portions of the plasma membrane invaginate to form a small membrane-bound vesicle (endosome). The endosome is then combined with a primary lysosome to create a secondary lysosome. Secondary lysosomes can also form when primary lysosomes fuse with phagasomes (where particles are enveloped by the plasma membrane and internalized). Finally, aged mitochondria are removed by a process known as autophagy—here an autophagosome combines with a primary lysosome to make a

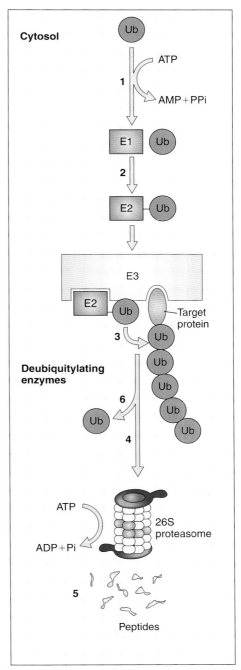

Fig. 1-38. Proteosomal degradation of cellular protein. Ubiquitin (Ub) is added to enzyme E1 (ubiquitin-activating enzyme) in an ATP-dependent process (1); Ubiquitin is transferred to protein E2 (ubiquitin-carrier protein) (2). This is then complexed to ubiquitin ligase (3). E3 binds E2/ubiquitin and the target protein that is destined for polyuquitination and destruction. This allows ubiquitin to be transferred to the polyubiquitin chain. The polyubiquitinated protein is then proteolysed in a 26S proteosome in an ATP-dependent process.

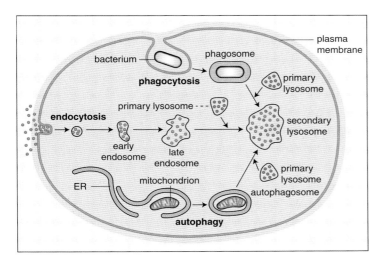

Fig. 1-37. Lysosomes degrade ingested extracellular (e.g., bacterium) and intracellular particles. This shows three main pathways that deliver material to lysosomes.

secondary lysosome. Lysosomes then release enzymes (termed acid hydrolases) that work at acid pH to denature the lysosome contents (e.g., proteins). An ATP-dependent pump generates the acid pH, and lysosomal enzymes work best in acid (pH 4.8) conditions and not in neutral cytosolic pH.

PROTEIN UBIQUITINATION

Ubiquitin (ubiquitous immunopoietic peptide) is a highly conserved 76 amino acid 8.5 KD peptide that is used to mark proteins for destruction. Ubiquinated proteins are targeted to the proteosome (a macromolcular structure that cleaves proteins) that cleaves ubiquitin-tagged proteins in an ATP-dependent process to yield peptides and intact ubiquitin. Ubiquitin is added by a conjugating enzyme (ubiquitinating complex). First, ubiquitin is activated and bound to the enzyme E1 and then is transferred to the enzyme E2. E2 binds the ubiquitin ligases E3 (there are many different types of E3 ligase) (Fig. 1-38). The protein targeted for destruction is recognized by internal sequences. Successive conjugation of ubiquitin moieties (at least four) usually to a lysine residue is required for proteosome targeting. The ubiquitin-proteosome pathway is a central process in controlling protein turnover in the cell. There are hematologic diseases associated with this pathway, including forms of Fanconi anemia (mutations in genes for a large E3 ligase) (Chapter 17) and Chuvash polycythemia (encodes another E3 ligase) (page 263).

CELLULAR BASIS OF HEMATOPOIESIS

Hematopoiesis is the process by which blood cells are made. This occurs in waves and at multiple discrete anatomic sites that change through development (Fig. 2-1). In humans, like other vertebrates, the initial wave of hematopoiesis occurs in the extraembryonic yolk sac (YS) blood islands (Fig. 2-2). The yolk sac primarily produces primitive erythroid cells that express embryonic globins (see Chapter 5) that deliver oxygen to tissues in the rapidly growing embryo. Primitive erythropoiesis is transient and is replaced by adult or definitive hematopoiesis that sustains blood production throughout development and postnatal life. Hematopoietic activity is then detected within the embryo, in a region around the ventral wall of the dorsal aorta called the aorta-gonad mesonephros (AGM) (Fig. 2-3). In early development blood cells arise in close connection with the vascular structures (both in the yolk sac and the dorsal aorta), giving rise to the notion that there may be a common precursor cell population that gives rise to both blood and blood vessel cells called a *hemangioblast*. Though there is good evidence that such a cell is likely to exist, formal proof of this is still awaited. More recent data suggests that blood cells are derived from endothelial cells surrounding vascular structures like the yolk sac and the dorsal aorta.

In mice and other animals, studies have shown that definitive hematopoietic stem cells (HSCs) with serially transplantable activity together with long-term engraftment capacity are found in the AGM. Additional hematopoietic activity can also be detected in the embryo in the umbilical arteries, allantosis, and placenta. It is still a matter of much debate whether HSCs arise from the embryo proper from the

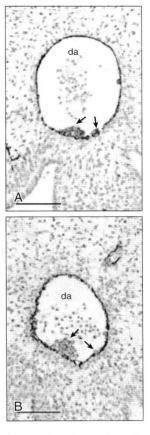

Fig. 2-2. Yolk sac blood islands in a human fetus. **A,** Transverse section in a 3 somite human embryo (21 days) at the truncal level stained with anti-CD34 antibody. Paired dorsal aorta (da) ventrolateral to the neural tube (nt) and above the yolk sac (ys) and blood islands (bi). **B,** Higher magnification of a solid hemangioblastic mesodermal cluster of CD34 expressing cells in a blood island of the yolk sac (brown). (Adapted from Tavian M et al: *Development* 126:793-803, 1999, Fig. 1 A, B.)

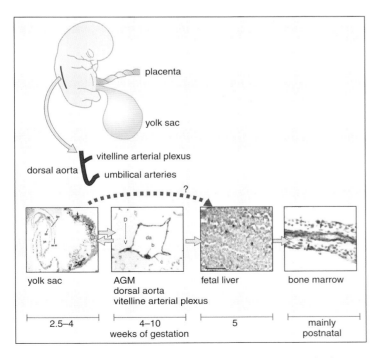

Fig. 2-1. Changing anatomic locations of hematopoiesis through development. Hematopoiesis is initially detected in the extraembryonic yolk sac, in a region known as the aorta-gonad mesonephros (AGM) in the embryo, the placenta, the umbilical arteries, and vitelline vessels. It then shifts to the fetal liver and finally to the bone marrow. See text for further details.

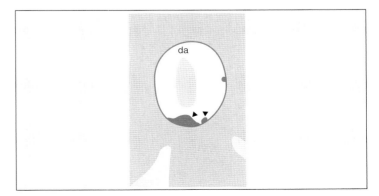

Fig. 2-3. Transverse section through the human fetal dorsal aorta at embryonic day 32 showing hematopoietic CD34+ cells clusters (arrowheads) associated with ventral wall. CD34+ cells (hematopoietic and endothelial cells) are stained brown. (Adapted from Tavian M et al: *Development* 126:793-803, 1999, Fig. 5, c.)

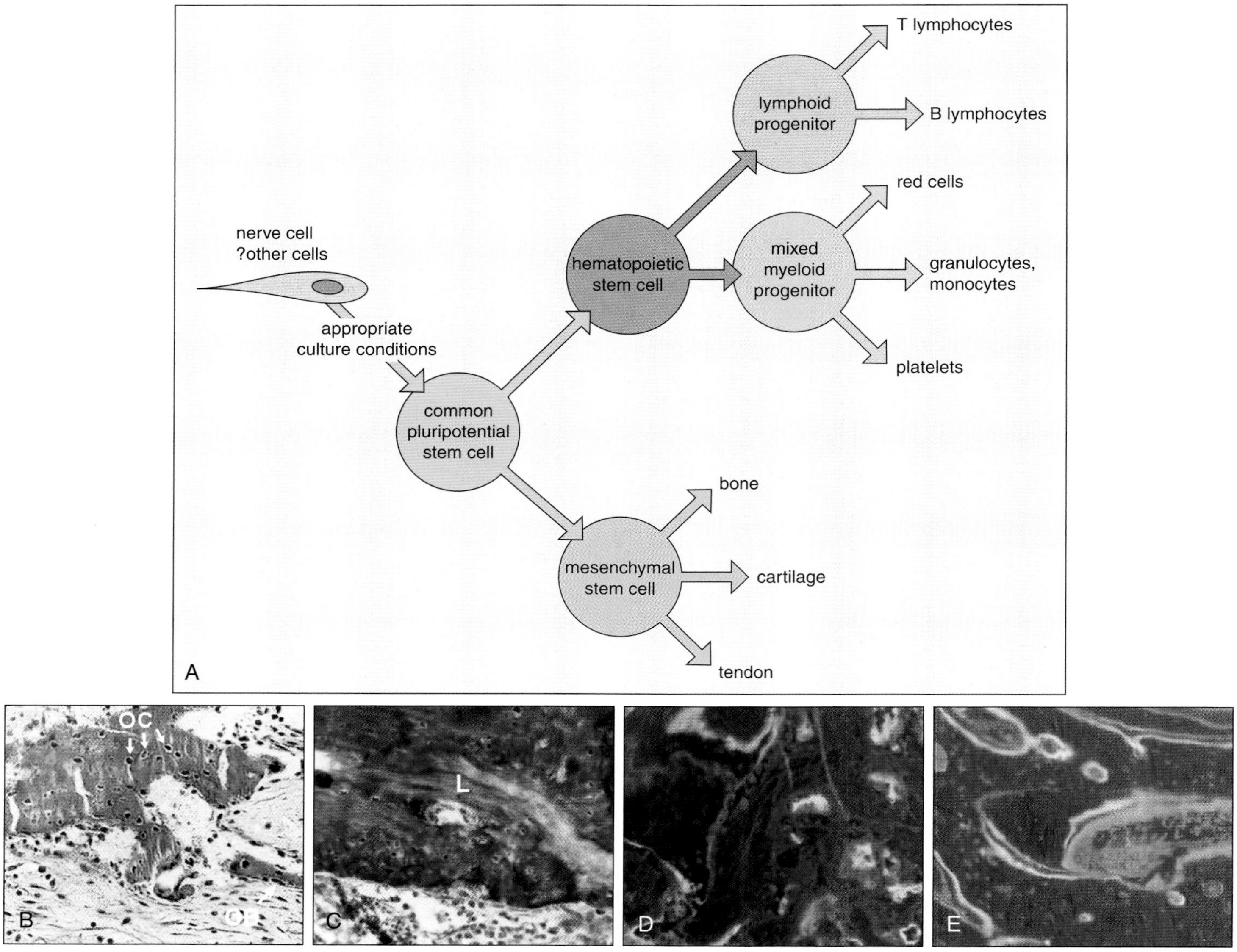

Fig. 2-4. **A,** Mensenchymal cells: these cells and hematopoietic cells probably have a common precursor pluripotential cell. Under appropriate culture conditions, muscle cells (and nerve sheath cells) may be transformed into common pluripotential hematopoietic stem cells. **B–E,** Differentiation of mesenchymal stem cells in culture: **(B)** undifferentiated human MSCs; **(C)** bone formation by osteoblasts and osteocytes into which human MSCs have differentiated when grown on ceramic tubes and placed in severe combined immunodeficiency mice; **(D)** cartilage derived from human MSCs grown from a cell platelet; **(E)** rabbit MSCs form tendon when placed in a ruptured tendon sheath. (Reproduced with permission from Gerson SL: Mesenchymal stem cells: no longer second class marrow citizens, *Nature Med* 5:262-264, 1999.)

AGM or by colonization from the yolk sac. It is also unclear if HSCs from the AGM migrate and colonize the other embryonic sites or whether they arise de novo at these other sites.

Subsequently, hematopoiesis is detected in the fetal liver, spleen, thymus, and ultimately bone marrow (see Fig. 2-1). It is thought that AGM HSCs (or possibly yolk sac HSCs) migrate to the fetal liver. In the fetal liver, expansion and differentiation of HSCs allows for development of definitive red cells, myeloid cells, and lymphoid cells (T cells that develop in the thymus and B cells in the marrow).

Bone marrow also contains multipotential cells and mesenchymal stem cells (MSCs) that can produce a variety of mesenchymal cell types: osteoblasts (to make bone), chrondocytes (to make cartilage), connective and synovial tissue (to make tendon), and possibly skeletal muscle (Fig. 2-4). There is active research into these and other mesoendodermal bone marrow cell populations as they provide the prospect that bone marrow could be used to purify and expand these populations for therapeutic benefit. It is unclear how MSCs are derived from mesoderm and if they are present only in postnatal marrow.

ROAD MAPS OF HEMATOPOIESIS: CELLULAR PATHWAYS AS HSCs DIFFERENTIATE INTO TERMINALLY MATURE CELLS

At the apex of hematopoiesis HSCs sustain all the hematopoietic lineages throughout the lifetime of the individual. Considerable progress has been made over the last two to three decades in prospectively isolating HSCs and the different downstream multipotential (MPPs) and unilineage progenitors from humans and rodents. These studies allowed isolation of relative pure populations of cells of defined functionality. It has allowed one to begin to dissect the relationships between different blood cell populations. This is essential in describing the cellular basis of normal hematopoiesis. In turn this is critical when trying to understand how cells in hematologic diseases arise by genetic and epigenetic change from normal hematopoietic cells.

Central to isolation of HSCs and MPPs has been the identification of combinations of cell surface markers that allow separation of

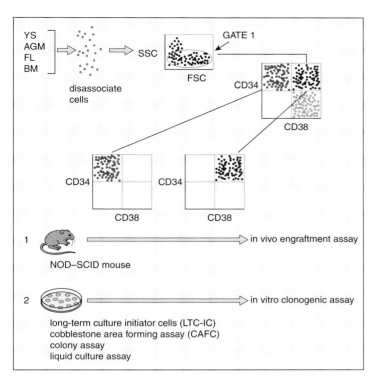

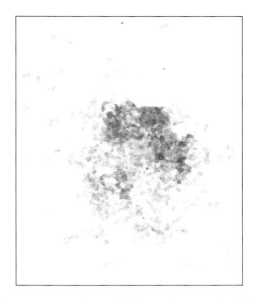

Fig. 2-6. Bone marrow culture: mixed granulocyte-erythroid (GE) colony. Hemoglobin-containing cells are stained with o-dianisidine (reddish brown). The neutrophils stain only with the hematoxylin counterstain. (Courtesy of Dr. G. E. Francis.)

Fig. 2-5. This shows how hematopoietic stem cells can be isolated from different sources. Cells are initially disassociated and stained with multiple antibodies. They are then analyzed and then sorted using a fluorescent-activated cell sorter (FACS). Here mononuclear live cells are separated in Gate 1. These live cells are then analyzed for CD34 and CD38 expression. Those live cells that are CD34+CD38− are enriched for stem cell potential. Further purification can be undertaken on the basis of additional cell surface markers such as CD90 (Thy1), SLAM markers, and N-cadherin. To test the functionality of isolated (sorted) cells, the cells can be tested in in vivo assays (transplanted into immunodeficient mice such as the NOD-SCID mouse model) and in vitro in long-term culture (long-term culture initiating cell culture assay and cobblestone-area forming assay), clonogenic colony assays, and liquid culture assays.

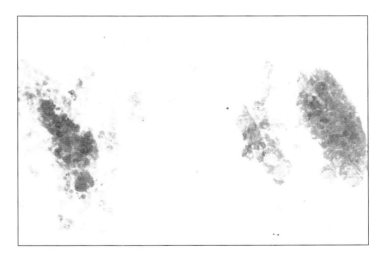

Fig. 2-7. Bone marrow culture: mixed GE colony adjacent to an eosinophil colony. (Luxol-fast blue stain.) (Courtesy of Dr. G. E. Francis.)

HSCs, MPPs, and unilineage progenitors by florescent-activated cell sorting (FACS). Fig. 2-5 schematically illustrates how HSCs (and progenitors) are isolated and tested for function. Hematopoietic tissues are isolated, cells disassociated, and then labeled with panels of fluorescently conjugated antibodies. The cell populations can then be analyzed and then separated on an FACS sorter. For example, human HSC populations express the cell surface antigen CD34. CD34 cells make up approximately 1% of bone marrow mononuclear cell population. Within CD34+ cells, HSCs principally reside in the CD38− population, which are only 1% of the CD34 population. Within the CD34+CD38− population, HSCs are enriched in cell populations that express the cell surface marker CD90+ and do not express CD45RA. This progressive purification scheme allows greater and greater enrichment of a cell population with HSC activity. These highly purified populations can then be tested functionally in in vitro assays that serve as surrogate assays for stem/early progenitor cells such as long-term culture initiating cell assay and cobblestone area forming assay. The most stringent test for stem cell activity is the ability of a cell population to serially engraft a whole animal and produce all hematopoietic cells. For human cells, this has involved transplanting cell populations into immunodeficient mice (such as NOD-SCID or NOG mice) that will allow human cells to engraft. Though there are limitations with this assay, it is the "gold standard" assay. Progenitor activity of populations can be tested either in vitro in colony (Figs. 2-6 and 2-7) or liquid culture assays or in vivo in xenograft studies.

These studies have allowed one to construct roadmaps of the cellular intermediates as an HSC differentiates into mature terminally differentiated blood cells (Fig. 2-8, *A*). These cellular intermediates have distinctive expression of cell-surface antigens (immunophenotypes) (Fig. 2-8, *B*). This is still a very active topic of research, and it is likely that the current view of how hematopoiesis proceeds is likely to be modified as more information becomes available. It is also important to bear in mind that some of the information about these cellular pathways comes from studies in rodents and not all the findings in rodents may apply to human hematopoiesis.

HSC pools have been divided into long-term HSCs (LT-HSCs) (that provide long-term engraftment and will serially engraft irradiated mice) and short-term HSCs (ST-HSCs) that have more limited self-renewal capacity in a serial transplant assay. After this, the pathways of differentiation are still under debate. One model suggests that an HSC gives rise to a multipotential progenitor (MPP) capable of giving rise to all blood cells but lacking the ability to serially transplant mice. The MPP then differentiates into the myeloid

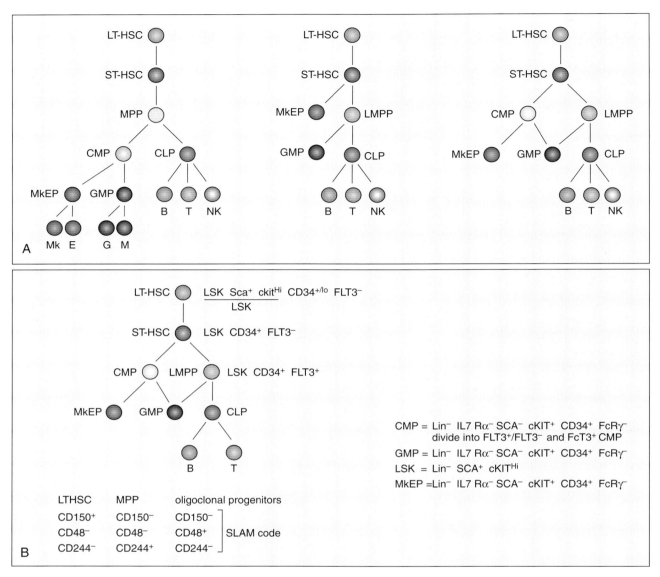

Fig. 2-8. A, Schematic representation of alternative views on the hierarchy of cellular intermediates (stem/progenitor cells) produced during differentiation of rodent long-term hematopoietic stem cell (LT-HSC) and short-term HSC (ST-HSC). MPP, multipotential progenitor; CMP, common myeloid progenitor; CLP, common lymphoid progenitor; MkEP, megakaryocyte-erythroid progenitor; GMP, granulocyte-macrophage progenitor; Mk, megakaryocyte; E, erythroid; G, granulocyte; M, macrophage/monocyte; **B,** B cell; T, T cell; NK, natural killer cell; LMPP, lymphoid-primed multipotential progenitor. **B,** The cell surface antigen expression that allows different HSC and progenitor populations to be prospectively isolated from human hematopoietic tissue.

and lymphoid lineages. The common myeloid progenitor (CMP) gives rise to all myeloid cells. Similarly, the common lymphoid progenitor (CLP) can differentiate into B and T lymphocytes and natural killer (NK) cells. The CMP further differentiates into progenitors with more restricted differentiation potential, the megakaryocyte-erythroid progenitor (MkEP) and a granulocyte-macrophage progenitor (GMP).

More recently, a modification of this model suggests that the first lineage commitment step from the HSC pool may not be a lymphoid-myeloid differentiation decision step, but one that allows the megakaryocyte-erythroid lineage to split off, leaving a progenitor that has both lymphoid and myeloid (granulocyte-macrophage) potential termed a *lymphoid primed multipotential progenitor* (LMPP). The LMPP then differentiates into the granulocyte-macrophage and lymphoid lineages. There is mounting evidence that early cell intermediates with combined myeloid/lymphoid potential exist. T-cell/myeloid progenitors and B-cell/myeloid progenitors have been isolated. Moreover, mixed myeloid/lymphoid leukemias also support the notion that there may be a normal counterpart of this malignant population. It may be that both models operate as shown in the third panel in Fig. 2-8, *A.*

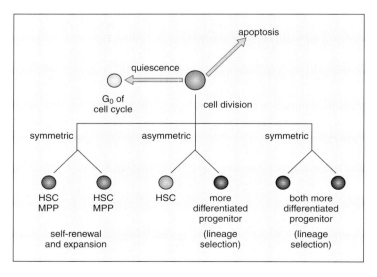

Fig. 2-9. Cell fate options for a hematopoietic stem cell (HSC). It can enter G_0 (quiescence), apoptose, or divide symmetrically or asymmetrically. MPP, multipotential progenitor.

What has also become clear is that the passage from one cellular compartment to another that results in a change of cellular potential (e.g., from ST-HSC to MPP or ST-HSC to MkEP and LMPP) is gradual process. It is also clear that genetic changes (such as mutations) or epigenetic changes, either in disease states or experimentally induced, can alter the progress of cells through these compartments. This can allow abnormal, accelerated, or even reverse differentiation. In the past the dogma has suggested that differentiation can only proceed in one direction, but we are now realizing that the whole process of hematopoiesis has much more plasticity than was appreciated.

Once specified, HSCs have a number of cell options (see Fig. 2-9). The key features of HSCs are their ability to self-renew throughout the lifetime of the individual and their ability to maintain their multipotentiality. Most of the time they remain quiescent and are in G_0 of the cell cycle. If they divide, they can undergo three types of cell division. In the first, they can generate two more HSCs. This type of division promotes expansion of HSC numbers at the expense of differentiation and ultimate production of lineage-affiliated cells. If this was the only type of HSC cell division, it would lead to cytopenias from arrested differentiation, a situation akin to hematopoietic malignancy. Second, HSCs can divide asymmetrically to produce an HSC and a more differentiated progeny that will eventually give rise to one or more lineage. This is a "balanced division," maintaining HSC numbers but allowing blood cell production. Third, HSCs can divide symmetrically to produce two differentiated progeny. If this was the only type of cell division undertaken by HSCs, it would lead to exhaustion of HSCs and eventually aplasia. Finally, HSCs can undergo apoptosis. The sum of all the HSC cell fate divisions determines the quality and quantity of hematopoietic activity.

As HSCs differentiate into progenitors and then terminal mature cells, the cell fate options that cells can make, change (Fig. 2-10). Progenitors have reduced self-renewal potential and this further declines with differentiation. In contrast to HSCs, progenitors spend much less time in G_0 and are highly proliferative. They provide much of the amplification in cell numbers required to satisfy the enormous daily demand for blood cells. In an adult human, approximately 10^{10} new blood cells are made daily. Finally, as progenitors enter terminal differentiation, the proliferative capacity is slowly lost and cells enter more progressively restricted pathways of differentiation that eventually lead to unilineage differentiation. Terminally mature cells are often postmitotic (e.g., red cells and granulocytes) and express the proteins required for function of terminally mature cells (see Chapter 4).

TRANSCRIPTIONAL CONTROL OF HEMATOPOIESIS

One crucial class of proteins that helps control hematopoiesis are transcription factors (TFs) (see Chapter 1) that are expressed either exclusively in blood cells or have restricted tissue-specific patterns of expression. The function of these critical TFs has often come to light as the genes encoding these TFs have acquired mutations in hematologic diseases such as lymphoma and leukemia (see Chapters 12, 13, and 18 through 20). The importance of these TFs is also underscored by the conserved role they play in hematopoiesis through evolution. Over the last two decades, this attribute has allowed the function of these TFs to be extensively investigated in animal models. In these models, genes encoding critical TFs have been deleted, modified, overexpressed, and misexpressed. A summary of the site of action of some of these TFs is shown in Fig. 2-11. A thorough description of the function of these proteins is not possible here. Some of the key points that arise from these studies are as follows:

1. TFs are divided into families that have similar protein domains.
2. They often bind DNA and interact with other proteins (other TFs and proteins that control transcription) via specific domains.
3. TFs work in combinations to both activate and repress the expression of a large number of genes.
4. TFs are required at discrete stages of hematopoiesis, and any one TF often functions at multiple stages within one lineage and can function in more than one lineage.
5. Ultimately, TFs work in complicated networks that can be modeled much like semiconductor/computing networks. TFs work in negative feedback loops, feed-forward loops, and cross-antagonistic loops, to mention just three such types of interaction.
6. The function of TFs helps regulate the cell's potential to make blood cells of different lineages, proliferate, undergo apoptosis, and self-renew.

More specifically, the TFs SCL/TAL1 and LMO2 are required to specify HSCs from mesoderm. The TFs RUNX1 (AML1), TEL1, MLL, and GATA2 are required to maintain stem cells once they have been specified. In myelopoiesis the TFs Pu.1, the C/EBP family (C/EBPα and C/EBPε), GFI-1, EGR-1, and NAB2 all promote the granulocyte-macrophage lineage programs. GATA2 is required in

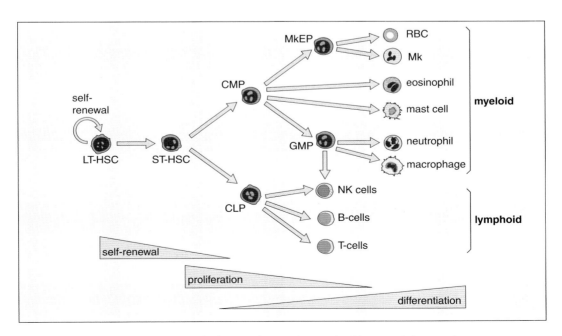

Fig. 2-10. A simplified schematic showing the cascade of hematopoietic progenitors and the relationship between these cell populations and their ability to self-renew, proliferate, and differentiate.

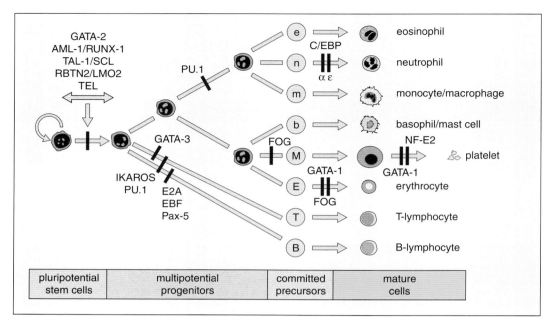

Fig. 2-11. A schematic representation of hematopoiesis and where key hematopoietic-specific transcription factors have nonredundant functions as revealed by gene deletion studies in mice. Thus, for example, the transcription factors GATA2, AML1/RUNX1, TAL-1/SCL, LMO2/RBTN2, and TEL are all critically required in hematopoietic stem cells (HSCs), and loss of function of these genes causes a block (as indicated by the red bar) in hematopoietic differentiation at the HSC level. Similarly, deletions of the other transcription factors cause blocks later in hematopoiesis as indicated by the red bars.

stem/early progenitor cells but is also required for mast cell differentiation and in the early phases of megakaryocyte-erythroid lineage maturation. Working with GATA2 to promote erythropoiesis and megakaryopoiesis are GATA1, FOG1, SCL, EKLF, p45NF-E2, and FlI-1. In early lymphopoiesis the TF Ikaros is required. In B-lymphopoiesis, the TFs E2A (and its family members), EBF, and PAX5 are required, and finally the TF BLIMP1 is necessary for plasma cell formation. In T-cell maturation, Notch signaling activates the TF CSL, which works with the TFs GATA3, T-BET, NFATc, and FOXP3.

Of note, the TFs SCL/TAL1, MLL, RUNX1, LMO2, PU.1, C/EBPα, PAX5, E2A, and GATA1 are all implicated in the pathogenesis of human leukemia.

THE HEMATOPOIETIC NICHE

It has been long appreciated that hematopoietic stem/progenitor cells require specialized anatomic locations called niches to survive and exercise their cell fate options. Niches are likely to exist in all hematopoietic organs. Most of the work has concentrated on the bone marrow niche, and lessons have been learned from a number of organisms, especially from mice. In the niche a number of extrinsic inputs influence hematopoietic cells (Fig. 2-12). The niche consists of a physical architecture: the cells surrounding hematopoietic cells (such as stromal cells, adipocytes, endothelial and perivascular cells of the vasculature, and osteoblasts) and the extracellular matrix (Table 2-1). Humoral inputs include cytokines. Paracrine signaling inputs (molecules that act over a short range) include chemokines such as CXCL12 that interact with the receptor CXCR4 on hematopoietic cells, soluble Wingless-related (WNT) proteins, NOTCH modulators, fibroblast growth factors (FGFs), and members of the Hedgehog family (Fig. 2-14). The role of cytokines, paracrine factors, and the downstream signaling pathways in hematopoiesis are discussed in Chapters 3 and 4.

More recently, it is being appreciated that metabolic inputs (such as ionic calcium levels regulated in part by surrounding osteoblasts) and neural inputs (signaling from autonomic nervous system) may also regulate hematopoietic stem/early progenitor behavior. The regulation of stem/progenitor cells is in part controlled by cell-cell contacts that are mediated by cell surface adhesion molecules (Table 2-2) that regulate the interaction of hematopoietic cells with surrounding niche cells and are important in the retention and release of hematopoietic

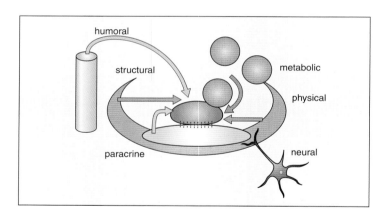

Fig. 2-12. Stem cells are thought to reside in specialized regions of the bone marrow, or "niches." The factors that regulate stem cell biology include the architectural space, physical engagement of the cell membrane with tethering molecules on neighboring cells or surfaces, signaling interactions, at the interface of the stem cell and its niche, paracrine and endocrine signals from local or distant sources, neural inputs, and metabolic products of tissue activity. (Adapted from Scadden DT: *Nature* 441, 1075-1079, 2006, Fig. 3.)

TABLE 2-1. THE STROMAL CELLS AND EXTRACELLULAR MATRIX: HEMATOPOIESIS DEPENDS ON THESE

Cells	Extracellular matrix/bone
Macrophages	Fibronectin
Fibroblasts	Hemonectin
Reticulum ('blanket') cells	Laminin
Fat cells	Collagen
Endothelial cells	Proteoglycans (acid mucopolysaccharides; e.g., chondroitin, heparan)

TABLE 2-2.   CELL ADHESION MOLECULES

Adhesion molecule	CD number	Ligand	Function
Integrin family			
Very late acting antigens			
$\alpha_1\beta_1$ (VLA-1)	CD49a/29	Collagen I, IV, laminin	Cell adherence to ECM
$\alpha_2\beta_1$ (VLA-2)	CD49b/29	Collagen I, IV, laminin	
$\alpha_3\beta_1$ (VLA-3)	CD49c/29	Collagen I, laminin, fibronectin	Cell adherence to ECM
$\alpha_4\beta_1$ (VLA-4)	CD49d/29	Fibronectin, VCAM-1	Cell adherence to ECM
			Cell–cell adhesion
$\alpha_5\beta_1$ (VLA-5)	CD49e/29	Fibronectin	Cell adherence to ECM
$\alpha_6\beta_1$ (VLA-6)	CD49f/29	Laminin	Cell adherence to ECM
Leukocyte integrins (LFA-1 family)			
$\alpha_D\beta_2$	CD18	?	
$\alpha_L\beta_2$ (LFA-1)	CD11a/18	ICAM-1, ICAM-2, ICAM-3	Cell–cell adhesion
			Cell–matrix adhesion
Cytoadhesins			
$\alpha_V\beta_3$ (vitronectin receptor)	CD51/61	Vitronectin, fibronectin, collagen, thrombospondin, vWF	Cell adherence to ECM
$\alpha_R\beta_3$ (leukocyte response integrin)		Vitronectin, fibronectin, collagen, thrombospondin, vWF	Cell adherence to ECM
$\alpha_V\beta_5$	CD51/–	Vitronectin, fibronectin	Cell adherence to ECM
$\alpha_V\beta_7$	CD51/–	?	
Immunoglobulin superfamily			
ICAM-1	CD54	$\alpha_L\beta_2$ $\alpha_M\beta_2$	Cell–cell adhesion
ICAM-2	CD102	$\alpha_L\beta_2$	Cell–cell adhesion
ICAM-3	CD50	$\alpha_L\beta_2$	Cell–cell adhesion
VCAM-1	CD106	$\alpha_R\beta_1$	Recruitment
PECAM-1	CD31	CD31, $\alpha_V\beta_3$	Transmigration
HCAM	CD44	Collagen I, IV, fibronectin	Extravasation
Selectin family			
L-selectin	CD62L	Carbohydrate determinants on EC	Migration, rolling on vessel wall
E-selectin	CD62E	Mo, neut, eos	Migration, rolling on vessel wall
P-selectin	CD62P	Mo, neut, eos	Adhesion to activated platelets and EC

Adapted from *Postgraduate Haematology*, ed. 5, Oxford, 2005, Blackwell Publishing: Table 17.1.

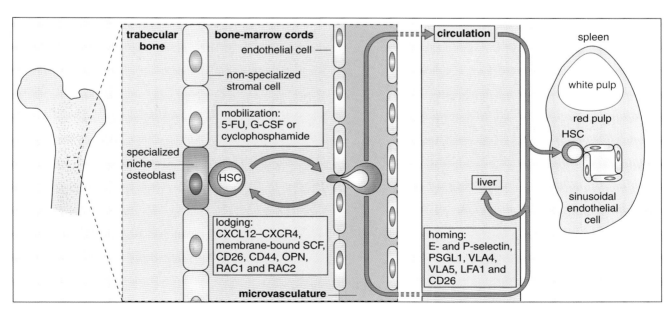

Fig. 2-13. Mobilization, homing, and lodging. Schematic diagram showing some of the factors implicated in these processes. Hematopoietic stem cells (HSCs) bound to the niche are mobilized into peripheral blood by growth factor therapy (G-CSF) or chemotherapy (cyclophosphamide or other regimens). Once in the blood-stream they migrate to all hematopoietic organs, including the spleen (as shown). They home to the bone marrow and bind to a number of cell surface molecules, including endothelial- (E-) and platelet- (P-) selectin, P-selectin glycoprotein ligand 1 (PSGL1), very late antigen 4 (VLA4) and VLA5, and lymphocyte function associated antigen 1 (LFA1). After entering the marrow they lodge in the niche, a process that is regulated by membrane-bound stem cell factor (SCF), CXC-chemokine ligand 12 (CXCL12) and its receptor CXC-chemokine receptor 4 (CXCR4), osteopontin (OPN), hyaluronic acids, and their corresponding receptors. (Adapted from Wilson A & Trumpp A: *Nature Review: Immunology* 6, 93-106, 2006, Fig. 4.)

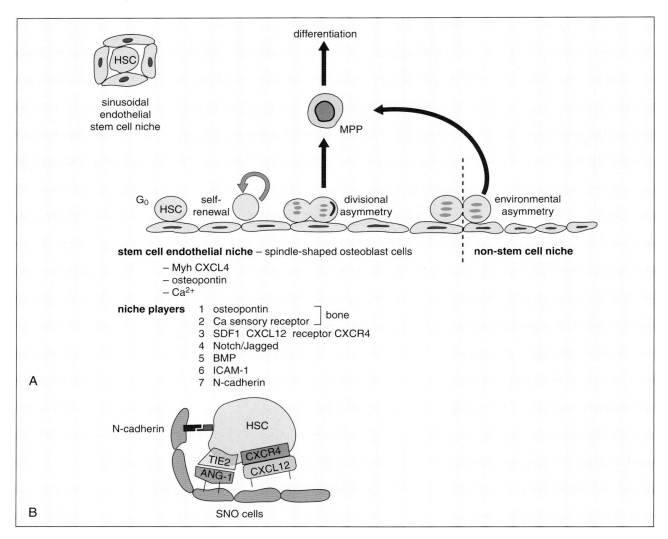

Fig. 2-14. A, The bone marrow niche, which, in part, consists of sinusoidal endothelial cells, helps control hematopoietic stem cell (HSC) fate. HSCs can be in G_0 or can enter cycle to divide symmetrically or asymmetrically (divisional asymmetry) to self-renew and/or to produce more differentiated cells such as multipotential progenitors (MPP). HSCs can also migrate into and out of the niche (environmental asymmetry). The components of the niche are shown below. **B,** This shows an HSC anchored into the niche via TIE-2/TEK binding to its ligand angiopoietin-1 on sinusoidal endothelial cells (SNO cells) and CXC-chemokine ligand 12 on SNO cells binding to its receptor CXCR4.

stem/progenitor cells. This is important in controlling the trafficking of hematopoietic stem/progenitor cells both normally and also in situations such as therapeutic stem/progenitor cell mobilization (Fig. 2-13).

In addition to the marrow niche there are likely to be other niches, but we know even less about them. For example, in development the fetal liver is a critical site of hematopoiesis and it is likely the niche here will be different from that in the bone marrow. In addition, there is increasing work studying how modifying the niche may modify the nature of cell divisions (symmetric-versus-asymmetric, Fig. 2-9) that HSCs undergo (Fig. 2-14).

GROWTH FACTORS

Blood cells, like other cells, receive signals that influence how they proliferate, differentiate, and apoptose (i.e., the cell fate). These signals also affect the functions of mature cells and are involved in the amplification of production of leukocytes in response to infection, red cells in response to anemia, and platelets in response to thrombocytopenia. In this chapter we review the biology of the signaling ligands, the receptors they interact with, and aspects of how these signals are transduced by cells. There are families of signaling pathways that share features in common. Often a signaling molecule will act at more than one stage in hematopoiesis and have different effects at different stages of hematopoiesis.

Signaling molecules that bind to cells are also termed cytokines. They are protein molecules. They can regulate cell growth and in this case are also termed growth factors. There are also cytokines that suppress cell growth. Signaling inputs can be transmitted in a number of different ways (Fig. 3-1). Cytokines or growth factors are released systemically into the bloodstream by organs (e.g., the kidneys release erythropoietin and the liver produces thrombopoietin) or other bone marrow cells: stromal cells (fibroblasts and endothelial cells), lymphocytes, and macrophages. Hematopoietic cytokines include colony-stimulating factors (CSFs), interleukins (ILs), monokines, chemokines, and interferons (IFNs). Signaling molecules can also act more locally, for example, just within the bone marrow. These molecules may also target cells at long range or just affect target cells nearby (paracrine), for example, within a local niche (see Chapter 2). In some cases paracrine signaling requires cell-to-cell contact. Finally, a cell may release signaling molecules that it can detect and that affect its own behavior (autocrine signaling).

SIGNALING AT DIFFERENT STAGES OF HEMATOPOIESIS

One way of demonstrating which cytokines, growth factors, and local signaling molecules function at different stages of hematopoiesis is by documenting the different complements of cell surface receptors that detect and respond to external signaling molecules in stem/progenitor and mature blood cells (Fig. 3-2).

In vitro culture systems have shown that although some cytokines support specific lineages, others affect multiple lineages. This has led to the notion that like hematopoiesis itself, signaling molecules can be arranged in a hierarchic manner. Some, such as stem cell factor (SCF, that binds the receptor c-KIT), Fms-like tyrosine kinase 3 (FLT3), thrombopoietin (TPO), and IL-3, act on the hematopoietic stem cells (HSCs) and multipotential cells. Others have a more restricted action and act on specific lineages, although they may also affect earlier cells (see pages 33 and 35). Examples include erythropoietin (EPO), which functions on erythroid cells; granulocyte-CSF (G-CSF), which is required for neutrophils; granulocyte macrophage-CSF (GM-CSF), which promotes granulocyte and monocyte production; IL-5, which is a central cytokine for eosinophils; and IL-4, interferon γ and IL-7, required for lymphocytes. TPO is a good example of a cytokine that acts on multiple cell types and promotes HSC growth but also has a critical role in megakaryocyte proliferation and maturation. The action of different cytokines and signaling molecules on all the different cell intermediates in granulopoiesis (Fig. 3-3), erythropoiesis

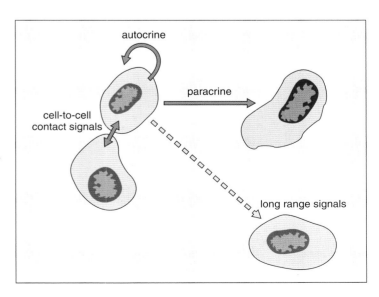

Fig. 3-1. Cells receive signals by a number of means. Cells can signal to themselves (autocrine), by cell-to-cell contact (juxtacrine), via short-range signals (paracrine), and via long-range signals.

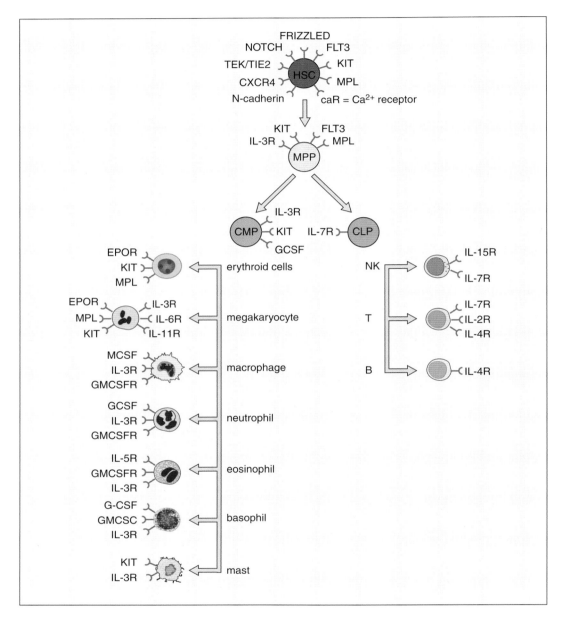

Fig. 3-2. The main cell surface receptors on hematopoietic stem cells (HSCs) and progenitor cells. MPP, multipotential progenitor; CMP, common myeloid progenitor; CLP, common lymphoid progenitor; TIE2/TEK, TEK tyrosine kinase (ligand is angio-poietin-1); Notch, NOTCH receptor family members including NOTCH-1, NOTCH-2, and TAN-1 (ligands are Jagged and Delta family members); Frizzled receptor (ligands are WNT family members, especially WNT 5a); FLT3, fms-related tyrosine kinase 3 (ligand is FLT3 ligand); c-KIT, also known as stem cell factor receptor (ligand is stem cell factor, SCF); TPO-R, thrombopoietin receptor (ligand is thrombopoietin, TPO); CaR, calcium sensing receptor (ligand is calcium); IL, interleukin (specific interleukins have a specific numeral; EPO-R, erythropoietin receptor (ligand is erythropoietin, EPO); MCSF, monocyte/macrophage receptor, GMCSFR, granulocyte-macrophage receptor.

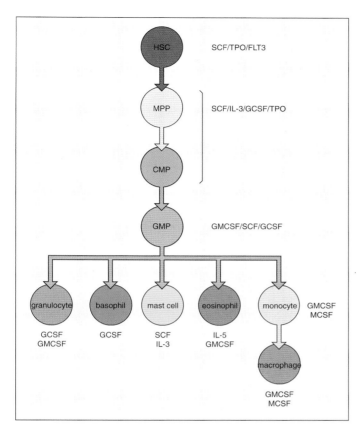

Fig. 3-3. The growth factors that act on the sequence of myeloid progenitors and granulocytic cells that differentiate from an HSC. See text for details.

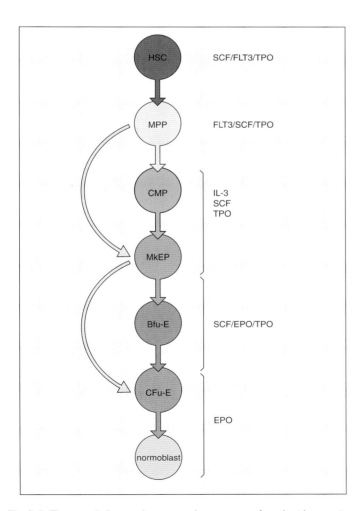

Fig. 3-4. The growth factors that act on the sequence of erythroid progenitors and differentiated erythroid cells (normoblasts) that differentiate from an HSC. See text for details.

(Fig. 3-4), megakaryopoiesis (Fig. 3-5), and lymphopoiesis (Fig. 3-6) is shown.

Some of the complexity of the signaling interplay between hematopoietic cells and cells in their microenvironment is shown in Fig. 3-7, *A*. Endotoxin stimulates monocytes to release IL-1 and tumor necrosis factor (TNF), which in turn induces marrow stromal cells (fibroblasts, endothelial cells), as well as T lymphocytes and macrophages, to produce a number of cytokines.

In Fig. 3-7, *B*, the interaction between the environment, body oxygen tension, organs that release EPO, and erythropoiesis is shown. Blood oxygen tension is sensed by mesangial cells in the kidney and, to a lesser extent, by hepatocytes. At high oxygen tension a family of oxygen-sensitive prolylhydroxylase enzymes hydroxylates the transcription factor HIF-1α (hypoxia inducing factor α) on prolyl residues. This leads to ubiquitination of HIF-1α by a ubiquitin ligase complex that contains the tumor suppressor von Hippel-Lindau protein. Ubiquitinated HIF-1α is then degraded. Lower levels of HIF-1α lead to lower transcription of EPO in renal mesangial cells. Thus, there is autocrine/paracrine regulation of EPO levels in the kidneys. (See also Chapter 4.)

By contrast, in response to hypoxia caused, for example, by anemia or high altitude, the prolylhydroxylases are inhibited and HIF-1α levels are high, and this upregulates EPO production. EPO stimulates erythropoiesis largely at the committed CFU-E stage; also, a proportion of BFU-E progenitors and more mature cells (up to the reticulocyte stage) are sensitive to EPO. The action of EPO is to increase the overall red cell mass leading to increased hemoglobin.

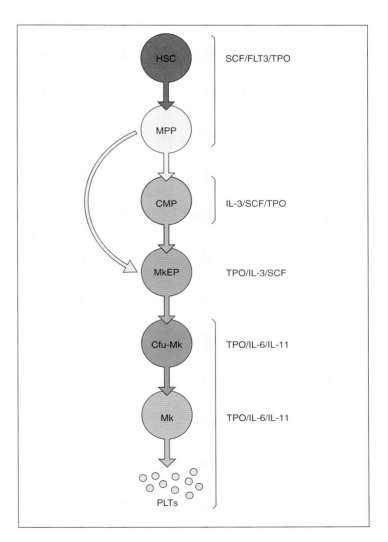

Fig. 3-5. The growth factors that act on the sequence of megakaryocyte progenitors and differentiated megakaryocytes that differentiate from an HSC. See text for details.

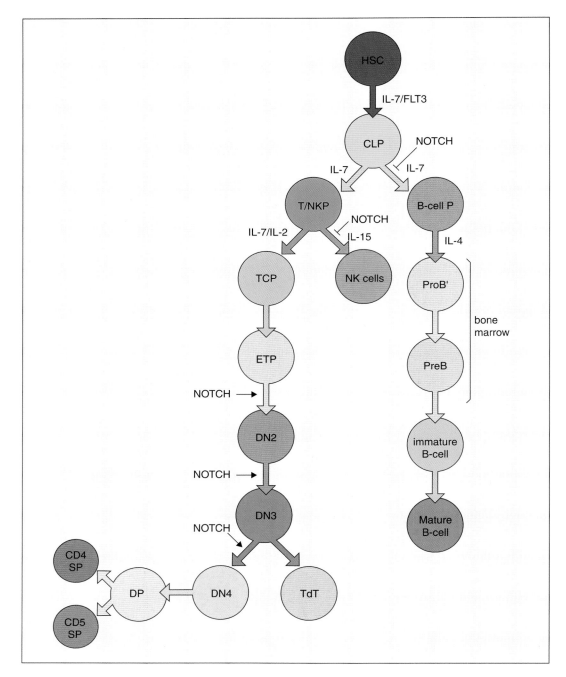

Fig. 3-6. The cytokines that act on the sequence of lymphocyte progenitors and differentiated lymphocytes that differentiate from an HSC. T/NKP, T and NK cell progenitor; TCP, T cell progenitor; ETP, early thymic progenitor; DN2, DN3, DN4, different types of double negative D4⁻ CD8⁻ T cells; DP, double positive CD4⁺ CD8⁺ T cells; SP single positive T cell; B cell, B cell progenitor; NK, natural killer cell. TdT, terminal deoxynucleotidyl transferase.

However, over time, and with increasingly refined analysis of genetically modified animal models, it has become apparent that cytokines such as TPO, G-CSF, and GM-CSF can regulate stem/progenitor cells as well as lineage-specific cells. Furthermore, it is likely some of these cytokines will have effects outside hematopoiesis. For example, EPO is thought to protect central nervous system neurons against hypoxic stress. The pleiotropic effects of cytokines are likely to be due to the level of cell-specific cytokine receptor expression, the availability of cytokines, synergistic interactions between cytokines, and the differential attenuation of cytokine signals in a cell-type-specific manner by negative regulators such as the SOCS (suppressor of cytokine signaling) proteins. Importantly, identification of cytokines such as EPO, G-CSF, and GM-CSF has led to their use therapeutically to increase erythrocyte and neutrophil production, respectively, in bone marrow transplantation and treatment of congenital and acquired cytopenias. They are also used to mobilize multipotent progenitors into the peripheral blood to improve the harvest of these cells before autologous stem cell transplantation.

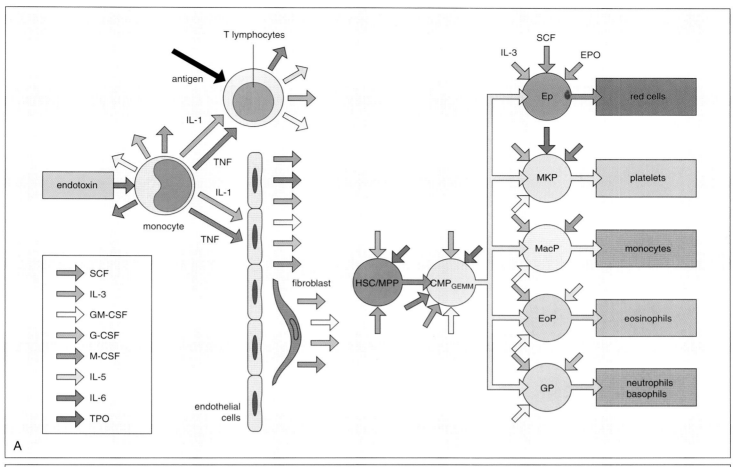

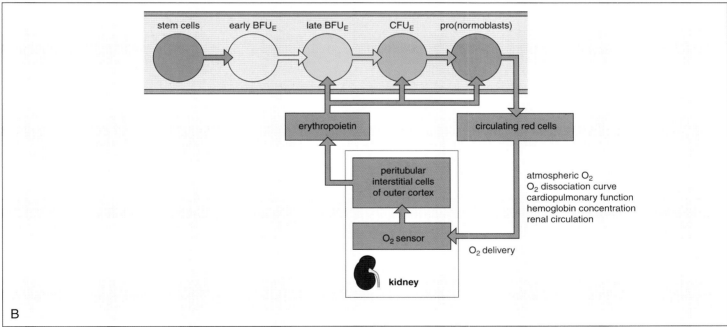

Fig. 3-7. Regulation of hematopoiesis. **A,** Pathways of stimulation of leukopoiesis by endotoxin (e.g., from infection). It is likely that endothelial and fibroblast cells release basal quantities of GM-CSF and G-CSF in the normal resting state and that this is enhanced substantially by the monokines TNF and IL-1 released in response to infection. Also, IL-1 and TNF stimulate T cells, and antigen may stimulate T cells directly. The action of IL-3 on human HSCs has not been proved (TPO, thrombopoietin). **B,** The production of erythropoietin by the kidney in response to its oxygen (O_2) supplies is shown. Erythropoietin stimulates erythropoiesis and so increases O_2 delivery; O_2 delivery may also be affected by other factors, as shown. (From Erslev AJ, Gabuzda TG: *Pathology of blood,* ed 3, Philadelphia, 1985, WB Saunders.) (See also Chapter 4.)

CYTOKINE RECEPTORS

Cytokines bind to their receptors with high picomolar affinity leading to receptor homodimerization (e.g., erythropoietin receptor, EPOR—see below) or heterodimerization/oligomerization of receptor subunits (e.g., IL-2 receptor) or induction of a conformational change in preformed receptor dimers (EPOR) resulting in the activation of downstream signaling pathways.

Cytokine receptors are divided into a number of families (Fig. 3-8, A–D). Receptors can be composed of dimers of a single receptor chain (see Fig. 3-8, A). Examples include erythropoietin receptor (EPOR), thrombopoietin receptor (MPL), and granulocyte colony-stimulating factor receptor (G-CSFR).

Alternatively, receptors can be heterodimeric with a common signaling subunit and a unique ligand-binding chain. There are three categories of receptor here. One group of hematopoietic receptors shares a common 130KD glycoprotein signaling subunit (gp130) (see Fig. 3-8, B). They include IL-6 receptor (IL-6Rα/gp130), IL-11 receptor (IL-11Rα/gp130), IL-12 receptor (IL-12Rα/gp130) leukemia inhibitory factor receptor (LIFR β/gp130), and oncostatin M receptor (OSMRα/gp130). The second heterodimeric group of receptors shares a common 140KD β-chain (Fig. 3-8, C, and Fig. 3-9). These include IL-3 receptor (IL-3Rα/gp140), IL-5 receptor (IL-5Rα/gp140), and granulocyte-macrophage colony-stimulating factor receptor (GM-CSFRα/gp140). Finally, some receptors share a common γ_c-chain (see Fig. 3-8, C) and include the IL-2 receptor (IL-2Rα/β/γ_c), IL-4 receptor (IL-4Rα/γ_c), IL-7 receptor (IL-7Rα/γ_c), IL-9 receptor (IL-9Rα/γ_c), IL-13 receptor (IL-13Rα/γ_c), IL-15 receptor (IL-15Rα/γ_c), and IL-21 receptor (IL-21Rα/γ_c).

All of these homodimeric and heterodimeric receptor groups constitute the type 1 cytokine receptors family. They share four conserved cysteine residues, a tryptophan-serine-X-tryptophan-serine motif (WSXWS motif), and fibronectin type III domains in the extracellular part of the receptor. They also share a conserved membrane proximal intracytoplasmic domain called the Box1/Box2 domain that is important for signaling following ligand binding.

A separate class of receptors, the Type II family, includes the receptors for interferon (IFN) α/β and interferon γ (see Fig. 3-8, D). These receptors are composed of two distinct subunits (IFNR1/IFNR2). They contain Box1/Box2 domains but lack the WSXWS motif.

SIGNALING PATHWAYS DOWNSTREAM OF RECEPTORS

Once a ligand has engaged a receptor, an intricate series of complex molecular events transduce the signal to effect changes in nuclear gene expression. Here, we give examples of these pathways. These are often drawn as linear pathways. However, it is important to remember that any one ligand/receptor pair often signals through more than one intracellular signaling pathway. Moreover, if multiple ligand/receptor pairs are "seen" by a cell, a complex interaction between pathways is likely to occur in a cell. This is hard to accurately document, is often not shown in textbooks, and is likely to determine the in vivo consequences of hematopoietic cells interacting with extrinsic signaling molecules.

WNT PATHWAY

An example of an important signaling pathway for hematopoietic stem cell (HSC) self-renewal is the evolutionarily conserved standard WNT (Wingless-related) pathway that acts both in development and in adult homeostasis (Fig. 3-10). Multiple WNT ligands engage their cognate receptor complex consisting of a serpentine receptor of the Frizzled family and a member of the LDL receptor family, LRP5/6. When the receptor is occupied the receptor binds the cytoplasmic scaffold protein Axin and the Axin-binding protein Dishevelled.

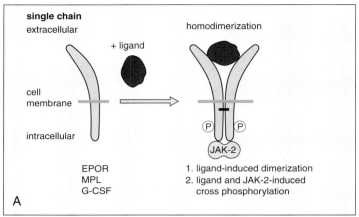

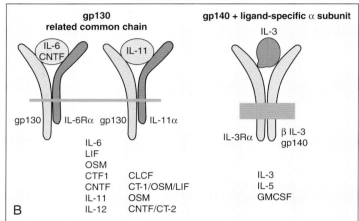

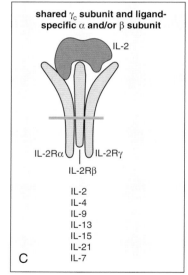

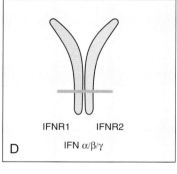

Fig. 3-8. A, EPO, TPO, and G-CSF receptors are all single-chain polypeptides that have an extracellular/transmembrane and intracellular portions *(left)*. On binding ligand, the receptor chains homodimerize, and recruit the downstream signal transduction molecule, the kinase JAK2, leading to cross phosphorylation of the receptor chains and JAK2 *(right)*. MPL, thrombo protein receptor; G-CSFR, G-CSFR receptor. **B,** IL-6, LIF (leukemia-inhibitory factor), OSM (oncostatin M), CTF1 (cardiotrophin 1), CNTF (ciliary neurotrophic factor), IL-11, IL-12 bind a unique receptor-specific chain that is complexed to a common chain called gp130. The combination of the unique receptor specific chain and gp130 creates a high-affinity receptor *(left)*. The cytokines IL-3, IL-5, and GM-CSF also bind a heterodimeric receptor, composed of unique receptor specific chain (the α chain of the receptor) that is complexed to a common chain called gp140. The genes encoding the unique chain are IL3RA (for IL-3 receptor), IL5RA (for IL-5 receptor), and CSF2RA (for GM-CSF receptor) *(right)*. **C,** Many interleukins (as indicated in the diagram) bind either a heterodimeric or heterotrimeric receptor that shares a common γ chain. **D,** Interferons α, β, and γ bind a heterodimeric receptor composed of two subunits. Interferons α and β bind the same receptor (genes encoding the polypeptides are called IFNAR1 and IFNAR2) whereas interferon γ binds a receptor with a similar structure but composed of related but distinct polypeptides encoded by the genes IFNGR1 and IFNGR2.

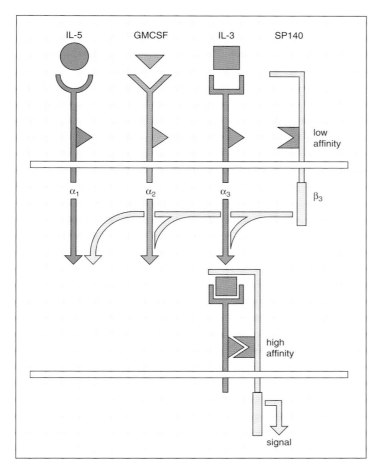

Fig. 3-9. Receptors for GM-CSF, IL-3, and IL-5: structures. These have different α chains but a common β chain (gp140) that, after binding to the α chain in the presence of the growth factor, forms a high-affinity receptor and is subsequently responsible for signal transduction to the cell interior. (Modified from Nicola NA, Metcalf D: Subunit promiscuity among haemopoietic growth factor receptors, *Cell* 67:1-4, 1991.)

Axin/Dishevelled then inhibits a protein destruction complex that contains the tumor suppressor protein adenomatous polyposis coli (APC) and the kinase GSK3-β (glycogen synthetase kinase 3 beta). B-catenin then accumulates in the cytoplasm and is transported into the nucleus. Here it binds the DNA-binding transcription factor TCF/LEF proteins. The β-catenin/TCF/LEF complex can then activate target genes. Target gene expression leads to HSC expansion and altered HSC function.

When the receptor is not engaged, the β-catenin is phosphorylated on conserved serine and threonine residues. Phosphorylated β-catenin is then ubiquitinated and degraded by a proteosome. Thus, β-catenin is not able to accumulate. LEF/TCF, without β-catenin, represses gene transcription. This leads to decreased ability of HSC to repopulate hematopoiesis in vivo. In addition to the standard WNT signaling, WNT also signals via an alternative calcium pathway and the c-Jun kinase pathway.

CYTOKINE SIGNALING PATHWAYS

Interaction of cytokines with the ligand-binding receptor subunit initiates oligomerization (see above) with other receptor subunits that triggers a web of intracellular signaling pathways that have distinct but also intercommunicating components (Fig. 3-11). The common finding of leukemia-associated mutations in these signaling pathways has suggested that they may be a required class mutation for leukemogenesis (see Chapter 12).

Common to most pathways are changes in protein phosphorylation on tyrosine, serine, and threonine residues (catalyzed by tyrosine and serine/threonine kinases respectively). In some cases (e.g., the receptors for SCF, M-CSF) the intracellular domain of the receptor acts as a tyrosine kinase, which phosphorylates itself on tyrosine residues following ligand binding. In all cases, the receptors activate important kinase pathways including the phosphatidyl-inositol-3-kinase (PI3K) pathway (see Figs. 3-11 and 3-13), the three mitogen-activated protein kinases pathways (MAPK)—extracellular-signal regulated kinases (ERK), c-jun N-terminal kinases/stress-activated protein kinases (JNK/SAPK), and p38 MAPK (see Figs. 3-11 and 3-13) together with the Janus-activated kinases (JAK) (see Figs. 3-11

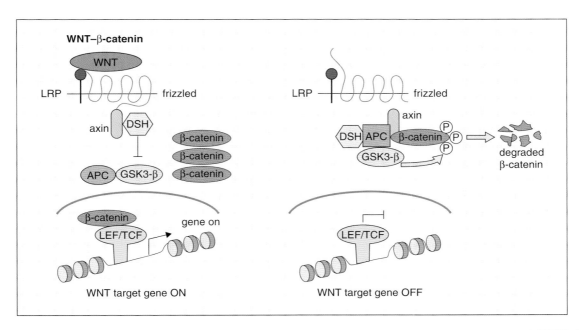

Fig. 3-10. Schematic pathway of the WNT-Frizzled receptor. On the left, when WNT is bound to its receptor—a heterodimer of Frizzled and its partner LRP. The receptor binds the Axin 1/dishevelled (DSH) complex. This complex inhibits APC (adenomatous polyposis coli gene) and the kinase GSK3-β (glycogen synthase kinase 3 beta). When GSK3-β is inhibited it fails to phosphorylate β-catenin, and β-catenin can then accumulate. β-catenin then translocates into the nucleus and binds to the transcription factor LEF/TCF. β-catenin/LEF/TCF then activates gene expression (WNT target gene are "on"). On the right, when LRP/Frizzled are not engaged by WNT, DSH/APC/Axin/GSK3-β forms an active complex that phosphorylates β-catenin. Phosphorylated β-catenin is then targeted for proteolysis. LEF/TCF fails to activate WNT target genes.

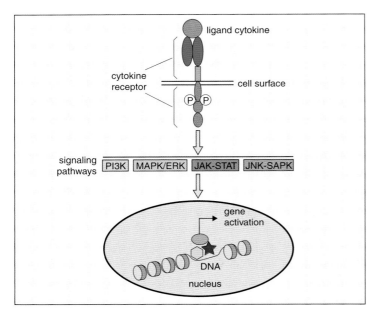

Fig. 3-11. Binding of cytokine to cytokine receptors leads to activation of intracellular signaling pathways (PI3K, MAPK/ERK, JAK-STAT, JNK-SAPK) that transmit messages from the cytoplasm to the nucleus where gene transcription is modulated. Ultimately this affects cell fate choice, cell cycle, and apoptosis machinery.

and 3-14). Other important signal transduction components include the STAT proteins (Signal Transducers of Activation and Transcription) (Fig. 3-14) that principally, but not exclusively, are activated by the JAK kinases.

THE RAS/MAPK KINASE PATHWAY

The RAS/MAPK kinase pathway (Figs. 3-12 and 3-13) has been one of the most intensively studied signal transduction pathways. The phosphotyrosine residues on receptors bind signal-transducing proteins that contain SRC homology 2 (SH2) domains, such as GAB1/SHC (see Fig. 3-13). These in turn bind a complex of proteins that includes Grb2 and SOS. This in turn leads to conversion of p21/RAS-GDP to p21/RAS-GTP. This occurs at the cell membrane. Farnesylation, a posttranslational modification consisting of the transfer of an isoprenoid moiety to the C-terminus of the protein, is required for localization of RAS to the cell membrane. Binding of RAS to the cell membrane is essential for function, including activation of downstream effectors in the MAP kinase pathway, and it is a prerequisite for its transforming activity. Farnesylation is inhibited by franesyl transferase inhibitors that are under investigation therapeutically in leukemia.

P21RAS-GTP then phosphorlyates and activates the kinase RAF-1, which in turn phosphorylates a series of MAP-kinases (ERKs) that have major roles in transmitting the signal to the nucleus and activating transcription factors (Fig. 3-13). In one related but separate pathway, the enzyme phospholipase Cγ (PLCγ), which cleaves phosphatidyl inositol bisphosphate, is activated to break down membrane lipid, releasing two secondary messengers, diacylglycerol (DG) and inositol triphosphate (IP3; see Fig. 3-12). Activation of PLCγ occurs by binding to phosphotyrosine residues of the activated receptor (see Fig. 3-12). The enzyme protein kinase C (PKC) is activated by DG and, in turn, phosphorylates proteins mainly on threonine and serine residues. Release of intracellular calcium ions is caused by IP3. The exact way in which these two biochemical changes subsequently cause signal transduction in the nucleus is unclear.

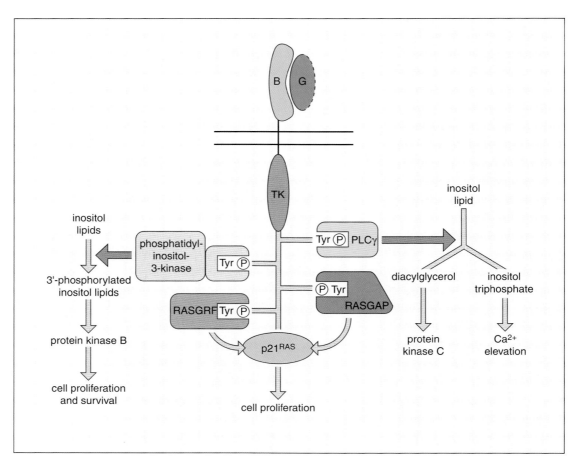

Fig. 3-12. SH2 domain-containing proteins. They bind to activated, tyrosine phosphorylated growth factor receptors. For clarity, only one partner of the receptor dimer is shown. (PLCγ, phospholipase Cγ; RASGAP, RAS GTPase-activating protein; RASGRF, guanine nucleotide releasing factor.) (Adapted with permission from Wickremasinghe RG, Hoffbrand AV: The molecular basis of leukaemia and lymphoma. In Hoffbrand AV, Lewis SM, Tuddenham EGD, editors: *Postgraduate haematology,* ed 4, Oxford, 1999, Butterworth-Heinemann, pp 354-372.)

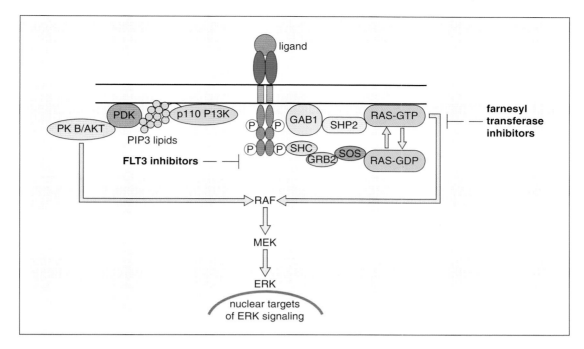

Fig. 3-13. Simplified relationship between the RAS and PI3 kinase pathways. After binding of ligand to the receptor the intracellular membrane becomes phosphorylated. This then binds a series of proteins that either activates the RAS pathway via the SH-containing adapter protein Shc (Src homology 2 domain containing transforming protein); GRB2 (growth factor receptor-bound protein 2); SOS (Son of Sevenless); GAB1 (GRB2-associated binding protein 1); PTPN11 (also called SHP2-protein tyrosine phosphatase, nonreceptor type 11). This leads to production of RAS-GTP that activates RAF1, which is a MAP kinase kinase kinase (MAP3K). RAF1 can also be activated by the PI3 kinase (phosphoinositol 3 kinase pathway) via membrane-bound p110 PI3K and PDK, which activates protein kinase B (AKT). PKB then activates RAF1. RAF1 phosphorylates MEK1/2 kinase, which phosphorylates ERK1/2 kinase. This leads to activation of nuclear ERK1/2 targets. The RAS pathway can be targeted by farnesyl transferase inhibitors (such as Tipfarnib). Also shown: the receptor itself can be targeted, and in this case an FLT3 receptor is targeted by FLT3 inhibitors. (See also Chapters 13 and 14.)

PI-3 KINASE PATHWAY

Phosphatidyl inositol 3′-kinase (PI-3 kinase) is also activated by binding to activated receptor. It phosphorylates inositol lipids in the cell membrane. Together with phosphoinositide-dependent protein kinase-1 (PDK-1) it then phosphorylates protein kinase B (also known as AKT), which can then interact with the RAF/MAPK pathway (see Figs. 3-11 and 3-12). Constitutive deregulated activation of this pathway has been shown to be oncogenic in human malignancy.

JAK-STAT PATHWAY

For those receptors that do not possess inherent protein kinase activity, the JAK-STAT system links cell surface receptors with transcription factor genes. The JAK kinase family includes JAK1, JAK2, JAK3, and TYK2. They are cytoplasmic, with molecular weight (MW) 130 kDa, and possess a conserved region at the N-terminal end, a kinase-like domain (J_H2 domain), and a tyrosine kinase domain (J_H1 domain) at the C-terminal end (Figs. 3-11, 3-14, and 3-15). The JAK kinases are activated by ligand binding and receptor

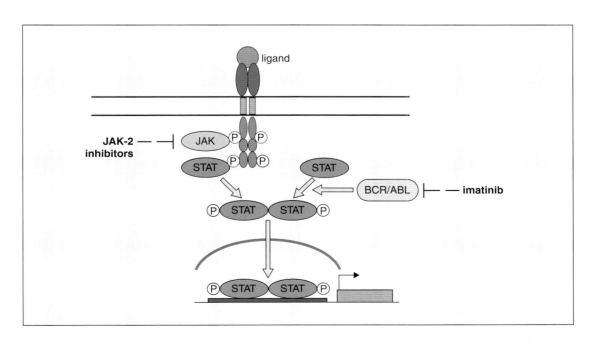

Fig. 3-14. Details of the JAK-STAT pathway. Ligand binding leads to receptor dimerization, cross phosphorylation of the receptor JAK, and STAT binding and phosphorylation of STAT proteins. Phospho-STAT proteins translocate to the nucleus where they bind critical DNA sequences to modulate gene expression. The modes of action of JAK2 inhibitors and imatinib are shown.

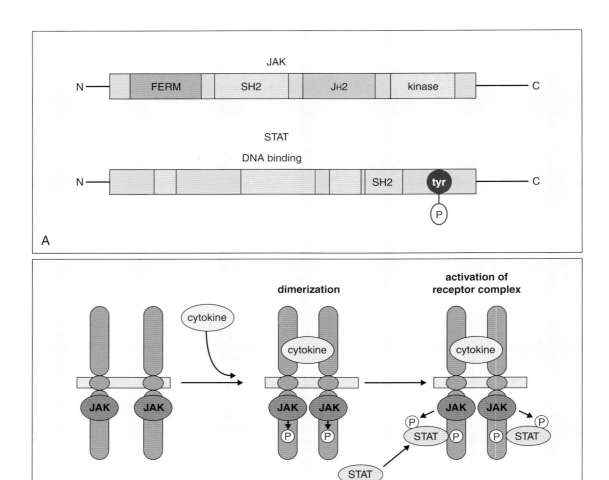

Fig. 3-15. **A,** Schematic structure of domains within the JAK protein; in this case JAK2 is shown. The FERM domain (required for binding to EPOR and other receptors), the SH2 domain (a protein interaction module), the JH2 domain (regulates activity of the kinase domain), and finally the kinase domain. **B,** The steps that lead to activation of the JAK-STAT pathway after binding of cytokine to the receptor. (See also Chapter 15.)

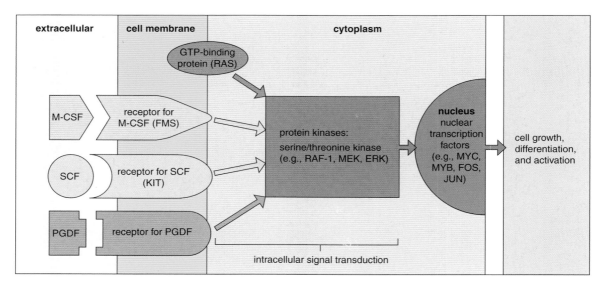

Fig. 3-16. Cellular proto-oncogene products: examples of those that act at different stages of the pathways that transduce growth signals from the cell membrane to the nucleus.

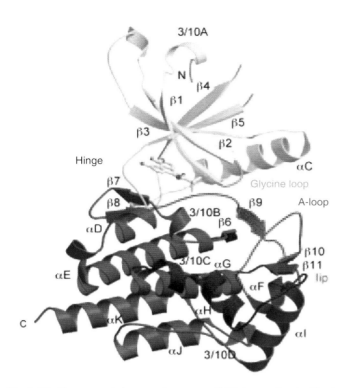

Fig. 3-17. Overview of the crystal structure JAK2 kinase domain. The kinase domain is divided into an amino portion (gray) and a C-terminal region (green) linked by a hinger (yellow). The catalytic region (blue) and activation loop (red) are centrally important for kinase activity. Structural studies such as these are important to design targeted therapies for diseases in which there is constitutively active JAK signaling.

dimerization. Box 1 and Box 2, conserved regions on the cytokine receptor intracytoplasmic regions, are involved in binding and activation of JAKs. The JAK kinases then phosphorylate tyrosine residues in latent cytokine transcription factors, the Signal Transducers, and Activators of Transcription (STATs). The STATs, of MW 80 to 100 kDa, are DNA-binding proteins with an SH2 domain and tyrosine phosphorylation sites at the C-terminal region (see Figs. 3-14 and 3-15). The activated STATs form a homodimer or heterodimer and translocate to the nucleus, where they bind to specific DNA motifs, positive promoter elements for cytokine-responsive genes. In addition to STAT activation, JAK kinases also phosphorylate additional proteins, including insulin-receptor substrate 1 and 2 (IRS-1, 2) and GAB2. The resultant phosphotyrosine residues serve as binding sites for SH2 domain-containing proteins, which activate signaling pathways that lead to ERK activation.

MUTATIONS IN SIGNALING COMPONENTS LEADING TO CLONAL HEMATOLOGIC DISORDERS

In hematologic malignancies, mutations are present in genes regulating intracellular signaling. These include cytokine receptors (e.g. mutations in *FLT-3* and *KIT* genes in acute myeloid leukemia, AML), intra-cellular signalling components (*JAK2* mutations in myeloproliferative disorders, T-cell acute lymphoblastic leukemia, Down Syndrome acute lymphoblastic leukemia, constitutive activation of ABL kinase by the *BCR-ABL* fusion gene in chronic myeloid leukemia, mutations in *RAS*, PTP11 genes in AML and myelodysplasia) (Fig. 3-16). Given the high frequency of such mutations and the fact that these mutations often deregulate enzymatic kinase function that is usually tightly controlled, much effort has gone into solving crystal structures of components of signaling pathways. In Fig. 3-17 the crystal structure of the JAK2 kinase domain is shown. These studies are important to help development of novel, potentially less toxic, targeted specific kinase inhibitors.

MATURATION OF BLOOD CELLS AND THEIR EXAMINATION IN PERIPHERAL BLOOD AND BONE MARROW

Every day the human marrow makes approximately 10^{10} new blood cells, the bulk of them mature erythrocytes, in a process called *erythropoiesis*. This massive undertaking ensures that there is adequate oxygen-carrying capacity in the body. A representation of the nuclear and cytoplasmic changes, the frequency in adult bone marrow, and the percentage in cycle of hematopoietic progenitor and precursor cells, produced as a hematopoietic stem cell (HSC) differentiates into erythroid cells, is shown (Fig. 4-1). Rare HSC cycle and commit to the myeloid lineage. The hierarchy of progenitors with erythroid potential (CFU-GEMM, BFU-E and CFU-E) are progressively amplified in number and cycle more actively. During terminal erythroid maturation, erythroid precursors (erythroblasts) mature through morphologically distinct maturation stages.

The main function of red cells is to carry oxygen to the tissues and return carbon dioxide from the tissues to the lungs. Hemoglobin is the critical protein constituent of red cells that is responsible for this gaseous exchange (Fig. 4-2, *A*). The principal adult hemoglobin molecule (Hb A) has a molecular weight (MW) of 68,000. It consists of α- and β-globin polypeptide chains (α2, β2). Each globin polypeptide chain has its own heme group that coordinates an iron molecule. The metabolism of iron and heme synthesis is set out in Chapter 5.

Control of erythroid production is principally regulated by varying the production of the cytokine erythropoietin (Epo) (Fig. 4-2B). In the kidney, oxygen is sensed in the cells of the kidney cortex. This is influenced by a number of factors, such as atmospheric oxygen, cardiopulmonary function, renal blood flow, and hemoglobin concentration. Hypoxia stimulates the peritubular interstitial cells to secrete erythropoietin (Epo), a 34 to 39 kDa protein (when fully glycosylated). The liver also produces a minor proportion of Epo. Epo promotes cell survival of the CFU-E and to a lesser extent BFU-E and erythroblasts that express the erythropoietin receptor (EpoR). Further discussion of erythropoietin receptor is set out in Chapter 3 and Figure 3-4. Epo stimulates these erythroid progenitor and precursor cells to proliferate and differentiate terminally. The level of Epo is principally controlled at the transcription level by the transcription factor HIFα (hypoxia inducing factor α). HIFα protein levels are controlled by ubiquination by an ubiquitin ligase complex that includes the tumor suppressor von Hippel-Lindau (VHL) protein (see Chapter 3 and Fig. 3-7, *B*). Germline mutations in the EpoR (associated with low or normal Epo levels) and VHL (Chuvash VHL mutation and other VHL mutations, associated with a high Epo level) are causes of familial erythrocytosis.

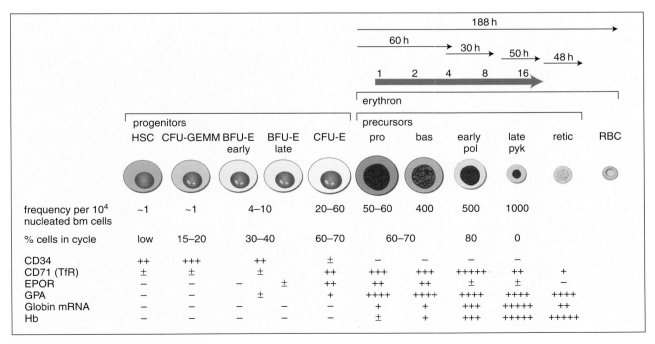

	HSC	CFU-GEMM	BFU-E early	BFU-E late	CFU-E	pro	bas	early pol	late pyk	retic	RBC
frequency per 10^4 nucleated bm cells	~1	~1	4–10		20–60	50–60	400	500	1000		
% cells in cycle	low	15–20	30–40		60–70	60–70		80	0		
CD34	++	+++	++		±	–	–	–	–		
CD71 (TfR)	±	±	±		++	+++	+++	+++++	++	+	
EPOR	–	–	–	±	++	++	++	±	±	–	
GPA	–	–	±		+	++++	++++	++++	++++	++++	
Globin mRNA	–	–	–	–	–	+	+	+++	+++++	++	
Hb	–	–	–	–	–	±	+	+++	+++++	+++++	

Fig. 4-1. The progression of cells through erythropoiesis from hematopoietic stem cells (HSCs) through multipotential myeloid cells (CFU-GEMM), to the earliest unilineage erythroid cells. Burst colony-forming erythroid cell (BFU-E), colony-forming erythroid (CFU-E), to maturing erythroblasts (proerythroblasts, pro; basophilic erythroblasts, bas; early polychromatic erythroblasts, early pol; late pyknotic erythroblasts, pyk), finally to enucleated reticulated cells (retic) and mature erythrocytes (RBCs). (Courtesy of Professor D. R. Higgs.)

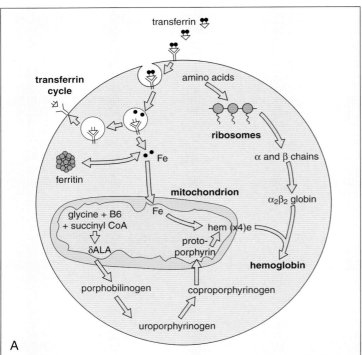

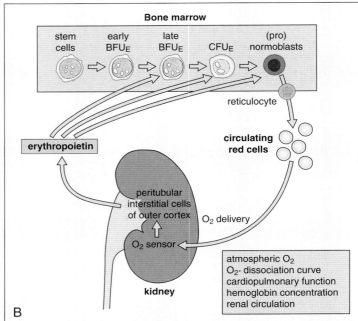

Fig. 4-2. A, A critical aspect of erythropoiesis is the production of hemoglobin. Iron is imported into erythroblasts via the transferrin receptor, enters mitochondria, and is incorporated into heme. Concurrently, globin chains are synthesized and the heme moiety and globin chains combine to form hemoglobin. **B,** Red cell production is controlled, in part, by serum erythropoietin levels. Erythropoietin is produced by the kidney, which senses blood oxygen levels. Decreased oxygen tension leads to increased erythropoietin production. Erythropoietin promotes survival of BFU-E and downstream erythroid cellular intermediates.

EXAMINATION OF PERIPHERAL BLOOD AND THE BONE MARROW

The usual initial diagnostic approach to blood disorders is blood counting (Table 4-1) and blood film examination and, if required, examination of the cytology and histology of the bone marrow (Table 4-2). Blood films are usually spread on glass slides stained with one of the Romanowsky stains (e.g., May-Grünwald/Giemsa or Wright's) (see Fig. 4-3). Bone marrow aspirates provide films on which the cytologic details of developing cells can be examined (Fig. 4-4, *A–C*). The proportions of different cells are assessed, appearances of the individual cells noted, and a search made for the presence of cells foreign to the normal marrow, such as metastatic deposits from carcinoma. Bone marrow trephine biopsies produce cores of bone and marrow, which are decalcified and processed for histologic assessment (Figs. 4-5 to 4-7). The trephine provides an excellent sample for examination of marrow architecture and cellularity. It is the most reliable method of detecting marrow infiltrates.

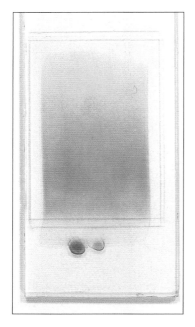

Fig. 4-3. Peripheral blood film: glass slide of a well-spread blood film stained by the May-Grünwald/Giemsa technique.

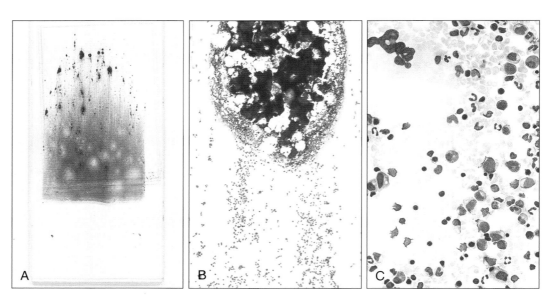

Fig. 4-4. A, Bone marrow aspirate: this normal aspirate has been spread, allowed to dry, and stained by the May-Grünwald/Giemsa technique. Bone marrow fragments are clearly visible at the tail end of the smear. Normal marrow fragment and cell trails: the marrow fragment **(B)** contains hematopoietic cells, supporting reticuloendothelial cells and some fat spaces. During the spreading procedure, representative cells of each hematopoietic cell line spill out into "trails" behind the marrow fragments; **(C)** higher magnification.

TABLE 4-1. NORMAL BLOOD COUNT

Hemoglobin (Hb)	male	13.5–17.5 g/dl
	female	11.5–15.5 g/dl
Red cells (RBC; erythrocytes	male	4.5–6.5 /l
	female	3.9–5.6 × 10^{12}/L
Packed cell volume (PCV; hematocrit)	male	40–50%
	female	36–48%
Mean corpuscular volume (MCV)		80–95 fl
Mean corpuscular hemoglobin (MCH)		27–34 pg
Mean corpuscular hemoglobin concentration (MCHC)		30–35 g/dl
Reticulocytes		0.5–2.0%; 50–60 × 10^9/L
White cells (WBC; leukocytes)	total	4.0–11.0 × 10^9/L
	neutrophils	2.5–7.5 × 10^9/L
	lymphocytes	1.5–3.5 × 10^9/L
	monocytes	0.2–0.8 × 10^9/L
	eosinophils	0.04–0.44 × 10^9/L
	basophils	0.01–0.1 × 10^9/L
Platelets		150–400 × 10^9/L

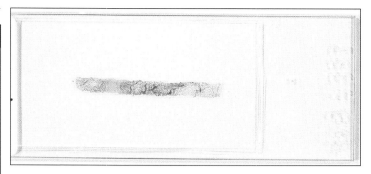

Fig. 4-5. Normal trephine biopsy: gross appearance of a section prepared from a trephine biopsy of the posterior iliac crest. (H & E stain.)

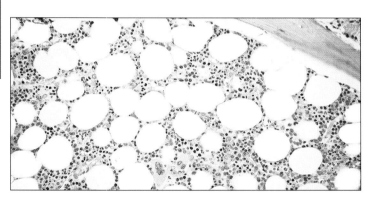

Fig. 4-6. Normal trephine biopsy: representative histology taken from the posterior iliac crest. Approximately half the intertrabecular space is occupied by hematopoietic tissue and half by fat. (H & E stain.)

TABLE 4-2. PERCENTAGE OF CELLS OF VARIOUS CATEGORIES IN BONE MARROW FILMS

Cells		Observed range	95% range (mean)
Blast cells		0.0–3.2	0.0–3.0 (1.4)
Promyelocytes		3.6–13.2	3.2–12.4 (7.8)
Neutrophil myelocytes		4.0–21.4	3.7–10.0 (7.6)
Eosinophil myelocytes		0.0–5.0	0.0–2.8 (1.3)
Metamyelocytes		1.0–7.0	2.3–5.9 (4.1)
Neutrophils	males	21.0–45.6*	21.9–42.3 (32.1)
	females	29.6–46.6*	28.8–45.9 (37.4)
Eosinophils		0.4–4.2	0.3–4.2 (2.2)
Eosinophils plus eosinophil myelocytes		0.9–7.4	0.7–6.3 (3.5)
Basophils		0.0–0.8	0.0–0.4 (0.1)
Erythroblasts	males	18.0–39.4*	16.2–40.1 (28.1)
	females	14.0–31.8*	13.0–32.0 (22.5)
Lymphocytes		4.6–22.6	6.0–20.0 (13.1)
Plasma cells		0.0–1.4	0.0–1.2 (0.6)
Manocytes		0.0–3.2	0.0–2.6 (1.3)
Macrophages		0.0–1.8	0.0–1.3 (0.4)
Myeloid: erythroid ratio	males	1.1–4.0†	1.1–4.1 (2.1)
	females	1.6–5.4†	1.6–5.2 (2.8)

Significance of difference between men and women: *$P < 0.001$; †$P < 0.01$.

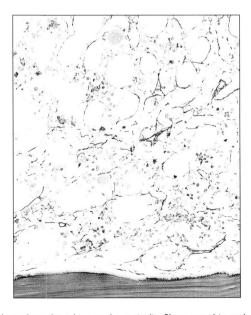

Fig. 4-7. Normal trephine biopsy: the reticulin fibers are thin and delicate, and form a network around the hematopoietic cells. (Silver impregnation stain.)

ERYTHROID CELLS IN THE BONE MARROW AND PERIPHERAL BLOOD

The earliest recognizable erythroid cell in the marrow is the proerythroblast, a large cell with dark blue cytoplasm and a primitive nuclear chromatin pattern (Fig. 4-8). The more differentiated erythroblasts are progressively smaller and contain increasing amounts of hemoglobin, to give a polychromatic cytoplasm; the nuclear chromatin becomes progressively more condensed. Basophilic (early), polychromatic (intermediate), and pyknotic (late) stages of erythroblast development are recognized (Figs. 4-9 and 4-10). Kinetic studies have identified four cell cycles between the proerythroblast and the late nondividing erythroblast (see Fig. 4-10, *C*). In the marrow,

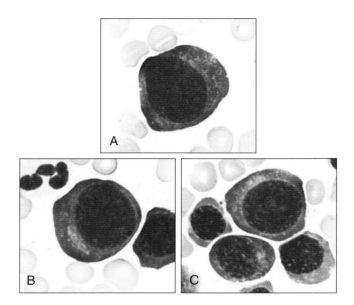

Fig. 4-8. Erythropoiesis. **A–C,** Proerythroblasts and smaller basophilic and polychromatic erythroblasts.

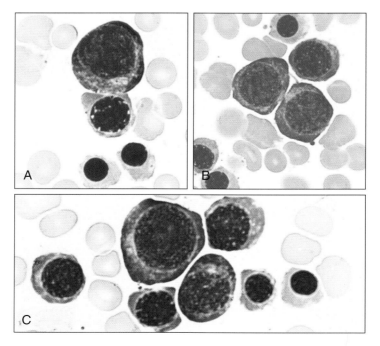

Fig. 4-9. Erythropoiesis: **(A)** from top to bottom, basophilic, polychromatic, and two pyknotic erythroblasts; **(B, C)** further examples of basophilic, polychromatic, and pyknotic erythroblasts.

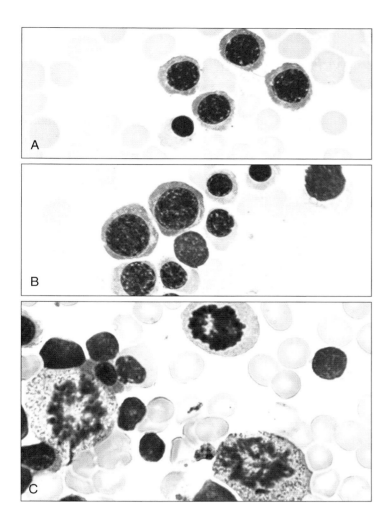

Fig. 4-10. Erythropoiesis. **A, B,** Polychromatic and pyknotic erythroblasts. **C,** Mitotic figures: three cells, a late basophilic erythroblast (upper field), and two myelocytes, in metaphase. Only a small fraction of the cells seen in normal marrow are undergoing mitosis.

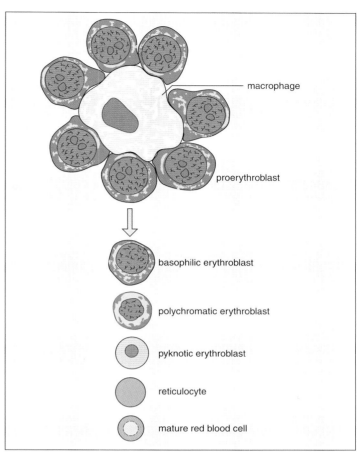

Fig. 4-11. In the bone marrow erythroblasts mature in close proximity to macrophages in an erythroid nest. It is thought that this may help erythroblasts access macrophage iron, allowing the iron to be incorporated into heme. Below are shown the stages of erythroblast maturation into a mature red cell.

erythroblasts are associated closely with their supportive macrophages (Figs. 4-11 to 4-13).

Finally, through a process that is probably an erythroid-specific variant of apoptosis, the nucleus is enucleated to produce a reticulocyte that still contains messenger ribonucleic acid (mRNA) capable of synthesizing hemoglobin and stains with supravital stains (Fig. 4-14). This cell spends 1 to 2 days in the marrow and then a further 1 to 2 days in the peripheral blood and spleen, in which the RNA is completely lost and an orthochromatic or pink-staining erythrocyte (red blood cell [RBC]) results. The mature red cell contains little or no mRNA.

In adults in normal steady-state conditions, only reticulocytes and red cells are present in peripheral blood. Red cells in normal peripheral blood are circular and fairly uniform in size with a mean cell diameter of 8 μm. For successful gaseous exchange, the flexible biconcave red cell, 8 μm in diameter, has to pass through the microcirculation, whose diameter is only 3.5 μm (Fig. 4-15). Important for normal erythropoiesis is the ability to incorporate iron. Bone marrow iron stores can be determined by staining for iron by Perls' reaction (Fig. 4-16). In the ideal part of the blood film for examination, which is where the red cells are just beginning to touch and overlap, their biconcave shape produces a central pallor. Only mild variations in size (anisocytosis) and shape (poikilocytosis) are seen (Fig. 4-17).

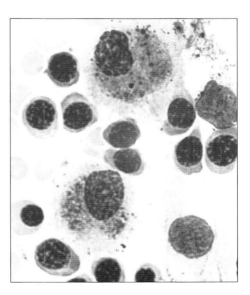

Fig. 4-12. Bone marrow macrophages: close association of polychromatic normoblasts with two pigmented macrophages.

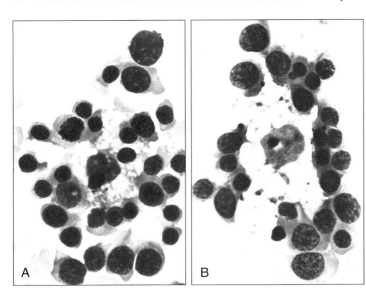

Fig. 4-13. Erythroblast-macrophage nests: **(A, B)** erythroblasts in tight clusters around central macrophages with lipid-laden cytoplasm.

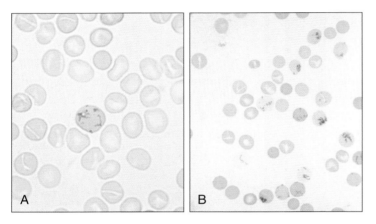

Fig. 4-14. Reticulocytes: reticular material (precipitated RNA and protein) is shown clearly **(A)** in normal blood by supravital staining with new methylene blue, and **(B)** in autoimmune hemolytic anemia.

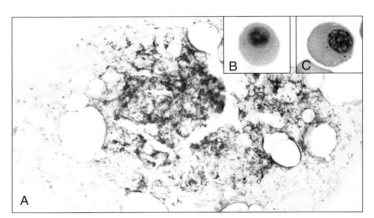

Fig. 4-16. Bone marrow iron assessment: bone marrow fragment stained for iron by the Perls' reaction. **A,** Abundant Prussian blue positivity indicates iron as hemosiderin in reticuloendothelial cell macrophages. **B, C,** In the cell trails, some of the erythroblasts contain one, two, or three Prussian blue–positive "siderotic" granules.

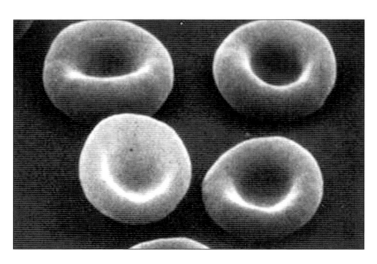

Fig. 4-15. Scanning electron micrograph of an erythrocyte.

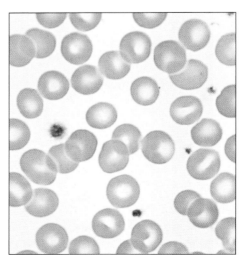

Fig. 4-17. Normal red cells: mean 8 μm in diameter with minor variations in size and shape. The majority show a central pale area of diminished staining. Platelets, 1 to 3 μm across, are also evident.

MEGAKARYOCYTE AND PLATELET PRODUCTION

The earliest small progenitor cells of the megakaryocytic line are not easily differentiated from myeloblasts. They may be identified by electron microscopic or immunologic techniques. Megakaryoblasts undergo nuclear and cytoplasmic maturation from progenitor cells (Fig. 4-18). The megakaryocyte matures through endomitotic synchronous nuclear replications, which enlarge the cytoplasmic volume as the number of nuclei increases in multiples of two. These polyploid cells contain the equivalent of 4, 8, 16, or 32 sets of chromosomes. At a variable stage of development, usually at the 4N, 8N, or 16N stage, further nuclear replication and cell growth cease (Figs. 4-19 and 4-20), the cytoplasm becomes granular, and platelets are produced. Platelets appear as granular basophilic forms with a diameter of 1 to 3 μm (Figs. 4-21 and 4-22). The volume of platelets diminishes as they mature and age in the circulation.

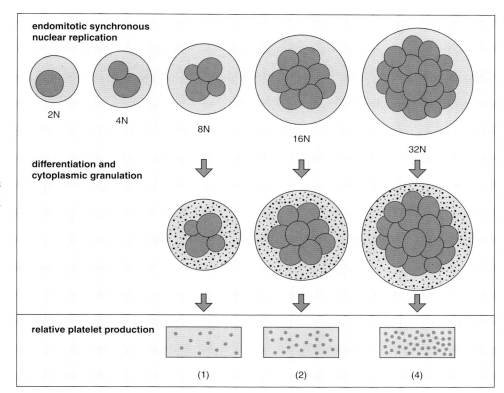

Fig. 4-18. Megakaryocyte development and platelet production: each nuclear unit has two sets of chromosomes. (*N*, number of sets of chromosomes or "ploidy.")

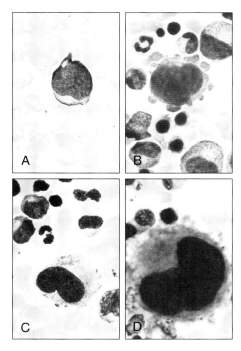

Fig. 4-19. Megakaryocyte development: **(A, B)** megakaryoblasts with nucleoli; **(C)** early bilobed megakaryocyte with no obvious cytoplasmic granulation; **(D)** larger megakaryocyte with obvious early granulation of cytoplasm.

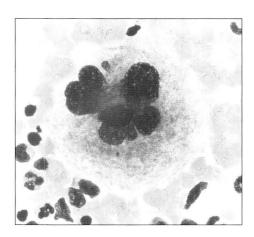

Fig. 4-20. Megakaryocyte: mature megakaryocyte with many nuclear lobes and pronounced granulation of its cytoplasm.

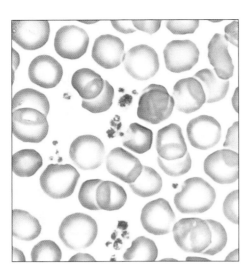

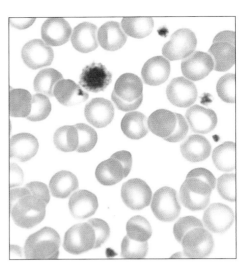

Fig. 4-21. Normal platelets: in this blood film, made from a finger-prick sample, the platelets have agglutinated into small clumps. This is a regular feature of blood films prepared from blood that has not been collected into an anticoagulant.

Fig. 4-22. Normal platelets: these platelets show more variation in size than those in Fig. 4-21, the largest measuring approximately 6 μm in diameter. Platelets of this size are seen only rarely in normal blood films.

GRANULOPOIESIS AND MONOCYTE PRODUCTION

During blood film examination, the white cell numbers and morphology are assessed and a differential count is performed, if this has not been provided by an electronic laboratory blood counter.

In granulopoiesis (Fig. 4-23), the first recognizable cell of the granulocytic series is the myeloblast. Following division and differentiation, the following sequence of cells may be seen (Figs. 4-24 to 4-27):
- Promyelocyte (which contains primary granules)
- Myelocyte
- Metamyelocyte
- Band cell
- Segmented or mature granulocyte

The distinction between immature myeloid precursors is dependent on the morphology of the nucleus and the cytoplasm. The most immature, the myeloblast, has immature nuclear chromatin with one or more nucleoli. The nuclear cytoplasmic ratio is high. Promyelocytes also have immature nuclear chromatin with nucleoli but they have more voluminous granulated cytoplasm with specific (secondary) granules (neutrophilic, eosinophilic, or basophilic) that remain

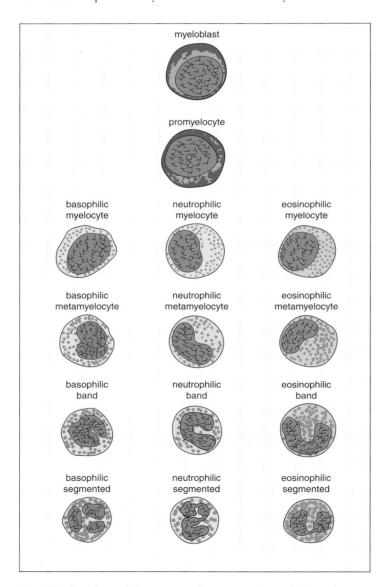

Fig. 4-23. Granulocyte differentiation and maturation: the myeloblast and promyelocyte give rise to three different cell lines, according to the type of secondary granules and nuclear morphology.

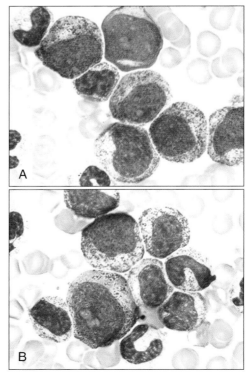

Fig. 4-24. Granulopoiesis: **(A)** a myeloblast, late promyelocytes, and myelocytes; **(B)** a promyelocyte, myelocytes, and metamyelocytes.

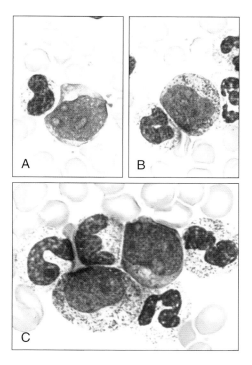

Fig. 4-25. Granulopoiesis: **(A)** myeloblast and **(B)** promyelocyte; **(C)** early promyelocyte, myelocyte, metamyelocyte, and band neutrophils.

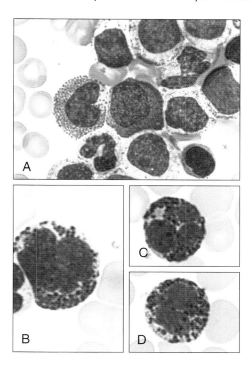

Fig. 4-27. Granulopoiesis: **(A)** eosinophilic myelocyte and metamyelocyte; **(B)** basophilic myelocyte; **(C, D)** more mature basophils.

from the promyelocyte stage onwards. Promyelocytes have a prominent paranuclear Golgi apparatus. Finally, myelocytes have more mature chromatin with granulated cytoplasm. All of these cells play a critical role in combating infection and generating an inflammatory response.

Osteoblasts and osteoclasts are occasionally seen during bone marrow examination (Figs. 4-28 and 4-29). They are derived from monocytic lineage cells and are important in laying down bone (osteoblast) and resorbing bone (osteoclast). When they are present in significant numbers, it is important not to confuse them with metastatic malignant cells.

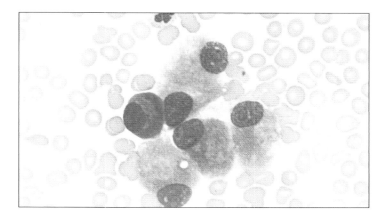

Fig. 4-28. Osteoblasts: a group of five osteoblasts and a plasma cell (on the left). The osteoblasts are large cells that resemble plasma cells, but their chromatin pattern is more open, their cytoplasm is less basophilic, and they tend to occur in clumps.

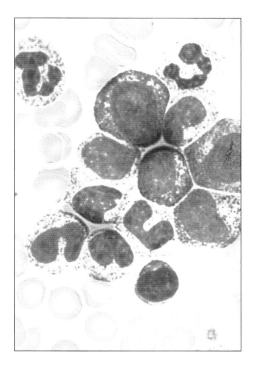

Fig. 4-26. Granulopoiesis: sequence of cells from myelocytes through metamyelocytes and band forms, and a single segmented neutrophil.

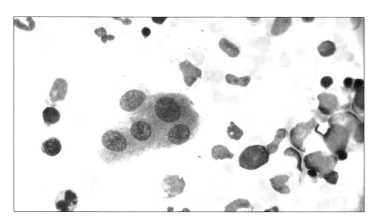

Fig. 4-29. Osteoclasts: these multinucleate cells are occasionally seen in normal marrow aspirates. In contrast to megakaryocytes, the nuclei of osteoclasts are usually discrete, round or oval, and often contain nucleoli.

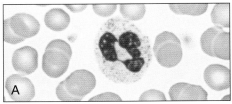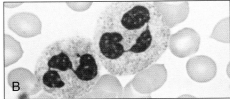

Fig. 4-30. Normal neutrophils. **A–B,** Mature forms showing typical nuclear lobe separation by fine filaments; normal segmented neutrophils may show up to five lobes.

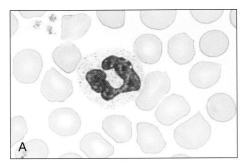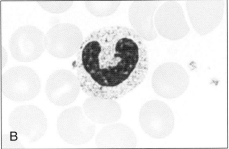

Fig. 4-31. Normal neutrophils: **(A, B)** stab or band forms. The nuclear segmentation of these less mature cells is incomplete.

NEUTROPHILS (POLYMORPHS)

The dominant granulocytic cells are neutrophils (Figs. 4-30 and 4-31), and neutrophil precursors account for the majority of granulocyte precursors in the marrow. Other rare appearances include neutrophil-platelet rosetting (Fig. 4-32) and neutrophil aggregation (Fig. 4-33), neither of which is usually of clinical significance.

Neutrophil production and differentiation takes 6 to 10 days. Ten to fifteen times the number of band and segmented neutrophils are present in the bone marrow compared with peripheral blood, where they serve as a "reserve pool." Once they enter the circulation, neutrophils have a half-life of only 6 to 12 hours before they migrate into tissues, usually via chemotaxis. In tissues they survive for only 2 to 4 days before they are destroyed or undergo senescence. Neutrophils destroy bacteria and fungi (Fig. 4-34). Organisms are ingested into

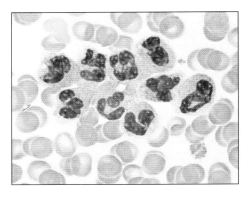

Fig. 4-33. Neutrophil agglutination: clusters of aggregated neutrophils are also an occasional and unexplained finding during blood film examination. The phenomenon is sometimes seen in patients with viral infections.

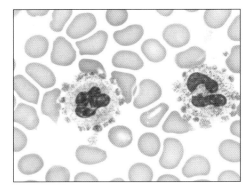

Fig. 4-32. Neutrophil-platelet adhesion: rosetting of platelets around neutrophils is an occasional interesting, but unexplained, finding in blood films. It only occurs in the presence of the anticoagulant ethylenediamine tetra-acetic acid.

phagosomes into which neutrophil granules (Table 4-3) are released and kill microbes by a number of mechanisms. Primary azurophilic neutrophil granules contain lysozyme, myeloperoxidase, and serine proteases. Moreover, microbes are killed by oxidant damage by superoxides generated by glucose metabolism. Finally, lactoferrin chelates iron that bacteria require.

There are far fewer eosinophil precursors (Figs. 4-35 and 4-36). They are derived from eosinophil myelocytes. Typically, mature cells have a bilobed nucleus and distinct eosinophilic granules. The granules are often membrane bound and have a crystalloid core. Basophil

Fig. 4-34. Phagocytosis and bacterial destruction: the neutrophil surrounds the bacterium with an invaginated surface membrane to form a phagosome by fusion with a primary lysosome. The lysosomal enzymes attack the bacterium. Secondary granules also fuse with the phagosomes, and new enzymes and lactoferrin attack the organism. Various types of activated oxygen generated by glucose metabolism also help to kill bacteria. Undigested residual bacterial products are excreted by exocytosis.

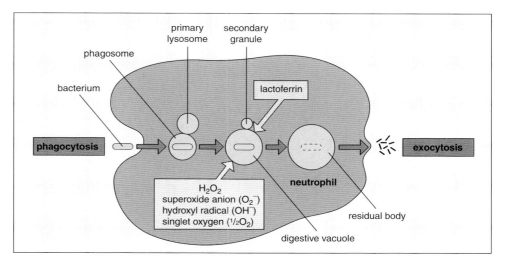

TABLE 4-3.   HUMAN NEUTROPHILS: GRANULE CONTENTS

Primary (azurophil) granules	Specific granules	Other organelles
Microbicidal proteins		
Myeloperoxidase		
Lysozyme	Lysozyme	Lysozyme
Bactericidal–permeability inducing factor/CAP57		
Defensins		
Serprocidins (serine proteases): cathepsin G proteinase 3 azurocidin/CAP37		
elastase	Collagenase	Alkaline phosphatase
	Gelatinase	Gelatinase
		Tetranectin
Acid hydrolases		
β-Glucuronidase		
β-Glycerophosphatase		
N-Acetyl-β-glucosaminidase		
α-Mannosidase		
Cathepsin B		
Cathepsin D	Other neutrophil gelatinase-associated lipocalin	
Aryl sulfatase	Lactoferrin	
	Transcobalamin I and III	
	Plasminogen activator	
	Histaminase	
	β₂-Microglobulin	
	Cytochrome b_{559}	
Receptors	**Receptors**	
$\alpha_{2M}\beta_2$ integrin = complement receptor 3 (C3bi)	$\alpha_M\beta_2$ integrin	
Bacterial tripeptide receptor (formyl-methionyl-leucyl-phenylalanine)	Complement receptor 1 = CD35	
Laminin receptor	FcγRIIIB	
$\alpha_2\beta_2$ integrin = Victronectin R		

Adapted with permission from Roberts PJ, Linch DC, Webb DKH: Phagocytes. In Hoffbrand AV, Lewis SM, Tuddenham EGD, editors: *Postgraduate haematology*, ed 4, Oxford, 1999, Butterworth-Heinemann, pp 235-266.

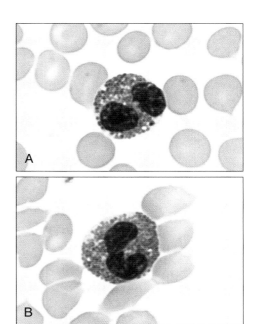

Fig. 4-35. Normal eosinophils.

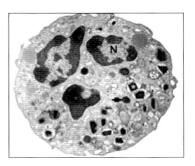

Fig. 4-36. Electron micrograph showing intracellular contents of an eosinophil. The nucleus and examples of large granules are shown.

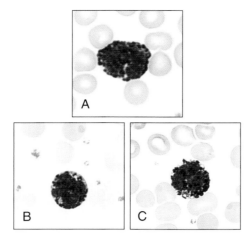

Fig. 4-37. Basophils. **A–C,** The coarse basophilic granules of these cells often overlie the nucleus, thus obscuring the detail of its segmented structure. Only small numbers of basophils are found in the normal blood film.

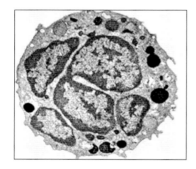

Fig. 4-38. Electron micrograph showing intracellular contents of a basophil. The nucleus and examples of large granules are shown.

(Figs. 4-37 and 4-38) and tissue mast cells are normally even rarer (Fig. 4-39). Basophils are distinctive with large basophilic granules occupying most of the volume of the cell. Mast cells have deep purple granules. All three of these specialized granulocytic cells have specific granules (Tables 4-3 and 4-5) that are especially important in providing protective immunity against parasites (Fig. 4-40) and are important in allergic responses. They combine with T and B lymphocytes and the antibody response (especially specific immunoglobulin E [IgE] antibodies) to release toxic granules that destroy parasites such as helminths. Mast cells and basophils also release pharmacologic mediators such as histamine, SRS-A, and heparin that in part cause the adverse symptoms in allergic response. Eosinophils, by contrast, release histaminase and aryl sulphatase, which inactivate histamine and SRS-A, respectively.

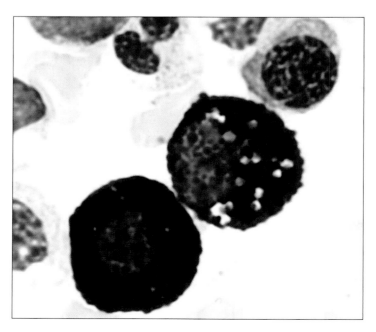

Fig. 4-39. Two mast cells.

TABLE 4-4.   EOSINOPHILS: GRANULE CONTENTS

Granule type/protein	Function	Downstream physiological role
Primary granule		
Charcot–Leyden crystal protein	Cleaves fatty acids from lysophospholipids (lysophospholipase)	Phospholipid mechanism
		Neutralizes pulmonary surfactants
Eosinophil peroxidase	Generates hypothiocyanous acid from H_2O_2	Kills microorganisms (*Escherichia coli*, schistosomes, microfilariae, trypanosomes, *Toxoplasma* spp., and mycobacteria)
		Toxic to mammalian cells – mast cells and tumours
	Allosteric inhibitor of muscarinic receptors	Bronchoconstriction
Specific/secondary granule		
Eosinophil peroxidase	As above	As above
Major basic protein (forms crystalline core of the granule)	Binds to acidic lipids, disrupts membranes (non-enzymatic activity)	Widespread toxicity to parasites
		Toxic to mammalian cells – desquamation and hypertrophy of lung epithelium (bronchospasm)
Eosinophil cationic protein	Forms transmembrane pores	Bactericidal – *E. coli* and *Staphylococcus aureus*
		Toxic to parasites
		Damage to lung epithelium (as above)
		Stimulates mast cell degranulation
	Ribonuclease	
	Neurotoxin (*in vitro*)	
	Neutralizes heparin	Effects on coagulation and fibrinolysis
Eosinophil-derived neurotoxin (eosinophil protein X)	Ribonuclease	Toxic to parasites
	Neurotoxin	
Gelatinase	Metalloproteinase	Damage to extracellular matrix

Adapted with permission from Roberts PJ, Linch DC, Webb DKH: Phagocytes. In Hoffbrand AV, Lewis SM, Tuddenham EGD, editors: *Postgraduate haematology*, ed 4, Oxford, 1999, Butterworth-Heinemann, pp 235-266.

TABLE 4-5. BASOPHILS AND MAST CELLS: GRANULE CONTENTS

Component	Function	Downstream physiological role	Other properties	Cell specificity
Protein				
Histamine	Binds to H1, H2, and H3 receptors	Major inducer of hypersensitivity reactions and inflammation		Basophils, mast cells
Proteoglycan				
Heparin	Packages basic proteins into granules		Binds and stabilizes proteases	Predominant in MC_{CT}
Chondroitin sulfates	Same function		Same function	Predominant in basophils
Enzymes: neutral proteases				
Chymase	Inactivates bradykinin	Affects microcirculation		MC_{CT}
	Injures lamina lucida of basement membrane at dermal–epidermal junction			
	Activates angiotensin I	Modulates microcirculation		
	Activates precursor IL-1b	Modulates skin inflammation		
Tryptase	Cleaves C3 into C3a + C3b	Proinflammatory; stimulates neutrophil chemotaxis and adherence	Tetrameric when bound to heparin; monomer active	Mast cells
	Cleaves C3a into inactive peptides		Restricted substrate specificity	
	Activates metalloproteinase 3	Regulates collagenase	Raised levels in mast cell disorders; anaphylaxis, mastocytosis	
	Inactivates fibrinogen	Attenuates fibrin deposition		
	Degrades calcitonin gene-related peptide			
Cathepsin G-like protease				MC_{CT}
Carboxypeptidase B				MC_{CT}
Other				
Charcot–Leyden crystal protein	Cleaves fatty acid from lysophospholipid (lysophospholipase)	Phospholipid mechanism		Basophils
		Neutralizes pulmonary surfactants		
Major basic protein		Disrupts membranes		
Sulfatase, exoglycosidase				

Mast cells = both connective tissue and mucosal mast cells; MC_{CT} = connective tissue mast cell.

Adapted with permission from Roberts PJ, Linch DC, Webb DKH: Phagocytes. In Hoffbrand AV, Lewis SM, Tuddenham EGD, editors: *Postgraduate haematology,* ed 4, Oxford, 1999, Butterworth-Heinemann, pp 235-266.

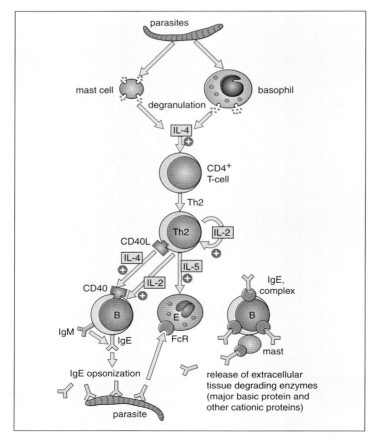

Fig. 4-40. T cells work with mast cells, basophils, and, most important, eosinophils to generate a protective immune response to parasites. Parasites trigger basophil and mast cell degranulation, release of IL-4, and activation of CD4+ and Th-2 T cells. Activated T cells promote protective antibody response (mainly IgE but also IgG and IgM) from B cells. IgE-opsonized parasites attract eosinophils that degranulate and release toxic granule components as shown.

MONONUCLEAR PHAGOCYTIC SYSTEM

Monocytes spend only a short time in the bone marrow, and normally few monocytes and their precursors, the monoblasts and promonocytes, are seen in normal marrow and peripheral blood (Fig. 4-41). Monoblasts and promonocytes can be difficult to distinguish from monocytes and occasionally from early myeloblasts. After circulating for 20 to 40 hours, monocytes migrate into tissues where they are known as macrophages (Fig. 4-42). The life span of macrophages can be months to years. Functionally, they phagocytose and remove particulate antigen and present antigen to lymphocytes.

Monocytes are phagocytes that will adhere to immunoglobulin G (IgG) and complement (e.g., C3b) coated microorganisms via the Fc portion of the IgG molecule. This process also facilitates ingestion of the microbes. Monocyte lysosomes contain hydrolases and peroxidase, which are important for microbial killing. Monocytes are also "factories" that release a number of mediators that help propagate the immune and inflammatory response.

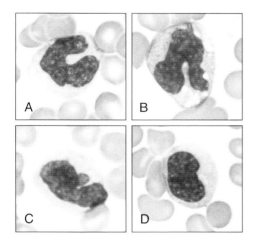

Fig. 4-41. Monocytes: **(A–D)** these cells are usually the largest white cells found in normal blood. The nucleus is usually folded or convoluted, with a moderately fine chromatin pattern. The cytoplasm typically has a gray "ground-glass" appearance with fine azurophilic granules. Some **(B)** have rather prominent cytoplasmic vacuoles.

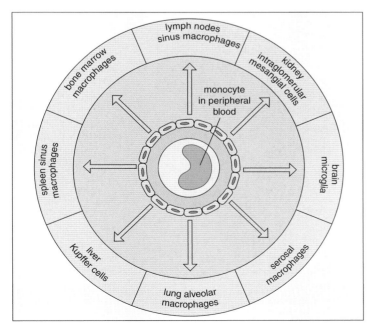

Fig. 4-42. Reticuloendothelial system: distribution of macrophages.

RETICULOENDOTHELIAL SYSTEM

This consists of phagocytic monocytes and tissue macrophages (including macrophages in bone marrow, spleen, lymph nodes, liver Kupffer cells, alveolar macrophages, macrophages of serosal surfaces, and mesangial cells of the kidney) (Fig. 4-42).

Dendritic cells (DCs) are specialized antigen-presenting cells (APCs) found in the skin, lymph nodes, spleen, and thymus (Fig. 4-43). They have an irregular shape, numerous cell-membrane processes, spiny dendrites, and bulbous pseudopods (Fig. 4-44). They have a paucity of intracellular organelles, lysosomes, endosomes, and prominent mitochondria (Figs. 4-45 and 4-46). They include myeloid- and lymphoid-derived DCs and Langerhans cells (Fig. 4-47). They process antigen and interact with and stimulate T cells. Myeloid-derived DCs originate from bone marrow and make up 1% to 2% of the blood mononuclear cells. They are negative for lineage markers, but are HLA-DR positive. A separate set of DCs is derived from CD34-positive cells and populates the skin epidermis (where they are called Langerhans cells), but also are found in the liver, lymph nodes, and the interstitial spaces in organs such as the kidney and the heart. Langerhans cells migrate to afferent lymphatics, following stimulation, into the paracortical areas of draining lymph nodes where they "interdigitate" with, and present antigen, to T cells (see Fig. 4-43). Lymphoid dendritic cells have yet a separate origin and within the thymus may be involved in tolerance induction to autoantigens.

Follicular dendritic cells (FDCs), also called germinal centrodenritic cell, form a dense network in germinal centers (GCs) of lymph nodes (B-cell areas). They are bone marrow derived and present retained antigen for prolonged periods (for several months), presumably to maintain B-cell activation and, indirectly, T-cell activation.

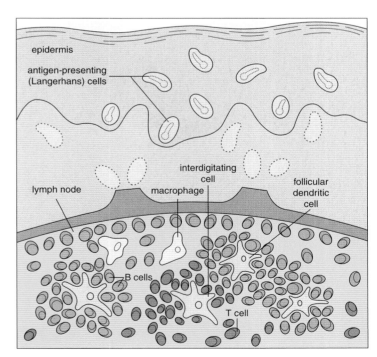

Fig. 4-43. Dendritic (antigen-presenting) (DC) cells in the skin and lymph nodes: Langerhans cells in the epidermis are characterized by the presence of Birbeck bodies (tennis racquet–shaped collections of granules). These antigen-carrying cells migrate via afferent lymphatics to the neighboring lymph nodes and become interdigitating cells in the T-cell paracortical zone. Follicular DCs are found in the B-cell germinal centers (GCs).

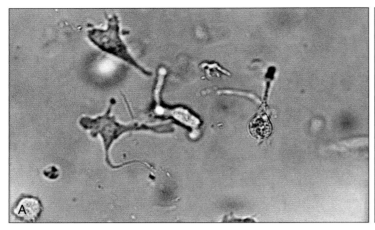

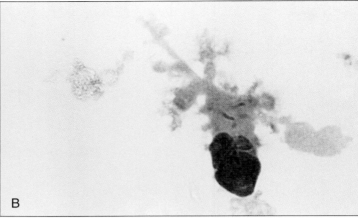

Fig. 4-44. Dendritic cells. **A,** DCs developing in methylcellulose culture from CD34+ bone marrow progenitors after 14 days in TNFa and GM-CSF. Note the fine, long dendritic processes characteristic of DCs under these conditions. These cells generally have the appearance and phenotype of skin Langerhans cells, are CD1a+, CD14–, and HLA-DR+, but lack Birbeck granules. **B,** Giemsa-stained DC from 14 day cultures of CD34+ as shown in **(A).** Note the fine, long dendritic processes and eccentric lobed nucleus characteristic of DCs under these conditions. (A, B, Courtesy of Dr. C. D. L. Reid.)

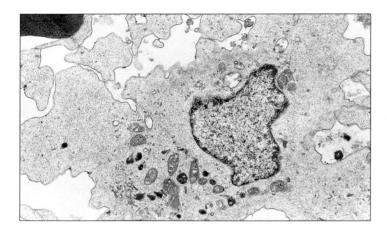

Fig. 4-45. Dendritic cells: electron microscopic appearances of DCs from 14-day cultures of CD34+ cells (as shown in Fig. 4-44, A). Note the many blunt pseudopodia and dendritic processes, the pale and rather featureless cytoplasm with little endoplasmic reticulum, and many free ribosomes and polyribosomes. (Courtesy of Dr. C. D. L. Reid.)

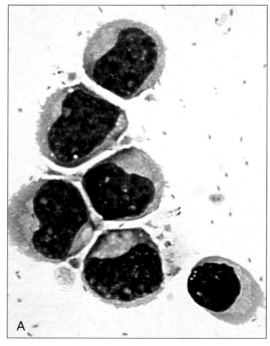

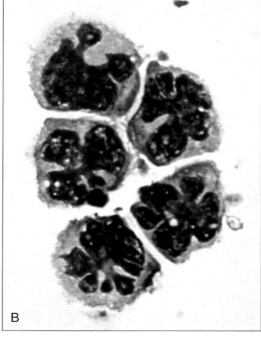

Fig. 4-46. Dendritic cells: **(A, B)** morphology of DC freshly isolated from peripheral blood. These cells are separated on the basis of strong Class II (HLA-DR) expression, but are lineage negative (CD3–, CD19–, CD20–, CD14–, CD16–, CD34–) and are allostimulatory in mixed lymphocyte cultures with T lymphocytes. The appearances of the two major subclasses of these cells differ according to their expression of the b2 integrin CD11c: **(A)** CD11c–; **(B)** CD11c+. (A, B, Courtesy of Dr. S. Robinson and Dr. C. D. L. Reid.)

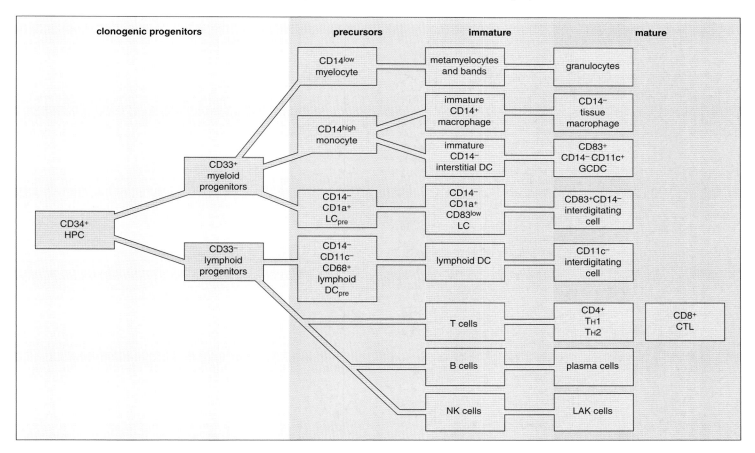

Fig. 4-47. Human dendritic cells: hematopoietic development. CD34+ hemato-poietic progenitor cells (HPCs) give rise to clonogenic myeloid or lymphoid pro-genitors. Regardless of the type of DC (myeloid versus lymphoid, monocyte-derived versus CD34+ hematopoietic progenitor cell derived, or Langerhans cell (LC)-like or interstitial type), DCs exist in both immature and mature, terminally differentiated forms. The CD34+ bipotential intermediate, generated in vitro from CD34+ HPCs, is the presumed equivalent of circulating monocyte precursors of DCs. (CD, cluster differentiation; CTL, cytolytic T lymphocyte; GCDC, germinal center dendritic cell; Th1, T helper 1; Th2, T helper 2.) (Adapted with permission from Young JW: Dendritic cells: expansion and differentiation with hematopoietic growth factors, *Curr Opin Hematol* 6:135-144, 1999.)

LYMPHOKINES, MONOKINES, CHEMOKINES

Central to the action of mononuclear cells is the action of the glyco-proteins, called lymphokines, monokines, and chemokines, that are released by lymphocytes and monocytes (macrophages) and stromal cells. They have wide-ranging effects on hematopoiesis, the immune response, and the response to infection and to invasion by tumors. They have a complex network of interactions and are described here only briefly. Thirty-three interleukins have been identified to date. Below, an outline is provided of the actions of some of the interleu-kins, monokines, and chemokines that are better characterized functionally.

INTERLEUKIN-1

Activated macrophages produce IL-1 in two forms, α and β, in the ratio 1:10, as do endothelial cells, astrocytes, fibroblasts, and T cells. Both α and β IL-1 are biologically active, with wide-spread participation in the recruitment and activation of cells in-volved in the inflammatory response, in wound healing, in the immune response, and in early stages of hematopoiesis. Figure 4-48 illustrates some of the functions of IL-1, which acts as an endogenous pyrogen; activates lymphocytes, neutrophils, other macrophages, and natural killer (NK) cells; induces proliferation of osteoclasts, fibroblasts, epithelial, endothelial, and synovial cells; and enhances major histocompatibility complex (MHC) Class II antigen expression.

Prostaglandin and collagenase synthesis is increased by IL-1. It plays an important role in hematopoiesis by stimulating marrow stromal cells to secrete colony-stimulating factors (CSFs).

INTERLEUKIN-2

The proliferation of T lymphocytes is promoted by IL-2, as is, to a lesser extent, that of B cells and monocytes. It promotes cytotoxic function by stimulating the proliferation and activity of NK cells. The IL-2 receptor consists of two proteins, one of which is detected by monoclonal antibodies of the CD25 group.

INTERLEUKIN-4

IL-4 has a wide variety of effects both in hematopoiesis and in devel-opment of both B and T cells. It is required for the development of B cells to switch expression of immunoglobulin (Ig) class.

INTERLEUKIN-6

Like IL-1, IL-6 has a wide variety of effects in hematopoiesis, the im-mune system, and as an acute phase protein (Fig. 4-49). It may have a particular role in platelet production, but is not essential for this.

INTERLEUKIN-7

IL-7 is secreted by bone marrow stromal cells and is critical for early B-cell development (pre-B cell) and for the proliferation and matura-tion of T cells an NK cells.

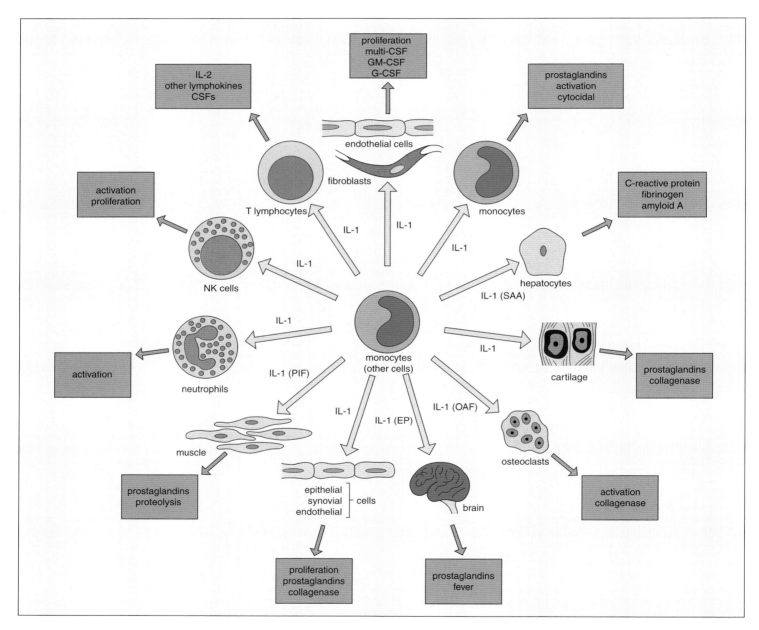

Fig. 4-48. Interleukin 1: some of its effects on target cells and tissues. Osteoclast activating factor (OAF) may be TNFa induced by IL-1. (SAA, serum amyloid A; PIF, proteolysis-inducing factor; EP, endogenous pyrogen.) (Modified from Oppenheim et al: *Immunol Today* 7:45-56, 1986.)

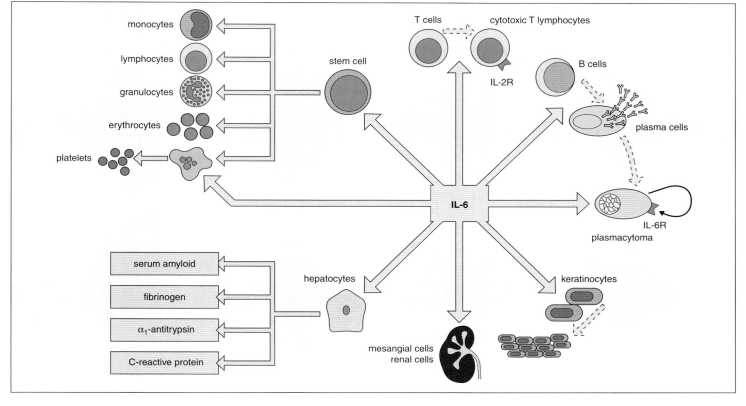

Fig. 4-49. Interleukin 6: pleiotropic functions. (Modified with permission from Hirano T, Akira S, Taga T, et al: Biological and clinical aspects of interleukin-6, *Immunol Today* 11:443-449, 1990.)

INTERLEUKIN-9

Secreted by CD4+ T cells (see below) and is thought to modulate T cells and myeloid cells. It is a candidate gene causal in asthma.

INTERLEUKIN-10, 12, AND 15

These cytokines are released by monocyte-macrophages primarily. They act to modulate T cell responses by regulating the types of T cells that are produced.

INTERLEUKIN-11

IL-11 is a multi-functional cytokine released by bone marrow stromal cells that promotes terminal megakaryopoiesis and osteoblast proliferation. It is also released by plasma cells. IL-11 promotes plasma cell survival by an autocrine mechanism.

CHEMOKINES

These are a class of cytokines with chemoattractant properties. There are two major groups based of different primary amino acid sequence. The CC chemokine family (Table 4-6) have two adjacent cysteine residues whereas the CXC chemokines (Table 4-7) have two cysteine residues that are separated by an intervening amino acid. Chemokines are detected by cells expressing chemokine receptors, seven membrane-spanning domain proteins coupled to G-proteins. Cells expressing chemokine receptors are attracted by increasing concentrations of chemokine molecules.

IL-8 is an example of a CXC chemokine, released by monocytes-macrophages and fibroblasts, that attracts neutrophils and T cells to sites of inflammation and is thought to be pro-angiogenic. For example, in the lung it is implicated in asthma and lung injury.

TABLE 4-6.	THE MAJOR CHEMOKINES CC SUBGROUP			
Chemokine	**Production**	**Receptors**	**Cells that are attracted**	**Effects**
MIP-1α	Monocytes T cells Fibroblasts	CCR1, 3, 5	Monocytes NK and T cells Dendritic cells	T_H1 immunity
MIP-1β	Monocytes Macrophages Neutrophils Endothelium	CCR1, 3, 5	Monocytes NK and T cells Dendritic cells	T_H immunity
MCP-1	Monocytes Macrophages Fibroblasts Keratinocytes	CCR2B	Monocytes NK and T cells Dendritic cells	T_H2 immunity
RANTES	T cells Endothelium Platelets	CCR1, 3, 5	Monocytes NK and T cells Dendritic cells	Inflammation T-cell activation
Eotaxin	Endothelium Monocytes Epithelium	CCR3	Eosinophils Monocytes T cells	Allergy

TABLE 4-7.   THE MAJOR CHEMOKINES C×C SUBGROUP

Chemokine	Production	Receptors	Cells that are attracted	Effects
Il-8? ? ?	Monocytes? Macrophages? Fibroblasts?	CXCR1? CXCR2? ?	Neutrophils? T?cells? ?	Inflammation Angiogenesis
β-TG?	Platelets?	CXCR2?	Neutrophils?	Inflammation
GROα,β,γ? ? ?	Monocytes? Endothelium? ?	CXCR2? ? ?	Neutrophils? T?cells? Fibroblasts	Inflammation Angiogenesis
IP-10? ? ? ?	Endothelium? Monocytes? T?cell? Fibroblasts?	CXCR3? ? ? ?	T?cells? NK?cells? Monocytes? ?	Promotes?T$_H$1?immunity ??? Immunostimulation
SDF-1? ?	Stromal?cells? ?	CXCR4? ?	Stem?cells? Lymphocytes?	Stem?cell?homing Hematopoiesis

LYMPHOCYTES AND PLASMA CELLS

Lymphocytes provide acquired immunity (Fig. 4-50). They have cell-surface receptors that bind specific antigens. They assist phagocytes in defense against infection and provide specificity. They are derived from stem cells (see Chapter 2). There are two types, B cells and T cells. B cells are so-called because in avians they differentiate in an organ called the bursa Fabricius. T cells are initially processed in the thymus. The majority of circulating lymphoid cells (mature T and B cells) are produced in peripheral lymphoid tissue—lymph nodes, spleen, thymus, and lymphoid tissues of the gastrointestinal and respiratory tracts. Lymphocytes usually make up less than 10% of the normal myelogram, and the progenitor lymphoblasts are difficult to differentiate from other blast cells.

T CELLS

Mature T cells, which make up 65% to 80% of the circulating lymphocyte population, carry a marker (antigen CD2) that binds sheep erythrocytes (Fig. 4-51). Early in T-cell development there is expression of nuclear terminal deoxynucleotide transferase (TdT) and the surface antigen CD7 followed by CD2 (Fig. 4-52). Rearrangement of the T-cell receptor genes occurs in the sequence δ, γ, β, and, finally, α. The CD2, CD5, and CD3 antigens are expressed on the surface later, although intracytoplasmic CD3 is one of the earliest markers. Surface markers may be defined by indirect immunofluorescence or by immunoperoxidase-linked specific antibodies (Fig. 4-53) or more routinely by fluorescent-activated cell sorting (FACS) analysis.

Finally, CD4 and CD8 antigens are expressed in medullary thymocytes after T-cell receptor gene rearrangement is complete (see Fig. 4-52). CD8+ cells, the major subpopulation of T cells in the marrow, include the suppressor and/or cytotoxic cells. CD8+ T cells can be seen after viral infection and have large granules (Fig. 4-54). CD4+ (helper) cells predominate in the peripheral blood. CD4+ cells are in turn subdivided into Th1 and Th2 cells, which secrete different cytokines in response to stimulation by IL-2 and IFN-γ or IL-4, respectively (Fig. 4-55).

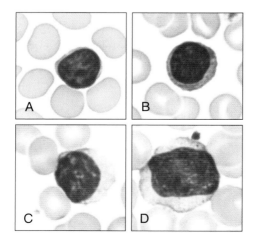

Fig. 4-50. T lymphocytes. **A, B,** Normal small lymphocytes are 7 to 12 μm in diameter with light blue scanty cytoplasm and a central round nucleus with a condensed amorphous chromatin pattern. **C, D,** Some lymphocytes have diameters up to 20 μm, and even larger forms are found during viral and other infections.

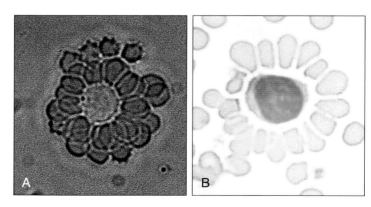

Fig. 4-51. T lymphocytes: following centrifugation together, human T lymphocytes and sheep red cells bind to each other in rosettes. **A,** Phase-contrast microscopy. **B,** May-Grünwald/Giemsa stain.

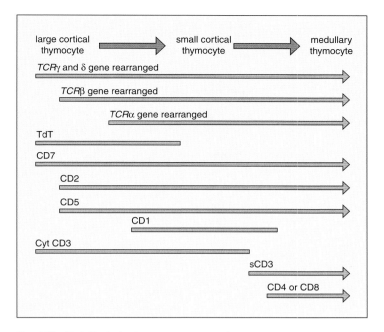

Fig. 4-52. Early T-cell development: sequence of T-cell receptor gene rearrangements and antigen expression (s, surface; cyt, cytoplasmic).

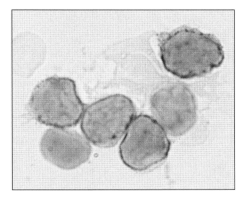

Fig. 4-53. T lymphocytes: human T cells identified by (brown) staining of surface antigen (four of the central cells are T cells). (Immunoperoxidase technique using anti-CD5 monoclonal antibody.)

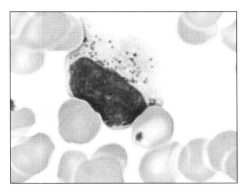

Fig. 4-54. Large granular lymphocyte: cells of lymphoid appearance with multiple azurophilic granules probably include cells of both lymphocyte (CD8+) and myeloid origin and have NK activity.

Fig. 4-55. CD4+ T helper cells: maturation pathways. CD4+ T cells that have been activated by antigen acquire the capacity to produce cytokines. The cytokines produced depend on the environment in which activation occurs. Two main types of cytokine-producing Th cell are recognized—Th1 and Th2 cells. The cytokines produced by Th1 cells tend to promote further Th1 cell formation and inhibit Th2 cell formation, and IL-4 produced by Th2 cells promotes further differentiation toward Th2 cells. Th1-promoting cytokines are also produced by activated macrophages, interdigitating cells, and NK cells, while mast cells also produce IL-4.

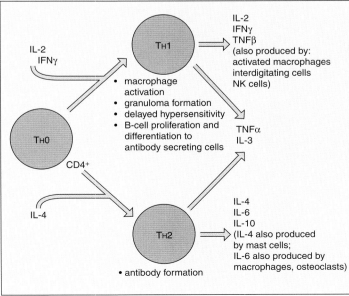

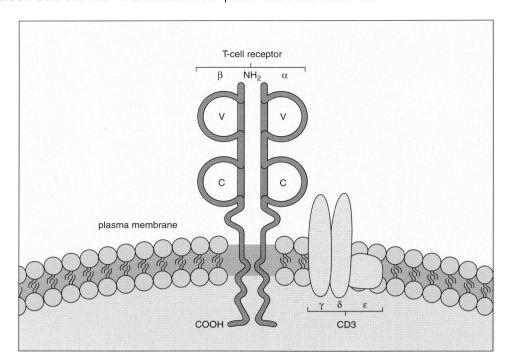

Fig. 4-56. The T-cell antigen receptor: this consists of α and β chains, each of which has a variable (V) and a constant (C) segment. The chains have transmembranous portions, but very short intracytoplasmic domains. The associated CD3 complex is involved in signal transduction to the cell interior.

The T-cell surface contains an antigen receptor that consists of α and β chains, each with variable and constant portions (Fig. 4-56). A receptor coded for by γ and δ genes exists in a minority of T cells. The genes for these polypeptide chains, on chromosomes 14 and 7 (Table 4-8; see Fig. 4-63), are rearranged in T cells in a manner similar to the rearrangement of Ig genes in B cells (see later), which results in a wide diversity among T lymphocytes. Close by the T-cell receptor on the cell surface membrane is a complex of proteins termed the *CD3 complex,* which consists of γ, δ, and ϵ chains (see Fig. 4-56). This complex is responsible for transducing signals derived from interaction of antigen with the T-cell receptor to the cell interior.

T cells also contain a number of lysosomal acid hydrolases, such as β-glucuronidase, and acid phosphatase, which may be detected cytologically as discrete masses in the Golgi zone in the cytoplasm (Fig. 4-57).

TABLE 4-8.   ANTIGEN RECEPTOR GENES: ORGANIZATION

Gene	Chromosome localization	V	D	J	C	Additional diversity	Complementarity determining region 3 diversity	Clonal rearrangement in (%) acute lymphoblastic leukemia	
								B lineage	T Lineage
IgH	14q32	~50	30	6	10	N regions	V-N1-D1-N2-J V-N1-D1-N2-D2-N3-J	100	15–20
IgLκ	2p12	~40	–	5	1	N regions	V-N-J/V-J	20	0
IgLγ	22q11	~29	–	6	6	None	V-J	5	0
TCRα	14q11	~70	–	~90	1	N regions	V-N-J	NT	70
TCRδ	14q11	~4	3	3	1	N regions	V-N1-D1-N2-D2-N3-J	40–50	95*
TCRγ	7p15	12	–	5	2	N regions	V-N-J	40–50	95
TCRβ	7q32	~50	2	13	2	N regions	V-N1-D-N2-J	0	80

*At least 30% of these cases show deletion of TCRd.

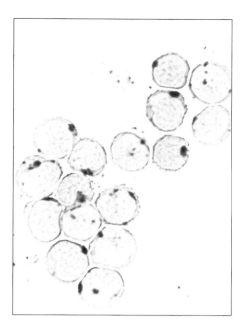

Fig. 4-57. T lymphocytes: using acid phosphatase, the cells show polar positive (red) staining in the Golgi zone.

B CELLS

The bone marrow remains the principal site of "virgin" B-lymphocyte formation. A schema of the B-cell maturation in the marrow and the periphery is set out in Figures 4-58 and 4-59, and this shows that the surface antigen profile allows identification of discrete stages of B-cell lymphopoiesis. As B cells mature in ontogeny there is a carefully co-ordinated program that leads to the production of nuclear (nuclear enzyme TdT), cytoplasmic, and surface markers (such as membrane-bound immunoglobulin molecules [Igs] that are antigen specific). Fluorescein-labeled specific antibodies may be used to demonstrate these surface-bound Igs (Fig. 4-60). Some surface antigens may be detected before surface Ig and others after Ig expression. They can be identified by monoclonal antibodies (e.g., CD10, CD19 [Fig. 4-61], CD20, and CD22). The majority of B cells carry HLA-DR antigens, which are important in the regulation of the immune response. Complement receptors for C3b and C3d are also found on more mature B cells.

The key hallmark of B cells is production of surface Ig (and eventually the ability to secrete Ig when they mature to cells called plasma cells—see later). Surface Igs are individual to each B-cell clone and are identical to those secreted as antibodies by the B lymphocyte or plasma cell. The Ig can be one of five classes—IgM, IgD, IgG (divided into four subtypes), IgE, and IgA (divided into two subtypes). Each Ig

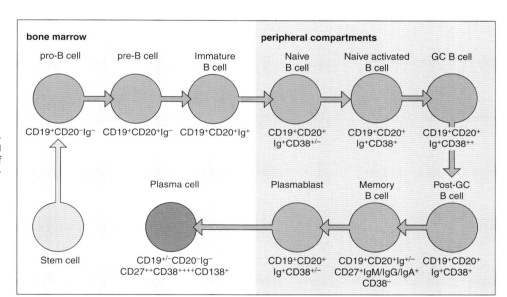

Fig. 4-58. Schematic pathway of cellular intermediates from a stem cell and the earliest recognized B cell (a pro-B cell) to more mature B cells. The location of the cell types is shown, as is the surface immunophenotype (below the cell).

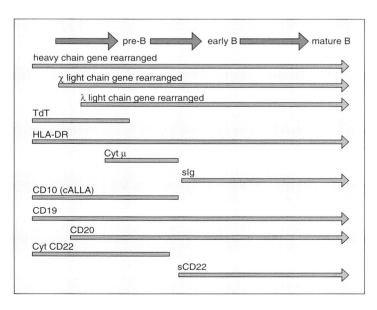

Fig. 4-59. Immunoglobulin gene: sequence of rearrangement, and antigen and Ig expression during early B-cell development. Intracytoplasmic CD22 is also a feature of very early B cells (s, surface; Cyt, cytoplasmic; cALLA, common acute lymphoblastic leukemia antigen).

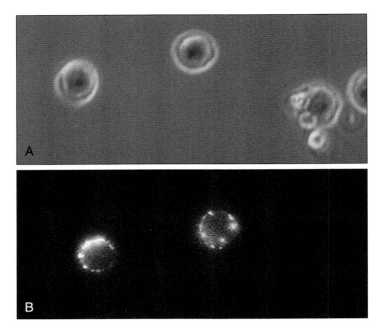

Fig. 4-60. B lymphocytes: **(A)** three peripheral blood lymphocytes seen by phase contrast microscopy; **(B)** patchy fluorescence under ultraviolet light using fluoresceinated anti-human Ig shows that only two of the cells carry surface Ig.

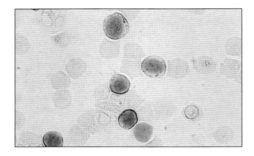

Fig. 4-61. B lymphocytes: identification by (brown) staining of antibody fixed to a surface antigen using the immunoperoxidase technique and CD19 monoclonal antibody.

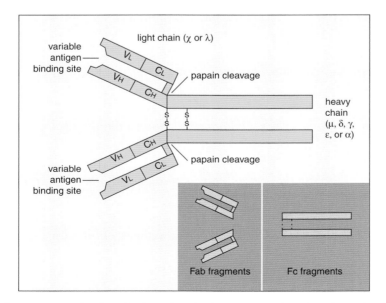

Fig. 4-62. Basic structure of an Ig molecule: each molecule is made up of two light (κ or λ) and two heavy chains, and each chain is made up of variable (V) and constant (C) portions; the V portions include the antigen binding site. The heavy chain (μ, δ, γ, ε, or α) varies according to the Ig class. IgA molecules form dimers, whereas IgM forms a ring of five molecules. Papain cleaves the molecules into an Fc fragment and two Fab fragments.

molecule consists of two light chains (κ or λ) and heavy chains (μ, δ, γ, ε, or α), which determine the class of Ig (Fig. 4-62). Both heavy and light chains contain constant and variable regions.

The heavy chain genes are on chromosome 14 and the light chain genes on chromosomes 2 (κ) and 22 (λ) (Fig. 4-63; see Table 4-8). The production of Igs requires a complex rearrangement of the immunoglobulin gene loci (Fig. 4-64). Diversity is produced by differences in the rearrangement of the genes for the variable (V), diversity (D), joining (J), and constant (C) regions of the Ig molecules they secrete (see Figs. 4-63 and 4-64), and also by insertions of a variable number of random bases in "N" regions of TdT. Gene rearrangement processes are mediated by a recombinase enzyme system, the RAG enzymes, that recognizes specific joining sequences, which consist of a palindromic heptamer and nonamer sequences separated by spacer regions of 12 or 23 base pairs. The sequence starts with the heptamers that border the 3 side of each V and D segment and the 5 side of each D and J segment. The gene rearrangement first requires back-to-back fusion of the heptamer-nonamer sequences. These sequences and a circular intervening sequence, including the sequences to be deleted, are excised and the ends of two gene segments joined up (Fig. 4-64). Class switching is achieved by deletion of the constant region genes upstream from the gene to be expressed. The process is similar to that of Ig variable gene rearrangement. The order of the heavy chain constant region genes downstream from the variable region genes is μ, δ, γ3, γ1, α1, γ2, γ4, ε, α2. Class switching is triggered by interactions between T and B cells in the T-cell zone of secondary lymphoid organs (see later). The Igs are initially expressed in the cytoplasm (in pre-B cells; Fig. 4-65) before they can be detected on the surface. Eventually mature B cells enter the peripheral circulation where they make up 5% to 15% of circulating lymphocytes.

NATURAL KILLER CELLS

A minor population of "lymphocytic" cells do not carry markers of either T or B cells and are known as "non-T, non-B" cells. The sequence of differentiation of these cells is given in Fig. 4-47. The majority of natural killer cells appear as large granular lymphocytes (see Fig. 4-54) in the peripheral blood. This population of cells contains the majority of NK cells, which can kill target cells without MHC restriction, and antibody-dependent cellular cytotoxic cells, which are able to kill tumor and virus-infected cells. They are also involved in graft rejection. Their proliferation is stimulated by IL-2 and interferon-γ.

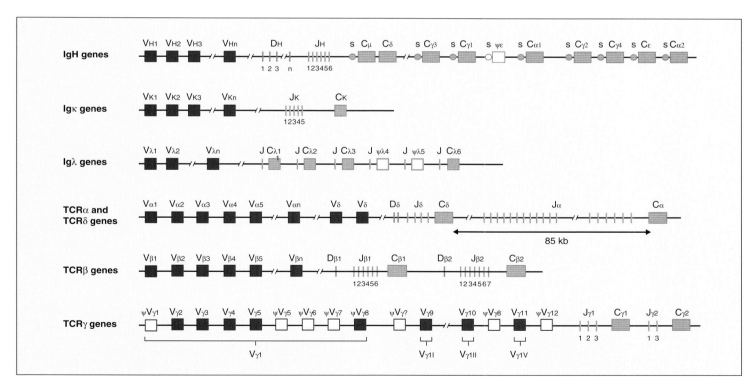

Fig. 4-63. Human Ig genes: the IgH genes consist of many V genes, at least 30 D genes, approximately 6 J genes, and 10 C genes for the various IgH classes and subclasses. Most C genes are preceded by a switch (s) gene, which plays a role in IgH (sub)class switch. The Igk gene complex consists of a series of V genes, approximately five J genes, and one C gene, while the Igl gene complex consists of many V genes and six C genes, all of which are preceded by a J gene. Pseudo genes (c) are indicated with open symbols. The TCRα genes consist of many V genes, a remarkably long stretch of J genes, and one C gene. The TCRβ gene complex consists of a series of V genes and two C genes, both of which are preceded by one D gene and six or seven J genes. The TCRγ genes consist of a restricted number of V genes (12 functional Vγ genes and seven pseudo genes) and two C genes, each preceded by two or three J genes. Interestingly, the TCRδ genes are located between the Vα and Jα genes and probably consist of a few V genes, three D genes, three J genes, and one C gene. (Modified with permission from Van Dongen JJM, Wolvers-Tettero ILM: Analysis of Ig and T-cell receptor genes. Part 1: basic and technical aspects, *Clin Chim Acta* 198:1-92, 1991.)

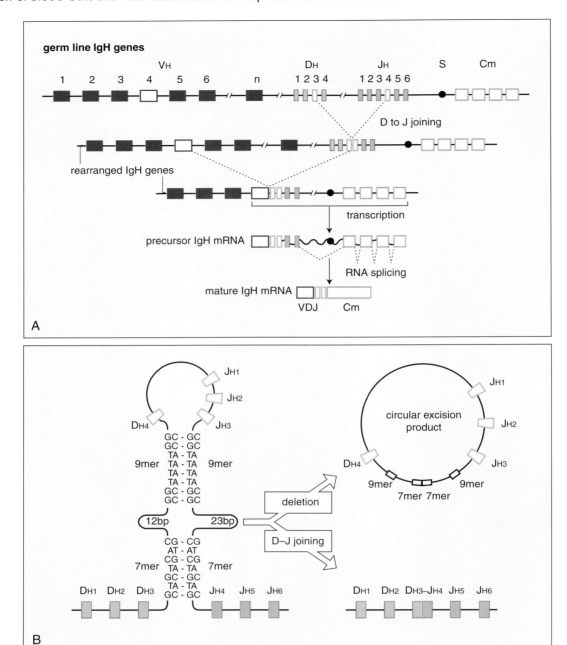

Fig. 4-64. Gene rearrangement. **A,** Rearrangement and transcription of IgH genes. First D to J joining occurs, followed by V to D–J joining. The rearranged genes can be transcribed into a precursor IgH mRNA, which becomes a mature IgH mRNA after splicing all noncoding intervening sequences. **B,** Function of the joining sequences during gene rearrangement. In this typical rearrangement the 3′ Dh3 and 5′ Jh4 heptamer-nonamer sequences fuse back to back. This is followed by a Dh3–Jh4 joining and the deletion of a circular excision product. The heptamer-nonamer sequences shown are not those exactly associated with Dh3 and Jh4, but represent consensus sequences well conserved in Ig as well as TCR genes. (Modified with permission from Van Dongen JM, Wolvers-Tettero ILM: *Clin Chim Acta* 198:1-92, 1991.)

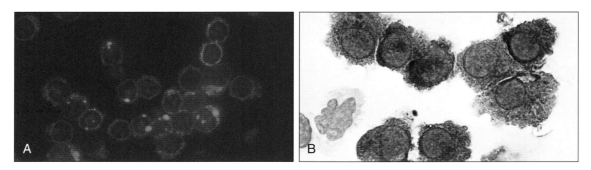

Fig. 4-65. Pre-B lymphoid cells: peripheral blood cells expressing intracytoplasmic IgM **(A)** seen with a crystal-line appearance using indirect immunofluorescence, from a patient with chronic lymphocytic leukemia, and **(B)** seen using the indirect immunoperoxidase method, from a case of hairy cell leukemia. (Courtesy of Dr. J. V. Melo.)

LYMPHOCYTE PROLIFERATION AND DIFFERENTIATION

T and B cells proliferate and develop in reactive lymphoid tissue (e.g., lymph nodes, and lymphoid tissues of the alimentary and respiratory tracts and spleen). Both T and B cells acquire receptors for antigens, which commit them to a single antigenic specificity, and are activated when they bind their specific antigen in the presence of accessory cells.

Provided there is MHC (see below) recognition (Class I for CD8+ and Class II for CD4+ cells), antigen-presenting cells (APCs) interact with T cells bearing the appropriate receptor for that particular antigen. B cells with the appropriate surface receptor (Ig) for the antigen are also stimulated (Fig. 4-66). Adhesion molecules are involved in the cell-cell binding (Fig. 4-67).

Subsequently, these stimulated T and B cells proliferate and differentiate under the stimulus of factors released from APCs (IL-l, IL-6, and IL-7) and activated T helper cells (IL-2, IL-4, IL-6, IL-10, IFN-γ, and tumor necrosis factor [TNF]; see Fig. 4-55). The B cells are also stimulated to secrete antibody. Clones of both effector and memory T and B cells are produced (Figs. 4-68 and 4-69). When the memory cells are stimulated at a later date by their specific antigen, they are able to proliferate again in an accelerated fashion (secondary response).

Activated Th1 cells become responsible for cell-mediated immunity (see Fig. 4-55). Other lymphokines activate killer T cells, enabling them to attack an invading organism or cell, and induce macrophages to stay at the site of infection and help to digest the cells they have phagocytosed. They may also have a direct action on organisms by inhibiting proliferation or activating apoptosis.

Fig. 4-66. The immune response: there is interaction between an APC and a CD4+ (helper) T cell, with MHC-II and antigen T-cell receptor recognition, and both cells interact with a B cell, with recognition between its surface Ig and the antigen. T cells and B cells interact with different epitopes of the antigen. As a result, clones of T cells and B cells are stimulated to proliferate, the B cells becoming either plasma cells (secreting antibody to the antigen) or memory B cells. A phagocyte takes up the antigen-antibody complex.

Fig. 4-67. T-dependent B-cell activation in T zones: surface molecule involvement. B cells take up antigen, which they bind specifically through their surface Ig. This is internalized and broken down into peptides, which are presented on the B-cell surface, held in the peptide-binding grooves of MHC Class II molecules. Cross-linking of surface Ig by antigen induces endocytosis of the antigen-antibody complex and signals upregulation of CD40 expression and de novo B7.1 and B7.2 expression. If this B cell interacts with a primed T cell that recognizes the peptide complex with Class II MHC molecules, this can induce the T cell to express CD40 ligand (CD40L), CTLA4, or both transiently, and to start to secrete cytokines. Cytokine receptor expression by the B and T cells is initiated or upregulated. The arrows indicate that TCR engagement induces CD40-ligand and CTLA4 expression, and that engagement of these molecules by their counterstructures on the B cell delivers further signals to the T cell. CD40 ligation induces Ig class switching in the B cell and migration. (Adapted with permission from MacLennan ICM, Drayson MT: Normal lymphocytes and non-neoplastic lymphocyte disorders. In Hoffbrand AV, Lewis SM, Tuddenham EGD, editors: *Postgraduate haematology*, ed 4, Oxford, 1999, Butterworth-Heinemann, pp 267-308.)

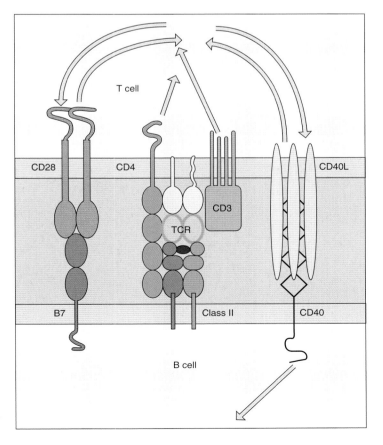

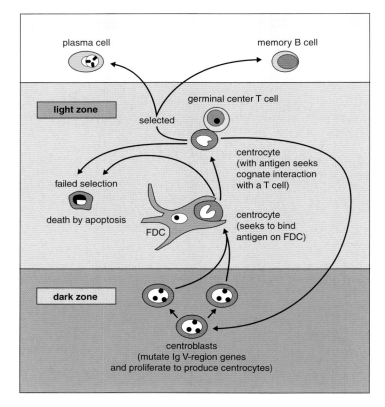

Fig. 4-68. Hypermutation: selection of cells that have undergone Ig V-region hypermutation in GCs. The hypermutation mechanism is active in centroblasts, which are the rapidly dividing cells of the dark zone that give rise to centrocytes. Centrocytes die by apoptosis unless they pick up and process antigen held on follicular dendritic cells (FDC), and find a T cell in the GC that recognizes the peptides from this antigen presented on centrocytes in association with self-MHC class II. The T-cell–dependent selection mechanism makes it unlikely that centrocytes with mutated Ig V-region genes that encode self-reactive antibody will be selected. Most B cells that are selected leave the GC either to migrate to distant sites of antibody production (the gut or bone marrow) where they differentiate to become plasma cells, or to differentiate into memory B cells. Some selected cells remain within the GC and return to the dark zone as centroblasts. (Adapted with permission from MacLennan ICM, Drayson MT: Normal lymphocytes and non-neoplastic lymphocyte disorders. In Hoffbrand AV, Lewis SM, Tuddenham EGD, editors: *Postgraduate haematology,* ed 4, Oxford, 1999, Butterworth-Heinemann, pp 267-308.)

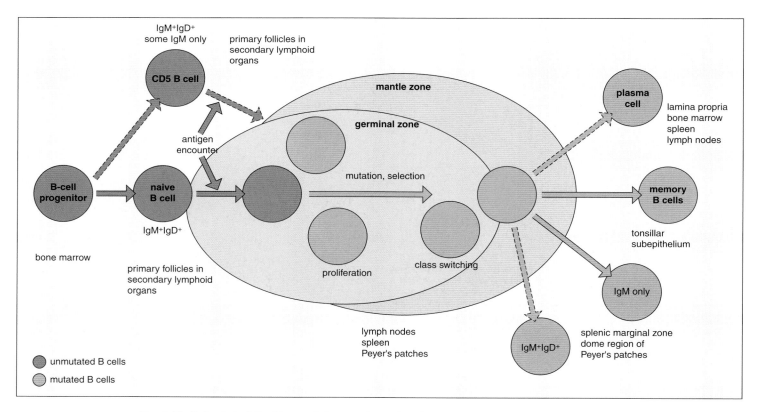

Fig. 4-69. Molecularly defined human B-lineage subsets: these have been characterized by V-gene sequence analysis, and their location in the human body is shown. Hypothetical differentiation pathways are indicated by dashed arrows. (PB, peripheral blood.) (Adapted with permission from Klein U, Goossens T, Fischer M, et al: Somatic hypermutation in normal and transformed human B cells, *Immunol Rev* 162:261-280, 1998.)

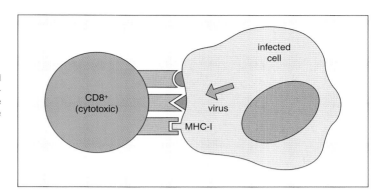

Fig. 4-70. Interaction between a CD8+ (cytotoxic) T cell and a virus-infected cell: when there is MHC-I recognition between the two cells, as well as correspondence between the antigens of the virus expressed on the cell surface and the T-cell antigen receptor on the surface of the CD8+ cell, the CD8+ cell kills the virus-infected cell.

Thus, T helper cells are important in the initiation of a B-cell response to antigens; T suppressor cells reduce the B lymphocytic response; and T cytotoxic cells are capable of directly damaging cells recognized as foreign or virus infected (Fig. 4-70).

Activated B cells are responsible for humoral immunity. Many B-cells mature into plasma cells, which produce and secrete antibodies of one specificity and Ig class (Figs. 4-71 to 4-74). B lymphocytes at different stages of differentiation and activation are shown in Fig. 4-75.

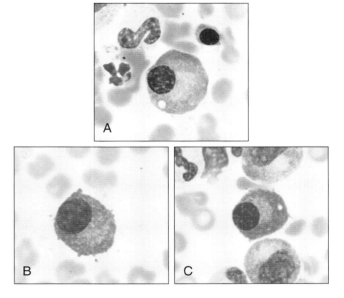

Fig. 4-73. Plasma cells. **A–C,** These occur in bone marrow and in other tissues of the reticuloendothelial system, including the intestine. They are not found in normal peripheral blood. The cells are usually oval. They show a deeply basophilic cytoplasm with a perinuclear halo, and an eccentric nucleus with coarse chromatin condensation ("clock-face" pattern).

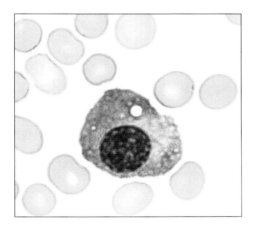

Fig. 4-71. Plasma cell: typical eccentric nucleus with basophilic cytoplasm, prominent perinuclear clearing, and a single vacuole.

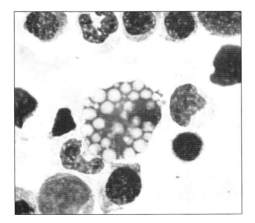

Fig. 4-72. Plasma cell: this type contains many spherical cytoplasmic inclusions and is sometimes referred to as a "Mott" cell.

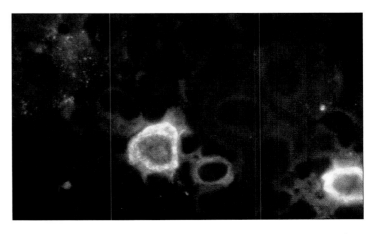

Fig. 4-74. Plasma cells: two plasma cells from a bone marrow aspirate show intense intracytoplasmic fluorescence. (Fluoresceinated anti-IgG, Evans blue counterstain.)

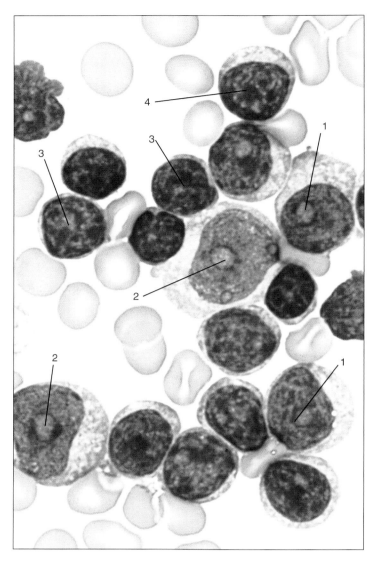

Fig. 4-75. B lymphocytes: peripheral blood film of a patient with chronic lymphocytic leukemia with prolymphocytoid transformation shows B cells at various stages of development (1, prolymphocytes; 2, immunoblasts; 3, small lymphocytes; 4, large lymphocytes). Prolymphocytes probably represent a stage of activated B cell. (Courtesy of Professor J. V. Melo.)

SOMATIC HYPERMUTATION IN NORMAL B CELLS

B cells released from the bone marrow into the peripheral blood have generated a functional non-autoreactive antigen receptor. They remain "naïve" until they encounter antigen, whereupon the antibody expressed by the B cell may be modified, both by class-switch recombination and somatic hypermutation (see Figs. 4-68 and 4-69). Somatic hypermutation is restricted to B cells that proliferate in the GC microenvironment. Somatically mutated V-region genes therefore characterize GC B cells or post-GC B cells. B-lineage–derived lymphoma can thus be characterized as arising from GC or post-GC somatically hypermutated cells.

LYMPHOCYTE CIRCULATION

Lymphocytes from the primary lymphoid organs of the marrow and thymus migrate via the blood through postcapillary venules into the substance of lymph nodes, into unencapsulated lymphoid collections of the body, and into the spleen. T cells home to the paracortical areas of these nodes and to the periarteriolar sheaths of the spleen. B cells accumulate selectively in germinal follicles of lymphoid tissue, in the subcapsular periphery of the cortex, and in the medullary cords of the lymph nodes (Figs. 4-76 and 4-77). Lymphocytes return to the peripheral blood by the efferent lymphatic system and the thoracic duct. The median duration of a complete circulation is about 10 hours. The majority of recirculating cells are T cells. B cells are mainly sessile and spend long periods in lymphoid tissue and the spleen. Many lymphocytes have long life spans and may survive as memory cells for several years.

MESENCHYMAL CELLS

Bone marrow contains precursors of mesenchymal tissues including bone, cartilage, and muscle. This has been demonstrated in humans by allogeneic bone marrow transplantation, which has been shown to correct the mesenchymal disorder osteogenesis imperfecta (Fig. 4-78).

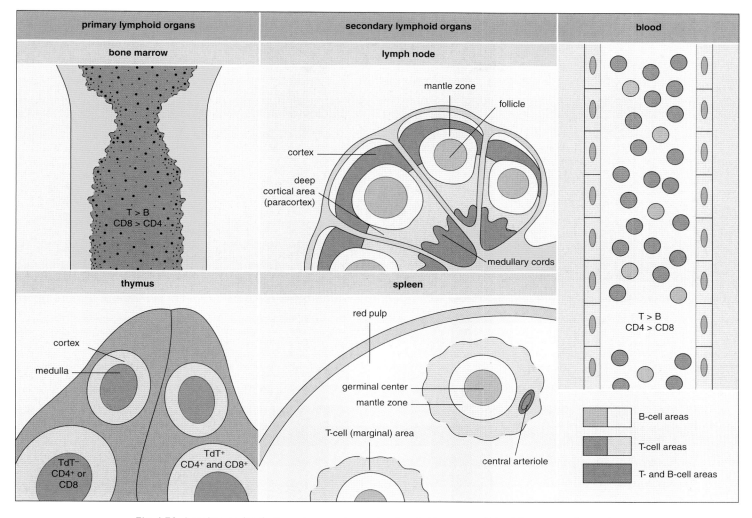

Fig. 4-76. Lymphocyte distribution: primary and secondary lymphoid organs and blood. Aggregates of secondary lymphoid tissue are found elsewhere in the body (e.g., Peyer's patches of the small intestine). The mantle zones of the lymph nodes and spleen also contain macrophages and APCs, and the paracortex also contains many interdigitating reticulum cells.

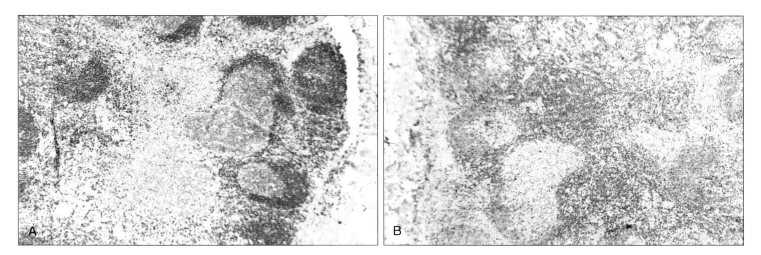

Fig. 4-77. B- and T-lymphocyte distribution: lymph node section showing **(A)** B cells in the GCs, their coronas (heavy staining) in the subcapsular cortex and medullary cords; **(B)** T cells, most numerous in perifollicular areas of the deeper cortical region. Immunoperoxidase technique using **(A)** pan-B monoclonal antibody (anti-CD19) and **(B)** pan-T (anti-CD3) monoclonal antibody.

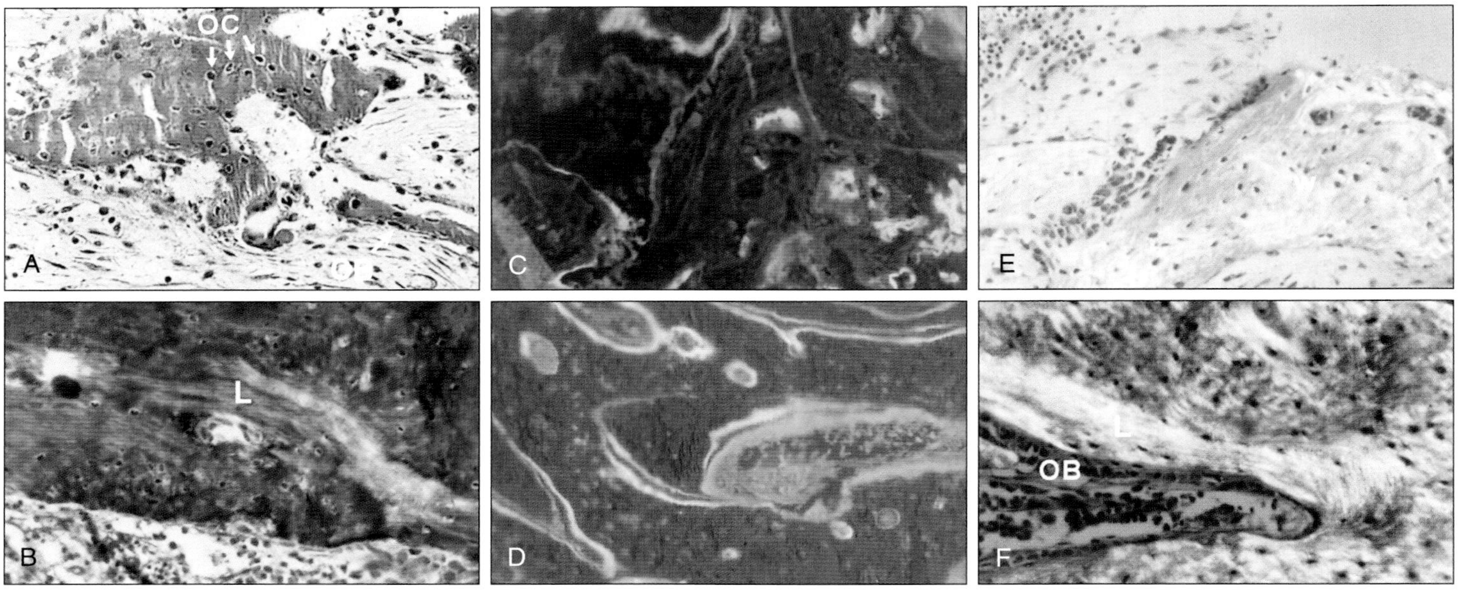

Fig. 4-78. Mesenchymal cells: allogeneic bone marrow transplantation in osteogenesis imperfecta. **A,** Biopsy specimen of trabecular bone before transplantation. The calcified tissue appears blue-green and the uncalcified tissue is red-brown. Numerous, randomly arranged osteocytes (OCs) are present in large lacunae. Peritrabecular marrow fibrosis is also present, and there is a paucity of osteoblasts (OBs) relative to the specimens after transplantation and an incompletely calcified area of bone marrow. **B,** A specimen after transplantation taken near the site shown in **(A).** Osteocytes are fewer, and a small section of lamellar bone (L) indicates normalization of the remodeling process. **C,** Fluorescence photomicrograph of the trabecular bone specimen, from the same section as shown in **(A).** The poorly defined labeling indicates disorganized formation of new bone and abnormal mineralization. **D,** A contrasting specimen to that shown in **(C)** after transplantation, with definitive, crisp, single and double tetracycline labeling, indicative of considerably improved new bone formation and mineralization. **E,** Trabecular bone specimen before transplantation that shows the woven (w) texture of the bone, a characteristic feature of patients with osteogenesis imperfecta. **F,** Bone specimen after transplantation that demonstrates lamellar (L) bone formation and linearly arranged osteoblasts (OBs) in areas of active bone formation along the calcified trabecular surface. (See also Fig. 2-4.) (A, B, Goldners-Masson trichrome; C, D, fluorescent tetracycline labeling; E, F, toluidine blue under polarized light. (Reproduced with permission from Horwitz EM, Prockop DJ, Fitzpatrick LA, et al: Transplantability and therapeutic effects of bone marrow-derived mesenchymal cells in children with osteogenesis imperfecta, *Nature Med* 5:309-313, 1999.)

In this disorder, mutation occurs of one of the two genes that encode Type I collagen, the main structural protein of bone, which results in generalized osteopenia with bone deformities, pathologic fractures, and short stature. In culture, depending on the conditions, mesenchymal stem cells (MSCs) can differentiate into osteoblasts and osteocytes, cartilage, or tendon. It is likely that a common pluripotential stem cell can give rise either to mesenchymal stem cells or to hematopoietic stem cells. Also, recent evidence suggests that, given the correct culture conditions, certain types of nerve cells, muscle cells, and other body cells can transform into hematopoietic stem cells.

HYPOCHROMIC ANEMIAS

The hypochromic anemias are characterized by hypochromic cells in the peripheral blood with a mean cell hemoglobin (MCH) of <27 pg. The cells are also usually microcytic, with a mean cell volume (MCV) of <80 fl.

The hypochromasia is caused by failure of hemoglobin synthesis, the mechanism of which is shown in Fig. 5-1. This failure occurs most commonly as a result of iron deficiency, but it may also arise from a block in iron metabolism as in the anemia of chronic disorders; from failure of protoporphyrin and heme synthesis as in the sideroblastic anemias; from failure of globin synthesis as in the thalassemias (see Chapter 9); or from crystallization of hemoglobin in some of the other hemoglobin disorders, for example, hemoglobin C (see Chapter 9). Lead inhibits both heme and globin synthesis and may cause a hypochromic anemia, but it also causes hemolysis, probably because of failure of ribonucleic acid (RNA) breakdown.

IRON METABOLISM

Most body iron, present in hemoglobin, is found in circulating red cells (Fig. 5-2). The macrophages of the reticuloendothelial system store iron released from hemoglobin as ferritin and hemosiderin. They also release iron to plasma where it attaches to transferrin, which takes it to tissues with transferrin receptors, especially the bone marrow where the iron is incorporated by erythroid cells into hemoglobin. There is a small loss of iron each day in urine, feces, skin, and nails and in menstruating females via blood. This loss (1–2 mg daily) is replaced by iron absorbed from the diet.

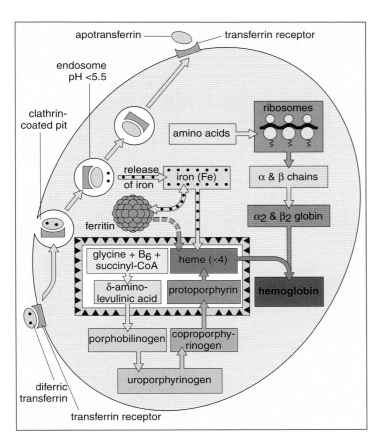

Fig. 5-1. Hemoglobin synthesis in the developing red cell: Iron enters the cell with transferrin and is combined with protoporphyrin, synthesized largely from glycine and succinyl-CoA in mitochondria, to form heme. One molecule of heme attaches to one of the globin polypeptide chains to form a unit of hemoglobin, and one hemoglobin molecule is made up of four hemoglobin units. Transferrin together with its receptor enters the cell by receptor-mediated endocytosis. Iron is released by a fall in pH, and the apotransferrin and receptor are recycled to plasma and membrane, respectively. Hypochromic anemias arise from lack of iron or failure of heme synthesis for other reasons.

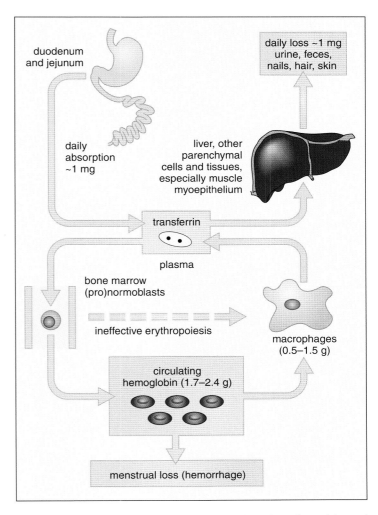

Fig. 5-2. Iron metabolism: Normal iron content of circulating hemoglobin and macrophages is indicated, as well as the approximate amount of iron absorbed and lost from the body each day.

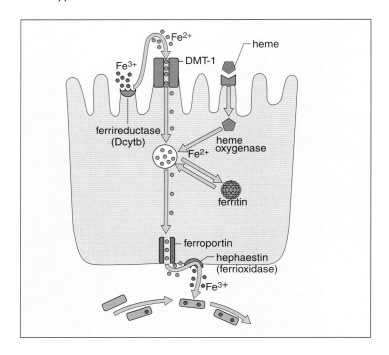

Fig. 5-3. Iron absorption: Inorganic iron is reduced to the Fe^{2+} form and transported into the cell by DMT-1 and out by ferroportin. It is reoxidized to Fe^{3+} as it exits the enterocyte. Heme iron is now thought to be absorbed by a separate receptor.

IRON ABSORPTION

Entry of inorganic iron into the duodenal enterocyte is via the protein receptor DMT-1 (Fig. 5-3). Levels of DMT-1 are regulated by the iron-responsive element (IRE) mechanism (see the following), iron deficiency leading to increased DMT-1. Exit of iron into portal plasma is controlled by ferroportin. The levels of this protein are regulated by hepcidin, which is discussed next. Heme iron is absorbed via a heme receptor at the cell surface, heme being subsequently digested in the enterocyte by heme oxygenase and other enzymes.

HEPCIDIN

This is a large polypeptide, produced by the liver, that controls iron metabolism by inhibiting its absorption and release from macrophages (Fig. 6-12). Hepcidin causes degradation of the messenger RNA (mRNA) for ferroportin, a protein that promotes iron release from enterocytes into portal plasma and from macrophages into peripheral blood. Synthesis of hepcidin is controlled by three proteins: HFE, hemojuvelin (HJV), and transferrin receptor 2 (TFR2). Low levels of HFE or HJV or low iron saturation of TFR2 lead to reduced hepcidin levels, resulting in increased iron absorption.

Interleukin-6, produced in response to inflammation, stimulates hepcidin production. Anoxia, on the other hand, a protein (GDF15) produced by erythroblasts and matriptase-2 (also called TMPRSS6), a transmembrane serine protease in liver and other tissues, downregulate hepcidin secretion (see page 97). Rare genetic defects of TMPRSS6 are associated with a familial, hypochromic, microcytic anemia, low serum iron and low saturation of transferrin, normal or raised serum hepcidin and ferritin, and poor hematological response to oral iron. The autosomal recessive disease has been termed IRIDA (iron refractory iron deficiency anemia).

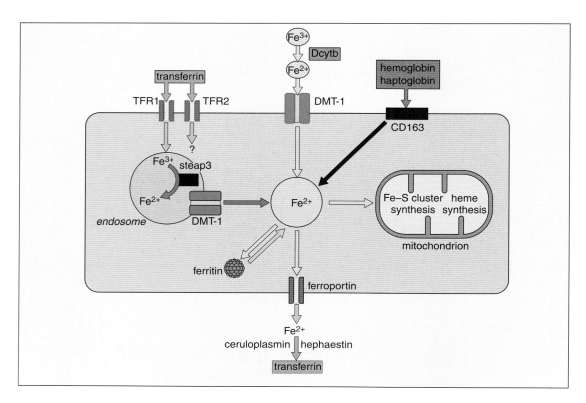

Fig. 5-4. Cellular iron metabolism: Similar proteins are involved as in iron absorption. Steap 3 is an intracellular ferrireductase. Dcytb is also a ferrireductase. *TFR*, Transferrin receptor. FLCVR (not shown) is a protein which exports heme iron from the cell. Mitoferrin (not shown) is involved in the transport of iron into the mitochondrion. (Modified from Hentze MW et al: *Cell* 117:285–297, 2004.)

IRON HOMEOSTASIS

Metabolism of iron in body cells involves similar proteins to those involved in iron absorption (Fig. 5-4). Iron uptake via the transferrin receptor, intracellular storage of iron in ferritin, and the incorporation of iron into heme in mitochondria are all coordinated in response to iron supply at the transcriptional and translational levels. This is achieved partly by the presence of IREs located in the upstream untranslated regions of the mRNAs for ferritin, ferroportin, m-aconitase, and the erythroid heme synthetic enzyme δ-aminolevulinic acid synthase (ALA-S), or in the downstream region for transferrin receptor (TFRI) and the iron transporter DMT-1 in untranslated regions of the mRNAs (Fig. 5-5). The IREs consist of both a double-stranded stem and a single-stranded loop RNA structure. Iron regulatory proteins (IRPs) bind to IRE and exist in two isoforms, IRP1 and IRP2. Increased iron levels result in conversion of IRP1 to an iron-sulfur cluster containing acotinase, which lacks IRE-binding activity. Increased iron also leads to degradation of IRP2; low levels of iron have the opposite effects.

IRON-DEFICIENCY ANEMIA

Iron deficiency usually results from hemorrhage because most body iron is present in circulatory hemoglobin. The symptoms of iron deficiency are caused by anemia (if sufficiently severe), as well as damage to epithelial tissues in some cases. Also, symptoms of the underlying disease may be present. On rare occasions, a patient has a bizarre craving to eat items such as ice, chalk, or paper. This is known as *pica*. In infants, impairment of psychomotor development and cognitive function may occur, especially in the first 2 years of life.

A patient with iron-deficiency anemia may show pallor of the mucous membranes, which is usually only recognized clinically if the hemoglobin is less than about 9 g/dl. There is pallor of the conjunctivae, lips, palm creases, and nail beds (Figs. 5-6 to 5-8). Skin color,

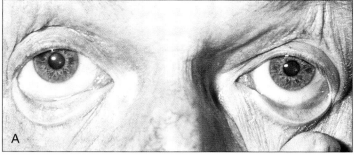
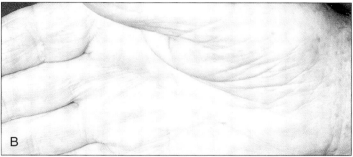

Fig. 5-6. Iron-deficiency anemia. **A,** Pallor of conjunctival mucosa; mucous membrane pallor becomes clinically apparent when the hemoglobin concentration is below 9 g/dl. **B,** Pallor of palmar skin creases.

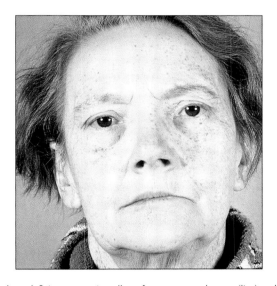

Fig. 5-7. Iron-deficiency anemia: pallor of mucous membranes (lips) and skin in a 69-year-old woman. (Hb, 8.1 g/dl; RBC, 4.13 × 10^{12}/L; PCV, 26.8%; MCV, 65 fl; MCH, 19.6 pg.)

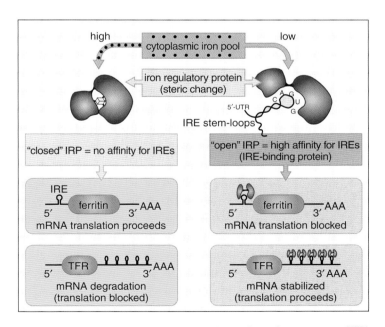

Fig. 5-5. Cellular iron homeostasis: The synthesis of transferrin receptor (TFR), DMT-1, ferritin, erythroid δ-aminolevulinic acid synthase (ALA-S), ferroportin, and m-acotinase is regulated at the level of ribonucleic acid (RNA) translation by cytoplasmic iron regulatory proteins (IRP). These proteins can bind to messenger RNAs (mRNAs) that contain a stem and loop structure—an iron-responsive element (IRE). When iron is plentiful, it has a low affinity for IRE, resulting in less transferrin receptor and DMT-1 but more ferritin, erythroid ALA-S, ferroportin, and m-acotinase synthesis. When iron supply is low, binding to the IRE is increased with increased synthesis of transferrin receptor and DMT-1 and less ferritin, ALA-S, ferroportin, and m-acotinase synthesis. (Courtesy of Dr. D. Girelli.)

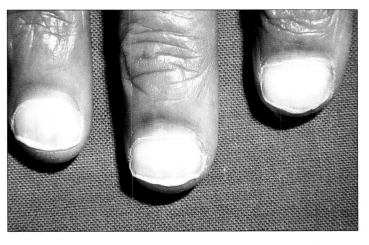

Fig. 5-8. Iron-deficiency anemia: marked pallor of the nail beds in a dark-skinned patient. The nails are flattened.

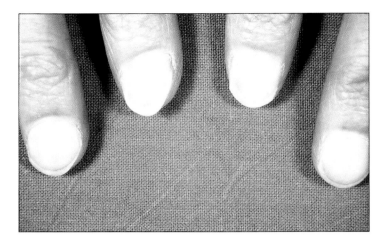

Fig. 5-9. Iron-deficiency anemia: Although there is no obvious concavity, these nails are flattened and brittle with marked pallor of the nail beds.

however, is not a reliable sign of anemia because it depends on the state of the skin circulation, as well as on the hemoglobin content of the blood. A patient's nails are frequently ridged and brittle (Fig. 5-9) or may show spoon nails, known as *koilonychia* (Fig. 5-10). There

may be angular cheilosis (stomatitis; cracking at the corners of the mouth), especially in those with badly fitting false teeth (Fig. 5-11).

In severe cases, especially in older patients, an atrophic glossitis with loss of filiform papillae (Fig. 5-12) may be present.

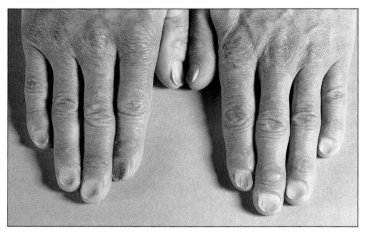

Fig. 5-10. Iron-deficiency anemia: koilonychia. The nails are concave, ridged, and brittle. This patient's anemia had been rapidly corrected by blood transfusion before an operation for cecal carcinoma. The cause of the nail changes in iron deficiency is uncertain but may be related to the iron requirement of many enzymes present in epithelial and other cells. (Courtesy of Dr. S. M. Knowles.)

Fig. 5-11. Iron-deficiency anemia: angular cheilosis. There is fissuring and ulceration at the corners of the mouth. The biochemical mechanism is uncertain but may be similar to that for nail, mucosal, and pharyngeal changes.

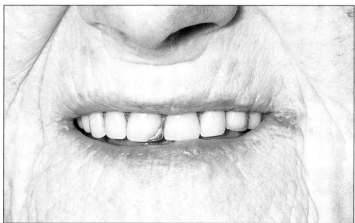

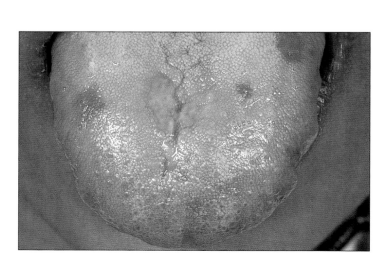

Fig. 5-12. Iron-deficiency anemia: glossitis. The bald, fissured appearance of the tongue is caused by flattening and loss of papillae.

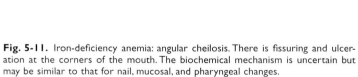

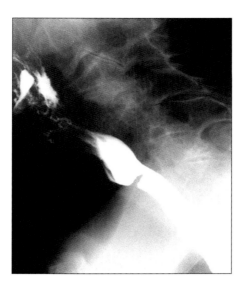

Fig. 5-13. Iron-deficiency anemia: barium swallow radiograph showing a postcricoid web causing a filling defect in a 50-year-old woman with the Plummer-Vinson (Paterson-Kelly) syndrome who complained of dysphagia.

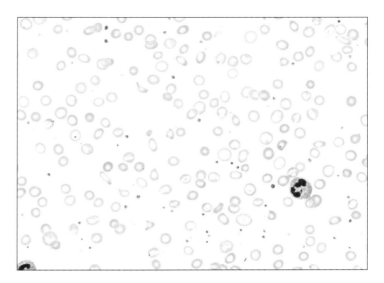

Fig. 5-15. Iron-deficiency anemia: low-power view of peripheral blood film. The red cells are hypochromic and microcytic. Some poikilocytes are present, including thin elongated ("pencil") cells and occasional target cells. Platelets are plentiful. (Hb, 7.5 g/dl.)

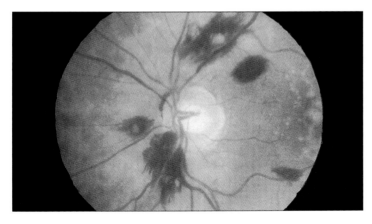

Fig. 5-14. Iron-deficiency anemia; multiple retinal hemorrhages in a 25-year-old woman with chronic iron deficiency because of severe hemorrhage (menorrhagia; Hb, 2.5 g/dl). These appearances may occur in other severe anemias.

Fig. 5-16. Iron-deficiency anemia: High-power view of peripheral blood film shows hypochromic cells and poikilocytes.

There may also be dysphagia resulting from postcricoid webs (Plummer-Vinson or Paterson-Kelly syndrome), especially in middle-aged women (Fig. 5-13).

The biochemical explanation for these epithelial cell abnormalities is unclear; they may be related to a reduction in heme-containing enzymes (e.g., cytochromes, cytochrome c oxidase, succinic dehydrogenase, catalase, peroxidase, ribonucleotide reductase, xanthine oxidase, and aconitase). When anemia is very severe and of rapid onset, there may be retinal hemorrhages (Fig. 5-14).

BLOOD AND BONE MARROW APPEARANCES

A blood film shows the presence of hypochromic microcytic red cells (Figs. 5-15 to 5-17) with abnormally shaped cells ("pencil" or cigar-shaped poikilocytes) and occasional target cells. The severity of the blood film changes and of the fall in MCH and MCV is related to the degree of anemia. Platelet count is often raised, particularly if hemorrhage is occurring.

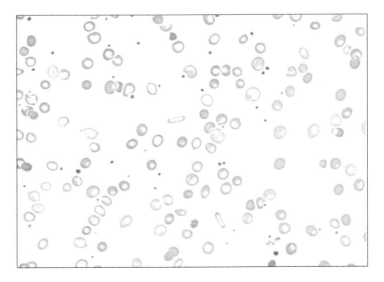

Fig. 5-17. Iron-deficiency anemia: low-power peripheral blood film taken during therapy with oral iron. There is a dimorphic population of hypochromic microcytic cells and target cells and well-hemoglobinized cells of normal size, but there are some large polychromatic cells (newly formed well-hemoglobinized reticulocytes).

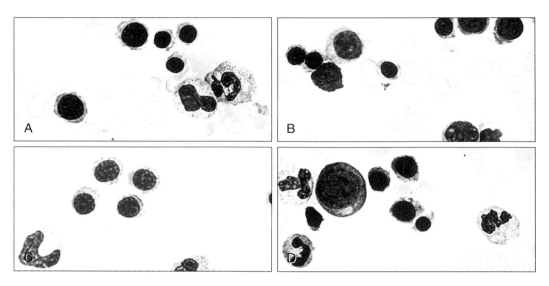

Fig. 5-18. Iron-deficiency anemia: bone marrow aspirate. **A–D,** The cytoplasm of polychromatic and pyknotic erythroblasts is scanty, vacuolated, and irregular in outline. This type of erythropoiesis has been described as *micronormoblastic.*

Bone marrow is of normal cellularity, sometimes with normoblastic hyperplasia, and the developing erythroblasts show a ragged vacuolated cytoplasm (Fig. 5-18). Perls' staining shows a complete absence of iron stores (Fig. 5-19) and of siderotic granules from developing erythroblasts (Fig. 5-20).

CAUSES OF IRON DEFICIENCY

The causes of iron-deficiency anemia are listed in Table 5-1. About two thirds of body iron is circulating in red cells as hemoglobin, 1 L of blood containing about 500 mg of iron. The next biggest store, which varies between 0 and 2 g, is within the macrophages of the reticuloendothelial system in the form of the storage proteins hemosiderin (visible on light microscopy) and ferritin (seen only by electron microscopy). The absence of iron stores, with a fall in serum iron and serum ferritin and a rise in total iron-binding capacity (transferrin) but without anemia and without a fall in red cell indices, is termed *latent iron deficiency.* Iron in myoglobin and a variety of enzymes make up the rest of the body iron.

Daily iron losses and, thus, requirements for iron in adults are normally small in relation to body stores, about 1 mg daily in men and in postmenopausal women, and 1.5 to 3.9 mg in menstruating women. Requirements are also increased in children (to provide for growth and increase in red cell mass) and during pregnancy (for transfer to the fetus).

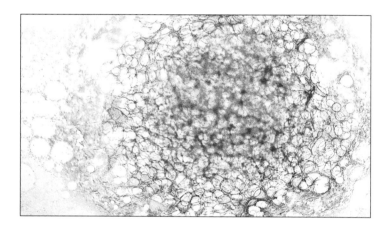

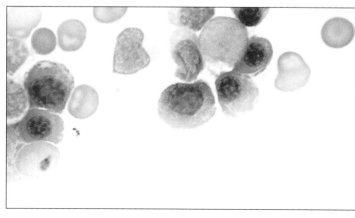

Fig. 5-19. Iron-deficiency anemia: bone marrow aspirate showing absence of stainable iron in a bone marrow fragment. The appearances are similar in iron-deficiency anemia and latent iron deficiency (absent iron stores without anemia). Compare with the appearances of normal iron stores in Fig. 4-56 (Perls' stain, methyl red counterstain).

Fig. 5-20. Iron-deficiency anemia: bone marrow aspirate showing lack of siderotic granules in developing erythroblasts. Compare with the normal appearance of isolated Prussian blue–positive granules in the erythroblast cytoplasm in Fig. 4-56 (Perls' stain, methyl red counterstain).

TABLE 5-1.   IRON-DEFICIENCY ANEMIA: CAUSES

Hemorrhage	Gastrointestinal	Pulmonary	Transfer to fetus	Pregnancy
	hiatus hernia	pulmonary hemosiderosis		
	esophageal varices		Hemosiderinuria	Chronic intravascular hemolysis
	peptic ulcer	Uterine		paroxysmal nocturnal hemoglobinuria
	aspirin ingestion	menorrhagia		heart valve hemolysis
	hookworm	ante- and postpartum		
	neoplasm		Malabsorption	Atrophic gastritis
	ulcerative colitis	Renal tract		Gluten-induced enteropathy
	telangiectasia	hematuria		Partial gastrectomy
	angiodysplasia	chronic dialysis		
	diverticulosis		Poor diet	Poor-quality diet,
	hemorrhoids	Self-induced		especially if mostly vegetable
				Infants fed on cows' milk with late
				weaning

Iron deficiency is usually the result of hemorrhage, the most common cause in many countries being hookworm infestation (Fig. 5-21); the loss is related to the worm load. In women, menorrhagia or repeated pregnancy without iron supplementation is a frequent cause.

In men and in postmenopausal women, iron deficiency is usually caused by chronic gastrointestinal blood loss, which in Western countries is often the result of hiatus hernia (Fig. 5-22), peptic ulceration (Fig. 5-23), chronic aspirin ingestion, colonic or cecal carcinoma

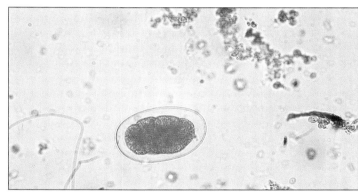

Fig. 5-21. Iron-deficiency anemia: an ovum of the hookworm. Ancylostoma duodenale, a frequent cause of iron-deficiency anemia in many parts of the world, is present. Blood loss and therefore severity of anemia are related to the degree of parasitization.

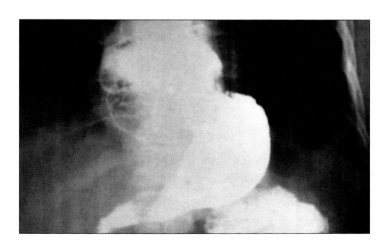

Fig. 5-22. Iron-deficiency anemia: barium meal radiograph showing a gross hiatus hernia in a 55-year-old patient. Endoscopy showed a small, ulcerated area of bleeding.

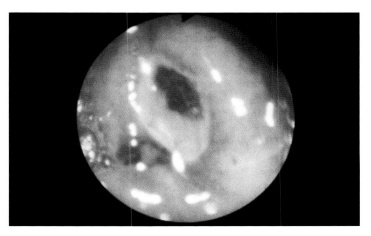

Fig. 5-23. Iron-deficiency anemia: endoscopic appearance of a bleeding duodenal ulcer in a 45-year-old man with symptoms of anemia. (Courtesy of Professor R. E. Pounder.)

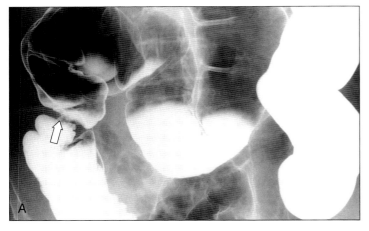

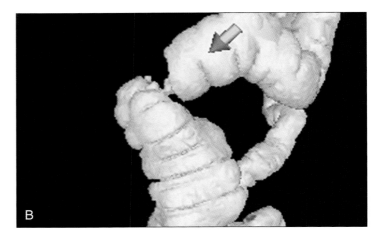

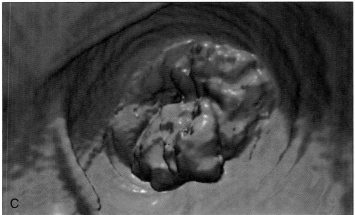

Fig. 5-24. Iron-deficiency anemia. **A,** Barium enema radiograph showing an annular filling defect *(arrow)* of the ascending colon due to adenocarcinoma. **B,** Virtual colonoscopy: annular ("apple-core") narrowing of the colon 126 cm from the anal verge. **C,** Luminal views reveal fungating adenocarcinoma (same case as **B**). (*B* and *C,* Courtesy of Dr. J. Bell.)

Fig. 5-25. Iron deficiency anemia. **A,** Pill camera. This is swallowed and transmits images to a camera worn as a belt. The camera is not reused. **B,** Pill camera image: bleeding angioma present in small intestine. **C,** Pill camera image: angiodysplasia present in small intestine. **D,** Pill camera image: angiodysplasia bleeding in small intestine. (*A–D,* Courtesy of Professor O. Epstein and Dr. M. Caplin.)

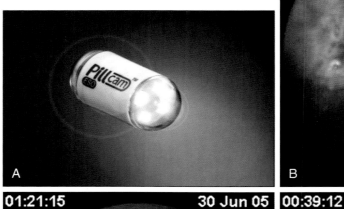

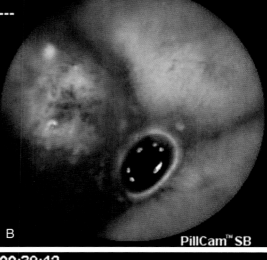

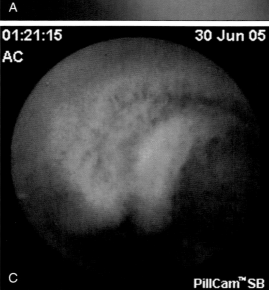

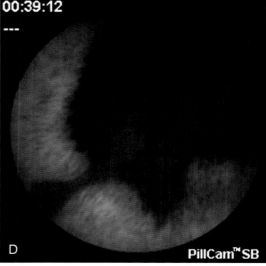

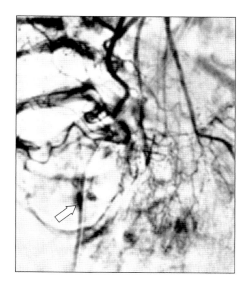

Fig. 5-26. Iron-deficiency anemia: angiogram of coeliac axis showing numerous "blushes" *(arrow)* that result from angiodysplasia of the terminal ileum and ascending colon. (Courtesy of Dr. R. Dick.)

(Fig. 5-24), angiodysplasia (Figs. 5-25 and 5-26), colonic diverticulosis (Fig. 5-27), or hemorrhoids. Rare causes of iron deficiency are pulmonary hemosiderosis (Fig. 5-28), chronic intravascular hemolysis as in paroxysmal nocturnal hemoglobinuria, and self-inflicted venesection.

A normal Western diet contains 10 to 15 mg of iron daily, of which 5% to 10% is absorbed. Iron absorption is increased in iron deficiency but reduced by some food substances, such as phytates and phosphates. Poor dietary intake of iron may be the sole cause of iron deficiency if present for many years. However, more often poor diet provides a background of reduced iron stores on which other causes of iron deficiency, such as heavy menstrual loss or increased requirements for pregnancy or for growth in infants and children, may lead to iron-deficiency anemia.

Malabsorption alone is also an unusual cause of iron deficiency. Even in patients with atrophic gastritis or gluten-induced enteropathy, loss resulting from an increased turnover of cells and exudation of transferrin iron may be as important as the malabsorption. Following gastrectomy, the two main factors are blood loss and malabsorption, more marked for food iron than for inorganic iron.

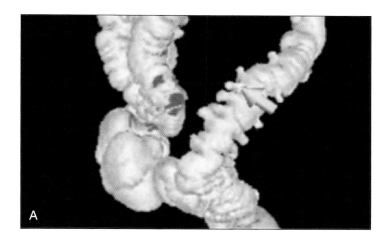

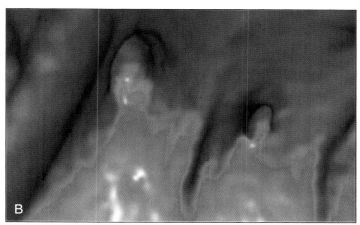

Fig. 5-27. Iron-deficiency anemia: virtual colonoscopy. **A,** Multiple diverticula, one arrowed of the sigmoid colon. **B,** Luminal view shows the mouths of two diverticula. (Courtesy of Dr. J. Bell.)

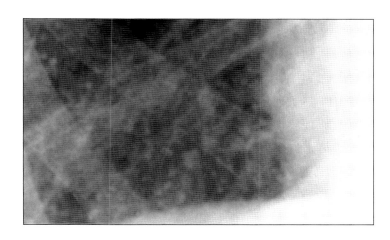

Fig. 5-28. Iron-deficiency anemia: chest radiograph showing diffuse mottled appearance caused by pulmonary hemosiderosis. The lesions consist of aggregates of iron-laden macrophages with surrounding fibrosis. (Courtesy of Dr. R. Dick.)

SIDEROBLASTIC ANEMIA

Sideroblastic anemia is characterized by the presence of ring sideroblasts (>15% of erythroblasts) in the bone marrow. The iron is deposited in the mitochondria of the erythroblasts. Mitochondrial iron uptake, metabolism, and release into the cell cytoplasm is described in Fig. 5-29. The disorder is classified into congenital and acquired types; the acquired type is further subdivided into primary and secondary types, including some types associated with other bone marrow disorders (Table 5-2). In the secondary types, the proportion of ring sideroblasts is usually <15% and the anemia has other causes.

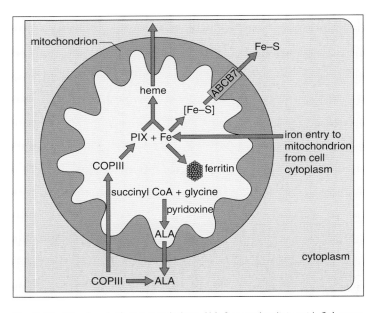

Fig. 5-29. Mitochondrial iron metabolism. *ALA,* δ-aminolevulinic acid; *CoA,* coenzyme A; *COP,* coproporphyrin; *Fe-S,* iron-sulfur cluster; *PIX,* protoporphyrin IX.

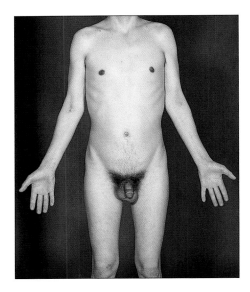

Fig. 5-30. Sideroblastic anemia: This 18-year-old male with hereditary (congenital) sideroblastic anemia had symptoms of anemia at age 16 and was found to have a microcytic hypochromic anemia (Hb, 9.8 g/dl; MCV, 75 fl; MCH, 23.1 pg) with many ring sideroblasts in the bone marrow. His height (1.75 m) and sexual development are normal. Pallor of the mucous membranes and early melanin skin pigmentation resulted from iron overload arising from blood transfusions given over a 2-year period and commenced soon after presentation because his hemoglobin had fallen spontaneously to <6 g/dl. He subsequently died of infection with *Yersinia enterocolitica,* having received over 500 units of blood. The patient's older brother was also affected (see Figs. 5-32 and 5-33).

The congenital type usually occurs in males (Fig. 5-30), indicating a sex-linked pattern of inheritance, but it is also seen, though rarely, in females (Fig. 5-31). The blood film is hypochromic and microcytic, or dimorphic of varying severity (Fig. 5-32). About one third of congenital cases respond to pyridoxine (vitamin B₆), a greater percentage than in the other types of sideroblastic anemia.

The congenital type of sideroblastic anemia includes a group with mutations in the gene on the X-chromosome coding for the erythroid specific enzyme, ALA-S (Fig. 5-33). It usually affects men and manifests in the third decade of life. Women are rarely affected.

TABLE 5-2.   SIDEROBLASTIC ANEMIA: CLASSIFICATION

Hereditary	
X-linked	– mutations in erythroid-specific ALAS2 (Xp11.21) – with spinocerebellar degeneration and ataxia; mutations of mitochondrial ABCB7
Mitochondrial	– DNA deletions, for example, Pearson and Kearns–Sayre syndromes – mutation in subunit 1 of mitochondrial cytochrome oxidase
Autosomal	– thiamine-responsive mutations of gene SLC19A2 that encodes thiamine transporter THTR-1 (1q23.3)
Acquired	
Primary	– myelodysplastic syndromes

Secondary	– associated with malignant marrow disorders
	  acute myeloid leukemia
	  polycythemia vera
	  myelofibrosis
	  myeloma
	– drugs (isoniazid, pyrizinamide, cycloserine, chloramphenicol, penicillamine, fusidic acid)
	– toxins (lead, alcohol)
	– megaloblastic anemia, hemolytic anemia, pregnancy, rheumatoid arthritis, carcinoma

DNA, Deoxyribonucleic acid.

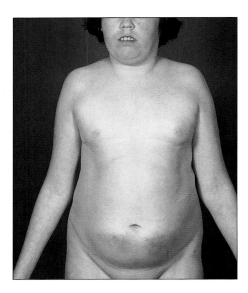

Fig. 5-31. Sideroblastic anemia: a 17-year-old girl with congenital sideroblastic anemia, a rare occurrence. Iron overload developed because of the need for regular blood transfusions from 3 years of age. She failed to commence menstruation and shows delayed puberty, absence of axillary and pubic hair, and minimal breast development. She also has a thalassemic facies with a bossed skull, prominent maxilla, and abnormally widened spaces between the teeth. The lower abdominal bruising is from the regular insertion of needles for subcutaneous desferrioxamine infusions.

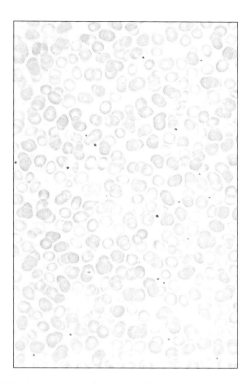

Fig. 5-32. Sideroblastic anemia (hereditary): Peripheral blood film from a 19-year-old man shows a dimorphic anemia with a mixture of poorly hemoglobinized microcytic cells and well-hemoglobinized normocytic cells. (Hb, 11.5 g/dl; MCV, 78 fl; MCH, 22.3 pg.)

Manifestation in both sexes in old age has been described. The mutations identified have been missense, affecting exons 5, 7, 8, and 9. Pyridoxine responsiveness correlates with mutations affecting exon 9, the region that codes for the pyridoxal-5-phosphate binding site. Exon 5 may also code for sequences involved in pyridoxal-5-phosphate binding.

Some of the congenital types are now thought to result from a fault in mitochondrial deoxyribonucleic acid (DNA), including that

in Pearson or Kearns-Sayre syndromes, which causes a defect in one or more enzymes in the respiratory chain generating adenosine triphosphate (ATP) and coded for by mitochondrial DNA (Fig. 5-34).

Pearson syndrome consists of neutropenia, thrombocytopenia, sideroblastic anemia, exocrine pancreatic dysfunction, and hepatic dysfunction. There is vacuolation of marrow erythroid and myeloid precursors (Fig. 5-35, A). The syndrome may be accompanied by neurologic and muscle disorders. The bone marrow and skeletal muscle findings of a 42-year-old man with the combination of congenital sideroblastic anemia and a proximal myopathy are shown in Figs. 5-35, B, and 5-36. The bone marrow shows ring sideroblasts and vacuolation of normoblasts (see Fig. 5-35, B). Electron microscopy of a skeletal muscle biopsy shows crystalline deposits in mitochondria (see Fig. 5-36). The exact defect is unclear despite analysis of ALA-S and mitochondrial DNA. This patient did not fit precisely into any clear phenotype.

DIDMOAD (Wolfram) syndrome consists of Diabetes Insipidus, Diabetes Mellitus, Optic Atrophy, and sensorineural Deafness. It may be accompanied by megaloblastic and sideroblastic anemia, in some cases responding to thiamine. As in other forms of sideroblastic anemia, there is iron loading of erythroblast mitochondria (Fig. 5-37). A less common triad of thiamine-responsive megaloblastic anemia, diabetes mellitus, and sensorineural deafness has been described. A defect in thiamine phosphorylation resulting from mutation of the gene *SLC19A2* on chromosome 1q23.3 encoding the thiamine transporter THTR-1 has been identified. The patient illustrated in Fig. 5-38 resembles one with the DIDMOAD syndrome most closely.

A rare form of inherited sideroblastic anemia is due to mutations in ABCB7, an ATP-binding cassette protein involved in transport of iron-sulfur clusters from the mitochondria (see Fig. 5-29). There is usually non-progressive ataxia.

In primary acquired sideroblastic anemia (refractory anemia with ring sideroblasts), there is usually macrocytosis and gross anisocytosis and poikilocytosis (Fig. 5-39). This disease is classified by the World Health Organization (WHO) as a type of myelodysplasia (see Chapter 14). In a proportion of patients the disease transforms into acute myeloid leukemia after a variable number of years. In many cases careful examination reveals white-cell or platelet abnormalities in the peripheral blood or in their precursors in the bone marrow. These cases with trilineage dysplasia have a much higher incidence of transformation to acute myeloid leukemia.

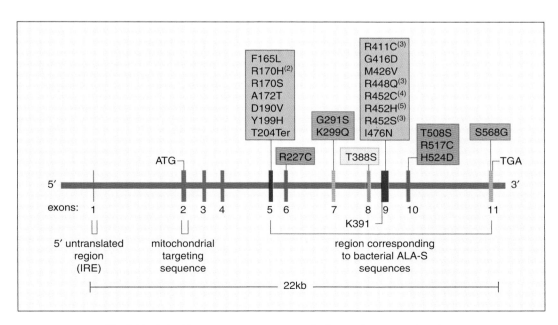

Fig. 5-33. Sideroblastic anemia: mutations in the δ-aminolevulinic acid synthase (ALA-S) gene in patients with X-linked sideroblastic anemia. *IRE,* Iron-responsive element. (The superscript numbers in parentheses refer to the number of cases described at the time of writing; courtesy of Professor D. F. Bishop.)

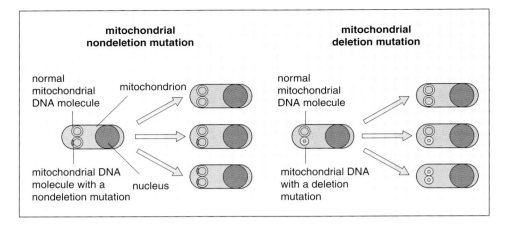

Fig. 5-34. Mitochondrial deoxyribonucleic acid (DNA): This consists of a circular loop of DNA coding for enzymes in the mitochondrial respiratory chain. Mitochondrial DNA is inherited from the cytoplasm of the maternal ovum. Multiple copies (50–1000) are present in each cell. The relative proportions of a mutant (deletional or nondeletional) and wild-type mitochondrial DNA that occur in the individual cells of a particular tissue determine the phenotype when a mitochondrial defect is inherited.

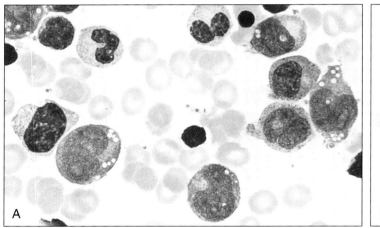

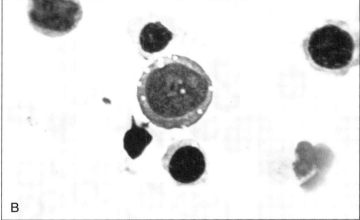

Fig. 5-35. Congenital sideroblastic anemia. **A,** Bone marrow of a baby with Pearson syndrome showing vacuolated proerythroblasts and dysplastic neutrophils. **B,** Bone marrow of a 42-year-old man showing vacuolation of blast cells.

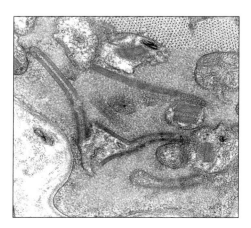

Fig. 5-36. Congenital sideroblastic anemia: Electron micrograph of skeletal muscle of a 42-year-old man showing bizarrely shaped mitochondria with abnormal cristae and intramitochondrial paracrystalline inclusions. The changes are typical of a mitochondrial respiratory chain defect. (Courtesy of Professor A. H. V. Schapira.)

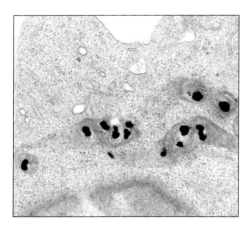

Fig. 5-37. Hereditary sideroblastic anemia: Electron microscopy of erythroblast showing iron-laden mitochondria. The patient, a 13-year-old male, had diabetes mellitus, deafness, and optic atrophy (Hb, 10.3 g/dl; RBC, 3.47 × 10¹²/L). Peripheral blood showed macrocytes and hypochromic and microcytic red cells; bone marrow showed megaloblastic and dyserythropoietic changes and ringed sideroblasts. There was no response to folic acid or pyridoxine, but a reticulocytosis with a rise in hemoglobin to 12.9 g/dl occurred in response to thiamine therapy. (From Haworth C, Evans DJ, Mitra J, et al: Thiamine responsive anemia: a study of two further cases, *Br J Hematol* 50:549–561, 1982. Courtesy of Professor S. N. Wickramasinghe.)

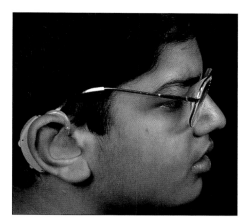

Fig. 5-38. Sideroblastic anemia: an 11-year-old boy with congenital deafness, optic atrophy, diabetes mellitus, and megaloblastic and sideroblastic anemia (a variant of DIDMOAD syndrome). His older sister showed the same syndrome, but in her case the anemia responded to thiamine. In this patient the anemia is refractory to thiamine, pyridoxine, and folic acid, and regular blood transfusions are needed. (Courtesy of Dr. J. Z. Wimperis.)

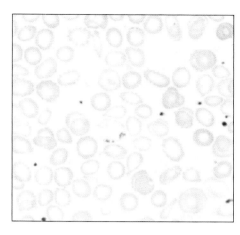

Fig. 5-40. Refractory anemia with ring sideroblasts: peripheral blood film following splenectomy showing Pappenheimer bodies in the red cells. Their iron content is demonstrated by Perls' staining (siderotic granules). In addition, Howell-Jolly bodies (deoxyribonucleic acid [DNA] remnants) were present and the platelet count was raised (652×10^9/L).

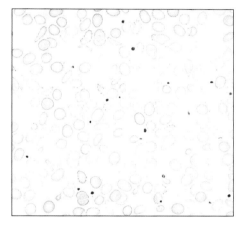

Fig. 5-39. Refractory anemia with ring sideroblasts: peripheral blood film from a 65-year-old man with a predominantly hypochromic anemia with numerous poikilocytes. In most such cases, the anemia is dimorphic with an overall increase in MCV to above normal. (Hb, 7.2 g/dl; MCV, 82 fl; MCH, 26.8 pg.)

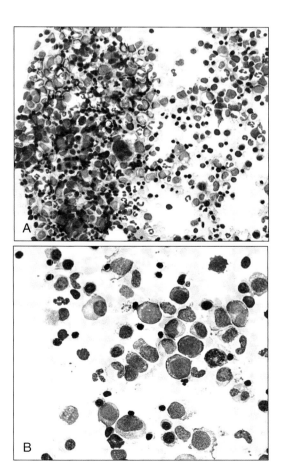

Fig. 5-41. Refractory anemia with ring sideroblasts. **A,** Low-power view of bone marrow aspirate shows increased cellularity of the fragment and trails. **B,** At higher power, erythroid hyperplasia is also seen.

Siderotic granules are frequently seen in the peripheral blood red cells following splenectomy (Fig. 5-40). The bone marrow shows erythroid hyperplasia (Fig. 5-41) with vacuolated erythroblasts (Fig. 5-42).

In contrast to the inherited form, in refractory anemia with ring sideroblasts, the erythroblasts are megaloblastic in about 50% of cases (Fig. 5-43). Iron staining shows many ring sideroblasts (Fig. 5-44), and iron stores may be increased (Fig. 5-45). In refractory anemia with ring sideroblasts, 15% or more of the erythroblasts show partial or complete rings. In the secondary forms, ring sideroblasts are usually less common.

Sideroblastic anemia, especially the inherited form, occasionally responds to vitamin B_6 (pyridoxine) therapy. Other therapy may include folic acid, blood transfusion, and iron chelation. Thiamine may produce a response in rare inherited cases (see above). In refractory anemia with ring sideroblasts, treatment resembles that for other myelodysplastic syndromes.

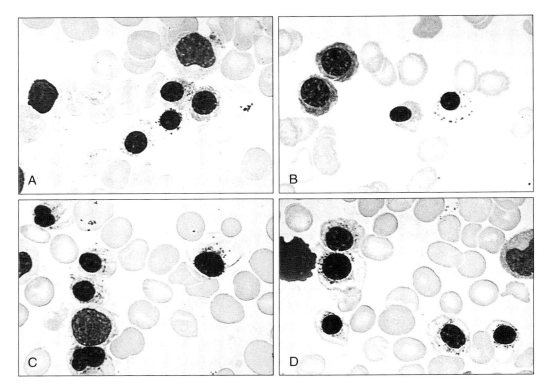

Fig. 5-42. Refractory anemia with ring sideroblasts. **A–D,** Bone marrow aspirate showing vacuolation of erythroblasts with intact cytoplasmic margins. In some cells the vacuoles are surrounded by heavily stained cytoplasmic granules (punctate basophilia). Contrast the appearances with those in iron-deficiency anemia (see Fig. 5-18) and thalassemia major (see Fig. 9-21).

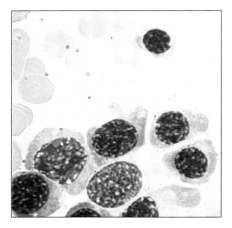

Fig. 5-43. Refractory anemia with ring sideroblasts: bone marrow showing mildly megaloblastic erythroblasts. Serum vitamin B_{12} and folate levels were normal; the deoxyuridine suppression test was normal; giant metamyelocytes and hypersegmented polymorphs were absent. Megaloblastic change is found in 50% of patients with this type of anemia. The biochemical mechanism is uncertain.

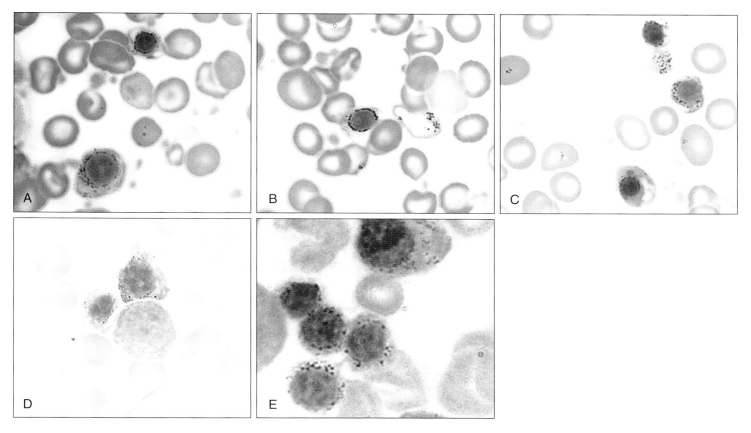

Fig. 5-44. Refractory anemia with ring sideroblasts. **A–E,** Bone marrow aspirate showing erythroblasts with complete or nearly complete rings (or collars) of iron granules around their nuclei. The rings are best seen in late erythroblasts but in severe cases also occur in the earliest recognizable erythroblasts (Perls' stain).

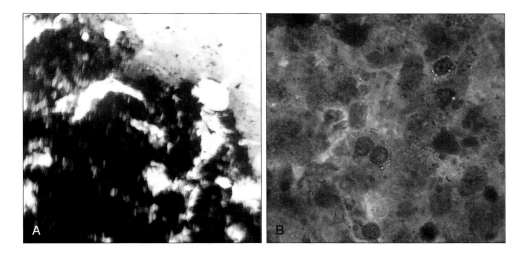

Fig. 5-45. Sideroblastic anemia (hereditary): Bone marrow fragments stained for iron **(A)** show a gross increase in iron in a patient who had been transfused for many years before the diagnosis was made. Treatment with pyridoxine allowed a satisfactory rise in hemoglobin, enabling subsequent venesections for reduction of iron overload. The high-power view **(B)** shows multiple ring sideroblasts and increased iron (hemosiderin) in macrophages.

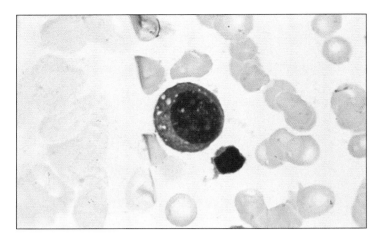

Fig. 5-46. Alcohol-related bone marrow toxicity: Vacuolation of a pronormoblast can be seen.

ALCOHOL

Excessive ingestion of alcohol may cause a variety of hematologic abnormalities, including macrocytosis, megaloblastic and sideroblastic changes, and thrombocytopenia. In some cases vacuolation of erythroblasts is apparent (Fig. 5-46).

LEAD POISONING

Clinically, lead poisoning causes abdominal colic and constipation, a peripheral neuropathy and anemia. Two important enzymes in heme synthesis, δ-aminolevulinic acid (ALA) dehydratase and ferrochelatase, are inhibited. There may be a lead line visible in the gums (Fig. 5-47), marked punctate basophilia in the peripheral blood (Fig. 5-48, *A*), a mild hypochromic anemia with hemolysis, and ring sideroblasts in the marrow (Fig. 5-48, *B*). Lead poisoning may result from excessive exposure to lead paint or to lead in industry. It may also occur because of ingestion of herbal medicines containing excess lead. The punctate basophilia is caused by aggregates of undegraded RNA, a result of inhibition of the enzyme pyrimidine 5′-nucleotidase (Table 5-3).

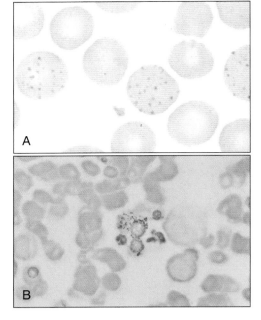

Fig. 5-48. Lead poisoning. **A,** Peripheral blood film showing punctate basophilia. This is caused by precipitates of undegraded ribonucleic acid (RNA), the result of inhibition by lead of pyrimidine 5′-nucleotidase, one of the enzymes responsible for RNA degradation. Similar appearances occur in hereditary pyrimidine 5′-nucleotidase deficiency (see Fig. 8-36). **B,** Bone marrow aspirate showing coarse siderotic granules in a ring around the nucleus of an erythroblast (Perls' stain).

TABLE 5-3. PUNCTATE BASOPHILIA: CAUSES
Thalassemia (α and β)
Acquired sideroblastic anemia and other myelodysplasias
Lead poisoning
Severe megaloblastic anemia
Pyrimidine 5′-nucleotidase deficiency
Congenital dyserythropoietic anemia

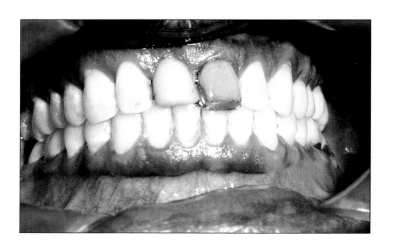

Fig. 5-47. Lead poisoning: a lead line in the gums of a young man with abdominal colic. The poisoning was from prolonged occupational exposure to molten lead.

TABLE 5-4.   DIFFERENTIAL DIAGNOSIS OF HYPOCHROMIC MICROCYTIC ANEMIA

	Iron deficiency	Chronic inflammation or malignancy	Thalassemia trait (α or β)	Sideroblastic anemia
MCV MCH	Reduced in relation to severity of anemia	Normal or mild reduction	Reduced: very low for degree of anemia	Usually low in congenital type but MCV often raised in acquired type
Serum iron	Reduced	Reduced	Normal	Raised
TIBC	Raised	Reduced	Normal	Normal
Serum transferrin receptor	Raised	Normal/low	Variable	Normal
Serum ferritin	Reduced	Normal or raised	Normal	Raised
Bone marrow iron stores	Absent	Present	Present	Present
Erythroblast iron	Absent	Absent	Present	Ring forms
Hemoglobin electrophoresis	Normal	Normal	Hb A$_2$ raised in β form	Normal

MCH, Mean corpuscular hemoglobin; *MCV*, mean corpuscular volume; *TIBC*, total iron-binding capacity.

DIFFERENTIAL DIAGNOSIS OF HYPOCHROMIC MICROCYTIC ANEMIAS

The causes of hypochromic microcytic anemia include iron deficiency, thalassemias and other genetic disorders of hemoglobin, the anemia of chronic disorders, sideroblastic anemia, and lead poisoning (Table 5-4). These causes may be differentiated by special tests, including measurement of serum iron, total iron-binding capacity, or serum ferritin; by hemoglobin electrophoresis or high-performance liquid chromatography (HPLC) examination; or if necessary, by DNA analysis. Bone marrow examination is necessary to diagnose sideroblastic anemia. In thalassemia trait, the disorders may be suspected from the presence of a high red cell count (more than 5.5×10^{12}/L) with low MCV and MCH values (see Chapter 9). Serum hepcidin is raised in chronic inflammation or malignancy but low in iron deficiency. Iron refractory iron deficiency anemia (IRIDA) is discussed on page 76.

THE PORPHYRIAS AND IRON OVERLOAD

Table 6-1 shows the pathways of porphyrin synthesis. The main types of inherited defect of porphyrin synthesis associated with light sensitivity, which affect the hematopoietic system: are congenital erythropoietic porphyria (CEP; known as Günther's disease) and congenital erythropoietic protoporphyria (CEPP). Although not associated with a hypochromic anemia, they are discussed here for convenience.

CONGENITAL ERYTHROPOIETIC PORPHYRIA

Inherited as an autosomal recessive trait, CEP is characterized by excessive production of uroporphyrinogen I, which forms the pigments uroporphyrin I and coproporphyrin I. There is deficiency of the heme synthetic enzyme uroporphyrin III cosynthase. The plasma and erythrocytes contain excessive quantities of uroporphyrin I, coproporphyrin I, and protoporphyrin.

The patient shown in Fig. 6-1 has bullous ulcerating lesions on light-exposed skin, hirsutism, and a hemolytic anemia associated with splenomegaly. The urine is red and fluorescent (Fig. 6-2), and the bones and teeth are discolored and also fluorescent (Fig. 6-3). The nucleated red cells fluoresce when exposed to ultraviolet light (Fig. 6-4).

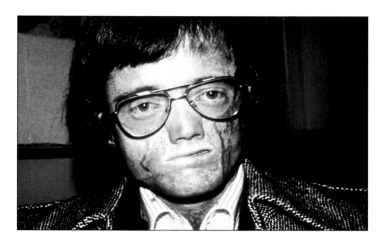

Fig. 6-1. Congenital erythropoietic porphyria (CEP): This 22-year-old man was first diagnosed with this condition (Günther's disease) at 6 years of age, although skin changes had been noted from 2 years of age, especially in the summer. These changes of blistering and susceptibility to mechanical injury were found on exposed areas of skin and led to mutilation of the extremities, including the nose, ears, and hands. He has erythrodontia, splenomegaly, and increased erythropoiesis with red cells that fluoresce. Hemolysis increased with age and is associated with a reticulocytosis. In this case, increased activity of ALA-S and decreased activity of uroporphyrinogen cosynthase were demonstrated, with increased excretion of uroporphyrin I and coproporphyrin I in the urine, together with increased concentrations of these porphyrins in erythrocytes and plasma. (Courtesy of Dr. M. R. Moore.)

TABLE 6-1.   PORPHYRIN METABOLISM

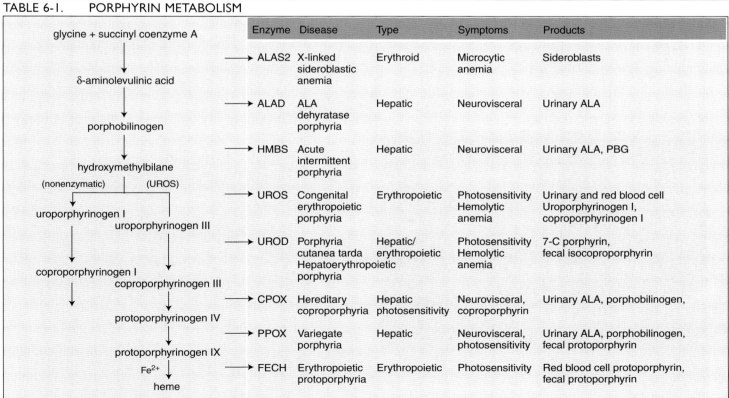

	Enzyme	Disease	Type	Symptoms	Products
glycine + succinyl coenzyme A → δ-aminolevulinic acid	ALAS2	X-linked sideroblastic anemia	Erythroid	Microcytic anemia	Sideroblasts
δ-aminolevulinic acid → porphobilinogen	ALAD	ALA dehyratase porphyria	Hepatic	Neurovisceral	Urinary ALA
porphobilinogen → hydroxymethylbilane	HMBS	Acute intermittent porphyria	Hepatic	Neurovisceral	Urinary ALA, PBG
(nonenzymatic) (UROS) → uroporphyrinogen I / uroporphyrinogen III	UROS	Congenital erythropoietic porphyria	Erythropoietic	Photosensitivity Hemolytic anemia	Urinary and red blood cell Uroporphyrinogen I, coproporphyrinogen I
coproporphyrinogen I / coproporphyrinogen III	UROD	Porphyria cutanea tarda Hepatoerythropoietic porphyria	Hepatic/ erythropoietic	Photosensitivity Hemolytic anemia	7-C porphyrin, fecal isocoproporphyrin
→ protoporphyrinogen IV	CPOX	Hereditary coproporphyria	Hepatic photosensitivity	Neurovisceral, coproporphyrin	Urinary ALA, porphobilinogen,
→ protoporphyrinogen IX	PPOX	Variegate porphyria	Hepatic	Neurovisceral, photosensitivity	Urinary ALA, porphobilinogen, fecal protoporphyrin
Fe²⁺ → heme	FECH	Erythropoietic protoporphyria	Erythropoietic	Photosensitivity	Red blood cell protoporphyrin, fecal protoporphyrin

Adapted from Sassa S: Modern diagnosis and management of porphyrias. *Br J Haematol* 135:282–292, 2006.

For contrast, a patient with porphyria cutanea tarda is shown (Fig. 6-5). A bullous eruption occurs on exposure to sunlight. There is a defect of hepatic uroporphyrinogen decarboxylase, which may be genetic or acquired as a result of alcohol, iron, or estrogen in excess. Iron loading may be a result, as well as a cause, of the syndrome.

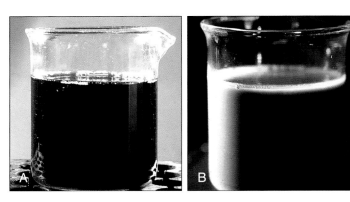

Fig. 6-2. Congenital erythropoietic porphyria (CEP): urine sample in daylight **(A)** and in ultraviolet light **(B).** (A, B, Courtesy of Dr. M. R. Moore.)

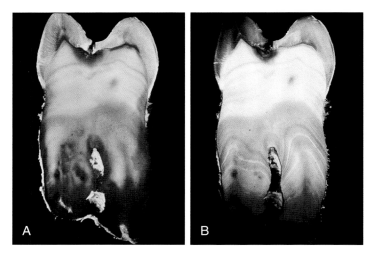

Fig. 6-3. Congenital erythropoietic porphyria (CEP): molar tooth in ordinary light **(A),** with brown discoloration, and ultraviolet light **(B),** with fluorescence most marked in the cortical bone. (A, B, Courtesy of Dr. M. R. Moore.)

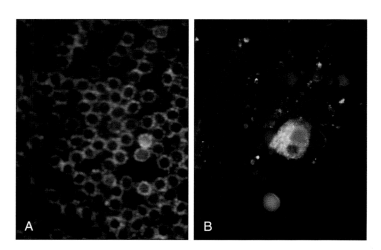

Fig. 6-4. Congenital erythropoietic porphyria (CEP): Peripheral blood film **(A)** and bone marrow aspirate **(B)** viewed in ultraviolet light show nuclear fluorescence of erythroblasts caused by the presence of large amounts of uroporphyrin I. (A, B, Courtesy of Dr. I. Magnus.)

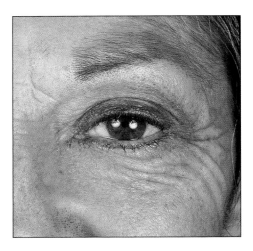

Fig. 6-5. Porphyria cutanea tarda: This 55-year-old woman had bullous eruptions on exposed skin surfaces. (Courtesy of Dr. M. Rustin.)

CONGENITAL ERYTHROPOIETIC PROTOPORPHYRIA

In CEPP, which is inherited as autosomal dominant, the underlying defect is one of ferrochelatase (heme synthase), the final enzyme in heme synthesis. There is excess production of protoporphyrin, which accumulates in erythrocytes, the liver, and other tissues. The erythroblasts fluoresce when exposed to ultraviolet light.

Patients with CEPP are also light sensitive and develop pruritus, swelling, and reddening of the skin. The urine and teeth are of normal color and nonfluorescent, and hemolytic anemia is not present. Cholestasis, hepatitis, and cirrhosis may lead to death from liver failure.

IRON OVERLOAD

PRIMARY (GENETIC) HEMOCHROMATOSIS

The main causes of increased storage of iron are listed in Table 6-2. Transfusional iron overload is discussed in detail in conjunction with thalassemia major in Chapter 9, and porphyria cutanea tarda was discussed previously in this chapter. The genetic basis for most cases of primary hemochromatosis has now been established (Table 6-3), and these diseases are discussed briefly here.

TABLE 6-2.   IRON OVERLOAD: CAUSES

Increased iron absorption
From diets of normal iron content
Primary (genetic) hemochromatosis
Iron loading anemia (refractory anemias with increased bone marrow erythroid cells)
Chronic liver disease (cirrhosis, porto-caval shunt)
Porphyria cutanea tarda
Rare congenital defects (atransferrinemia, aceruloplasminemia, Friedreich's ataxia, hyperferritinemia with autosomal dominant congenital cataracts, other diseases)
From diets with increased iron content
African diet overload*
Medicinal iron

Transfusional iron overload

*A genetic abnormality may play a role

TABLE 6-3.   GENETIC HEMOCHROMATOSIS: GENES
             AND PROTEINS

Gene	Protein	Protein class	Expression	Interaction
HFE	HFE	HLA class I	Ubiquitous	TFR1
TFR2	TFR2	TFR family	Hepatocytes	Transferrin
HAMP	Hepcidin	Antimicrobial peptide	Hepatocytes, skeletal muscle, heart	Ferroportin
HJV	Hemojuvelin	RGM homologue	Heart, liver, skeletal muscle	Neogenin
SLC40A1	Ferroportin	Iron exporter	Ubiquitous	Hepcidin

Adapted from Camaschella C: Understanding iron homeostasis through genetic analysis of hemochromatosis and related disorders. *Blood* 106:3710–3717, 2005.
HJV, Hemojuvelin-encoding gene; *RGM,* repulsive guidance molecule; *SLC40,* solute carrier family 40; *TFR,* transferrin receptor.

The clinical features of the most common type of genetic hemochromatosis are largely similar to those of transfusional iron overload and include hyperpigmentation of the skin (Fig. 6-6) and endocrine abnormalities: diabetes mellitus; gonadal, pituitary, thyroid, and parathyroid dysfunction. Liver parenchymal iron overload is invariable (Fig. 6-7), and fibrosis, cirrhosis, and hepatocellular carcinoma may develop. Computed tomography (CT) scans (Fig. 6-8) can be used to diagnose and measure iron overload. Magnetic resonance imaging (MRI) is now preferred to measure liver and cardiac iron (Fig. 6-9). T_2^* measures the speed of relaxation of the tissue after a magnetic field; the more rapid the relaxation, the higher the iron content. A cardiomyopathy may occur with arrhythmia, pericarditis, or congestive heart failure. An asymmetric arthropathy principally affecting the distal interphalangeal joints with calcium pyrophosphate deposition is characteristic of primary hemochromatosis (Fig. 6-10) and is not seen in transfusional iron overload.

The gene, *HFE,* responsible for the most common type of genetic hemochromatosis (type I) is located on the short arm of chromosome 6, close to the human leukocyte antigen (HLA) locus, and has an association with HLA-A3 and, to a lesser extent, with B7. About a

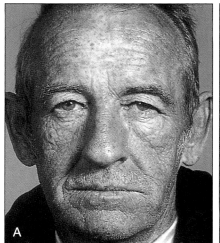
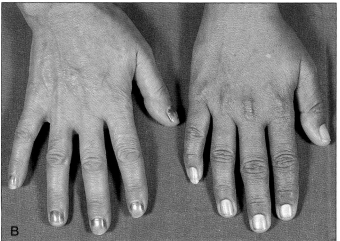

Fig. 6-6. Hemochromatosis. **A,** The appearance of an adult male patient with primary hemochromatosis is shown. Note the characteristic bronze appearance. The hyperpigmentation results from melanin deposition in the skin. The patient also showed hepatic cirrhosis and diabetes mellitus. **B,** For comparison, the hand *(on the right)* of a 16-year-old patient with thalassemia major shows heavy melanin pigmentation; in contrast, his mother's hand *(on the left)* shows normal coloration. (*A,* Courtesy of Dr. R. Britt.)

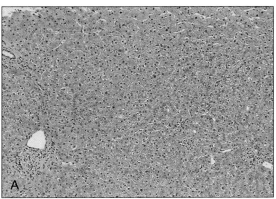
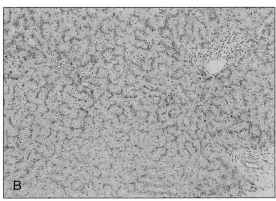

Fig. 6-7. Primary hemochromatosis. **A,** Needle biopsy of the liver in a 30-year-old woman. H & E stain showing normal architecture with golden brown deposits (hemosiderin) in parenchymal cells. **B,** Perls' stain confirming heavy siderosis of parenchymal cells with sparing of Kupffer cells.

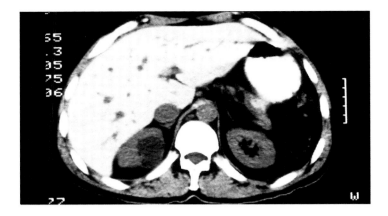

Fig. 6-8. Primary hemochromatosis: axial computed tomography (CT) scan showing increased density of the liver caused by iron overload. The patient, a 50-year-old man, has diabetes mellitus and also pyruvate kinase deficiency for which splenectomy had been performed.

Fig. 6-9. Transfusional iron overload: T_2^* magnetic resonance imaging appearances of liver and spleen **(B)** compared with normal **(A)**. (Courtesy of Professor D. J. Pennell.)

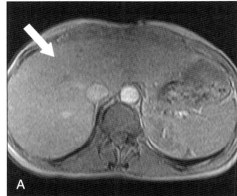
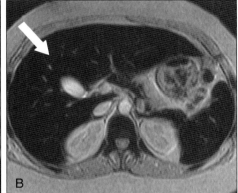

quarter of all men but only 1% of women homozygous for the mutation show iron overload–related disease. The HLA class 1–like gene, *HFE,* is located 3 mb telomeric to the HLA-A locus. It contains seven exons; the putative protein structure is shown in Fig. 6-11. A homozygous missense G to A mutation at nucleotide 845 resulting in a cysteine to tyrosine substitution at amino acid 282 has been found in 83% to 100% of cases in most series studied. A second mutation, C to G in exon 2, results in a histidine to aspartic acid substitution at amino acid 63, and a small percentage of patients are compound heterozygotes. HFE is one of the proteins controlling synthesis of hepcidin (Fig. 6-12).

Hemochromatosis can also result from genetic defects of hemojuvelin (HJV) and hepcidin itself, in which case the clinical presentation is usually earlier in life and more severe, often with an iron-induced cardiomyopathy. In all types the serum hepcidin is low. A membrane-bound serine protease, TMPRSS6, has been found to be a powerful down-regulator of hepcidin, blunting the stimulating effects of IL6, HJV, Smad 4, and BMP. Erythroblasts secrete a protein, GDFI5, that inhibits hepcidin synthesis, explaining the low serum hepcidin levels and increased iron absorption found in thalassemia major despite iron overload.

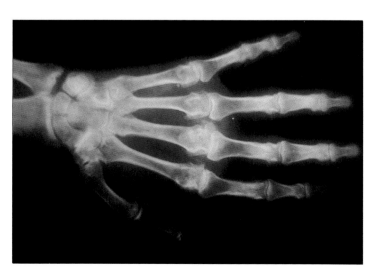

Fig. 6-10. Primary hemochromatosis: radiographs of a hand showing degenerative arthritis (caused by calcium pyrophosphate deposition) affecting the interphalangeal joints.

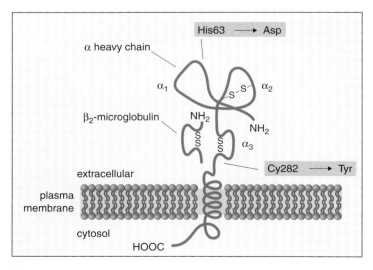

Fig. 6-11. Primary hemochromatosis: hypothetical model of the protein derived from the *HFE* gene based on its homology to the HLA class 1 molecule. The sites of the mutations found in primary hemochromatosis are shown. (Adapted with permission from Feder JN, Girke A, Thomas W, et al: A novel MHC class I–like gene is mutated in patients with hereditary hemochromatosis, *Nat Genet* 13: 399–408, 1996.)

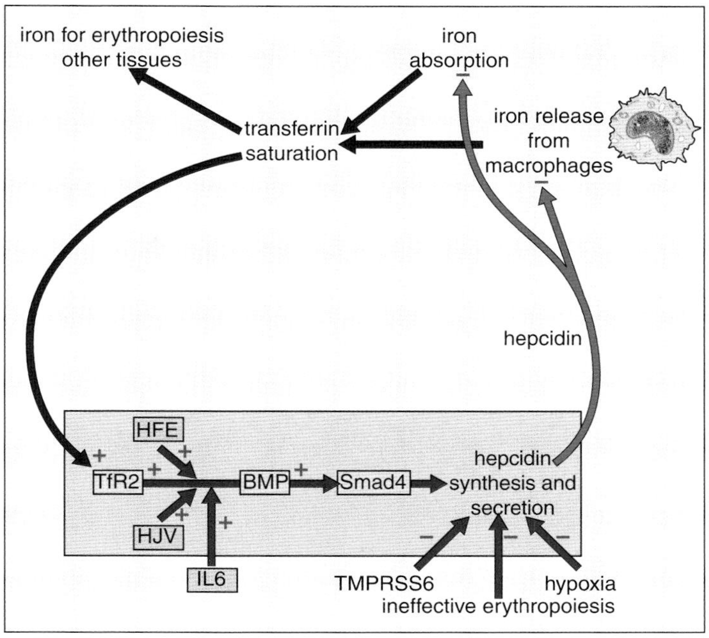

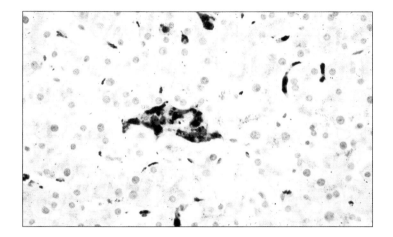

Fig. 6-12. Hepcidin metabolism. *BMP,* Bone morphogenetic protein; *Smad 4* is a transcription factor; *HJV, TMPRSS6* (codes for matriptase-2), *TfR,* see text.

Fig. 6-13. Primary hemochromatosis, type 4: ferroportin defect. Iron is increased in the reticuloendothelial cells but not usually in parenchymal cells. (Courtesy of Dr. J. Dooley.)

Ferroportin deficiency is a rare genetic defect resulting from different mutations of the gene *SLC40A1.* There is iron accumulation in macrophages and a raised serum ferritin, but parenchymal iron is usually but not always normal (Fig. 6-13). There is, however, phenotypic variation depending on the mutation involved. Recently, iron overload and sideroblastic anemia resulting from a genetic defect in an iron-sulfur cluster protein, glutaredoxin 5, has also been described. Management of types I through III hemochromatosis consists of venesection to remove iron and appropriate treatment for dysfunction of damaged organs.

RARE CAUSES OF IRON OVERLOAD

Porphyria cutanea tarda (see Fig. 6-5) is associated with iron loading in the liver. In the rare autosomal recessive disorder atransferrinemia, there is a microcytic, hypochromic anemia with excess iron deposition in the reticuloendothelial cells (Table 6-4). In aceruloplasminemia, also autosomal recessive, retinal and basal ganglia degeneration occurs with iron loading in the liver, pancreas, brain, and other organs. Serum iron is low, total body iron content normal, and serum

TABLE 6-4.   RARE CAUSES OF IRON OVERLOAD

Disease	Inheritance	Gene	Clinical features
Hypotransferrinemia	AR	TF	Anemia, iron overload
Aceruloplasminemia	AR	CP	Anemia, iron overload
DMT-1 defects	AR	SLC11A2	Anemia, iron overload, neurological symptoms
Friedreich's ataxia	AR	Frataxin	Spino-cerebellar ataxia, cardiomyopathy
Hyperferritinemia-cataract	AD	L-ferritin	Bilateral cataracts
Hemochromatosis	AD	H-ferritin	Iron overload
Hemochromatosis, sideroblastic anemia	?	Glutaredoxin 5	Iron overload
Neonatal hemochromatosis	?	?	Liver failure, iron overload

Adapted from Camaschella C: *Blood* 106:3710–3717, 2005.
AD, Autosomal dominant; *AR,* autosomal recessive.

ferritin raised. Mutation of DMT-1 has been described in a human. The patient had a hypochromic-microcytic anemia with liver iron overload. This could be due to increased up-regulation of the heme-iron absorption pathway, bypassing the DMT-1 defect in the intestine. Friedreich's ataxia manifests in middle age with spinocerebellar ataxia and a cardiomyopathy. There is a mutation in the gene for frataxin, a mitochondrial protein. This leads to a decrease in biosynthesis of iron-sulfur clusters and heme and in oxidative damage to mitochondrial DNA, proteins, and membranes. Excess iron deposition is found in the heart.

HEREDITARY HYPERFERRITINEMIA WITH AUTOSOMAL DOMINANT CONGENITAL CATARACT SYNDROME

Hereditary hyperferritinemia–cataract syndrome (HHCS) manifests with early-onset cataract (caused by ferritin deposition in the lens; Fig. 6-14) and elevated serum ferritin (1000–2500 μg/L). Serum ferritin, normally composed of molecules with either light (L; molecular weight 19 kDa, coded for on chromosome 19) or heavy (H; molecular weight 21 kDa, coded for on chromosome 11) subunits (24 in total), is of L type only, the type mainly found in

normal tissues of iron storage (e.g., liver and spleen). The H type is dominant in organs, not normally iron storage sites (e.g., heart). There are mutations in the iron-response element (IRE) of the L-ferritin messenger ribonucleic acid (mRNA) (Fig. 6-15) that affect its binding to the iron-regulatory protein (IRP). Iron stores, serum iron, and transferrin levels are normal.

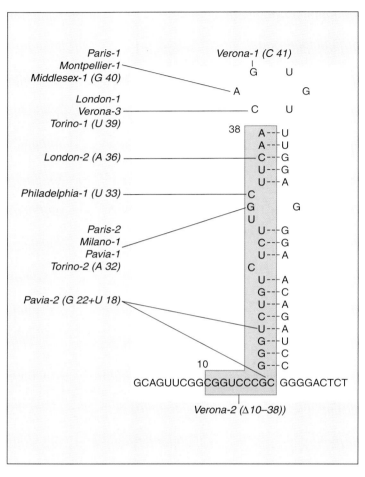

Fig. 6-15. Hereditary hyperferritinemia–cataract syndrome (HHCS): representation of the iron-response element (IRE) located in the 5′ untranslated region (UTR) of L-ferritin messenger ribonucleic acid (mRNA) and of the mutations associated with HHCS showing evidence for genetic heterogeneity of the disease. (Courtesy of Dr. D. Girelli and Professor R. Corrocher.)

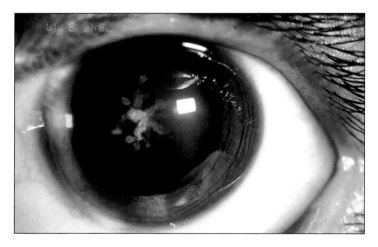

Fig. 6-14. Hereditary hyperferritinemia–cataract syndrome (HHCS): The "starring" lens opacity is characteristic. (Courtesy of Dr. D. Girelli and Professor R. Corrocher.)

MEGALOBLASTIC ANEMIAS

The megaloblastic anemias are a group of disorders characterized by a macrocytic blood picture and megaloblastic erythropoiesis; causes are listed in Table 7-1. The underlying biochemical defect appears to be a fault in deoxyribonucleic acid (DNA) synthesis, which may result from a lesion at some point in pyrimidine or purine synthesis or from inhibition of DNA polymerization. The anemia is usually caused by deficiency of vitamin B_{12} or cobalamin (referred to simply as B_{12} hereafter) or folate. In most cases the site of the biochemical defect in DNA synthesis is known. In some types, however, particularly in myeloblastic leukemia and myelodysplasia in which megaloblastic changes are unresponsive to B_{12} and folate therapy, the exact site of the defect remains obscure.

B_{12} is involved in only two reactions in human tissues (Figs. 7-1 and 7-2) whereas folate coenzymes are involved in many reactions involving one carbon unit transfer. The roles of B_{12} and folate in DNA biosynthesis are shown in Fig. 7-1. Folate deficiency affects thymidylate synthesis, a rate-limiting step in pyrimidine synthesis, because a folate coenzyme, 5,10-methylene tetrahydrofolate–polyglutamate, is necessary for this reaction. Folate coenzymes are also required in two reactions in purine synthesis, but these are not normally considered rate limiting for DNA synthesis in humans.

B_{12} is not required directly for DNA synthesis. It is needed as methylcobalamin to convert 5-methyltetrahydrofolate (methyl-THF), which enters cells from plasma, into other folate coenzyme forms (including all the polyglutamate derivatives) through its involvement in the methionine synthase reaction in which homocysteine is methylated to methionine. In this reaction the removal of the methyl group from methyl-THF forms THF, which can be converted into folate polyglutamates by the addition of glutamate moieties. Methyl-THF cannot act as a substrate for the enzyme responsible for polyglutamate formation. The role of folate in the metabolism of homocysteine is shown in Fig. 7-10.

B_{12} in food is released from protein binding by proteolytic enzymes and attached to a so-called R-binder (Fig. 7-3). B_{12} is released from this binding by pancreatic enzymes and transferred to intrinsic factor (IF) secreted by the parietal cells of the stomach. B_{12} in bile also attaches to intrinsic factor. Intrinsic factor–bound B_{12} is carried to the ileum, where it attaches to specific receptors formed by a cubilin/amnion complex; the IF is digested and B_{12} appears in the portal blood attached to a polypeptide protein, transcobalamin II. In peripheral blood, most B_{12} is attached to the glycoprotein transcobalamin I (derived from granulocytes, monocytes, and their precursors),

TABLE 7-1.   MEGALOBLASTIC ANEMIA: CAUSES

Causes of megaloblastic anemia I	Causes of megaloblastic anemia II		Causes of megaloblastic anemia III	
Vitamin B_{12} deficiency	Folate deficiency		Abnormalities of	
Inadequate diet	Inadequate diet	Malabsorption	Vitamin B_{12} metabolism	DNA synthesis
Veganism	Poverty	Gluten-induced enteropathy	Congenital:	Congenital:
Maternal deficiency	Institutions	Dermatitis herpetiformis	transcobalamin II deficiency	orotic aciduria
Malabsorption	Goats' milk	Tropical sprue	homocystinuria with methylmalonic aciduria	Lesch–Nyhan syndrome
Gastric:	Special diets	Congenital specific		dyserythropoietic anemia
pernicious anemia, acquired (autoimmune), and congenital, IF deficiency partial, or total gastrectomy	Excess losses	Systemic infections	Acquired:	thiamine-responsive
	Dialysis	Increased utilization	nitrous oxide anesthesia	Acquired:
Intestinal:	Congestive heart failure	Pregnancy	Folate metabolism	drugs (e.g., hydroxyurea, cytosine arabinoside, 6-mercaptopurine, 5-azacytidine)
stagnant-loop syndrome (e.g., jejunal diverticulosis, ileocolic fistulae)	Drugs	Prematurity	Congenital:	
	Anticonvulsants	Excess marrow turnover (e.g., in hemolytic anemias)	inborn errors (e.g., 5-methyltetra-hydrofolate transferase deficiency)	
chronic tropical sprue	Barbiturates	Malignancy (e.g., myeloma, carcinoma)	Acquired:	
ileal resection and Crohn's disease	Mixed	Inflammatory disease (e.g., Crohn's, rheumatoid arthritis, widespread eczema)	antifolate drugs (e.g., methotrexate, pyrimethamine)	
congenital-specific malabsorption with with proteinuria (Imerslund–Gräsbeck)	Alcohol			
	Liver disease			
fish tapeworm				
drugs (e.g., metformin)				

IF, instrinsic factor

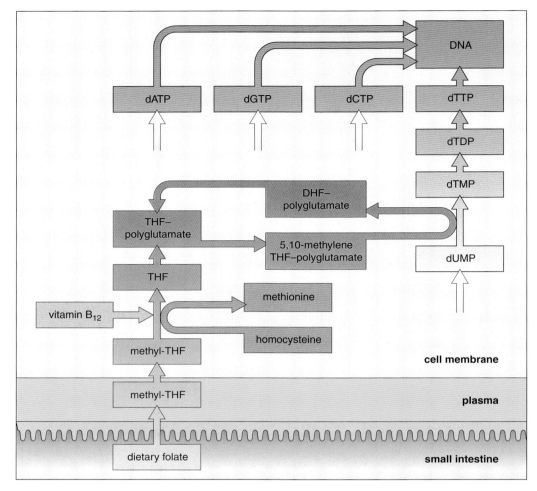

Fig. 7-1. Megaloblastic anemia: suggested roles of B_{12} and folate in DNA biosynthesis. *ATP,* Adenosine triphosphate; *CTP,* cytosine triphosphate; *d,* deoxyribose; *DHF,* dihydrofolate; *GTP,* guanosine triphosphate; *TDP,* thymidine diphosphate; *THF,* tetrahydrofolate; *TMP,* thymidine monophosphate; *TTP,* thymidine triphosphate; *UMP,* uridine monophosphate.

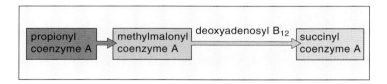

Fig. 7-2. Megaloblastic anemia: Deoxyadenosyl B_{12} acts as a coenzyme in the metabolism of methylmalonyl coenzyme A.

but it is transcobalamin II that is responsible for delivery of the vitamin to the tissues.

Dietary folate is deconjugated to the monoglutamate form, fully reduced, and methylated in the upper intestinal epithelial cells so that it is all absorbed in the form of methyl-THF (see Fig. 7-1).

CLINICAL FEATURES

Megaloblastic anemia is usually of insidious onset, progressing so slowly that the patient has time to adapt. A patient may therefore not seek treatment until the anemia is quite severe, unless diagnosed early through an incidental blood examination for other reasons. There is jaundice of varying degree in combination with anemia, giving the

patient's skin a lemon-yellow tint (Fig. 7-4). The jaundice is caused by unconjugated bilirubin produced in excess because of severe intramedullary death of nucleated red cell precursors *(ineffective erythropoiesis)* with reticuloendothelial breakdown of their hemoglobin. Also, a marked rise in serum lactate dehydrogenase concentration occurs because of excessive cell breakdown.

Severe cases show features of intravascular breakdown of hemoglobin with methemalbuminemia and hemosiderinuria; pancytopenia often occurs and the patient may have bruising from thrombocytopenia (Fig. 7-5). The white cell and platelet counts are rarely as low as in severe aplastic anemia.

Disordered proliferation of the epithelial cell surfaces gives rise to glossitis (Fig. 7-6) and angular cheilosis (Fig. 7-7) and can also be seen microscopically in the buccal, bronchial, bladder, and cervical mucosae.

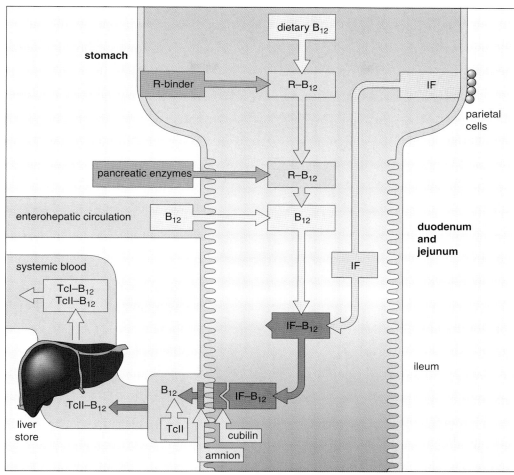

Fig. 7-3. Megaloblastic anemia: absorption of B_{12}. *IF*, intrinsic factor; *R*, R-binder; *TcI*, transcobalamin I; *TcII*, transcobalamin II.

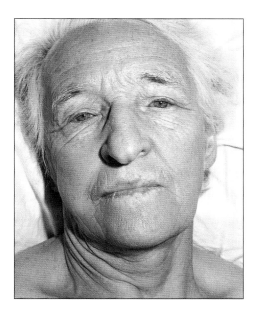

Fig. 7-4. Megaloblastic anemia: typical lemon-yellow appearance of a 69-year-old woman with pernicious anemia and severe megaloblastic anemia (Hb, 7.0 g/dl; MCV, 132 fl). The color is from the combination of pallor (from anemia) and jaundice (from ineffective erythropoiesis).

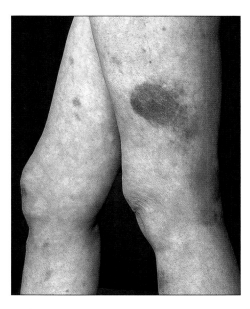

Fig. 7-5. Megaloblastic anemia: spontaneous bruising on the thigh of a 34-year-old woman with widespread purpura and menorrhagia. She was found to have megaloblastic anemia as a result of nutritional folate deficiency and alcoholism. (Hb, 8.1 g/dl; MCV, 115 fl; platelet count, 2×10^9/L.)

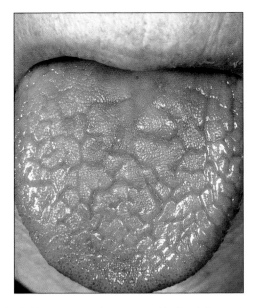

Fig. 7-6. Megaloblastic anemia: glossitis caused by B₁₂ deficiency in a 55-year-old woman with untreated pernicious anemia. The tongue is beefy red and painful, particularly with hot and acidic foods. An identical appearance occurs in folate deficiency because of impaired DNA synthesis in the mucosal epithelium.

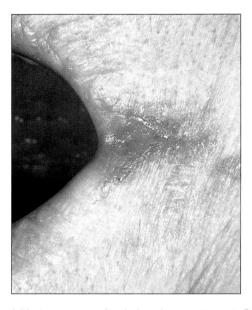

Fig. 7-7. Megaloblastic anemia: angular cheilosis (same patient as in Fig. 7-5). This is also thought to result from impaired proliferation of epithelial cells. It is unusual for this abnormality to be so marked.

In a small proportion of cases, melanin pigmentation of the skin is present (Fig. 7-8). A neuropathy of varying severity may occur with B₁₂ deficiency, such as subacute combined degeneration of the spinal cord that includes posterior and lateral column demyelination (see Fig. 7-27) and peripheral or optic neuropathy. The patient has bilaterally symmetric symptoms that are usually most marked in the lower limbs and comprise tingling, unsteadiness of gait, falling over in the dark, altered sensation, and reduced strength. Visual and psychiatric disturbances are less frequent.

Folic acid therapy before conception and in early pregnancy has been shown to reduce the incidence of babies with neural tube defect (NTD). The lesions may be spina bifida (Fig. 7-9), anencephaly, or encephalocoele. This occurs even if the mother is not folate deficient, assessed hematologically or by serum or red cell folate (although the lower the serum folate or B₁₂ or red cell folate, the higher the incidence, even when the levels are in the accepted normal range). An association between NTD and a common mutation (nucleotide

677C → T) in the gene for the enzyme 5,10-methylene-THF reductase (Fig. 7-10) has been found. The mutated enzyme is thermolabile. It is considered that prophylactic folic acid overcomes this or other as yet unidentified abnormalities of folate or B₁₂ metabolism. The mutation is associated with a raised homocysteine level. Folate or B₁₂ deficiency aggravates the tendency for a rise in homocysteine level to occur in maternal plasma. It is unclear exactly how disturbed homocysteine metabolism leads to NTD.

Raised plasma homocysteine levels are also associated with an increased incidence of arterial and venous thrombosis (see Chapter 26). The levels may be raised because of B₁₂, folate, or vitamin B₆ deficiency or through smoking or excess alcohol consumption. The levels are higher in males and postmenopausal women than in premenopausal women or those on hormone replacement therapy and rise with age. Congenital homocystinuria that results from an inherited defect of one of three enzymes, cystathionine synthase, methionine synthase, or 5,10-methylene-THF reductase (Fig. 7-10) is associated with the onset of cardiovascular disease in childhood or early adult life.

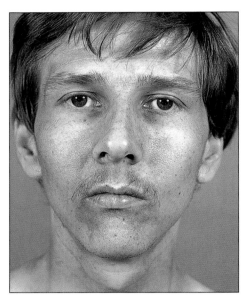

Fig. 7-8. Megaloblastic anemia: melanin pigmentation of the skin in a 24-year-old man with B₁₂ deficiency caused by pernicious anemia. Similar pigmentation affected the nail beds, skin creases, and periorbital areas. Such pigmentation also occurs in patients with folate deficiency. In both, the pigmentation rapidly disappears with appropriate vitamin therapy. The biochemical basis for the melanin excess is unknown.

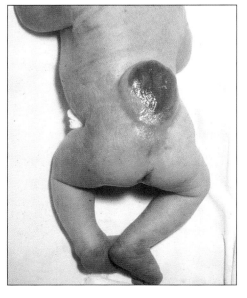

Fig. 7-9. Baby with spina bifida. (Courtesy of Professor C. J. Schorah.)

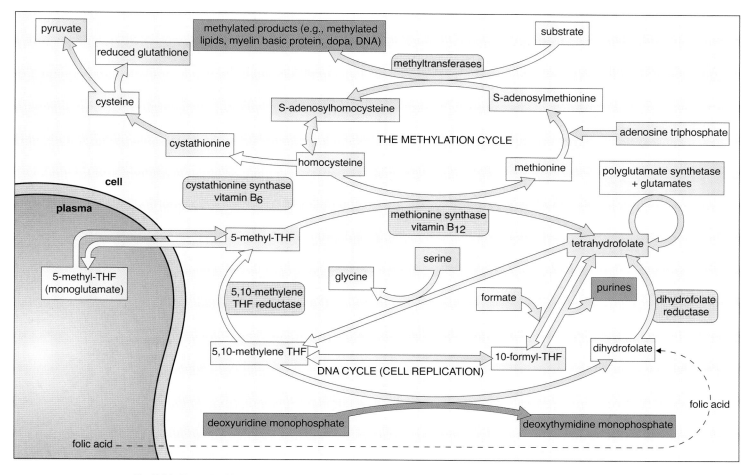

Fig. 7-10. The role of folate coenzymes and vitamins B$_{12}$ and B$_6$ in the metabolism of homocysteine and in DNA synthesis. (Courtesy of Professor J. Scott.)

BLOOD COUNT AND BLOOD FILM APPEARANCES

The blood film shows oval macrocytes, fragmented cells, poikilocytes of varying shapes (Figs. 7-11 to 7-13), and hypersegmental neutrophils (showing more than five nuclear lobes, some of which may be macropolycytes; Fig. 7-14). The severity of these changes depends on the degree of anemia. In the most anemic patients, megaloblasts may circulate because of extramedullary hematopoiesis in the liver and spleen (Fig. 7-15).

Cabot rings, which are acidophilic and arginine rich and contain nonhemoglobin iron, may also be seen (see Fig. 7-15, *inset*). If the spleen has been removed, as with a gastrectomy, or has atrophied, as in 15% of adult cases with gluten-induced enteropathy (adult celiac disease), changes caused by hyposplenism in the peripheral blood are particularly marked (Fig. 7-16). In some extremely anemic patients, the mean cell volume is normal because of excessive fragmentation of red cells.

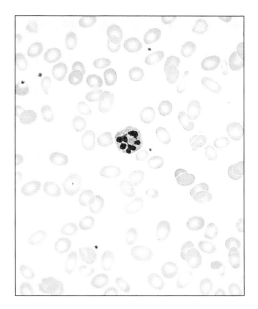

Fig. 7-11. Megaloblastic anemia: peripheral blood film in a severe case, showing oval macrocytes, marked anisocytosis, and poikilocytosis. There is a neutrophil with a hypersegmented nucleus (more than five lobes). (Hb, 5.1 g/dl; MCV, 129 fl.)

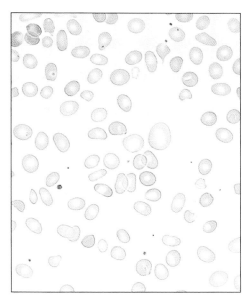

Fig. 7-12. Megaloblastic anemia: peripheral blood film showing marked oval macrocytosis, anisocytosis, and poikilocytosis. (Hb, 5.4 g/dl; MCV, 130 fl.)

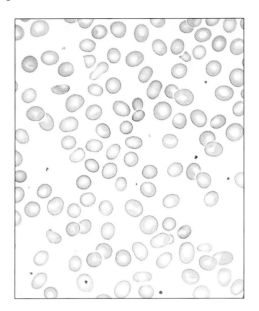

Fig. 7-13. Megaloblastic anemia: peripheral blood film in a mild case showing moderate red cell macrocytosis, anisocytosis, and poikilocytosis. (Hb, 10.5 g/dl; MCV, 112 fl.)

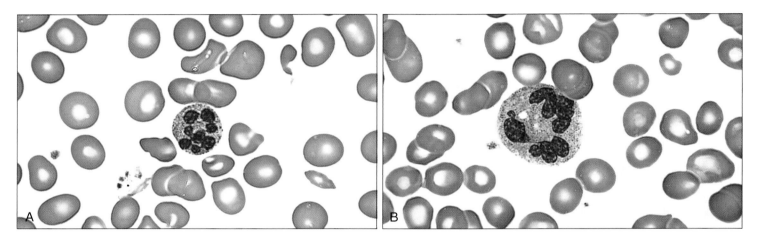

Fig. 7-14. Megaloblastic anemia: higher-power views showing a hypersegmented neutrophil **(A)** and a hyper-diploid neutrophil or "macropolycyte" **(B).**

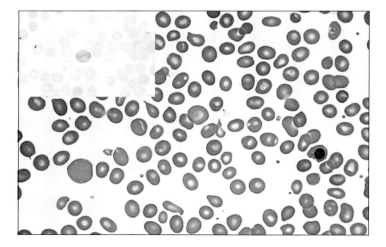

Fig. 7-15. Megaloblastic anemia: peripheral blood film in a severe case showing a circulating orthochromatic nucleated red cell. The presence of such circulating megaloblasts may be the result of extramedullary hemopoiesis in the spleen and liver. The *inset (upper left)* shows a Cabot ring, which is occasionally seen in the peripheral blood in severe megaloblastic anemia.

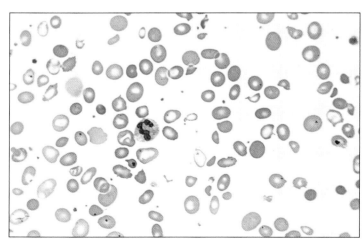

Fig. 7-16. Megaloblastic anemia and splenic atrophy: peripheral blood film showing Howell-Jolly bodies (DNA remnants) and Pappenheimer bodies (iron- and protein-containing bodies). The patient had severe folate deficiency and splenic atrophy caused by adult celiac disease.

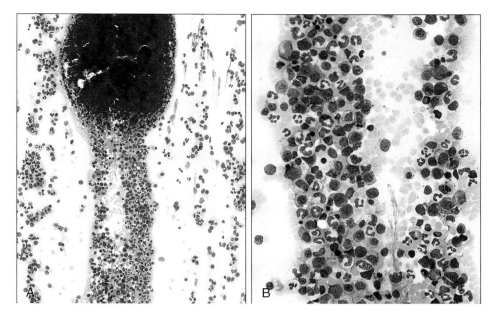

Fig. 7-17. Megaloblastic anemia. **A,** Low-power view of bone marrow fragments showing an increased cellularity with loss of fat spaces. **B,** Higher-power view of cell trails showing accumulation of early cells, an increased proportion of erythroid precursors, and the presence of giant metamyelocytes and hypersegmented neutrophils.

BONE MARROW APPEARANCES

In severe cases, the bone marrow is markedly hypercellular with a relative increase in early erythroblasts caused by death of later cells (Fig. 7-17). The myeloid-to-erythroid ratio may be reversed, with an excess of erythroid precursors. Developing erythroblasts show asynchrony of nuclear and cytoplasmic maturation, the nucleus retaining an open, lacy, or stippled appearance while the cytoplasm matures and hemoglobinizes normally. The developing (nucleated) red cells also show a variety of dyserythropoietic features with an excess of multinucleate cells, nuclear bridging, and Howell-Jolly bodies; dying cells are also present (Fig. 7-18).

Giant and abnormally shaped metamyelocytes are found (Fig. 7-19), and the megakaryocytes show hypersegmented nuclei with an open chromatin network (Fig. 7-20).

In milder cases, megaloblastic changes in the red cell precursors are only identified in late erythroblasts with mild asynchrony of nuclear-cytoplasmic development (Fig. 7-21). This is termed *mild, transitional,* or *intermediate* megaloblastic change.

Where iron deficiency and megaloblastic anemia coexist, a dimorphic anemia occurs with two red cell populations in the peripheral blood, one of well-hemoglobinized macrocytes and the other of hypochromic microcytes (Fig. 7-22, *A*). Megaloblastic changes may be masked in the erythroblasts, even though giant metamyelocytes are seen in the bone marrow (Fig. 7-22, *B*). In patients with normal iron stores, there is usually excessive iron granulation of erythroblasts; in some cases, especially in association with alcohol, ring sideroblasts are frequent but disappear with appropriate therapy (Fig. 7-23). Trephine biopsy confirms the accumulation of early cells and excess mitoses (Fig. 7-24). It is of interest that erythropoiesis in early fetal life is also megaloblastic (Fig. 7-25).

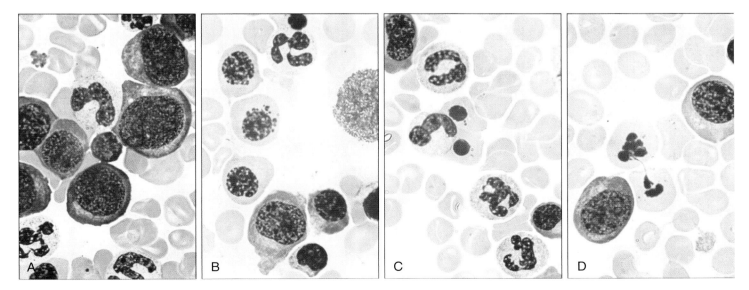

Fig. 7-18. Megaloblastic anemia: high-power views showing accumulation of early cells, mainly promegaloblasts **(A)**; megaloblasts at all stages (the nuclei have primitive open [lacy] chromatin patterns despite maturation of the cytoplasm with hemoglobinization [pink staining] and two cells have nuclear [DNA] fragments [Howell-Jolly bodies] in their cytoplasm) **(B)**; two late megaloblasts with fully orthochromatic (pink-staining) cytoplasm (two large band-form neutrophils are also present) **(C)**; and the central orthochromatic cells have karyorrhectic pyknotic nuclei linked by a thin chromatin bridge **(D)**.

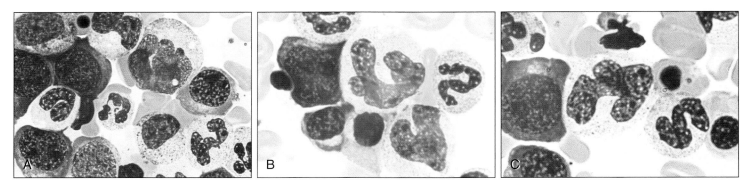

Fig. 7-19. Megaloblastic anemia. **A–C,** High-power views showing a number of giant abnormally shaped meta-myelocytes.

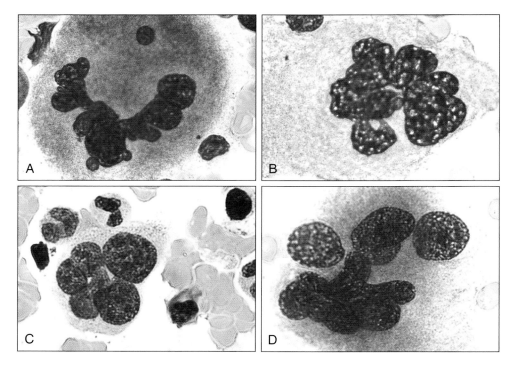

Fig. 7-20. Megaloblastic anemia: megakaryocytes of variable maturity. **A–D,** All show nuclei with abnormal open chromatin patterns.

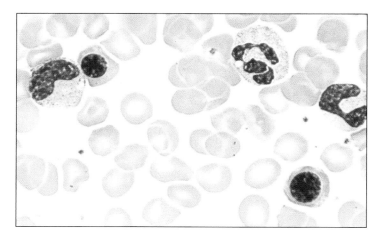

Fig. 7-21. Megaloblastic anemia: mild marrow changes in B$_{12}$ deficiency following partial gastrectomy. The nucleated red cells show mild asynchrony of nuclear-cytoplasmic development with delay of nuclear maturation *(lower right)*. Iron stores were present. (Hb, 12.4 g/dl; MCV, 105 fl; serum B$_{12}$, 80 ng/L [normal, 160 to 925 ng/L]; serum folate, 10.3 μg/L [normal, 6.0 to 21.0 μg/L].)

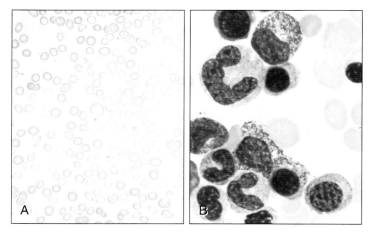

Fig. 7-22. Megaloblastic anemia. **A,** Dimorphic peripheral blood film in iron and B$_{12}$ deficiencies following partial gastrectomy. There is a mixed population of microcytic hypochromic cells and well-hemoglobinized macrocytes (Hb, 8.0 g/dl; MCV, 87 fl; MCH, 27 pg). **B,** In the bone marrow aspirate from the same case, giant metamyelocytes are present but megaloblastic changes in the erythroblasts are masked.

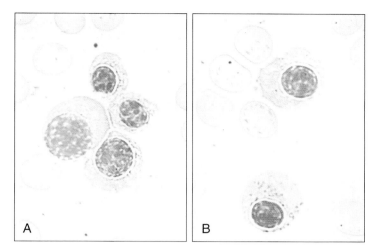

Fig. 7-23. Megaloblastic anemia. **A** and **B,** Bone marrow aspirates in alcoholism and folate deficiency showing partial ring sideroblasts, which rapidly disappeared on alcohol withdrawal and folic acid therapy (Perls' stain).

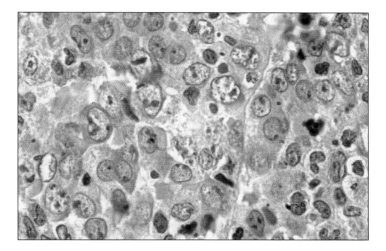

Fig. 7-24. Megaloblastic anemia: Trephine biopsy of iliac crest in untreated pernicious anemia shows many megaloblasts with a fine open chromatin pattern and a number of mitotic figures.

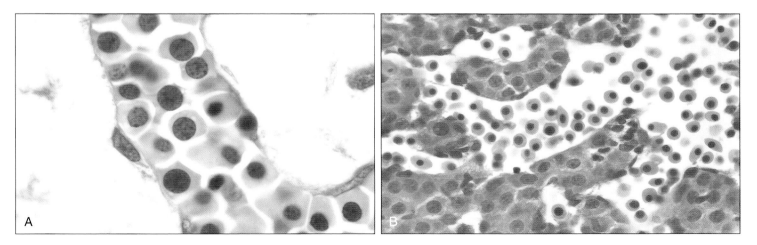

Fig. 7-25. Fetal erythropoiesis: sections of placenta showing circulating erythroblasts with a nuclear morphology similar to megaloblasts **(A)**; and liver, showing extramedullary megaloblastic erythropoiesis **(B)**.

CAUSES OF MEGALOBLASTIC ANEMIA

VITAMIN B₁₂ DEFICIENCY

Because B_{12} is stored in amounts of 2 to 3 mg, and daily losses and requirements are 1 to 2 μg, it takes 2 to 4 years for B_{12} deficiency to develop from dietary lack or malabsorption. Deficiency resulting from excessive losses or breakdown of B_{12} has not been described. The anesthetic gas nitrous oxide may rapidly inactivate body B_{12} from the fully reduced cobalamin I state to the oxidized cobalamin II and cobalamin III forms; if exposure is prolonged, megaloblastic changes occur (Fig. 7-26).

While folate occurs in most foods, including fruit, vegetables, and cereals, as well as animal products, B_{12} occurs only in foods of animal origin. Veganism may lead to B_{12} deficiency, found most frequently in Hindus. Liver has the highest concentration of both folate and B_{12} because it is the main storage organ.

Although not necessarily associated with severe anemia, severe B_{12} deficiency, assessed by serum B_{12} levels, may cause demyelination of the posterior and lateral columns of the spinal cord (Fig. 7-27). It is often associated with a peripheral neuropathy and is

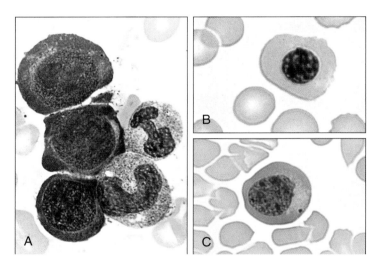

Fig. 7-26. B_{12} oxidation. **A–C,** Bone marrow aspirate showing megaloblasts in a patient receiving prolonged nitrous oxide anesthesia in intensive care following cardiac surgery.

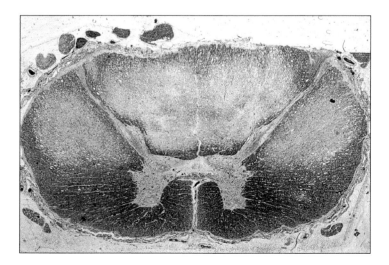

Fig. 7-27. Pernicious anemia: cross-section of spinal cord of a patient with severe B_{12} neuropathy who died (subacute combined degeneration of the spinal cord). There is demyelination of the lateral (pyramidal) and posterior columns (Weigert-Pal stain).

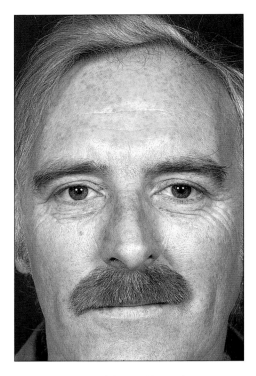

Fig. 7-28. Pernicious anemia: This 38-year-old man shows premature graying and has blue eyes and vitiligo, three features that are more common in patients with pernicious anemia than in control subjects.

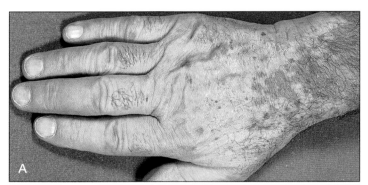

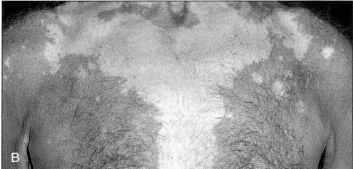

Fig. 7-29. Pernicious anemia. **A** and **B,** Marked vitiligo in a 67-year-old man.

found more frequently in males than in females; yet pernicious anemia, the most common cause of severe B_{12} deficiency, is more common in females.

Addisonian pernicious anemia is the dominant cause of B_{12} deficiency in Western countries. Although particularly common in northern Europe, it occurs in all races and countries. It is associated with early graying of the hair (Fig. 7-28), vitiligo (Fig. 7-29), and thyroid disorders (Fig. 7-30), as well as with other organ-specific

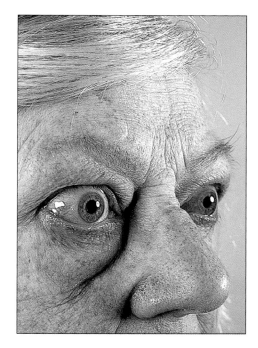

Fig. 7-30. Pernicious anemia: exophthalmic ophthalmoplegia in a patient who developed myxoedema while receiving maintenance B_{12} therapy. She had presented with megaloblastic anemia 6 years earlier.

Fig. 7-31. Pernicious anemia: sections of stomach. **A,** Normal; **B,** in pernicious anemia. There is atrophy of all coats, loss of gastric glands and parietal cells, and infiltration of the lamina propria by lymphocytes and plasma cells. (*A* and *B*, Courtesy of Dr. J. E. McLaughlin.)

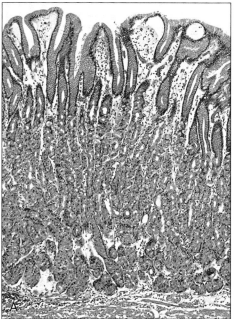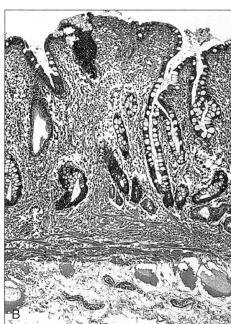

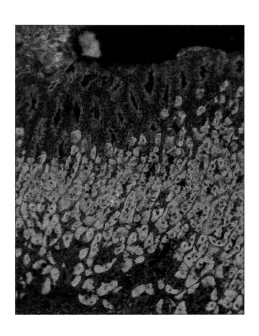

Fig. 7-32. Pernicious anemia: positive indirect immunofluorescent test for parietal cell autoantibody. A frozen section of gastric mucosa (rat) has been layered with the patient's serum and washed, followed by the addition of rabbit antihuman immunoglobulin G conjugated with fluorescein.

autoimmune diseases, such as Addison's disease and hypoparathyroidism. Specific variants of the gene *NALP1* on chromosome 17p13 coding for NACHT leucine-rich repeat protein 1, a regulator of the innate immune system, show association with vitiligo and autoimmune diseases, including pernicious anemia. There is gastric atrophy (Fig. 7-31) with achlorhydria; also, parietal cell autoantibodies are present in the serum of 90% of patients (Fig. 7-32) and IF autoantibodies in 50%. Gastric carcinoma develops two to three times more frequently than in control populations (Fig. 7-33).

Small intestinal causes of B_{12} deficiency include the stagnant-loop syndrome (e.g., jejunal diverticulosis (Fig. 7-34), ileocolic fistula (Fig. 7-35), and ileal resection).

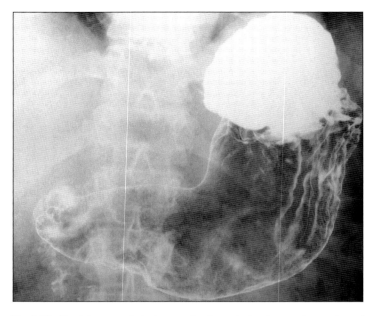

Fig. 7-33. Pernicious anemia: barium meal radiograph showing gastric atrophy and carcinoma. There is thinning of the gastric wall and lack of mucosal pattern and an ulcerated filling defect in the horizontal part of the greater curve.

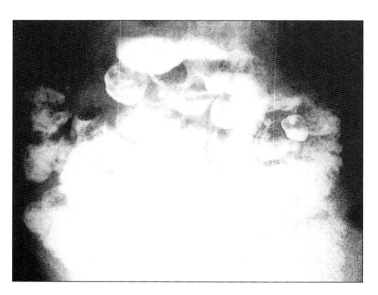

Fig. 7-34. Jejunal diverticulosis: barium meal radiograph showing multiple jejunal diverticula in a 71-year-old patient with megaloblastic anemia caused by B$_{12}$ deficiency. (Courtesy of Dr. D. Nag.)

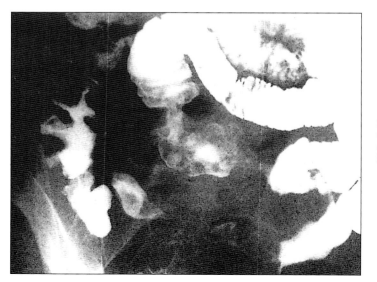

FOLATE DEFICIENCY

Because adult daily requirements of folate are about 100 μg, body stores (10 to 15 mg) are sufficient for only a few months, a period that can be reduced in conditions of increased turnover and, hence, breakdown of folates.

Folate deficiency may result from inadequate dietary intake or malabsorption, as in gluten-induced enteropathy (celiac disease) (Figs. 7-36 to 7-40) and tropical sprue (Fig. 7-41).

Dermatitis herpetiformis is associated with gluten-induced enteropathy and, hence, with folate deficiency. The duodenal mucosa may show only mild changes (e.g., infiltration of the mucosal epithelium by lymphocytes) (Fig. 7-42). The most common cause of deficiency is pregnancy, when folate requirements rise from the normal 100 μg daily to about 350 μg daily. However, the incidence of this complication is now reduced with prophylactic folic acid therapy. Other causes of increased folate utilization include diseases with increased bone marrow or other cell turnover (see Table 7-1). The excessive demands for folate in these conditions, combined with poor dietary intake, may lead to megaloblastic anemia.

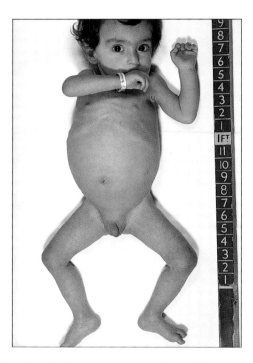

Fig. 7-36. Infantile celiac disease: wasting and abdominal distention in a 2-year-old boy who developed megaloblastic anemia as a result of folate deficiency. Celiac disease was diagnosed by jejunal biopsy.

Fig. 7-35. Intestinal stagnant-loop syndrome: barium follow-through radiograph in Crohn's disease showing defective filling of the terminal ileum with a blind loop clearly visible. There is early filling of the ascending colon. The patient had megaloblastic anemia caused by B$_{12}$ deficiency. (Courtesy of Dr. R. Dick.)

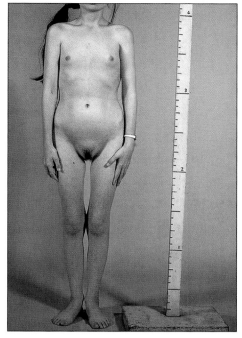

Fig. 7-37. Celiac disease: a 16-year-old girl with severe megaloblastic anemia as a result of folate deficiency who was found, on jejunal biopsy, to have celiac disease. There was no history of diarrhea. She had delayed puberty and menarche.

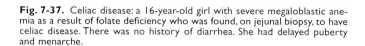

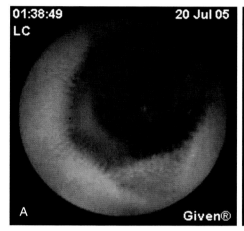
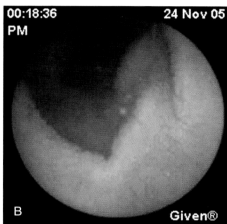

Fig. 7-38. Capsule camera appearance of duodenal mucosa. **A,** Normal showing multiple fine villi. **B,** Celiac disease showing absence of villi. (Courtesy of Dr. M. Caplyn.)

Fig. 7-39. Adult celiac disease: low- and medium-power dissecting microscope views of jejunal biopsies showing normal villi in finger and leaf patterns **(A** and **B)** and abnormal mosaic pattern with obvious crypt openings **(C** and **D).** (A–D, Courtesy of Dr. J. S. Stewart.)

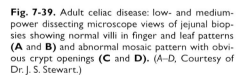
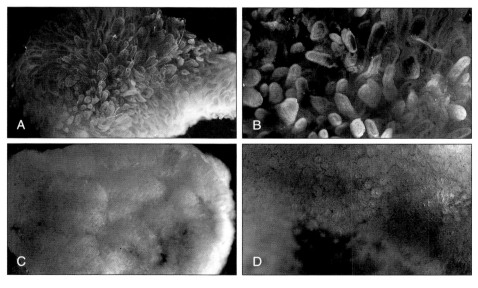

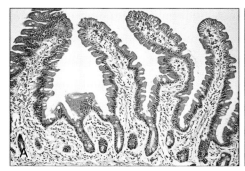
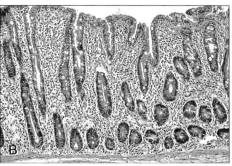

Fig. 7-40. Celiac disease: histologic sections of jejunal biopsies showing normal mucosa with finger-like villi **(A)** and subtotal villous atrophy with absence of villi and hypertrophy of the mucosal crypts **(B).** (B, Courtesy of Dr. A. Price.)

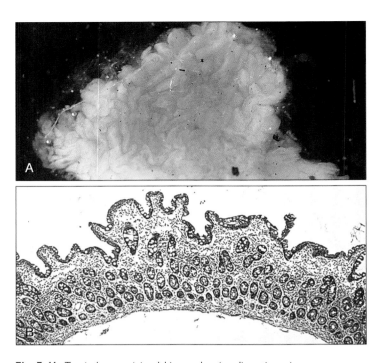

Fig. 7-41. Tropical sprue: jejunal biopsy showing dissecting microscope appearance with typical convoluted mucosal pattern **(A)** and partial villous atrophy **(B).** (*A* and *B,* Courtesy of Professor V. Chadwick.)

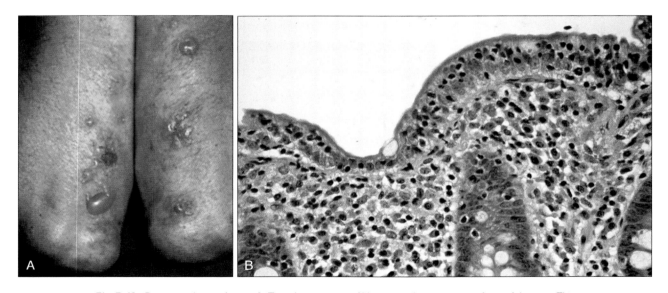

Fig. 7-42. Dermatitis herpetiformis. **A,** Typical appearance of blisters on the extensor surfaces of the arms. This skin condition is associated with gluten-induced enteropathy and folate deficiency. **B,** Duodenal biopsy showing intraepithelial lymphocytes. (Courtesy of Professor L. Fry.)

ABNORMALITIES OF VITAMIN B$_{12}$ OR FOLATE METABOLISM

These abnormalities may be inherited or acquired. Transcobalamin II deficiency is an autosomal recessive inherited trait leading, in the homozygous state, to megaloblastic anemia caused by failure of B$_{12}$ transport into bone marrow and other cells. It usually manifests in the first few months of life (Fig. 7-43). Nitrous oxide is discussed on page 108.

Rare abnormalities of intracellular B$_{12}$ are usually, but not always, associated with megaloblastic anemia (Fig. 7-44). A number of rare abnormalities of folate metabolism have been described, and megaloblastic anemia may also arise during therapy with the antifolate drugs that inhibit dihydrofolate reductase, such as methotrexate or pyrimethamine.

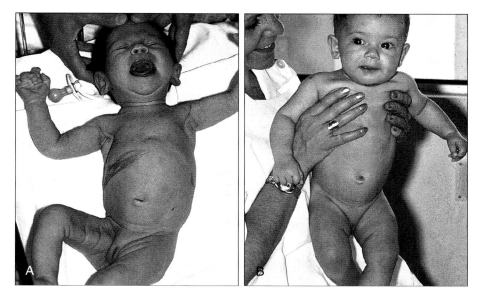

Fig. 7-43. Transcobalamin II deficiency: This child, before **(A)** and 6 months after **(B)** therapy, presented at 20 days with weight loss, irritability, pallor, glossitis, and hepatosplenomegaly. Tests showed a macrocytic anemia and megaloblastic bone marrow. Serum B_{12} and folate levels were normal, but chromatography of serum showed absence of transcobalamin II. Treatment was 1 mg of hydroxocobalamin intramuscularly twice weekly; the child remains well 18 years later. (*A* and *B*, Courtesy of Dr. M. C. Arrabel.)

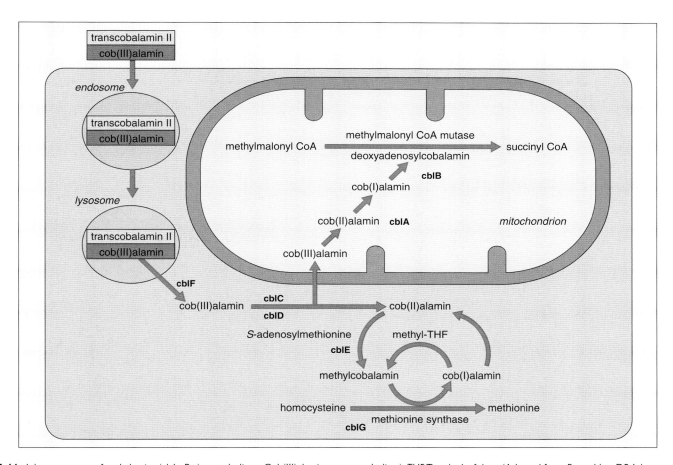

Fig. 7-44. Inborn errors of cobalamin (cbl, B_{12}) metabolism. Cob(III)alamin, cob(II)alamin, and cob(I)alamin are the cobalt in cobalamin in its trivalent, divalent, or monovalent oxidation state (cblA to cblG, sites of inborn errors in cobalamin metabolism). *THF,* Tetrahydrofolate. (Adapted from Rosenblatt DS: Inborn errors of folate and cobalamin metabolism. In Carmel R, Jacobsen DW, editors: *Homocysteine in Health and Disease,* Cambridge, 2001, Cambridge University Press, p 249.)

OTHER CAUSES

Megaloblastic anemia as a result of antimetabolite chemotherapy with, for example, hydroxyurea or cytosine arabinoside shows similar morphologic features to those that result from B_{12} or folate deficiencies. However, dyserythropoietic changes are often more marked.

In acute myeloid leukemia of the erythroblastic type or in myelodysplasia, megaloblastic changes are usually confined to the erythroid series. Giant metamyelocytes, hypersegmented polymorphs and other changes in leukopoiesis, or megakaryocytes seen in B_{12} or folate deficiency are not present.

Rare inborn errors of metabolism other than those affecting B_{12} or folate metabolism, such as orotic aciduria in which there is a fault in pyrimidine synthesis, may also occur in megaloblastic anemia (Fig. 7-45). A defect in thiamine phosphorylation may lead to megaloblastic and sideroblastic anemia responding to thiamine. This is discussed on page 85.

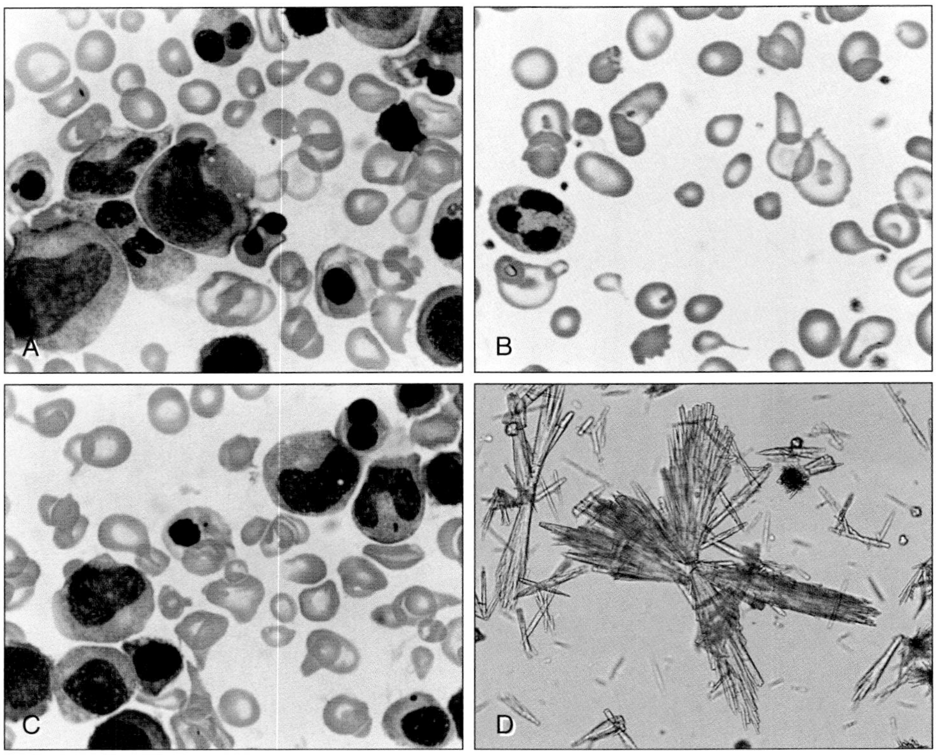

Fig. 7-45. Orotic aciduria: female who presented at 6 months with anemia (Hb, 6.0 g/dl; MCV, 110 fl) and normal white cell and platelet counts. The serum B$_{12}$ and folate levels were normal. **A** and **C,** Bone marrow shows megaloblastic erythropoiesis with a binucleate cell, Howell-Jolly body formation, and giant metamyelocytes. **B,** The peripheral blood film shows marked anisocytosis and poikilocytosis with macrocytic and microcytic cells. **D,** Crystals of orotic acid are present in the urine. The child responded hematologically to treatment with uridine 50 mg/kg daily orally with a reduction in orotic acid excretion. (A–D, Courtesy of Dr. J. Price.)

TREATMENT OF MEGALOBLASTIC ANEMIA

B$_{12}$ deficiency is treated by intramuscular or subcutaneous hydroxo-cobalamin (e.g., six injections each of 1 mg). Maintenance is with similar injections at 3-month intervals.

Folate deficiency may be corrected with daily oral folic acid given for 4 months. Long-term folic acid therapy may be needed when the cause of the deficiency, for example, a severe hemolytic anemia or myelofibrosis, cannot be corrected. In patients with severe megaloblastic anemia who need urgent therapy, both vitamins may be given initially and continued until the cause of the anemia has been established. Dietary fortification with folic acid has been introduced in several countries, including the United States and Canada, to reduce the incidence of babies with NTD.

CAUSES OF MACROCYTOSIS OTHER THAN MEGALOBLASTIC ANEMIA

Macrocytosis may be caused by a number of marrow disorders that disturb erythropoiesis, cause lipid deposition on the red cell membrane, or affect red cell size by other mechanisms (Table 7-2). When the cause is alcohol excess, the MCV is often raised, even though the hemoglobin level is normal.

TABLE 7-2.   MACROCYTOSIS: CAUSES OTHER THAN MEGALOBLASTIC ANEMIA

Alcohol
Liver disease
Hypothyroidism
Myelodysplasia, including acquired sideroblastic anemia
Aplastic anemia and red cell aplasia
Raised reticulocyte count
Hypoxia
Myeloma and other paraproteinemias
Cytotoxic drugs
Pregnancy

HEMOLYTIC ANEMIAS

The dominant cause of the anemia in hemolytic anemias is an increased rate of red cell destruction. This red cell destruction is usually extravascular (taking place in the macrophages of the reticuloendothelial system, as in normal individuals), although in some types of acute or chronic hemolysis red cell destruction occurs intravascularly (Fig. 8-1). The clinical and laboratory features differ according to whether the main site of destruction is extravascular or intravascular.

In addition to the clinical feature of pallor, many patients show mild fluctuating jaundice (Figs. 8-2 and 8-3) and splenomegaly (Fig. 8-4). Increased bilirubin production may result in pigment gallstones (Figs. 8-5 and 8-6).

Laboratory findings in hemolytic anemia include raised unconjugated serum bilirubin and increased fecal stercobilinogen and urinary urobilinogen from accelerated red cell destruction; serum haptoglobins are absent. A reticulocytosis (Fig. 8-7) and bone marrow erythroid

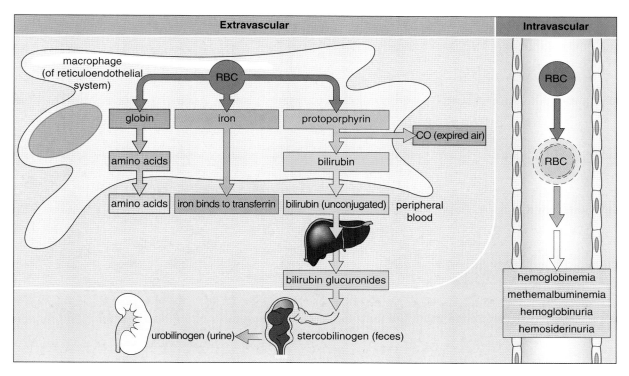

Fig. 8-1. Hemolytic anemia: extravascular and intravascular mechanisms of red blood cell (RBC) breakdown.

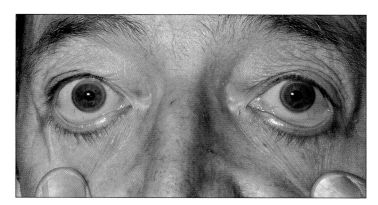

Fig. 8-2. Hemolytic anemia (autoimmune): scleral jaundice.

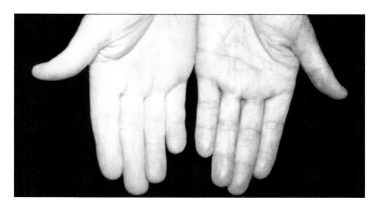

Fig. 8-3. Hemolytic anemia (autoimmune): jaundice of the palmar skin (on the *left*) contrasted with normal skin color.

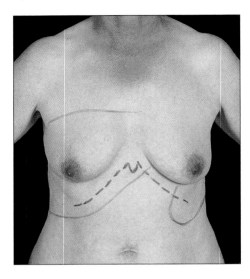

Fig. 8-4. Hemolytic anemia: mild splenomegaly and jaundice in a delayed hemolytic transfusion reaction.

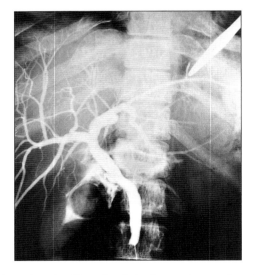

Fig. 8-5. Thalassemia major: Operative cholangiogram shows a distended biliary tree and failure of contrast to pass gallstone obstruction at the lower part of the common bile duct. (Courtesy of Dr. R. Dick.)

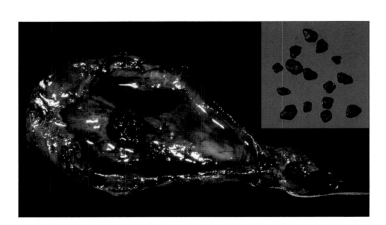

Fig. 8-6. Thalassemia major: opened gallbladder and its bilirubin gallstones *(inset)*.

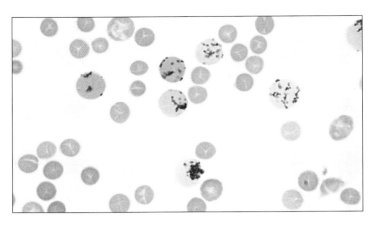

Fig. 8-7. Hemolytic anemia: reticulocytosis. Reticular (precipitated RNA) material is seen in the larger cells. New methylene blue stain (Giemsa counterstain).

hyperplasia (Fig. 8-8) are the result of compensatory increases in red cell production. Characteristic changes in red cell morphology occur in a number of hemolytic anemias and, in the most severe, the peripheral blood film shows red cell polychromasia (caused by reticulocytosis) and occasional erythroblasts (Fig. 8-9).

In those anemias caused by oxidant damage to hemoglobin and other red cell proteins, Heinz bodies may be found in reticulocyte preparations (Fig. 8-10). Intravascular red cell destruction is accompanied by hemoglobinemia, hemoglobinuria (Fig. 8-11), plasma methemoglobinemia, methemalbuminemia, and hemosiderinuria (Fig. 8-12). Jaundice is less common. Causes of intravascular hemolysis are listed in Table 8-1.

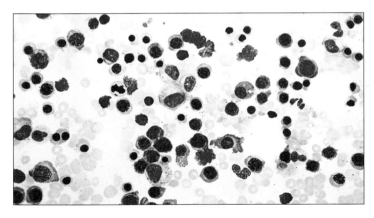

Fig. 8-8. Hemolytic anemia: This bone marrow cell trail with erythroid hyperplasia shows a dominance of erythroblasts.

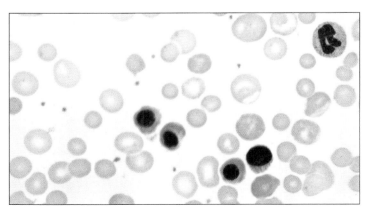

Fig. 8-9. Hemolytic anemia (autoimmune): peripheral blood film showing erythroblasts, red cell polychromasia, and spherocytosis.

Fig. 8-10. Deficiency of glucose-6-phosphate dehydrogenase: peripheral blood film showing Heinz bodies in red cells and a single reticulocyte. (Supravital new methylene blue stain.)

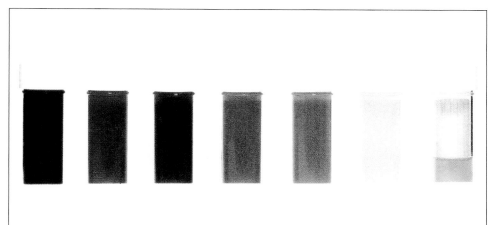

Fig. 8-11. Glucose-6-phosphate dehydrogenase deficiency: urine samples showing hemoglobinuria of decreasing severity following an episode of acute intravascular hemolysis.

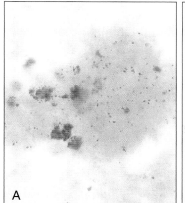
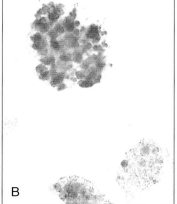

Fig. 8-12. Intravascular hemolysis in paroxysmal nocturnal hemoglobinuria (PNH): hemosiderinuria. Prussian-blue positive material seen in urinary deposit **(A)** and at higher magnification in individual renal tubular cells **(B)** (Perls' stain).

HEREDITARY HEMOLYTIC ANEMIA

The hereditary hemolytic anemias are usually the result of intrinsic red cell defects. A simplified classification is shown in Table 8-2; thalassemia and other genetic disorders of hemoglobin are discussed in Chapter 9.

NORMAL RED CELL MEMBRANE

Normal red cell membrane consists of a phospholipid bilayer, with hydrophilic phosphate residues on the external and inner surfaces and nonpolar fatty acid side chains projecting into the center (Fig. 8-13). The bilayer also contains a variable proportion of cholesterol. Proteins may be either transmembrane integral proteins, for example, band 3 and glycophorins A or B, or peripheral (extrinsic) proteins, such as spectrin, actin, and bands 2.1 (ankyrin), 4.1, and 4.2, which form a scaffolding structure on the inner surface of the membrane. The band numbers refer to the Coomassie blue bands on sodium dodecyl sulphate plus polyacrylamide gel electrophoresis (SDS-PAGE; Fig. 8-14).

TABLE 8-1.   CAUSES OF INTRAVASCULAR HEMOLYSIS

Mismatched blood transfusion (usually ABO)

G6PD deficiency with oxidant stress (e.g., drugs, fava beans, infections)

Red cell fragmentation syndromes

Some autoimmune hemolytic anemias

Some drug-induced hemolytic anemias: direct action (e.g., dapsone, salazopyrine) and immune complex types (e.g., phenacetin, quinidine, diclofenac)

Paroxysmal nocturnal hemoglobinuria

Unstable hemoglobins

Chemicals (e.g., sodium chlorate, nitrates, arsine)

Severe burns

Infections (e.g., *Clostridium perfringens*, malaria, babesiosis, bartonellosis, dengue fever)

Snake and spider bites

G6PD, Glucose-6-phosphate dehydrogenase.

TABLE 8-2.   HEREDITARY HEMOLYTIC ANEMIA: CAUSES

Membrane defects	Metabolic defects	Haemoglobin defects
Hereditary spherocytosis	Deficiency of:	Defective synthesis (e.g., thalassemia α or β)
Hereditary elliptocytosis	pyruvate kinase	
	triose phosphate isomerase	Abnormal variants (e.g., HbS, HbC, unstable)
Hereditary stomatocytosis	pyrimidine 5-nucleotidase	
South-east Asian ovalocytosis	glucose 6-phosphate dehydrogenase	
etc.	glutathione synthase	
	etc.	

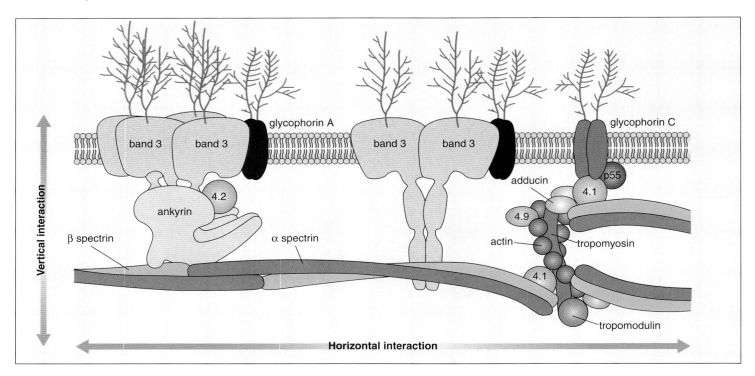

Fig. 8-13. Hereditary spherocytosis and hereditary elliptocytosis and/or pyropoikilocytosis: the red cell membrane with vertical and horizontal interactions of its components. Estimated frequencies of mutations in different membrane proteins are as follows:

- Vertical interaction—hereditary spherocytosis: band 3, about 20%; protein 4.2, about 5%; ankyrin, about 45%; β spectrin, about 30%.

- Horizontal interaction—hereditary elliptocytosis and/or pyropoikilocytosis: β spectrin, about 5%; α spectrin, about 80%; protein 4.1, about 15%.

The relative positions of the various proteins are correct, but the proteins and lipids are not drawn to scale. (Adapted with permission from Tse WT, Lux SE: Red blood cell membrane disorders [review], *Br J Hematol* 104:2–13, 1999.)

The phospholipids or proteins on the external surface may carry sugars that determine blood groups or may act as viral receptors. Spectrin consists of two forms, α and β, joined to form a heterodimer with a hairpin structure. The protein 2.1 (ankyrin) binds the spectrin β chains to band 3, a large integral membrane protein, while the tail end of spectrin binds to protein 4.1, thus forming spectrin tetramers. Protein 4.1 also binds to glycophorin A or aminophospholipids to serve as secondary attachment sites of the cytoskeleton to the inner surface of the bilayer.

RED CELL BLOOD GROUP ANTIGENS

The red cell plasma membrane contains a large number of different antigens. Many of these have sugar residues attached to membrane proteins or lipids. The structure of the most important antigens, those of the ABO system, is discussed in Chapter 29.

Over 600 different antigens exist; the best characterized are listed in Fig. 29-1. Blood group antigens are important in blood transfusion, and autoantibodies may be directed against them in autoimmune hemolytic anemias (e.g., against specific Rhesus antigens in warm-type autoimmune hemolytic anemia, and against the i antigen in infectious mononucleosis).

HEREDITARY SPHEROCYTOSIS

Hereditary spherocytosis may result from a variety of abnormalities of the cytoskeletal proteins involved in vertical interactions of the red cell membrane. Defects of ankyrin, spectrin, band 3, or other proteins have been described in various kindreds (Table 8-3). The cells are excessively permeable to sodium influx; glycolysis and adenosine triphosphate (ATP) turnover are increased. The marrow produces red cells of normal biconcave shape, but these lose membrane during passage through the spleen and the rest of the reticuloendothelial system. The resultant rigid and spherical cells have a shortened life span, the spleen being the principal organ of red cell destruction.

The condition is characterized by a dominant inheritance pattern. Typically, anemia, jaundice, and splenomegaly are present. The blood film from a patient with hereditary spherocytosis shows microspherocytes (Fig. 8-15); red cell osmotic fragility is characteristically increased (Fig. 8-16), and tests for autohemolysis show increased lysis of red cells at least partly corrected by glucose (Fig. 8-17).

In most patients with hereditary spherocytosis there is loss of Rh-related membrane proteins and fluorescence activated cell sorting (FACS) screening shows reduced binding of eosin-labeled maleiamide (Fig. 8-18). The blood film in many of patients with band 3 deficiency

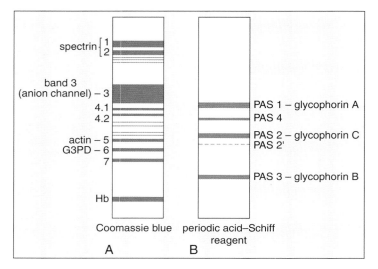

Fig. 8-14. Red cell membrane: separation of proteins by electrophoresis in sodium dodecyl sulphate (SDS) gels. **A,** Staining for protein. **B,** Staining for carbohydrate. (Adapted with permission from Contreras M, Lubenko A: Immunohematology: introduction. In Hoffbrand AV, Lewis SM, Tuddenham EGD, editors: *Postgraduate hematology,* ed 4, Oxford, 1999, Butterworth-Heinemann.)

TABLE 8-3.   HEREDITARY SPHEROCYTOSIS, HEREDITARY ELLIPTOCYTOSIS,
AND SOUTHEAST ASIAN OVALOCYTOSIS: CAUSES

Hereditary spherocytosis (vertical interactions)	Hereditary elliptocytosis (horizontal interactions)
Ankyrin deficiency (>50%) Amino acid substitution Frame shift and nonsense mutations δ Untranslated region/promoter mutations Splicing defects Gene deletions Balanced translocations	*Spectrin abnormalities* α Chain defects (80%) β Chain defects (5%)
Spectrin deficiency α Chain defects (rare) β Chain defects (uncommon)	*Protein 4.1 deficiency (15%)* *South-east Asian ovalocytosis* Band 3 defect (deletion of nine amino acids at junction of cytoplasmic and transmembrane domains)
Pallidin (protein 4.2) abnormalities (5%)	
Band 3 deficiency (20%)	

The figures given in parentheses indicate the approximate percentages of patients with hereditary spherocytosis or hereditary elliptocytosis with that abnormality.

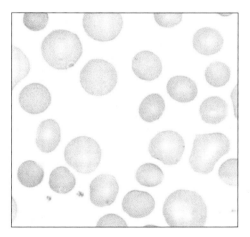

Fig. 8-15. Hereditary spherocytosis: peripheral blood film showing smaller spherocytes among larger polychromatic red cells.

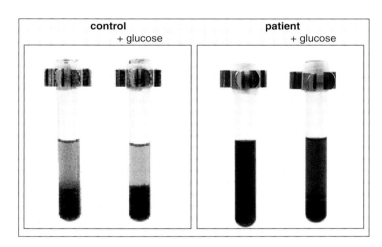

Fig. 8-17. Autohemolysis test: Red cells are incubated in saline at 37° C for 48 hours with and without additional glucose and the amount of lysis is determined. Autohemolysis, particularly in the absence of an energy supply (glucose), is markedly increased in hereditary spherocytosis.

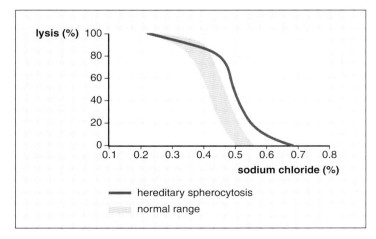

Fig. 8-16. Osmotic fragility test: comparison of red cell lysis in severe hereditary spherocytosis and in normal blood. The curve is shifted to the right of the normal range, but a tail of osmotically resistant cells (reticulocytes) is present.

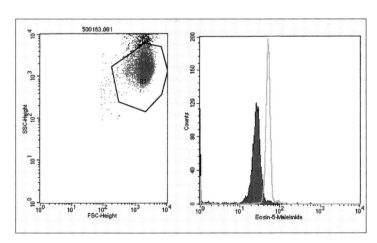

Fig. 8-18. Hereditary spherocytosis: fluorescence overlay plot of eosin-5-maleimide (EMA) screening test. In hereditary spherocytosis (purple histogram) there is reduced binding of EMA due to reduced levels of band 3 membrane protein. The histogram of normal EMA-treated cells is shown in green. Normal control set to mean cell fluorescence (MCF) of 53; patient shows MCF of 24.9.

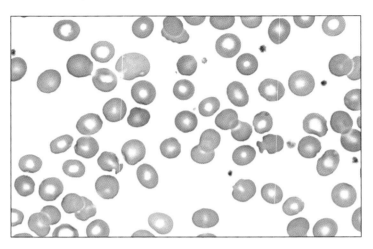

Fig. 8-19. Hereditary spherocytosis: blood film in band 3 deficiency. In addition to spherocytes, two "mushroom" or "pincered" cells are shown.

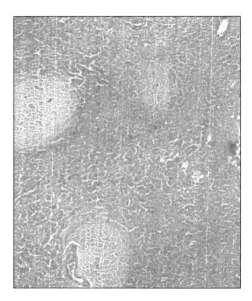

Fig. 8-20. Hereditary spherocytosis: section of spleen showing marked hyperplasia of reticuloendothelial cordal tissue and entrapment of large numbers of red cells.

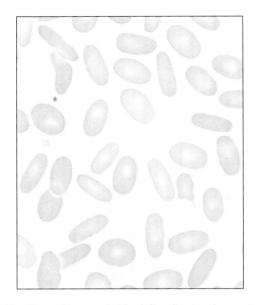

Fig. 8-21. Hereditary elliptocytosis: blood film showing characteristic elliptical red cells.

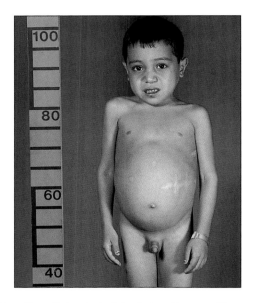

Fig. 8-22. Hereditary elliptocytosis: abdominal swelling caused by massive splenomegaly in a homozygous patient. The facies indicates expansion of hemopoietic tissue in the skull bones, particularly in the maxilla.

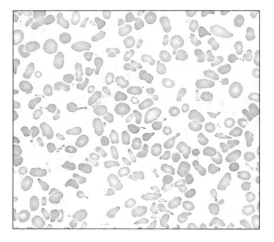

Fig. 8-23. Hereditary pyropoikilocytosis: blood film showing red cell anisocytosis, microspherocytosis, and micropoikilocytosis (MCV, 61 fl).

may show mushroom-shaped "pincered" red cells (Fig. 8-19). Splenectomy produces a considerable improvement in red cell survival and is associated with a rise in hemoglobin levels to normal. Sections of splenic tissue reveal many spherocytic red cells trapped in the splenic cords (Fig. 8-20).

HEREDITARY ELLIPTOCYTOSIS

The characteristic feature in hereditary elliptocytosis is the presence of elongated red cells in the peripheral blood (Fig. 8-21). A number of inherited protein defects that affect horizontal interactions, especially of spectrin or band 4.1, may produce this condition (see Table 8-3). A defective spectrin dimer-dimer interaction results in an increased proportion of dimers in relation to spectrin tetramers. The clinical expression in heterozygotes (elliptocytosis trait) is variable: while some have anemia and splenomegaly, the majority have only minimal or no reduction in red cell survival with little or no anemia. In rare homozygous patients, and occasional heterozygotes, there is severe anemia with marked hemolysis and splenomegaly (Fig. 8-22) and bizarre red cell morphology termed *pyropoikilocytosis* (Fig. 8-23). Heterozygous patients with an additional inherited red cell defect may also have bizarre red cell changes (Fig. 8-24).

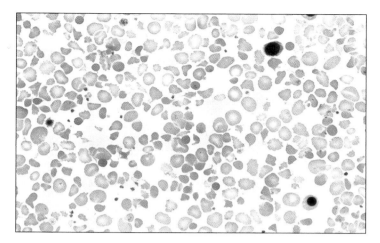

Fig. 8-24. Hereditary elliptocytosis: the blood film in an infant heterozygous for both hereditary elliptocytosis and hemoglobin Hagley Park showing marked red cell anisocytosis, poikilocytosis, and polychromasia. Two erythroblasts are seen.

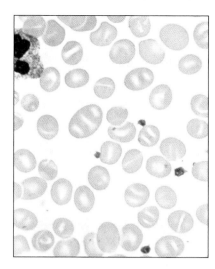

Fig. 8-26. Hereditary stomatocytosis: peripheral blood film showing many cells with the characteristic loosely folded appearance of the membrane. The membrane has increased passive permeability allowing excess sodium entry.

Southeast Asian Ovalocytosis (Stomatocytic Hereditary Elliptocytosis)

Southeast Asian ovalocytosis (Fig. 8-25) is an asymptomatic trait found in 30% of subjects in some coastal areas of New Guinea and Malaysia. The inheritance, whether dominant or recessive, is unclear. Homozygosity is probably lethal; heterozygotes are relatively protected from malaria.

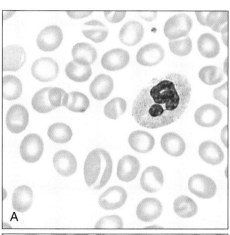

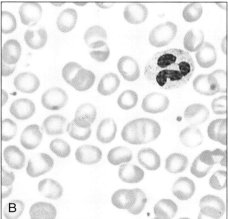

Fig. 8-25. Southeast Asian ovalocytosis. **A** and **B,** Peripheral blood films showing ovalocytes and stomatocytes, some with a longitudinal or Y-shaped slit and others with a transverse ridge. The red cell membrane is rigid, conferring resistance to malaria. The cells may form abnormal rouleaux and have reduced deformability. The genetic defect is in band 3 protein in which there is deletion of nine amino acids and which binds tightly to ankyrin. (Courtesy of Professor B. A. Bain.)

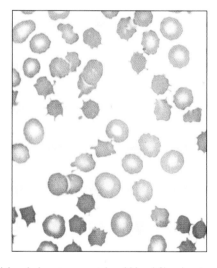

Fig. 8-27. McLeod phenotype: peripheral blood film showing marked acanthocytosis of red cells associated with the rare McLeod blood group. There is lack of the Kell antigen precursor (Kx).

Other Rare Inherited Defects of the Red Cell Membrane

Other rare inherited defects of the red cell membrane include hereditary stomatocytosis (Fig. 8-26) and acanthocytosis associated with the McLeod blood group system (Fig. 8-27).

NORMAL RED CELL METABOLISM

Normal red cells maintain themselves in a physiologic state for about 120 days by metabolizing glucose through the glycolytic (Embden-Meyerhof) and pentose phosphate (hexose monophosphate shunt) pathways (Fig. 8-28). In this way the cells are able to generate the energy needed to maintain cell shape and flexibility, as well as cation and water content through the action of sodium and calcium pumps. Although ATP acts as an energy store, it may also act as a substitute for 2,3-diphosphoglycerate (2,3-DPG) in maintaining the position of the oxygen dissociation curve. The most abundant red cell phosphate, 2,3-DPG is generated by the Rapoport-Luebering shunt of the glycolytic pathway (Fig. 8-29). The higher the 2,3-DPG content of red cells, the more easily is oxygen liberated from hemoglobin. Reducing power is also generated as the reduced forms of nicotinamide-adenine dinucleotide (NADH) and NAD phosphate (NADPH) and reduced glutathione (GSH), which protect the membrane, hemoglobin, and other cell structures from oxidant damage.

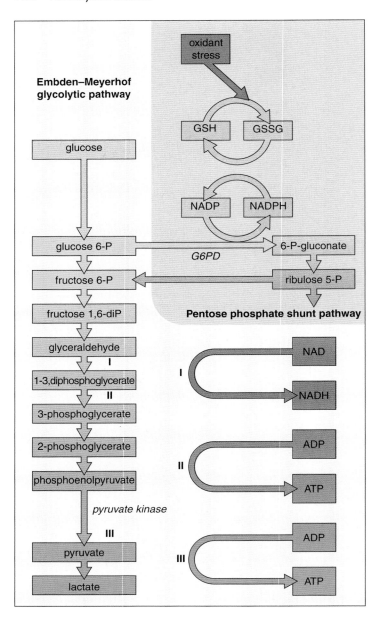

Embden–Meyerhof glycolytic pathway

Pentose phosphate shunt pathway

Fig. 8-28. Normal red cell metabolism: Embden-Meyerhof (glycolytic) and pentose phosphate (hexose monophosphate shunt) pathways. *ADP,* Adenosine diphosphate; *GSSG,* oxidized glutathione; *P,* phosphate; for other abbreviations see text.

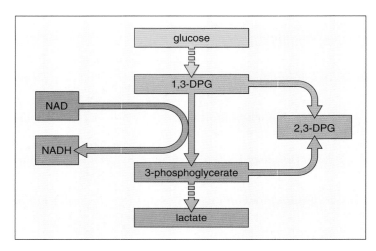

Fig. 8-29. Normal red cell metabolism: the Rapoport-Luebering shunt pathway for maintenance of red cell 2,3-DPG levels.

GLUCOSE-6-PHOSPHATE DEHYDROGENASE DEFICIENCY

Glucose-6-phosphate dehydrogenase (G6PD) deficiency is a "housekeeping gene" needed in all cells. Deficiency affects the red cells most severely, perhaps because they have no alternative source of NADPH and as a result of their long nonnucleated life span. The activity of G6PD diminishes as red cells age. The normal G6PD enzyme is genetically polymorphic and the most common form is type B. In Africa, up to 40% of the population carry an electrophoretically different normal form, type A.

Many of the several hundred inherited variants of the enzyme (Fig. 8-30) show less activity than normal. Worldwide, 400 million people are thought to be deficient (Fig. 8-31). The World Health Organization has classified G6PD variants on the extent of the enzyme deficiency and on the severity of hemolysis (Table 8-4):

- Class I: severe deficiency associated with nonspherocytic hemolytic anemia (NSHA)

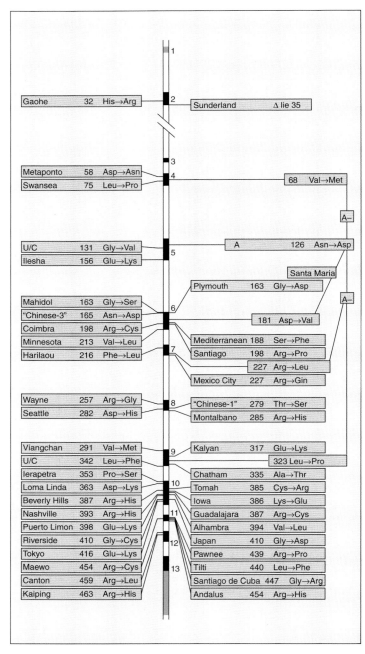

Fig. 8-30. G6PD deficiency: some of the G6PD mutations that may cause drug sensitivity *(green)* or, more rarely, chronic NSHA *(orange).* The exons are shown in *black bands,* except exon 1, which is noncoding and shown in *gray.* (Adapted with permission from Vulliamy TJ, Mason PJ, Luzzatto L: Molecular basis of glucose-6-phosphate dehydrogenase deficiency, *Trends Genet* 8:138–143, 1992.)

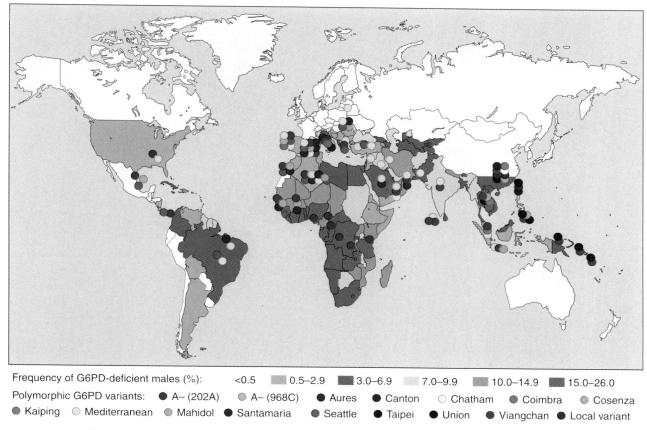

Frequency of G6PD-deficient males (%): <0.5 ▨ 0.5–2.9 ▨ 3.0–6.9 ▨ 7.0–9.9 ▨ 10.0–14.9 ▨ 15.0–26.0

Polymorphic G6PD variants: ● A– (202A) ● A– (968C) ● Aures ● Canton ○ Chatham ● Coimbra ● Cosenza
● Kaiping ○ Mediterranean ● Mahidol ● Santamaria ● Seattle ● Taipei ● Union ○ Viangchan ● Local variant

Fig. 8-31. World distribution of polymorphic G6PD-deficient mutants. The different shadings indicate the frequency of the G6PD-deficient phenotype in the respective population. (Modified from Postgraduate Haematology, 5th Ed. Fig 9.3 (From Luzzato and Notaro, 2001, Science 293: 442); Most recent modified map: Luzzato Lucio, *Haematologica/the hematology journal* 2006;91:1304.)

- Class II: less than 10% activity; includes the common Mediterranean and Asian variants not associated with NSHA
- Class III: 10% to 60% of activity; includes the common A– form
- Class IV: normal activity
- Class V: increased activity

Variants of the final two groups are of no clinical significance. The most frequent clinical syndrome is acute intravascular hemolysis caused by oxidant stress, drugs (Table 8-5), or fava beans or occurring during severe infection, diabetic ketoacidosis, or hepatitis. Marked changes occur in red cell morphology (Fig. 8-32) with Heinz bodies (see Fig. 8-10) and hemoglobinuria (see Fig. 8-11). Neonatal jaundice may also occur, and the most severe defects result in a chronic NSHA.

TABLE 8-4. WORLD HEALTH ORGANIZATION CLASSIFICATION OF G6PD VARIANTS AND DEFICIENCY

Class	Enzyme Activity (% normal)	Examples	Clinical effects
I	Severe (usually <20)	Santiago de Cuba (Gly447Arg)	Chronic nonspherocytic hemolytic anemia, acute exacerbations
II	<10	Mediterranean (Ser188Phe) Canton (Arg459Leu) Orissa (Ala44Gly)	Favism, drug-induced hemolytic anemia, neonatal jaundice
III	Moderate (>10, <60)	A– (Val68Met; Asn126Asp)	Drug-induced hemolytic anemia, neonatal jaundice
IV	100	B (wild type) A+ (Asn126Asp)	None None

TABLE 8-5. G6PD DEFICIENCY: DRUGS THAT CAUSE HEMOLYTIC ANEMIA IN ASSOCIATION WITH G6PD, AND THOSE THAT CAN BE GIVEN SAFELY TO SUBJECTS WITH G6PD DEFICIENCY WITHOUT NSHA

Drugs that may cause hemolytic anemia in subjects with G6PD deficiency	Drugs that can be given safely in therapeutic doses to subjects with G6PD deficiency without NSHA
Antimalarials Pyrimethamine with sulfadoxine (Fansidar) Pyrimethamine with dapsone (Maloprim) Primaquine ? Chloroquine	**Ascorbic acid** Aspirin Colchicine Isoniazid Menadiol Phenytoin
Sulfonamides Sulfamethoxazole Some other sulfonamides	Probenecid Procainamide Pyrimethamine Quinidine Quinine Trimethoprim
Sulfones Dapsone Thiazolesulfone	
Other antibacterial compounds Nitrofurans Nalidixic acid	
Anthelmintics Beta-naphthol	
Miscellaneous ? Vitamin K Naphthalene (moth balls) Methylene blue Doxorubicin	
? – there is some dispute with these compounds	

Adapted with permission from Beutler E: Glucose-6-phosphate dehydrogenase deficiency, *N Engl J Med* 324:169–178, 1991.

G6PD, Glucose-6-phosphate dehydrogenase; *NSHA*, nonspherocytic hemolytic anemia.

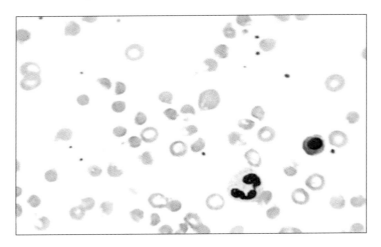

Fig. 8-32. G6PD deficiency: peripheral blood film following acute oxidant drug-induced hemolysis shows an erythroblast and damaged red cells, including irregularly contracted "blister" and "bite" cells.

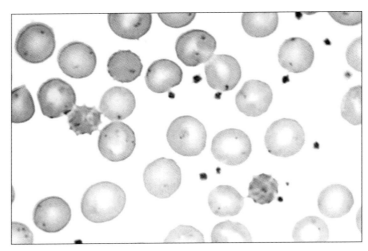

Fig. 8-34. Pyruvate kinase deficiency: peripheral blood film postsplenectomy with two small echinocytes or "prickle" cells.

The gene is located on the X chromosome and is fully expressed in males, but only one X chromosome is active in each female cell. As a result of X-chromosome inactivation, female heterozygotes for G6PD deficiency have two populations of cells (on average 50% of each), either with or without the enzyme. Because G6PD deficiency confers protection against *Plasmodium falciparum* malaria, it has a high frequency in areas of the world where malaria is or was common. Rarely, lack of G6PD may be responsible for decreased leukocyte function and for hyperbilirubinemia in some patients with neonatal jaundice or viral hepatitis.

PYRUVATE KINASE DEFICIENCY

Pyruvate kinase deficiency is the most frequently encountered hemolytic anemia due to an inherited defect in the Embden-Meyerhof glycolytic pathway. The majority of patients have red cells that show no particular diagnostic features (Fig. 8-33), although "prickle" cells may be found, especially following splenectomy (Fig. 8-34). The postsplenectomy reticulocyte count is often very high (Fig. 8-35). There is an abnormal autohemolysis test not corrected by glucose, and diagnosis is made by a specific enzyme assay.

PYRIMIDINE 5-NUCLEOTIDASE DEFICIENCY

This rare congenital hemolytic anemia is associated with basophilic stippling of the red cells (Fig. 8-36) caused by abnormal residual

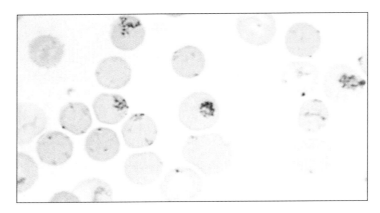

Fig. 8-35. Pyruvate kinase deficiency: gross reticulocytosis (over 90%) following splenectomy (supravital new methylene blue stain).

ribonucleic acid (RNA). This enzyme normally catalyzes the hydrolytic dephosphorylation of pyrimidine 5′-ribose monophosphates to freely diffusible pyrimidine nucleosides, an important step in the breakdown of RNA at the reticulocyte stage. The enzyme is also inhibited by lead.

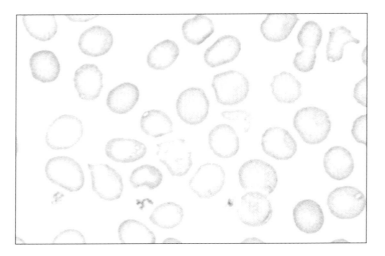

Fig. 8-33. Pyruvate kinase deficiency: peripheral blood film presplenectomy shows red cell anisocytosis and poikilocytosis.

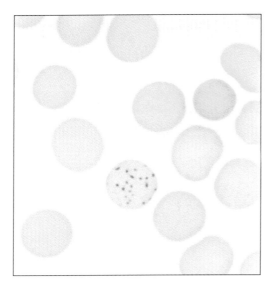

Fig. 8-36. Pyrimidine 5-nucleotidase deficiency: peripheral blood film showing basophilic stippling in the central red cell.

TABLE 8-6.   ACQUIRED HEMOLYTIC
ANEMIA: CAUSES

Immune
Autoimmune hemolytic anemia
Drug-induced immune hemolytic anemia
Isommune:
    hemolytic transfusion reaction
    hemolytic disease of the newborn

Red cell fragmentation syndrome

Hypersplenism

Paroxysmal nocturnal hemoglobinuria

Secondary
Renal disease, liver disease, etc.

Miscellaneous
Chemicals
Drugs
Infections
Toxins
Wilson's disease

TABLE 8-7.   AUTOIMMUNE
HEMOLYTIC ANEMIA:
CAUSES

Warm type	Cold type
Idiopathic	**Idiopathic**
Secondary	**Secondary**
Systemic lupus erythematosus, other connnective tissue disorders	Mycoplasma pneumonia
	Infectious mononucleosis
	Malignant lymphoma
Chronic lymphocytic leukemia	Ulcerative colitis
Malignant lymphoma	Paroxysmal cold hemoglobinuria:
Ovarian teratoma	rare; may be primary or associated with infection
Drugs (e.g., methyldopa, fludarabine)	

ACQUIRED HEMOLYTIC ANEMIA

The majority of acquired hemolytic anemias are caused by extracorpuscular or environmental changes. A simplified classification is given in Table 8-6.

AUTOIMMUNE HEMOLYTIC ANEMIAS

Autoimmune hemolytic anemias are characterized by a positive direct Coombs' (antiglobulin) test (Fig. 8-37) and are divided into "warm" and "cold" types, according to whether the antibody reacts better with red cells at 37° C or at 4° C. These acquired disorders occur at any age and produce hemolytic anemias of varying severity, often with associated disease (Table 8-7). In the warm type, the peripheral blood usually shows marked red cell spherocytosis (Figs. 8-38 and 8-39). In the cold type, the antibodies are usually immunoglobulin M (IgM) and may be associated with intravascular hemolysis. Marked autoagglutination of red cells may be seen in the blood film (Fig. 8-40). In many patients the hemolysis is aggravated

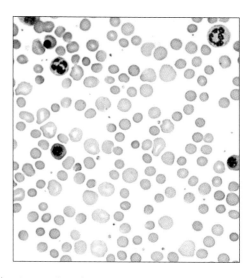

Fig. 8-38. Autoimmune hemolytic anemia: peripheral blood film showing erythroblasts, polychromatic macrocytes, and marked spherocytosis.

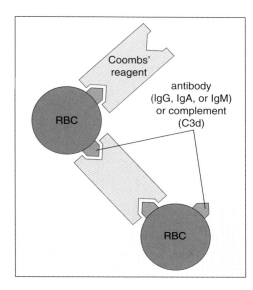

Fig. 8-37. Direct antiglobulin (Coombs') test: The Coombs' reagent may be broad spectrum or specifically directed against IgG, IgM, IgA, or complement (C3d). The test is positive if the red cells agglutinate. *RBC*, Red blood cell.

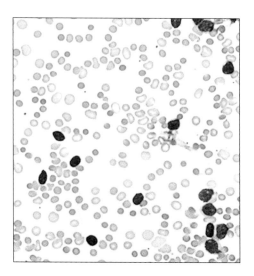

Fig. 8-39. Autoimmune hemolytic anemia with associated chronic lymphocytic leukemia: peripheral blood film showing red cell polychromasia spherocytosis and increased numbers of lymphocytes.

by cold weather, and it is often associated with Raynaud's phenomenon (Fig. 8-41). Rarely, the blood films show neutrophil–red cell rosettes (Fig. 8-42).

In warm autoimmune hemolytic anemia, high-dose corticosteroids often achieve a remission and splenectomy may be of value in those who do not respond satisfactorily. Patients with chronic cold autoimmune hemolytic anemia should avoid the cold, and some may benefit from therapy with alkylating agents.

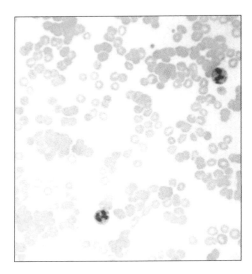

Fig. 8-40. Autoimmune hemolytic anemia (cold type): peripheral blood film showing autoagglutination of red cells.

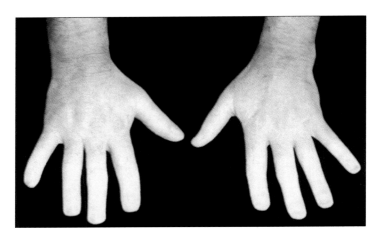

Fig. 8-41. Autoimmune hemolytic anemia (cold type): Raynaud's phenomenon manifested by marked pallor of the fingers.

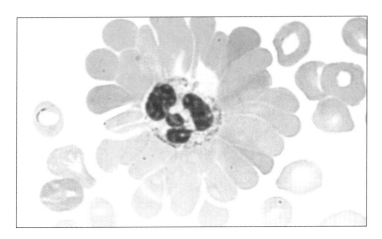

Fig. 8-42. Autoimmune hemolytic anemia: peripheral blood film showing a neutrophil–red cell rosette.

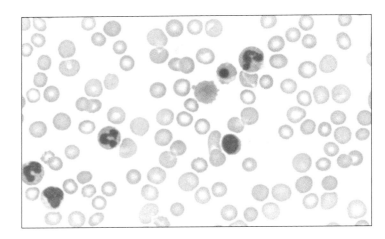

Fig. 8-43. Evans syndrome: The blood film shows an erythroblast, red cell spherocytosis, polychromasia, and a solitary giant platelet.

EVANS SYNDROME

In Evans syndrome, occasional patients with autoimmune hemolytic anemia also have an autoimmune thrombocytopenia. The blood film shows features of both conditions (Fig. 8-43). There is often an associated illness (e.g., lymphoproliferative disease or immunodeficiency).

DRUG-INDUCED IMMUNE HEMOLYTIC ANEMIA

Drugs cause immune hemolytic anemia by three mechanisms: antibodies may be directed against a red cell membrane–drug complex (e.g., with penicillin); there may be deposition of a protein-antibody-drug complex on the red cell surface (e.g., with quinine, rifampicin); or occasionally an autoimmune process is involved, as with methyldopa or fludarabine.

ISOIMMUNE HEMOLYTIC ANEMIA

Severe hemolysis follows transfusion of incompatible blood, particularly if the blood is of the wrong ABO group. There may be massive intravascular hemolysis, and the blood film usually shows both autoagglutination and spherocytosis (Fig. 8-44). The other major cause of isoimmune hemolytic anemia is hemolytic disease of the newborn, which may result from a number of different maternofetal blood group incompatibilities (Table 8-8 and Figs. 8-45 to 8-47; see also Chapter 29).

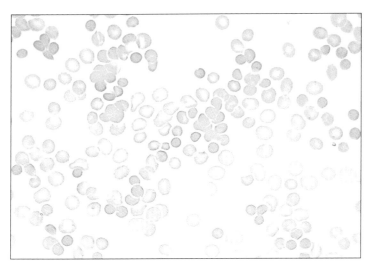

Fig. 8-44. ABO incompatibility transfusion reaction: peripheral blood film showing red cell autoagglutination and spherocytosis.

Blood group system	Frequency of antibodies	Hemolytic disease of newborn
ABO	Very common	Causal
Rhesus	Common	Causal
Kell	Occasional	Causal
Duffy	Occasional	Causal
Kidd	Occasional	Causal
Lutheran	Rare	Causal
Lewis	Rare	Not causal
P	Rare	Not causal
MNSs	Rare	Not causal
Ii	Rare	Not causal

TABLE 8-8. ISOIMMUNE HEMOLYTIC ANEMIA: THE MAIN BLOOD GROUP SYSTEMS AND THEIR ASSOCIATION WITH HEMOLYTIC DISEASE IN THE NEWBORN

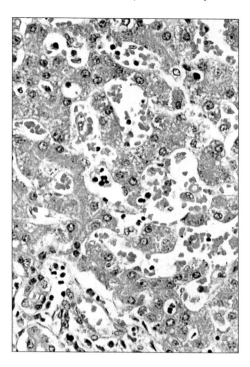

Fig. 8-46. Rhesus D hemolytic disease of the newborn: Histologic section of liver from a fatal case shows extramedullary hemopoiesis in the hepatic venous sinuses.

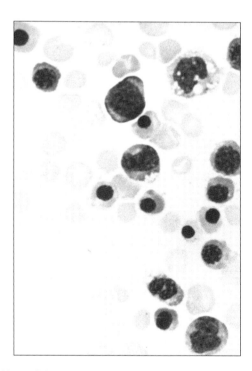

Fig. 8-45. Rhesus D hemolytic disease of the newborn (erythroblastosis fetalis): peripheral blood film from an infant born with severe anemia showing large numbers of erythroblasts, red cell polychromasia, and anisocytosis.

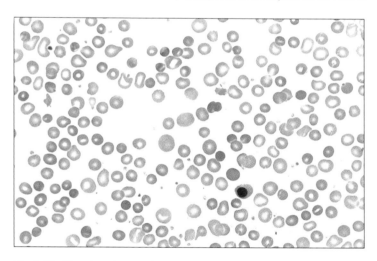

Fig. 8-47. Hemolytic disease of the newborn resulting from ABO incompatibility. The blood film shows an erythroblast, red cell polychromasia, and spherocytosis.

TABLE 8-9.   CAUSES OF FRAGMENTATION HEMOLYSIS

Cardiac hemolysis
Prosthetic heart valves
Patches, grafts
Paraprosthetic or perivalvular leaks

Arteriovenous malformations
Kasabach–Merritt syndrome
Malignant hemangioendotheliomas

Microangiopathic
TTP, HUS
Malignant disease
Vasculitis
Preeclampsia, HELLP
Renal vascular disorders
Disseminated intravascular coagulation

HELLP, Hemolysis, elevated liver enzymes low platelets; *HUS,* hemolytic uremic syndrome; *TTP,* thrombotic thrombocytopenic purpura.

RED CELL FRAGMENTATION SYNDROMES

The causes of red cell fragmentation syndrome are listed in Table 8-9. Fragmentation arises from direct damage to red cells, either on abnormal surfaces such as heart valves, or vascular malformations or changes in the microcirculation such as fibrin shearing in disseminated intravascular coagulation, vasculitis, and endothelial damage. Blood film changes in patients with mucin-secreting adenocarcinoma, thrombotic thrombocytopenic purpura, hemolytic-uremic syndrome, and gram-negative septicemia are shown in Figs. 8-48 to 8-51.

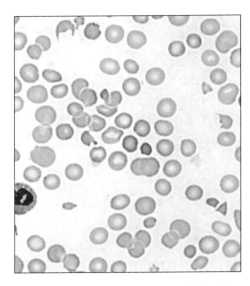

Fig. 8-48. Red cell fragmentation syndrome: peripheral blood film in widespread metastatic mucin-secreting adenocarcinoma showing deeply staining red cell fragments *(schistocytes)* and anisocytosis.

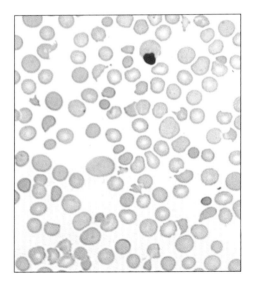

Fig. 8-49. Red cell fragmentation syndrome: peripheral blood film showing polychromatic and fragmented red cells in thrombotic thrombocytopenic purpura.

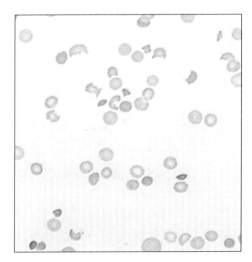

Fig. 8-50. Red cell fragmentation syndrome: peripheral blood film in hemolytic-uremic syndrome.

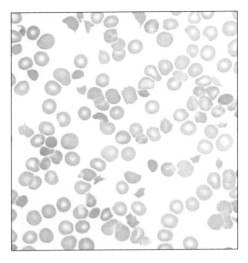

Fig. 8-51. Red cell fragmentation syndrome: peripheral blood film in gram-negative septicemia, showing red cell polychromasia, microspherocytes, and fragmentation.

SECONDARY HEMOLYTIC ANEMIAS

In a number of systemic disorders, hemolysis may contribute to observed anemia. In renal failure there may be crenated cells *(echinocytes),* including "burr" cells and acanthocytes (Fig. 8-52; see also Fig. 27-31). Red cell targeting is a feature of the hemolysis associated with liver disease, and with severe liver failure, there is often marked hemolysis with prominent red cell acanthocytosis (see Fig. 27-34).

PAROXYSMAL NOCTURNAL HEMOGLOBINURIA

In paroxysmal nocturnal hemoglobinuria (PNH), an acquired clonal disorder, the bone marrow produces red cells with defective cell membranes that are particularly sensitive to lysis by complement. There is chronic intravascular hemolysis with hemoglobinuria and hemosiderinuria (see Fig. 8-12). The defect that results in complement sensitivity is in the formation of phosphatidyl inositol, which anchors a number of proteins via an intervening glycan structure to the red cell membrane (Fig. 8-53). The proteins anchored by glycosylphosphatidyl inositol (GPI) include membrane inhibitor of reactive lysis (MIRL = CD59), decay accelerating factor (DAF = CD55), C8 binding protein (C8B)—these three proteins all react with complement—leukocyte function antigen (LAF-3 = CD58), acetylcholinesterase, alkaline phosphatase, and low-affinity immunoglobulin G (IgG)

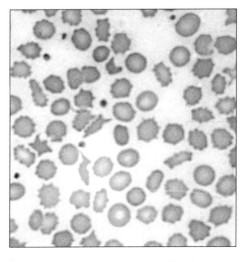

Fig. 8-52. Chronic renal failure: peripheral blood film showing red cell changes, including "burr" cells and acanthocytes (coarse crenated cells).

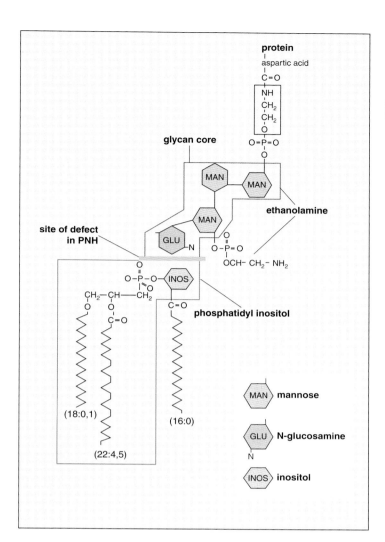

Fig. 8-54. Expression of GPI-linked molecules on the surface of blood cells. *AChE,* Acetylcholinesterase; *CD16,* FcRIII low-affinity receptor for IgG; *CD55,* DAF (see text); *CD59,* MIRL (see text); *Group-8,* monocyte activation antigen; *NAP,* alkaline phosphatase. (Adapted with permission from Rotoli B, Bessler M, Alfinito F, et al: Membrane proteins in paroxysmal nocturnal hemoglobinuria, *Blood Rev* 7:75–86, 1993.)

Fig. 8-53. The GPI anchor: structure and site of the defect in paroxysmal nocturnal hemoglobinuria (PNH). (Courtesy of Professor Wendell Rosse.)

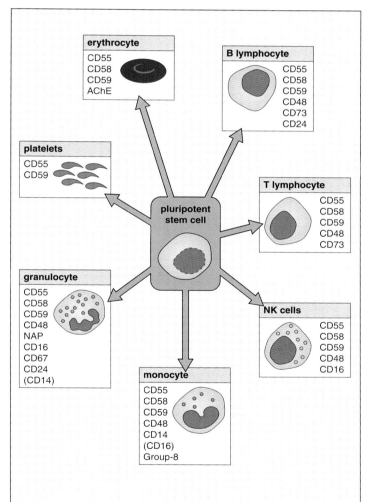

receptor (FcRIII; Fig. 8-54). Lack of MIRL appears to be responsible for the undue sensitivity to complement. The enzyme α-1,6-*N*-acetylglucosaminyltransferase is the enzyme involved in synthesis of the GPI anchor that is missing or defective because of different types of mutations in the *PIG-A* (phosphatidyl inositol glycan complementation class A) gene. The patients often develop iron deficiency. The bone marrow tends to be hypocellular and the reticulocyte count is lower than in other hemolytic anemias of equal severity. The white cell and platelet counts are also often low. Many patients develop recurrent

venous thromboses. Occasionally patients have the Budd-Chiari syndrome (Fig. 8-55). Traditional diagnosis of PNH is by finding a positive acid lysis test (Fig. 8-56). Flow cytometry using anti-CD59 (Fig. 8-57) is now preferred and provides an accurate estimate of the size of the PNH cell population. Recent trials with eculizumab, a humanized antibody that blocks the activation of the complement protein C5 and the terminal membrane attack phase of complement action (Fig. 8-58), have been effective in controlling hemolysis in patients with PNH who are transfusion dependent.

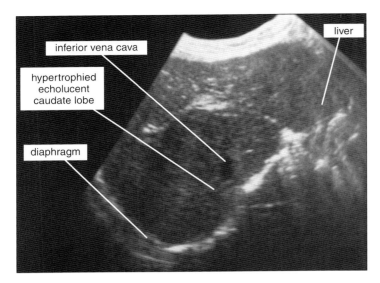

Fig. 8-55. Paroxysmal nocturnal hemoglobinuria: ultrasound study of liver in Budd-Chiari syndrome. The caudate lobe is hypertrophied and spongy, and the inferior vena cava is compressed in its passage through it. (Courtesy of Dr. L. Berger.)

Fig. 8-56. Paroxysmal nocturnal hemoglobinuria: acid lysis test. The affected red cells (on the *left*) show marked complement-dependent lysis in acidified fresh serum at 37° C. Preheating the acidified serum inactivates complement, preventing lysis of the affected cells.

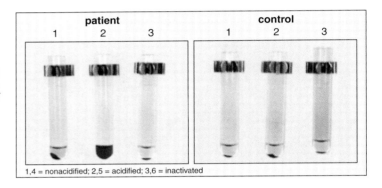

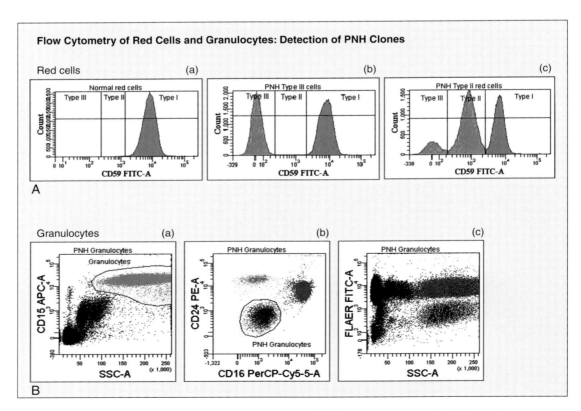

Fig. 8-57. Paroxysmal nocturnal hemoglobinuria (PNH): flow cytometry of red cells and granulocytes. **A,** Red cells. Analysis of CD59 expression on normal (*a*), and PNH red cells (*b* and *c*). Histogram *a* shows normal CD59 expression (type I cells). Plot *b* shows a major population of completely CD59-deficient red cells (46%, type III cells) and a population of normal red cells. Plot *c* shows a mixture of all three types of red cells: type III, 10%; type II (partial CD expression), 54%; and normal type I cells, 36%. **B,** Granulocytes. Granulocytes are identified on the basis of CD15 expression and variable SSC (plot *a*). Analysis of CD16 and CD24 (both GPI-linked antigens) for this population of cells shows a small population of PNH granulocytes that is deficient for both antigens and makes up 10% of total granulocytes. Plot *c* shows the same case also stained with FLAER (fluorescent aerolysin), a novel reagent that binds specifically to the GPI anchor. This is also an effective reagent for the detection of PNH cells by flow cytometry and can easily be used in combination with monoclonal antibodies. (Courtesy of Dr. Anita Hill.)

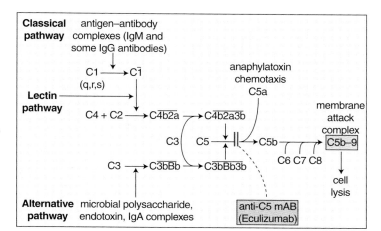

Fig. 8-58. Paroxysmal nocturnal hemoglobinuria: site of action of anti-C5 monoclonal antibody eculizumab. (Modified from Dr. Anita Hill.)

OTHER HEMOLYTIC ANEMIAS

Severe hemolytic anemia may be found during clostridial septicemia (Fig. 8-59) and in other infections, including malaria and bartonellemia (see Chapter 28). Hemolytic anemias may also be caused by extensive burns (Figs. 8-60 and 8-61), chemical poisoning, and snake and spider bites. Overdose with oxidizing drugs, such as sulfasalazine (Fig. 8-62) or dapsone (Fig. 8-63), may also cause severe hemolysis. Wilson's disease is also a cause of hemolysis, thought to result from oxidant damage to red cells caused by excess copper (Fig. 8-64).

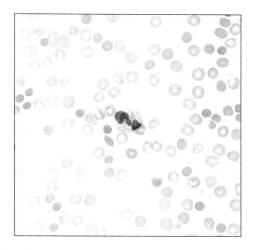

Fig. 8-59. Hemolytic anemia in clostridial septicemia: peripheral blood film showing red cell spherocytosis.

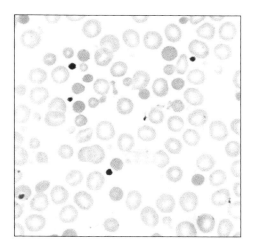

Fig. 8-61. Hemolytic anemia following extensive burns: peripheral blood film showing microspherocytes, ghost cells, cells with membrane projections, and "dumbbell" forms.

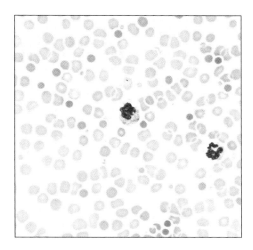

Fig. 8-60. Hemolytic anemia following extensive burns: peripheral blood film showing marked spherocytosis, including microspherocytic cells.

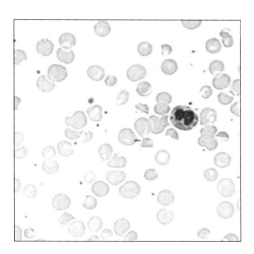

Fig. 8-62. Drug-induced hemolytic anemia: peripheral blood film associated with overdose of sulfasalazine. The red cells show polychromasia, irregular contraction, and some fragmentation.

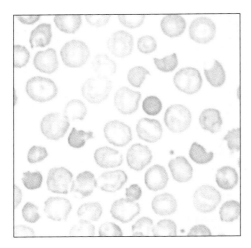

Fig. 8-63. Drug-induced hemolytic anemia: peripheral blood film in a case associated with high-dosage dapsone therapy for dermatitis herpetiformis. The red cells show irregular contraction, target cells, and cells with "bites" out of the membrane. There is a single "blister" cell in the *lower central area* of the field.

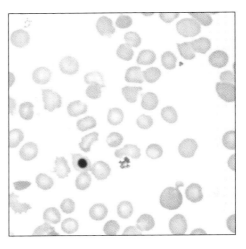

Fig. 8-64. Hemolytic anemia in Wilson's disease: peripheral blood film showing polychromasia, spur cells (acanthocytes), and a normoblast. (Courtesy of Dr. R. Britt.)

GENETIC DISORDERS OF HEMOGLOBIN

THALASSEMIA

Globin synthesis depends on two gene clusters situated on chromosomes 11 and 16 (Fig. 9-1). Different hemoglobins dominate in the embryo, fetus, and adult (Fig. 9-2). Each globin gene includes three coding regions, or exons, and two noncoding regions, called intervening sequences or introns. Globin molecules are synthesized from the appropriate genes via a ribonucleic acid (RNA) transcript. The genes all show two boxes, TATA and CCAAT, in the 5′ region, closely upstream in the flanking region, and further upstream sequences GGGGTG and CACCC; these all have important regulatory functions. There are promoter sequences involved in the initiation of transcription. At the 3′ noncoding region, there is a sequence AATAAA, which is the signal for the messenger RNA (mRNA) to be cleaved. Further upstream of the β-globin cluster, there is a key regulatory region, the locus control region (LCR) (see Fig. 9-1), which

performs two functions. It allows the β-globin cluster to transform from a transcriptionally inactive closed chromatin formation to an open transcriptionally active form. It also enhances transcription from the β-globin gene cluster. To do this, it binds erythroid-specific (e.g., GATA-I, NF-E2) and ubiquitous transacting factors. The α-globin clusters also include an LCR-like region designated HS40, but it differs from the β LCR. Following transcription, the RNA is processed (spliced) to remove redundant RNA derived from introns situated within the coding part of each gene (Fig. 9-3). The exon-intron junctions have the sequence GT at their 5′ end and AG at their 3′ end; these sequences are essential for correct splicing. The messenger is modified by addition of a CAP (start site for RNA transcription) structure at the 5′ end and a series of adenylic acid residues (the poly [A] tail) at the 3′ end. The processed message moves to the cytoplasm, attaches to ribosomes, and acts as a template for the addition of appropriate amino acids via their transfer RNAs. The amino acids link up to form the final polypeptide chain.

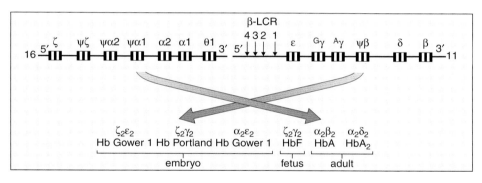

Fig. 9-1. Synthesis of hemoglobin: organization of the clusters of genes and their coding regions (exons, in black) for globin chain synthesis on chromosomes 11 and 16; noncoding regions (introns) occur between the exons. Gγ and Aγ are forms of the γ-globin gene that code for glutamic acid or alanine at position 136. *LCR,* Locus control region. (Adapted with permission from Weatherall DJ: Genetic disorders of haemoglobin. In Hoffbrand AV, Lewis SM, Tuddenham EGD: *Postgraduate haematology,* ed 4, Oxford, 1998, Butterworth Heinemann, pp 91–119.)

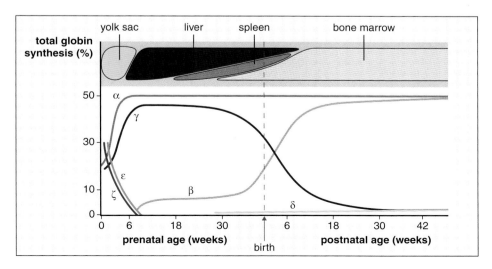

Fig. 9-2. Synthesis of hemoglobin: sites of globin chain synthesis in the embryo, fetus, and adult. (Adapted with permission from Hoffbrand AV, Pettit JE: *Essential haematology,* ed 3, Oxford, 1993, Blackwell Scientific.)

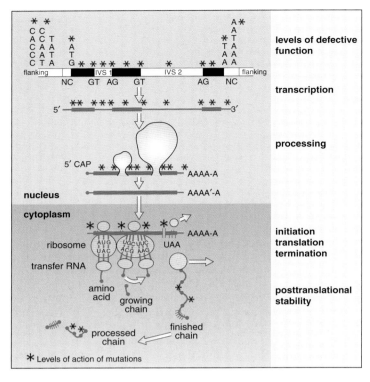

Fig. 9-3. Synthesis of hemoglobin: stages in the synthesis of β-globin from DNA to the final polypeptide chain. *A*, Adenine; *C*, cytosine; *G*, guanine; *IVS*, intervening sequence; *T*, thymine. (Adapted with permission from Weatherall DJ: Genetic disorders of haemoglobin. In Hoffbrand AV, Lewis SM, Tuddenham EGD: *Postgraduate haematology*, ed 4, Oxford, 1998, Butterworth Heinemann, pp 91–119.)

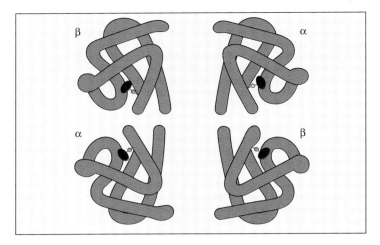

Fig. 9-4. Synthesis of hemoglobin: the hemoglobin tetramer—in this example, Hb A.

Each molecule of hemoglobin consists of four globin chains (Fig. 9-4). In normal adults, hemoglobin (Hb) A (α2,β2) forms 96% to 97% of the hemoglobin. The thalassemias are a group of disorders in which the underlying abnormality is reduced synthesis of either the α or β chains of hemoglobin A (Table 9-1). The global distribution of thalassemia and the frequency of different mutations in Mediterranean populations are shown in Fig. 9-5.

β-Thalassemia is divided into three types:
- A homozygous (major) form, in which there is complete or almost complete absence of β-globin chain synthesis
- A heterozygous (minor) or trait form, in which synthesis of only one β chain is reduced
- A clinically intermediate form, which can be a mild form of homozygous β-thalassemia, the result of interaction of β-thalassemia with other genetic disorders of hemoglobin synthesis, or an unusually severe form of β-thalassemia trait (see Table 9-2)

In general, β-thalassemias are the result of point mutations in or near the globin genes that cause, for example, defective transcription, processing of RNA, translation or posttranslation stability or splicing; internal intervening sequence (IVS); cryptic splice site; CAP and polyadenylation site changes or premature stop codons, nonsense lesions, and frameshift; and initiation site changes (Fig. 9-6). Gene deletion may also cause β-thalassemias (Fig. 9-7) but is more common in the

TABLE 9-1. CLASSIFICATION OF THE THALASSEMIA DISORDERS: CLINICAL, α-THALASSEMIAS, AND β-THALASSEMIAS

Classification of thalassemias I	Classification of thalassemias II			
Clinical	**α-Thalassemias**			
Thalassemia major	**Designation**	**Haplotype**	**Heterozygous**	**Homozygous**
Transfusion-dependent homozygous β⁰-thalassemia	α⁰-Thalassemia	– –/	α⁰-Thalassemia; MCH, MCV low	Hydrops fetalis
Homozygous β⁺-thalassemia (some types)	Dysfunctional α-thalassemia	– α⁰/	α⁰-Thalassemia; MCH, MCV low	Hydrops fetalis
Thalassemia intermedia	α⁺-Thalassemia	– α/	α⁺-Thalassemia; minimal, if any, haematological abnormality	As heterozygous α⁰-thalassemia
Mild forms of compound β⁺ α⁺ β⁰/β⁺ thalassemia	Nondeletion α-thalassemia	α α/	Variable	Hb H disease in some cases
Hemoglobin Lepore syndromes	Hb-Constant Spring (CS)	α α/	0.5%–1% Hb CS	More severe than heterozygous α⁰-thalassemia
Homozygous δβ-thalassemia and hereditary persistence of fetal haemoglobin				
Combinations of α- and β⁺-thalassemias	The combination of α⁰-thalassemia (or dysfunctional α-thalassemia) and α⁺-thalassemia gives rise to Hb H disease			
Heterozygous β-thalassemia with triplicated α genes	**Classification of Thalassemias III**			
Dominant β-thalassemia				
Heterozygosity for β-thalassemia and β chain variants (e.g., Hb E/β-thalassemia)	**β-Thalassemias**			
Hemoglobin H disease	**Type**	**Heterozygous**		**Homozygous**
Thalassemia minor	β⁰	Thalassemia minor; Hb A₂ >3.5%		Thalassemia major; Hb F 98%; Hb A₂ 2%; no Hb A
β⁰-Thalassemia trait	β⁺	Thalassemia minor; Hb A₂ >3.5%		Thalassemia major or intermedia; Hb F 70%–80%; Hb A 10%–20%; Hb A₂ variable
δβ-Thalassemia trait				
Hereditary persistence of fetal hemoglobin	δβ hereditary persistence of fetal hemoglobin	Thalassemia minor; Hb F >5%–20%; Hb A₂ normal or low		Thalassemia intermedia; Hb F 100%
β⁺-Thalassemia trait	Hb Lepore	Thalassemia minor; Hb A >80%–90%; Hb Lepore 10%; Hb A₂ reduced		Thalassemia major or intermedia; Hb F 80%; Hb Lepore 10%–20%; Hb A, Hb A₂ absent
α⁰-Thalassemia trait				
α⁺-Thalassemia trait				

Hb, hemoglobin; *MCH,* mean corpuscular hemoglobin; *MCV,* mean corpuscular volume.

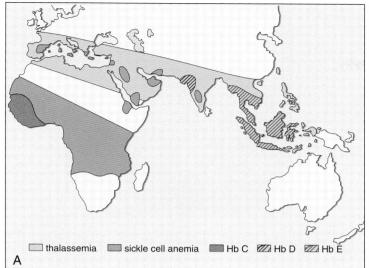

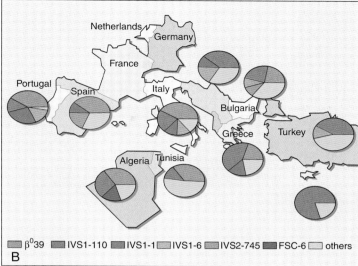

Fig. 9-5. Distribution of thalassemia disorders. **A,** The geographic distribution of thalassemia, sickle cell anemia, and the other common hemoglobin disorders. It is likely that the carriers of these disorders have a selective advantage against malaria compared with normal individuals. The disorders are also found in other parts of the world where emigrants from areas of higher incidence have settled. **B,** Frequency of different mutations of β-thalassemia in Mediterranean at-risk populations. *1, 6, 39, 110, 745,* Mutations of corresponding codons; *FSC-6,* frameshift mutation–6; *IVS 1, IVS 2,* introns 1 or 2 of β-globin gene. (Courtesy of Professor Anthony Cao.)

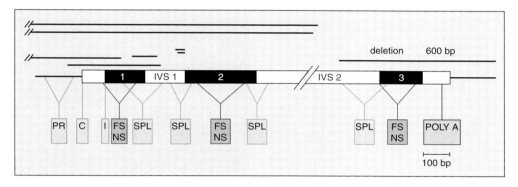

Fig. 9-6. β-Thalassemia: the classes of mutations that underlie β-thalassemia. The 600 base pair deletion may also cause β-thalassemia. Other rare deletions may occur that affect the β-globin gene, the β and δ genes, or the γ, δ, and β genes (see Fig. 9-7). *C,* CAP site; *FS,* frameshift; *I,* initiation codon; *NS,* nonsense (premature chain termination) mutation; *POLY A,* poly A addition site mutation; *PR,* promoter; *SPL,* splicing mutation. (Courtesy of Professor D. J. Weatherall.)

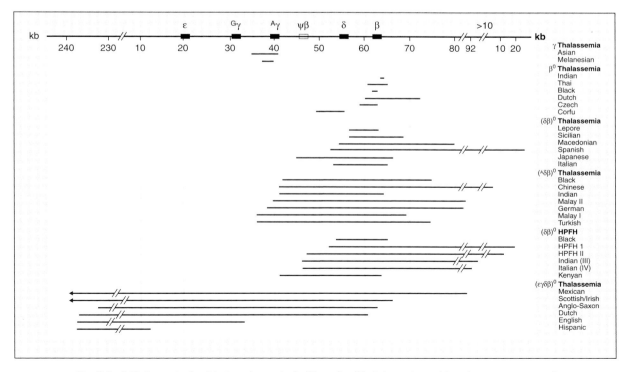

Fig. 9-7. β-Thalassemia: the deletions that underlie δβ- and εγδβ-thalassemias and hereditary persistence of fetal hemoglobin. (Adapted with permission from Weatherall DJ: Genetic disorders of haemoglobin. In Hoffbrand AV, Catovsky D, Tuddenham EGD: *Postgraduate haematology,* ed 5, Oxford 2005, Blackwell Publishing pp 85–103.

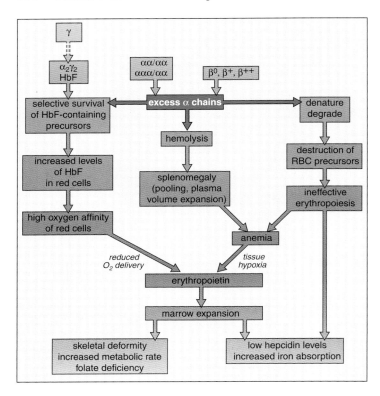

Fig. 9-8. Pathophysiology of β-thalassemia Adapted as Fig. 9-7.

α-thalassemias. Over 400 different genetic lesions have been detected in the β-thalassemias.

β-Thalassemia results in unbalanced synthesis of β chains and non-β (α and γ) chains. The greater the degree of imbalance, the more severe the anemia. Unpaired α chains pair and precipitate in the developing red cell, leading to ineffective erythropoiesis (Fig. 9-8).

β-THALASSEMIA MAJOR

The clinical features of β-thalassemia major result from a severe anemia combined with an intense increase in erythropoiesis, largely ineffective, with excessive bone marrow activity and extramedullary hemopoiesis. In the poorly transfused patient, there is expansion of the flat bones of the face and skull (Figs. 9-9 to 9-12) and expansion of the marrow in all bones (Fig. 9-13). There may be gross osteoporosis and premature fusion of the epiphyses (Fig. 9-14). Even in well-transfused and well-chelated patients, osteoporosis is frequent (Figs. 9-15 and 9-16), especially in males and in association with diabetes mellitus and failure of spontaneous puberty.

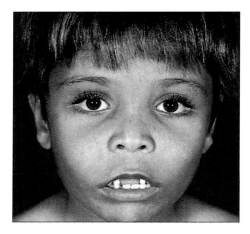

Fig. 9-9. β-Thalassemia major: characteristic facies of a 7-year-old Middle Eastern boy include prominent maxilla and widening of the bridge of the nose. There is also marked bossing of the frontal and parietal bones and zygomata, giving a mongoloid appearance.

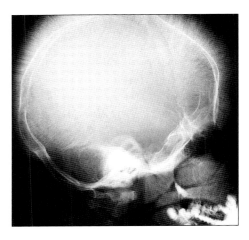

Fig. 9-10. β-Thalassemia major: Lateral radiograph of the skull (same case as shown in Fig. 9-9) shows the typical "hair-on-end" appearance, with thinning of the cortical bone and widening of the marrow cavity.

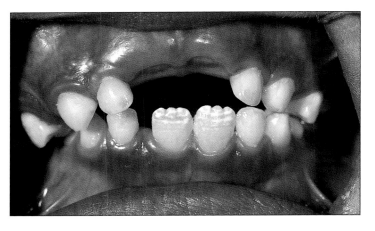

Fig. 9-11. β-Thalassemia major: The teeth (same case as shown in Fig. 9-9) are splayed because of widening of the maxilla and mandible.

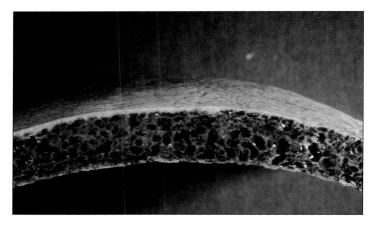

Fig. 9-12. β-Thalassemia major: Section through the skull at necropsy shows marked thinning of the cortices and an open porotic cancellous bone. The mahogany brown color results from extensive iron deposition (hemosiderin), in the marrow. (Courtesy of Dr. P. G. Bullough and Dr. V. J. Vigorita.)

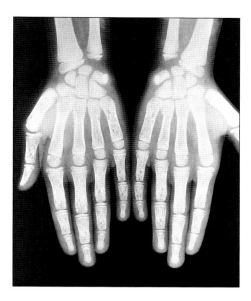

Fig. 9-13. β-Thalassemia major: radiograph of the hands of an undertransfused 7-year-old child. Thinning of the cortical bone results from expansion of the marrow space.

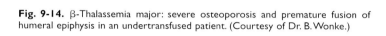

Fig. 9-14. β-Thalassemia major: severe osteoporosis and premature fusion of humeral epiphysis in an undertransfused patient. (Courtesy of Dr. B. Wonke.)

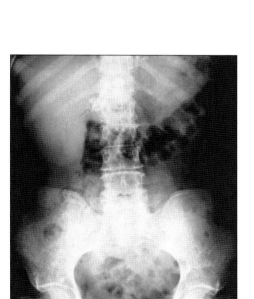

Fig. 9-15. β-Thalassemia major: severe osteoporosis in a patient 30 years of age. Osteoporosis is more common in males, in patients with diabetes mellitus, and in those with failed puberty. (Courtesy of Dr. B. Wonke.)

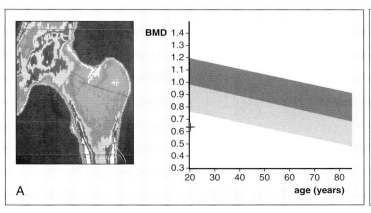

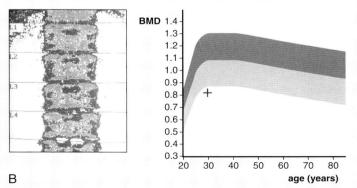

Fig. 9-16. β-Thalassemia major: bone density scans of hip **(A)** and lumbar vertebrae **(B).** The *bands* represent 1.5 standard deviation above and below the mean age-specific bone mineral density (BMD). The *red crosses* indicate the patient's results. (Courtesy of Dr. B. Wonke.)

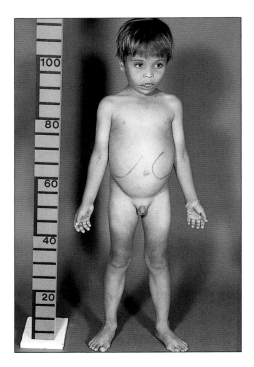

Fig. 9-17. β-Thalassemia major: overall view of the boy shown in Fig. 9-9, showing enlargement of the liver and spleen, and stunted growth. The child had been inadequately transfused since presenting with anemia at age 4 months.

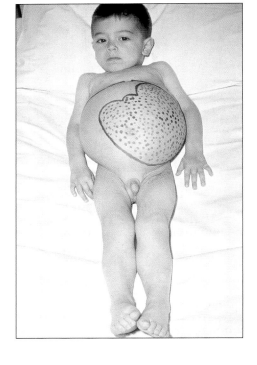

Fig. 9-18. β-Thalassemia major: This 4-year-old, inadequately transfused Cypriot boy has enlargement of the spleen to an unusual degree, which may be partly reversed by adequate transfusion. Splenectomy is usually required but should usually be delayed until the child is older than 6 years of age to reduce the incidence of postoperative fatal infection.

Spontaneous fractures may occur. Another feature is enlargement of the liver and spleen (Figs. 9-17 and 9-18), mainly because of extramedullary erythropoiesis but also from excessive breakdown of red cells and iron overload.

The peripheral blood in the poorly transfused patient shows the presence of hypochromic cells, target cells, and nucleated red cells (Fig. 9-19). Following splenectomy, red cell inclusions increase (e.g., iron granules and Howell-Jolly bodies) and the platelet count is high (Fig. 9-20). The bone marrow shows red cell hyperplasia with pink-staining inclusions of precipitated α-globin chains in the cytoplasm of erythroblasts (Fig. 9-21). Many of the erythroblasts die in the marrow and are digested by macrophages. There is increased iron in the macrophages and increased iron granules in developing erythroblasts (Fig. 9-22).

Much of the bone abnormality can be prevented by regular transfusions from the age of presentation (usually 6 months) to maintain the hemoglobin at all times at a level above 9 to 10 g/dl. However, these regular transfusions, together with increased iron absorption, lead to iron overload. Each unit of blood contains 200 to 250 mg of iron. After 50 units have been transfused, or earlier in children,

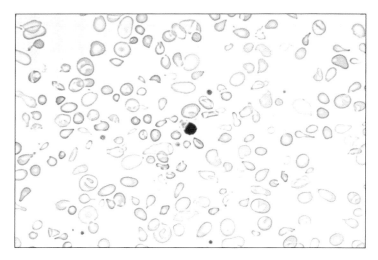

Fig. 9-19. β-Thalassemia major: peripheral blood film showing prominent hypochromic microcytic cells, target cells, and an erythroblast. Some normochromic cells are present from a previous blood transfusion.

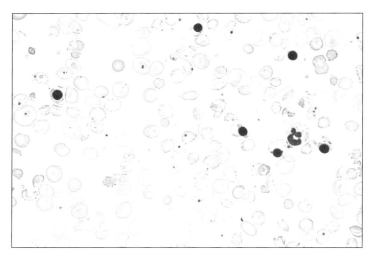

Fig. 9-20. β-Thalassemia major: peripheral blood film after splenectomy in which hypochromic cells, target cells, and erythroblasts are prominent. Pappenheimer and Howell-Jolly bodies are also seen, and the platelet count is raised.

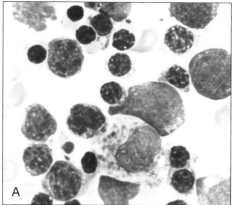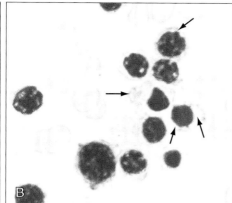

Fig. 9-21. β-Thalassemia major: bone marrow aspirates showing marked erythroid hyperplasia and erythroblasts with vacuolated cytoplasm; degenerate forms and a macrophage that contains pigment are present **(A)**. Erythroblasts with pink-staining cytoplasmic inclusions ("hemoglobin lakes," *arrows*), precipitates of excess α-globin chains **(B)**.

siderosis develops, with increased pigmentation of skin exposed to light (Fig. 9-23) and susceptibility to infection (Fig. 9-24), reduced growth, and delayed sexual development and puberty (Fig. 9-25). Iron overload is also a result of increased iron absorption because hepcidin levels are low due to increased production of a protein (growth differentiation factor 15) by erythroblasts, which inhibits hepcidin synthesis (Fig. 6-12).

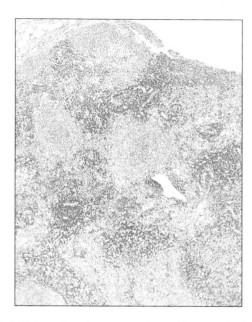

Fig. 9-24. β-Thalassemia major: mesenteric adenitis caused by *Yersinia enterocolitica* infection. The lymph node contains large numbers of granulomas with central necrosis. In keeping with the severity of the disease, the necrosis is more marked than that usually seen. The infection is particularly common in patients with iron overload. (Courtesy of Dr. J. Dyson.)

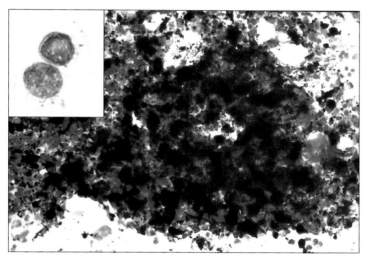

Fig. 9-22. β-Thalassemia major: low-power view of bone marrow fragment showing grossly increased iron stores, largely contained in macrophages as hemosiderin and (seen on electron microscopy) as ferritin. Bone marrow erythroblasts show prominent coarse iron granules *(inset)*. (Perls' stain.)

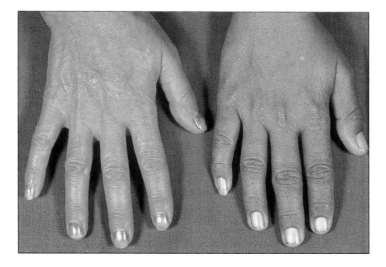

Fig. 9-23. β-Thalassemia major: The hand on the *right* is of a 16-year-old male patient and shows heavy melanin pigmentation; in contrast, his mother's hand (on the *left*) shows normal coloration. For comparison with the appearance of an adult male with genetic (primary) hemochromatosis, see Fig. 6-6.

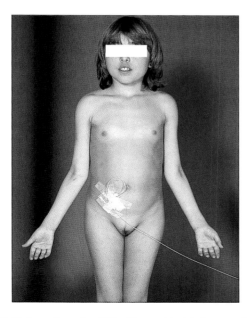

Fig. 9-25. β-Thalassemia major: This 17-year-old girl shows reduced stature (height 134 cm) and delayed pubertal development. Because circulating growth hormone levels are usually normal, the lack of growth results from "end-organ" failure. Subcutaneous infusion of desferrioxamine is in progress.

Bone development is delayed and abnormal (Figs. 9-26 to 9-28). Damage due to iron overloading occurs in the liver (Figs. 9-29 to 9-31) and myocardium (Figs. 9-32 and 9-33). Magnetic resonance imaging (MRI) studies show that the degree of iron loading in the liver and heart may not parallel each other (Fig. 9-34). There is also damage to the endocrine organs, including the pancreas (Figs. 9-35 and 9-36), hypothalamus, pituitary, thyroid, and parathyroids (Fig. 9-37). Iron deposition may occur in bone (Fig. 9-38). Liver damage may also occur because of viral hepatitis from repeated transfusions (Fig. 9-39).

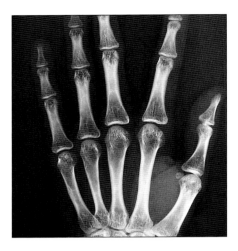

Fig. 9-26. β-Thalassemia major: radiograph of the hand of a 19-year-old man. The estimated bone age is 14 years and there is failure of epiphyseal closure. Widening of the marrow cavity and thinning of trabeculae and cortex are also seen.

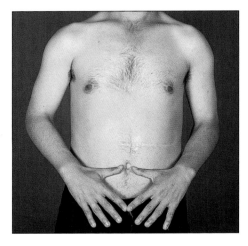

Fig. 9-27. β-Thalassemia major: shortening of the upper arms because of premature epiphyseal closure of the humeral heads.

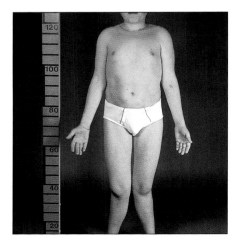

Fig. 9-28. β-Thalassemia major: genu valgum deformity.

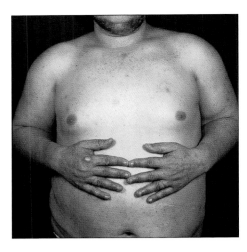

Fig. 9-29. β-Thalassemia major: patient age 37 years who followed an intermedia course for 25 years but then required regular blood transfusions. Heavy melanin pigmentation, a spider nevus, gynecomastia, and a splenectomy scar are seen. He had diabetes mellitus, cirrhosis, hypothyroidism, and hypoparathyroidism.

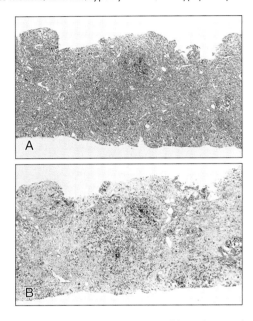

Fig. 9-30. β-Thalassemia major: needle biopsy of liver showing disturbances of normal architecture with fibrosis in portal tracts and nodular regeneration of hepatic parenchymal cells **(A)**; and grade IV siderosis with iron deposition in the hepatic parenchymal cells, bile duct epithelium, macrophages, and fibroblasts **(B)**. (A, H & E. B, Perls' stain.)

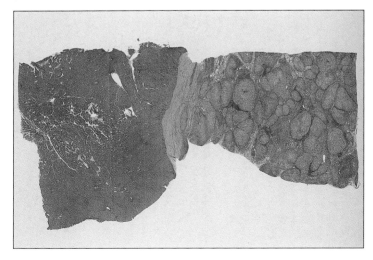

Fig. 9-31. β-Thalassemia major: postmortem section taken from the liver of a 27-year-old male patient dying of hepatocellular carcinoma (on the *left*), with preexisting hepatic cirrhosis (on the *right*) and hepatitis C infection. (Courtesy of Dr. B. Wonke.)

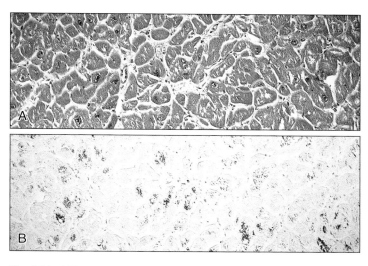

Fig. 9-32. β-Thalassemia major: postmortem sections of myocardium seen by H & E **(A)** and Perls' staining **(B).** The individual muscle fibers contain heavy deposits of iron pigment. In transfusional iron overload, iron deposition is most marked in the left ventricle (shown here) and interventricular septum.

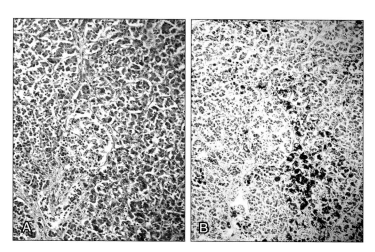

Fig. 9-35. β-Thalassemia major: postmortem sections of pancreas showing pigment (hemosiderin and lipofuscin) in acinar cells, macrophages, and connective tissue, with less obvious pigment in the islet cells **(A);** and gross iron (hemosiderin) deposits in all cell types, particularly marked in the acinar cells **(B).** (*A,* H & E. *B,* Perls' stain.)

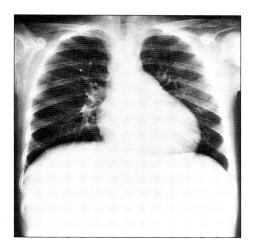

Fig. 9-33. β-Thalassemia major: chest radiograph showing cardiomegaly caused by chronic anemia and iron overload. Enlargement occurs mainly in the ventricles and interventricular septum.

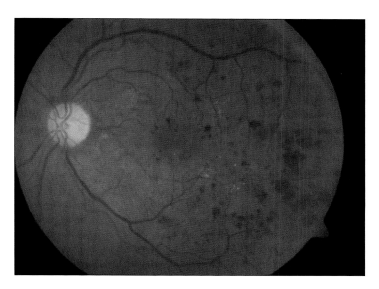

Fig. 9-36. β-Thalassemia major: diabetic retinopathy in a patient with iron overload.

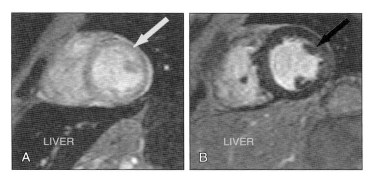

Fig. 9-34. T_2^* magnetic resonance imaging (MRI) studies. Lack of correlation between heart and liver iron. Case **A:** Liver iron overload, myocardial iron appears normal. Case **B:** Myocardial iron overload, liver iron appears normal. For normal appearances see Fig. 6-9. (Courtsey of Professor D. J. Pennell.)

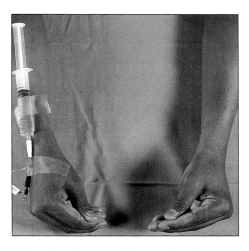

Fig. 9-37. β-Thalassemia major: tetany (Trousseau's sign) as a result of hypoparathyroidism caused by transfusional iron overload. An infusion of calcium is in progress. (Courtesy of Dr. B. Wonke.)

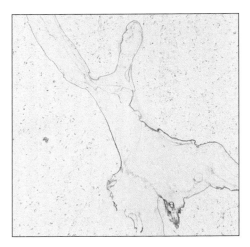

Fig. 9-38. β-Thalassemia major: section of bone showing iron deposition in the cement lines of the trabecula and in macrophages (as hemosiderin) throughout the bone marrow. (Courtesy of Dr. P. G. Bullough and Dr. V. J. Vigorita.)

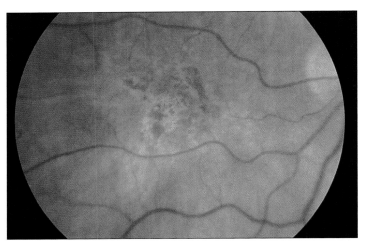

Fig. 9-40. Desferrioxamine toxicity: optic fundus of a 78-year-old man with primary acquired sideroblastic anemia (myelodysplasia) and transfusional iron overload receiving desferrioxamine (2 g) subcutaneously daily and intravenously with blood transfusions. He complained of night blindness and loss of visual acuity. There is degeneration with hyperpigmentation of the macula.

Iron overload may, however, be substantially reduced by iron chelation therapy. This may be achieved by daily subcutaneous desferrioxamine infusions (see Fig. 9-25). The iron is then excreted as ferrioxamine in the urine, which appears red, and in bile. Orally active iron chelators are now increasingly used.

Complications of desferrioxamine therapy may include ototoxicity with high tone deafness, retinal damage (Fig. 9-40), and, in children, pseudorickets, changes in the bones (Fig. 9-41), or spinal platyspondyly in some cases with intervertebral calcification (Fig. 9-42), which may be accompanied by reduced growth. Alternative orally acting iron chelators include 1,2-dimethyl-3-hydroxypyrid-4-one (deferiprone) (Fig. 9-43) and deferasirox (Exjade). Deferiprone is usually given three times daily. Side effects that have occurred include agranulocytosis, joint pains or effusions, and (rarely) zinc deficiency (Fig. 9-44). Deferasirox, which is given only once daily, causes mainly fecal iron excretion. Side effects include skin rashes and renal dysfunction.

Splenectomy may be needed to reduce transfusion requirements. Other supportive measures include folic acid, hepatitis immunization, and pneumococcal, hemophilus, and meningococcal immunization, plus regular prophylactic penicillin. Hormonal replacement therapy is needed in some cases, and calcium, vitamin D, and bisphosphonates for osteoporosis. Thalassemia major may also be cured by stem cell transplantation (Fig. 9-45).

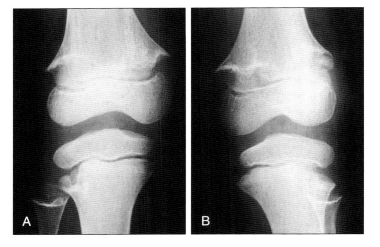

Fig. 9-41. Desferrioxamine toxicity. **A** and **B,** Pseudorickets in the knees of a child with β-thalassemia major who is receiving desferrioxamine therapy. There is flaring of the metaphyses and poor mineralization of the distal metaphyses with normal epiphyses. (Courtesy of Dr. V. DeSanctis.)

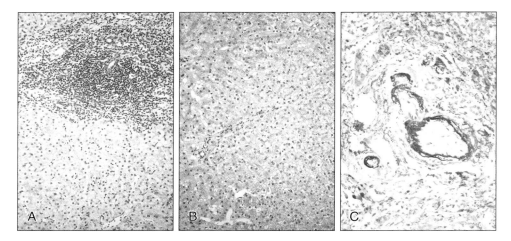

Fig. 9-39. β-Thalassemia major. **A,** Liver biopsy showing heavy infiltration of portal tracts by lymphocytes. The serum was positive for hepatitis C RNA. Following 6 months' therapy with α-interferon, there was considerable improvement in hepatic function and liver biopsy showed clearing of the lymphocyte infiltration **(B). C,** Liver biopsy showing heavy siderosis in parenchymal cells and in walls of vessels and sinuses (ferrocalcinosis). (A and B, H & E. C, Perls' stain.)

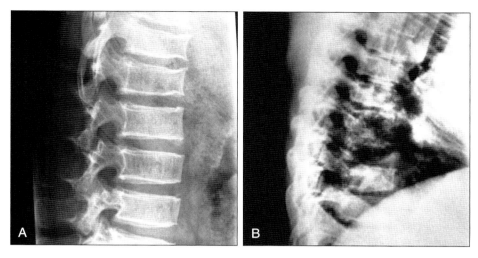

Fig. 9-42. Desferrioxamine toxicity: platyspondyly of the spine. (**A,** Courtesy of Dr. P. Tyler and *British Journal of Radiology.* **B,** Courtesy of Dr. B. Wonke)

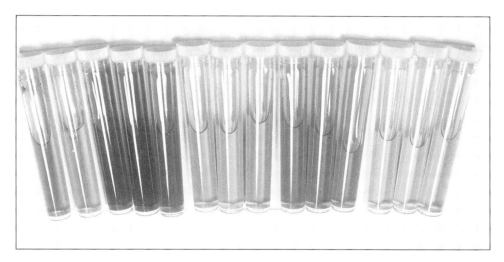

Fig. 9-43. Myelodysplastic syndrome: urine samples without (yellow) and with chelation therapy for transfusional iron overload. Subcutaneous desferrioxamine has resulted in orange urine, whereas oral deferiprone has resulted in a darker, red urine.

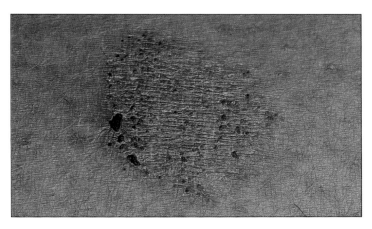

Fig. 9-44. Oral iron chelation: zinc deficiency causing raised, dry, itchy scaling patch in a patient receiving deferiprone (L1) long term.

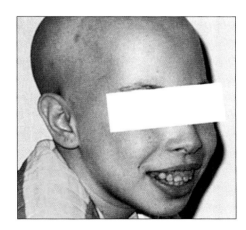

Fig. 9-45. β-Thalassemia major: A 14-year-old girl, after marrow transplantation from a human leukocyte antigen (HLA)–matched sibling, shows hair loss as a result of chemotherapy and bossing of the skull. (Courtesy of Professor C. Luccarelli.)

β-THALASSEMIA INTERMEDIA

The causes of β-thalassemia intermedia are listed in Table 9-2. One form results from homozygous hemoglobin Lepore (Fig. 9-46) or heterozygous Lepore in conjunction with another β chain abnormally. β-Thalassemia intermedia is compatible with normal growth and development (Fig. 9-47) but is characterized by bone deformities (Fig. 9-48), extramedullary hematopoiesis (Fig. 9-49), and iron overload. Ankle ulcers (Fig. 9-50), probably the result of anoxia caused by anemia and stasis of the local circulation, may arise as in thalassemia major, sickle cell anemia, and other hemolytic anemias. Unusually, thalassemia intermedia may cause a connective tissue pseudoxanthoma-elasticum–like syndrome with ocular changes (Fig. 9-51), arterial calcification (Fig. 9-52), and skin lesions (Fig. 9-53).

Iron overload in thalassemia intermedia because of increased absorption and blood transfusion is treated by chelation and possible gentle venesections.

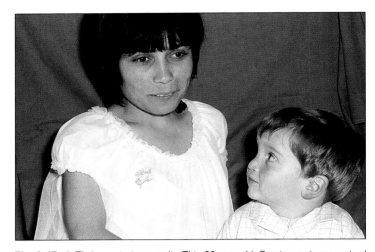

Fig. 9-47. β-Thalassemia intermedia: This 29-year-old Cypriot patient received occasional blood transfusions, with her hemoglobin ranging between 6.5 and 9.0 g/dl. She displays a thalassemic facies with marked maxillary expansion and also developed pigment gallstones. She has normal sexual development and fertility, as shown by her 2-year-old son.

TABLE 9-2.   CAUSES OF THALASSEMIA INTERMEDIA

Mild forms of β-thalassemia

Homozygosity for mild β+-thalassemia alleles
Compound heterozygosity for two mild β+-thalassemia alleles
Compound heterozygosity for a mild and more severe β-thalassemia allele

Inheritance of α- and β-thalassemia

β+-thalassemia with α⁰-thalassemia (− −/αα)
or with α+-thalassemia (−α/αα or −α/−α)
β+-thalassemia with genotype of HbH disease (− −/−α)

β-Thalassemia with elevated γ-chain synthesis

Homozygous β-thalassemia with heterocellular HPFH
Homozygous β-thalassemia with Gγ or Aγ promoter mutations
Compound heterozygosity for β-thalassemia and deletion forms of HPFH

Compound heterozygosity for β-thalassemia and β-chain variants

HbE/β-thalassemia
Other interactions with rare β-chain variants

Heterozygous β-thalassemia with triplicated α-chain genes (ααα)

Dominant forms of β-thalassemia

Interactions of β and (δβ)+ or (δβ)⁰-thalassemia

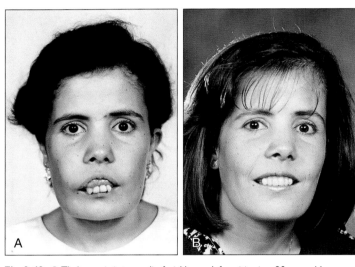

Fig. 9-48. β-Thalassemia intermedia: facial bone deformities in a 20-year-old woman. **A,** Before surgery. **B,** After surgical correction. (*A, B,* Courtesy Dr. B. Wonke.)

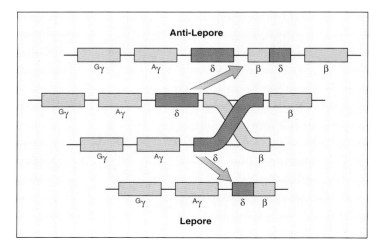

Fig. 9-46. Structure of hemoglobin-Lepore and anti-Lepore. These structural abnormalities are caused by crossing over of the δ- and β-globin genes at meiosis.

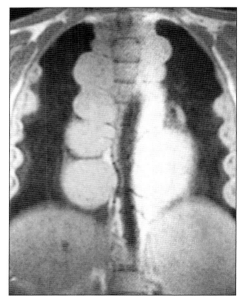

Fig. 9-49. β-Thalassemia intermedia: magnetic resonance imaging (MRI) scan from a 42-year-old Turkish patient with bossing of the skull bones, maxillary expansion, and splenomegaly (Hb, 9.7 g/dl; MCV, 78 fl; MCH, 23.5 pg; hemoglobin electrophoresis: Hb F, 98%; Hb A2, 2.0%). The scan shows masses of extramedullary hematopoietic tissue arising from the ribs and in the paravertebral region without encroachment of the spinal cord.

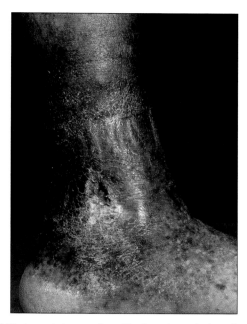

Fig. 9-50. β-Thalassemia intermedia: ankle ulcer above the lateral malleolus.

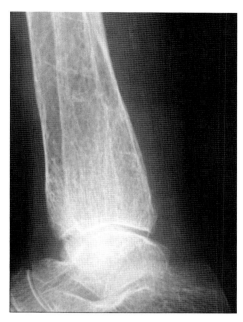

Fig. 9-52. Lateral x-ray of the tibia in a middle-aged patient with thalassemia intermedia showing calcification of the anterior and posterior tibial arteries. (With permission from Aessopos A et al: *Haematologica* 92:658–665, 2007.)

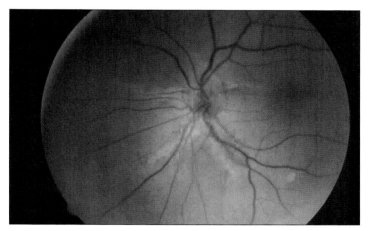

Fig. 9-51. Optic fundus of a thalassemia intermedia patient showing angioid streaks, the typical ocular manifestation of hemoglobinopathy-related pseudoxanthoma elasticum–like syndrome. (With permission from Aessopos A et al: *Haematologica* 92:658–665, 2007.)

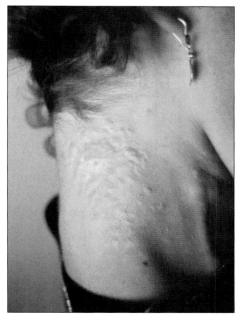

Fig. 9-53. Skin changes of thalassemia intermedia, typical manifestation of hemoglobinopathy-related pseudoxanthoma elasticum–like syndrome. (With permission from Aessopos A et al: *Haematologica* 92:658–665, 2007.)

β-THALASSEMIA TRAIT

In β-thalassemia trait there is a hypochromic microcytic blood picture with a high red cell count ($>5.5 \times 10^{12}$/L; Fig. 9-54) and raised hemoglobin A2 percentage on hemoglobin electrophoresis.

β-THALASSEMIA WITH A DOMINANT PHENOTYPE

β-Thalassemia with a dominant phenotype refers to a subgroup of β-thalassemias that result in a thalassemia intermedia phenotype in individuals who have inherited only a single copy of the abnormal β gene. Usually mutations affect exon 3 of the β-globin gene (Fig. 9-55). There is production of long unstable globin-gene protein, which, together with excess α chains, produces inclusions in normoblasts and red cells. The clinical features are those of a severe dyserythropoietic anemia associated with splenomegaly. The inclusion bodies are seen in the bone marrow and in peripheral red cells after splenectomy (Fig. 9-56). These inclusion bodies can be visualized after methyl violet staining of fresh blood. A spectrum of different mutations underlying these dominantly inherited forms of β-thalassemia have been identified, and it is now clear that the phenotype of these disorders overlaps both the β-thalassemias and the unstable hemoglobin variants.

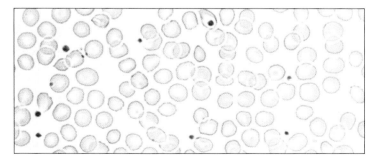

Fig. 9-54. β-Thalassemia trait: peripheral blood film from a 20-year-old Cypriot woman shows microcytic hypochromic red cells with occasional target cells and poikilocytes. The red cell indices show a much reduced MCV (60.3 fl) and MCH (18.6 pg), despite the levels of the hemoglobin (10.8 g/dl) and packed cell volume (PCV, 35%) being only slightly below normal. The red cell count was raised to 5.81 $\times 10^{12}$/L, and hemoglobin electrophoresis showed a raised hemoglobin A2 (4.5%) with a normal hemoglobin F (0.9%).

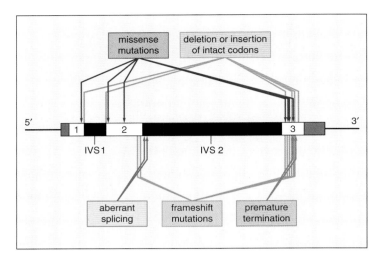

Fig. 9-55. β-Thalassemia: dominant phenotype. Dominantly inherited β-thalassemia. (Courtesy of Professor S. L. Thein.)

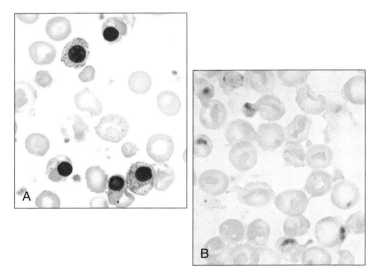

Fig. 9-56. β-Thalassemia: dominant phenotype. Peripheral blood postsplenectomy: **A,** May-Grünwald/Giemsa stain showing target cells, irregular contracted cells, punctate basophilia, and numerous erythroblasts; **B,** methyl violet stain showing inclusion bodies *(pink)* caused by precipitated α-globin chains. (*A* and *B,* Courtesy of Professor S. L. Thein.)

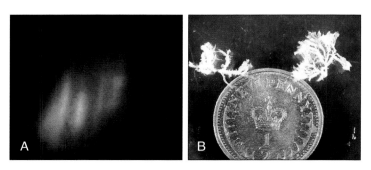

Fig. 9-57. Antenatal diagnosis. **A,** Fetal veins at 14 weeks, as seen through a fetoscope. **B,** Chorionic villus biopsy from a 12-week-old fetus. (*A,* Courtesy of C. Rodeck. *B,* Courtesy of J. W. Keeling.)

ANTENATAL DIAGNOSIS

If both parents are carriers of β-thalassemia or other genetic defects likely to lead to a severe hemoglobin defect in the child, fetal diagnosis is carried out. Initially it was performed using fetoscopy to obtain fetal blood (Fig. 9-57, *A*) and measuring the α/β chain synthesis ratio. It is now usually carried out by amniocentesis or trophoblast biopsy (Fig. 9-57, *B*) to obtain deoxyribonucleic acid (DNA) for analysis by one or other polymerase chain reaction (PCR) technique (Figs. 9-58 to 9-60). Restriction fragment length polymorphism (RFLP) analysis is used if the genetic defect is unknown (Fig. 9-61). Severely affected fetuses can then be aborted. The fall in incidence of the disease in Sardinia between 1975 and 1991 with the introduction of antenatal diagnosis is shown in Fig. 9-62.

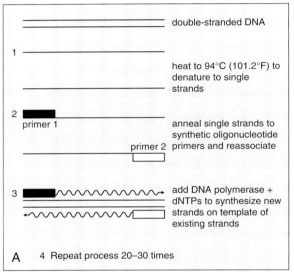

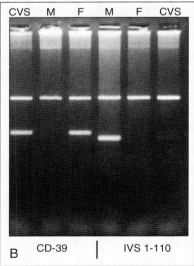

Fig. 9-58. α-Thalassemia: antenatal diagnosis. **A,** Polymerase chain reaction (PCR). Two primers are used, hybridizing to DNA on either side of the section of DNA to be amplified. Cycles of synthesis of new DNA using a heat-resistant DNA Taq polymerase and deoxynucleoside triphosphates (dNTPs), denaturation and synthesis of new DNA result in rapid amplification of the DNA over a million times. **B,** The rapid prenatal diagnosis of β-thalassemia by "mismatched PCR" amplification refractory mutation system (ARMS). One parent has the common Mediterranean codon 39 (CD-39) mutation, the other the IVS1-110 G→A mutation. The fetus is heterozygous for the CD-39 mutation. *CVS,* Fetal DNA from chorionic villus sampling; *F,* father; *M,* mother. (Courtesy of Dr. J. Old and Professor D. J. Weatherall and modified from Hoffbrand AV, Pettit JE: *Essential haematology,* ed 3, Oxford, 1993, Blackwell Scientific.)

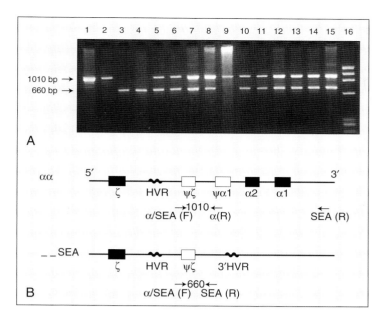

Fig. 9-59. α-Thalassemia: antenatal diagnosis for the Southeast Asian α⁰-thalassemia deletion mutation (_ _SEA) by gap-polymerase chain analysis. Two primers (α/SEA forward and α reverse) are used to amplify 1010 bp fragment of normal DNA across the gap of the deleted sequence, and two primers are used to amplify a 660 bp fragment across the gap of the deleted sequence of the (_ _SEA) allele (α/SEA forward and α/SEA reverse). The latter two primers are too far apart to produce a fragment from the normal DNA (αα). The pattern of amplified products designates the α-genotype of each DNA sample. Lanes 1 and 2 show normal DNA; lanes 3 and 4 show hydrops fetalis control DNA; lanes 5 to 8 show heterozygous control DNA samples; lanes 7 to 9 show a heterozygous chorionic villus sample (CVS) DNA sample at three different concentrations (note allele dropout in the most dilute sample in lane 9); lanes 10 to 12 show paternal DNA; lanes 13 to 15 show maternal DNA; and lane 16 shows marker fragments. (Courtesy of Dr. John Old.)

Fig. 9-61. α-Thalassemia: restriction fragment length polymorphism (RFLP) analysis. A new restriction enzyme site, resulting from a polymorphic change in DNA close to a gene to be studied, reduces the size of the fragment of DNA produced by a restriction enzyme. The DNA is separated in a gel and the smaller size fragment is detected after using a probe for the gene. The size of fragment may also be different if the DNA close to the gene and between restriction sites contains a region that is hypervariable in size between individuals. The PCR technique can also be used instead of Southern blotting to detect RFLPs, providing primers on either side of the segment to be analyzed are available. (Modified from Hoffbrand AV, Pettit JE: *Essential haematology*, ed 3, Oxford, 1993, Blackwell Scientific.)

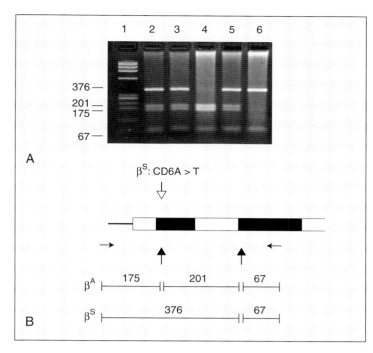

Fig. 9-60. Sickle cell disease: antenatal diagnosis by DdeI-PCR. Two primers are used to amplify a 433 bp fragment of DNA at the 5′-end of the β-globin gene. The amplified product is then digested with the restriction enzyme DdeI, which cuts the fragment at codon 6 and at the end of the intervening sequence I (IVSI). The presence of the sickle cell mutation changes the DNA sequence at codon 6, abolishing the DdeI site. Thus sickle cell DNA produces two fragments 367 and 67 bp long, and normal DNA produces three fragments 201, 175, and 67 bp long. The fragment pattern reveals the β-genotype of the DNA. Lane 1 has marker DNA fragments; lane 2, maternal DNA (Hb S trait); lane 3, CVS DNA (Hb S trait); lane 4, normal control DNA; lane 5, AS control DNA; and lane 6, SS control DNA. (Courtesy of Dr. John Old.)

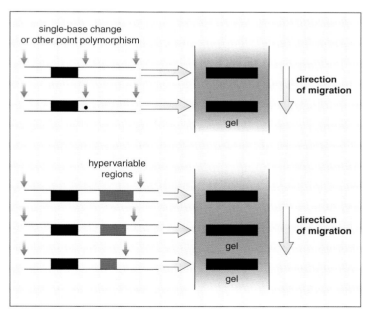

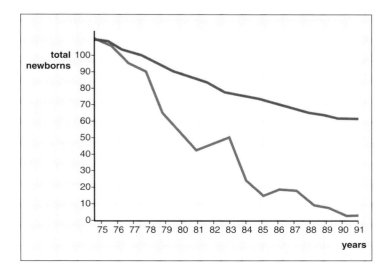

Fig. 9-62. β-Thalassemia: fall in the birth rate of homozygous β-thalassemia in Sardinia after the introduction of genetic counselling and antenatal diagnosis. The upper curve shows the predicted number of births without antenatal diagnosis, and the lower curve shows the actual number. (Courtesy of Professor Anthony Cao.)

α-THALASSEMIA

α-Thalassemia results from deletion or inactivation of one or more of the four α-globin genes (Fig. 9-63). The α-thalassemias are classified according to the number of genes affected. There is duplication of the α-globin genes. In the α^0 lesion, both α genes on one chromosome are deleted or ineffective; in the milder α^+ lesion, only one of the two genes is deleted or defective (Fig. 9-63).

The gene deletions that produce α-thalassemia are shown in Fig. 9-64. In its most severe form, in which all four genes are deleted, α-thalassemia is incompatible with life and the fetus is stillborn or critically ill with hydrops fetalis (Fig. 9-65). The blood shows gross hypochromasia and erythroblastosis (Fig. 9-66).

Deletion of three α-globin genes (hemoglobin H disease) manifests as a moderately severe anemia (Hb, 7.0 to 11.0 g/dl) with splenomegaly and a hypochromic, microcytic blood film appearance (Fig. 9-67). Hemoglobin H (β4) is demonstrable by special staining (Fig. 9-68) or hemoglobin electrophoresis.

α-Thalassemia trait may be caused by deletion of two genes (α^0 trait). The α^+ trait may result from deletion of one of the pair of linked α-globin genes. In others both α genes are present, but one has a mutation or other genetic effect that partly or completely inactivates it. α-Thalassemia trait shows a hypochromic, microcytic blood appearance of varying severity in adults. At birth, as much as 5% to 15% of Hb Bart's (γ4) may be detected in α^0 trait and up to 2% in α^+ trait. In α^0 trait, an occasional cell in the adult blood film may show Hb H bodies after incubation with a dye such as brilliant cresyl blue.

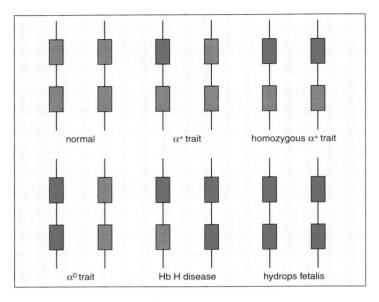

Fig. 9-63. α-Thalassemia: the different types of α-thalassemia. The *purple boxes* represent normal genes, and the *gray boxes* represent gene deletions or partially or completely inactivated genes.

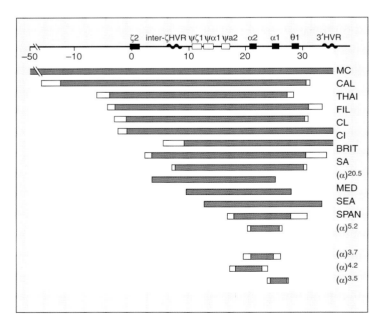

Fig. 9-64. α-Thalassemia: the deletions that produce α-thalassemia. The missing DNA is indicated by *black lines.* α^0-Thalassemia results from deletion of both linked α-globin genes or mutations that completely inactivate both (not shown). α^+-Thalassemia results from either deletion of one of the pair of linked α-globin genes or from a mutation that inactivates one of them partly or completely. One mutation affects the chain termination codon TAA and results in an elongated α chain (Hemoglobin Constant Spring), which is synthesized at a slower rate than normal. (Courtesy of Professor D. J. Weatherall.)

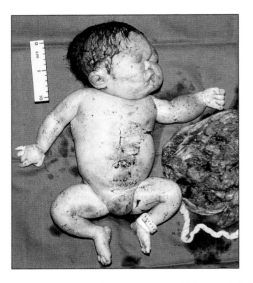

Fig. 9-65. α-Thalassemia: hydrops fetalis, the result of deletion of all four α-globin genes (homozygous α^0-thalassemia). The main hemoglobin present is Hb Bart's (g4). The condition is incompatible with life beyond the fetal stage. (Courtesy of Professor D. Todd.)

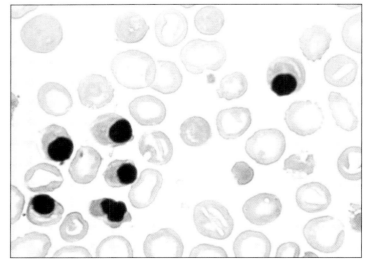

Fig. 9-66. α-Thalassemia: Peripheral blood film in homozygous α^0-thalassemia (hydrops fetalis) at birth shows marked hypochromasia, polychromasia, and many circulating erythroblasts.

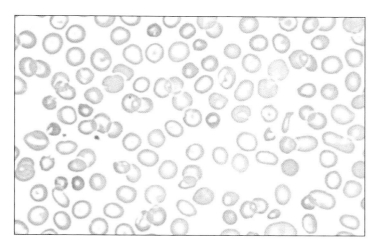

Fig. 9-67. α-Thalassemia: Peripheral blood film in hemoglobin H disease (three α-globin gene deletion or α^0/α^+-thalassemia) shows marked hypochromic and microcytic cells with target cells and poikilocytes. The patient was a normally developed 23-year-old man with a spleen enlarged to 6 cm below the costal margin, moderate anemia (Hb, 9.9 g/dl), and grossly reduced red cell indices. (MCV, 59 fl; MCH, 19 pg.) Electrophoresis showed Hb A, 76.6%; Hb A2, 2.5%; Hb F, 0.9%; Hb H (β4), 20%.

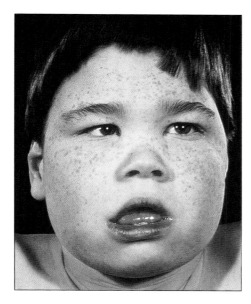

Fig. 9-69. α-Thalassemia/mental retardation syndrome: boy with characteristic dysmorphic facies. (Courtesy of Professor D. R. Higgs.)

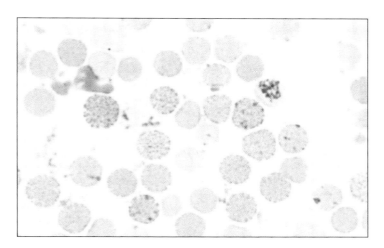

Fig. 9-68. α-Thalassemia: peripheral blood film in hemoglobin H disease stained supravitally with brilliant cresyl blue. Some of the cells show multiple, fine, deeply staining deposits, which are precipitated aggregates of α-globin chains ("golf ball" cells). Reticulocytes are also stained.

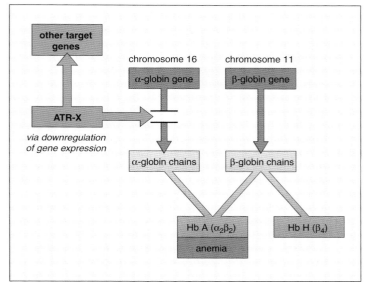

Fig. 9-70. α-Thalassemia/mental retardation syndrome: action of ATR-X (see text) on expression of α-globin and other genes. (Courtesy of Professor D. R. Higgs.)

X-LINKED α-THALASSEMIA AND MENTAL RETARDATION SYNDROME

The X-linked α-thalassemia and mental retardation (ATR-X) syndrome is characterized by a severe form of mental retardation associated with characteristic dysmorphic facies (Fig. 9-69), genital abnormalities, and an unusual, mild form of Hb H disease. In comparison with α-thalassemia caused by deletions or point mutations in the α-globin cluster on chromosome 16p13.3, hypochromia and microcytosis are less prominent and, in some affected individuals, the red cell indices may fall in the normal range. Red cells with Hb H inclusions can be demonstrated after incubation at room temperature in 1% brilliant cresyl blue solution. The frequency of such cells varies widely (0.001% to 40% red cells).

Carrier females are of normal appearance and intelligence. About 25% may exhibit very rare Hb H inclusions, and this reflects the very skewed pattern of X inactivation present, with the disease-bearing X chromosome being preferentially inactive.

The disease gene usually responsible for the syndrome has been identified and maps to Xq13.3. It is called the *ATR-X* gene and is a member of a family of proteins (SWI/SNF) with ATPase and putative helicase activity. Members of this group have a wide range of functions, but it is thought that they all act by interaction with chromatin. It seems likely that ATR-X acts on its target genes (including a-globin) as a transcriptional regulator (Fig. 9-70).

STRUCTURAL HEMOGLOBIN VARIANTS

SICKLE CELL ANEMIA

Sickle cell anemia is the most common of the severe structural hemoglobin variants (Table 9-3). It is the result of substitution of valine for glutamic acid in the sixth position of the β chain, caused by a single base change in the corresponding portion of DNA. Sickle

TABLE 9-3.   STRUCTURAL
HEMOGLOBIN
VARIANTS: DISEASES

Sickle syndromes
Sickle cell (SS) anemia
Sickle cell/hemoglobin C (SC)
Sickle cell/hemoglobin D (SD)
Sickle cell/β-thalassemia
Hemolytic anemia
Unstable hemoglobin
Polycythemia
High oxygen affinity hemoglobin
Methemoglobinemia
Hemoglobin M
Thalassemia syndromes
Hemoglobin Lepore
Chain-termination hemoglobins
Some unstable hemoglobins

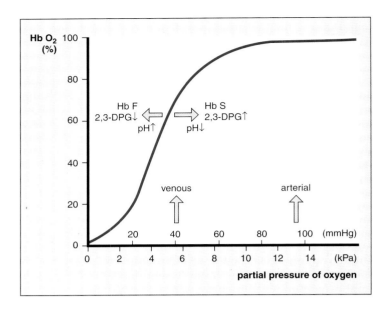

Fig. 9-72. Hemoglobin-oxygen dissociation. Normal sigmoid curve relating Hb saturation to the partial pressure of oxygen (PaO₂) to which it is exposed. The curve is shifted to the left (less oxygen is released at any given PaO₂) by a fall in 2,3-DPG, by a rise in pH (Bohr effect), or if Hb A is replaced by Hb F or by a high-affinity Hb. The curve is shifted to the right by a rise in 2,3-DPG attached to the Hb, by a fall in pH, if Hb A is replaced by Hb S or an Hb M (in which the heme iron is stabilized in the ferric form), or if the Hb is oxidized to methemoglobin.

hemoglobin (Hb S) is insoluble at low oxygen partial pressures and tends to crystallize (Fig. 9-71), which causes the red cells to assume a sickle-like appearance. The oxygen is given up to tissues relatively easily because the oxygen dissociation curve is shifted to the right (Fig. 9-72).

The patient has few symptoms of anemia, despite a hemoglobin level in the steady state of 6 to 8 g/dl, and has a chronic hemolytic anemia punctuated by sickle crises. Typically, the patient is of asthenic build (Fig. 9-73) and is mildly jaundiced. Ulcers around the ankle are common (Fig. 9-74).

Bone deformities may be present (Figs. 9-75 to 9-77). If the small bones of the hands and feet are affected, there may be unequal growth of the digits ("hand-foot" syndrome; Figs. 9-78 to 9-81).

As a result of infections together with infarcts, pneumonia (Fig. 9-82) may occur; it may be difficult to distinguish from the chest syndrome caused by blockage of small vessels and fat embolism from infarcted bones, especially the ribs (Figs. 9-83 and 9-84). The central nervous system may be damaged by infarction. Transcranial Doppler studies may help determine the risk of a stroke by showing increased blood flow due to arterial stenosis (Fig. 9-85). Ischemic damage in the

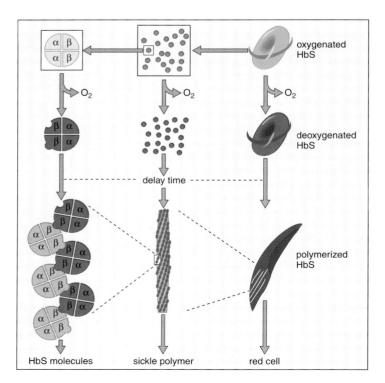

Fig. 9-71. Sickle cell anemia: pathophysiology. (Adapted from Bunn HF: *N Engl J Med* 337:762, 1997.)

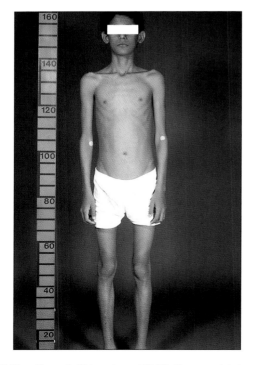

Fig. 9-73. Sickle cell anemia: This patient of Middle Eastern origin is tall with long thin limbs, a large arm span, and narrow pectoral and pelvic girdles. Sexual development is normal.

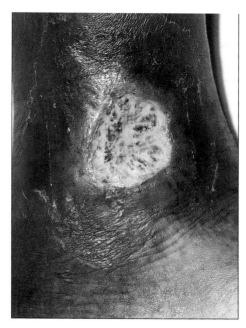

Fig. 9-74. Sickle cell anemia: ulcer above ankle.

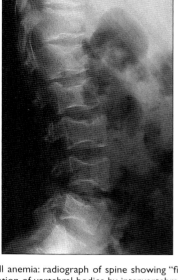

Fig. 9-77. Sickle cell anemia: radiograph of spine showing "fish bone" deformity as a result of indentation of vertebral bodies by intervertebral discs.

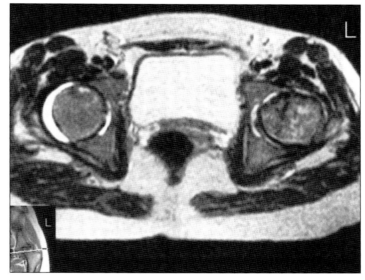

Fig. 9-75. Sickle cell/β-thalassemia: axial T₂-weighted magnetic resonance imaging (MRI) scan of the hips of a 17-year-old female showing a small area of high signal in the anterior portion of the right hip with a low-intensity rim. This is typical of early avascular necrosis. The irregular outline and signal in the left hip results from more advanced avascular necrosis.

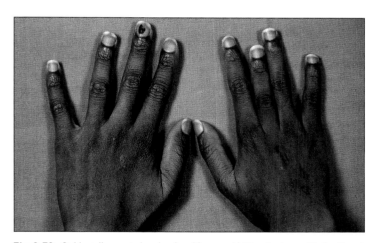

Fig. 9-78. Sickle cell anemia: hands of an 18-year-old Nigerian boy with the "hand-foot" syndrome. There is marked shortening of the right middle finger because the dactylitis in childhood affected the growth of the epiphysis.

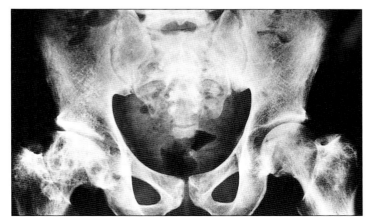

Fig. 9-76. Sickle cell anemia: Radiograph of the pelvis shows avascular necrosis with flattening of the femoral heads, more marked on the right; coarsening of the bone architecture; and cystic areas in the right femoral neck caused by previous infarcts.

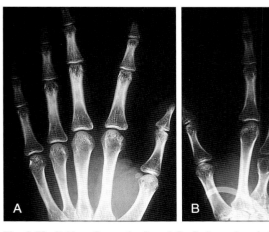

Fig. 9-79. Sickle cell anemia. **A** and **B,** Radiographs of the hands shown in Fig. 9-78. The right middle metacarpal bone is shortened because of infarction of the growing epiphysis during childhood. The patient was receiving intravenous rehydration during a painful crisis.

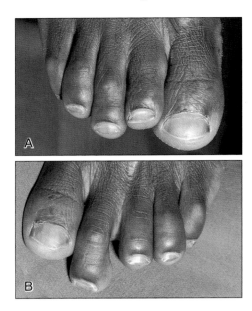

Fig. 9-80. Sickle cell anemia. **A** and **B,** The toes of the patient in Fig. 9-78 show irregularities in length.

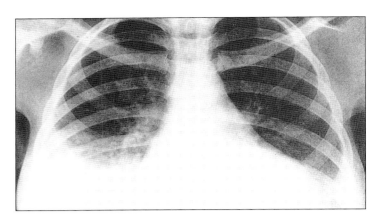

Fig. 9-82. Sickle cell anemia: chest radiograph of an 18-year old female admitted in crisis with a pulmonary syndrome. There is generalized cardiomegaly and increased vascularity of the lungs, typical of a chronic hemolytic anemia. In addition, there is shadowing, particularly in the right lower and middle lobes, which resolved slowly on antibiotic therapy and was considered to result from infection and small vessel obstruction.

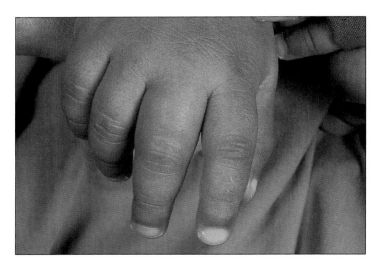

Fig. 9-81. Sickle cell anemia: hand of an 18-month-old child with painful, swollen fingers (dactylitis) caused by infarction of the metacarpal bones of the index and ring fingers. This acute syndrome rarely occurs after 2 years of age.

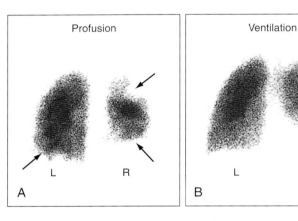

Fig. 9-83. Sickle cell anemia: Ventilation-perfusion lung scan of the patient in Fig. 9-82 shows perfusion measured with technetium 99m-aggregated albumin (50-mm particles) **(A)** and ventilation using krypton 81m **(B).** The ventilation defect at the base of the right lung *(R)* suggests infection only, but the multiple perfusion defects apparent in other areas of both lungs *(arrows)* suggest blockage of segmental and subsegmental arteries. (*A, B,* Courtesy of Dr. A. Hilson.)

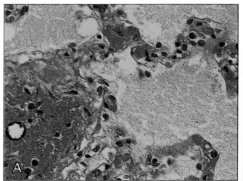

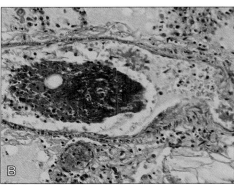

Fig. 9-84. Sickle cell anemia: chest syndrome. **A,** High-power view of lung showing alveolar edema, fat embolism within an arteriole surrounded by sickle cells, and microthrombi in the alveolar capillaries. Fat embolism is the white nonstaining hole (from which fat has dissolved out in processing). **B,** High-power view of an arteriole showing fat embolism with associated thrombus. (*A,* H & E. *B,* Martius scarlet blue with fibrin staining red.) (*A* and *B,* Courtesy of Professor S. Lucas.)

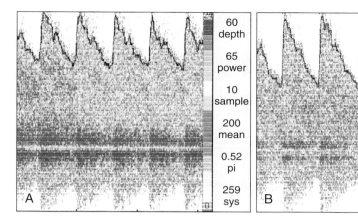

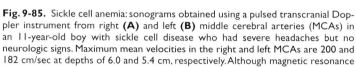

Fig. 9-85. Sickle cell anemia: sonograms obtained using a pulsed transcranial Doppler instrument from right **(A)** and left **(B)** middle cerebral arteries (MCAs) in an 11-year-old boy with sickle cell disease who had severe headaches but no neurologic signs. Maximum mean velocities in the right and left MCAs are 200 and 182 cm/sec at depths of 6.0 and 5.4 cm, respectively. Although magnetic resonance imaging (MRI) was normal, magnetic resonance angiography showed bilateral turbulence, suggestive of stenosis in both MCAs. For patients with an MCA velocity >200 cm/sec, the risk of stroke within 40 months is 40%; this child was therefore commenced on regular transfusions with resolution of his headaches. (*A* and *B*, Courtesy of Dr. J. P. M. Evans and Dr. F. Kirkham.)

brain occurs as a result of stenosis or occlusions of vessels in the circle of Willis and internal carotid arteries. Sometimes moyamoya disease with a plethora of small vessels in a damaged area of brain develops (Figs. 9-86 and 9-87). Osteomyelitis may also occur, usually from *Salmonella* spp. (Fig. 9-88), but sometimes from other organisms (Fig. 9-89). Parvovirus infection may cause an "aplastic" crisis. Infarcts may also occur in the kidney, and papillary necrosis is particularly common (Fig. 9-90). Priapism is a common problem in males.

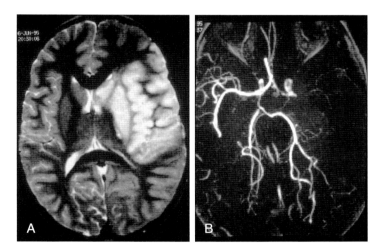

Fig. 9-86. Sickle cell anemia: right-sided frontal and temporal lobe infarction due to blocked middle cerebral artery. **A,** T2 weighted MRI; **B,** MR angiogram.

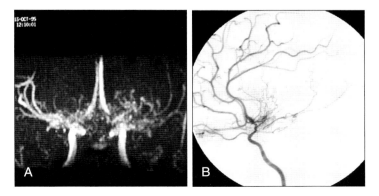

Fig. 9-87. Sickle cell anemia: moyamoya arterial deformation. There is revascularization with small vessels after a major arterial occlusion. **A,** MR angiogram; **B,** carotid angiogram.

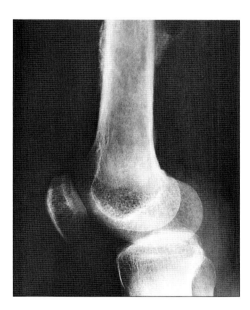

Fig. 9-88. Sickle cell anemia: lateral radiograph of the lower limb and knee in *Salmonella* osteomyelitis. The periosteum is irregularly raised in the lower third of the femur.

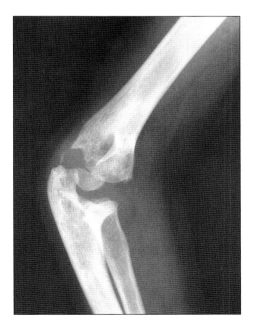

Fig. 9-89. Sickle cell anemia: Lateral radiograph of the elbow joint in *Staphylococcal* osteomyelitis shows destructive changes in the humerus and ulna.

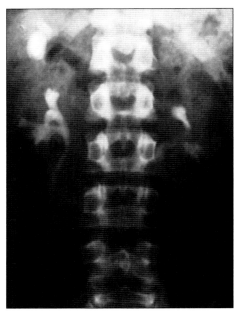

Fig. 9-90. Sickle cell anemia: intravenous pyelogram. There is clubbing of the caly-ceal outline in the left kidney. The patient, a 24-year-old man, also shows two large opaque pigment gallstones. The bone trabeculae in the ribs and vertebrae are fine because of expanded erythropoiesis.

Following occlusion of small vessels in the retina during sickle cell crises, there may be characteristic regrowth of blood vessels at the affected sites (Fig. 9-91). Infarction and atrophy of the spleen are usual after childhood (Fig. 9-92).

The blood film shows the presence of sickle cells and target cells (Fig. 9-93), as well as, in most adult cases, features of splenic atrophy (Fig. 9-94). The hematopoietic marrow expands down the long bones (Fig. 9-95), and the myeloid-to-erythroid ratio is reversed.

Laboratory diagnosis is made by measuring the hemoglobin S percentage in blood. The different types of hemoglobin may be separated and quantitated by electrophoresis in cellulose acetate (Fig. 9-96) or agar gel or by high-performance liquid chromatography (Fig. 9-97).

Sickle cell trait gives a normal blood appearance, possibly with an occasional sickle cell present, unless a crisis is induced, for example, by anoxia or severe infection. Recurrent hematuria because of renal papillary necrosis is an occasional problem. Usually combinations of sickle trait with other hemoglobin defects, such as β-thalassemia trait (Fig. 9-98) or C trait (Fig. 9-99), give rise clinically to mild forms of sickle cell disease. Antenatal diagnosis of sickle cell anemia is illustrated in Fig. 9-60.

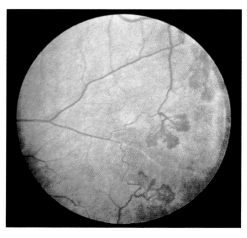

Fig. 9-91. Sickle cell anemia: retina showing peripheral vascular fronds resulting from formation of arteriovenous anastomoses.

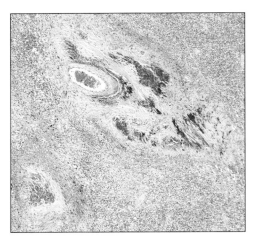

Fig. 9-92. Sickle cell anemia: section of atrophied spleen showing deposits of hemosiderin in nests of macrophages (Gamna-Gandy bodies) around the vessels. There is severe reduction of both red and white pulp. (H & E stain.)

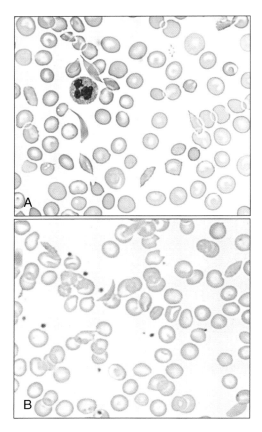

Fig. 9-93. Sickle cell anemia: peripheral blood films showing deeply staining sickle cells with target cells and polychromasia **(A)** and sickle, hypochromic, and target cells **(B).**

The main clinical problem in sickle cell anemia—recurring crises—is managed by rehydration, pain relief, antibiotic therapy as appropriate, and, in severe cases, exchange transfusion. Blood trans-fusions may also be needed in aplastic crises, during pregnancy, and preoperatively to reduce the hemoglobin S content of the blood and are sometimes used long term to "switch off" recurring crises. Patients with sickle cell disease, especially those with SC disease, tend to suffer thromboembolic problems and may require antiplatelet or anticoagulant therapy. Hydroxyurea therapy results in amelioration of sickle cell disease in many patients.

Fig. 9-94. Sickle cell anemia: peripheral blood film in a patient with splenic atrophy. Howell-Jolly and Pappenheimer bodies are seen in addition to the sickle and target cells.

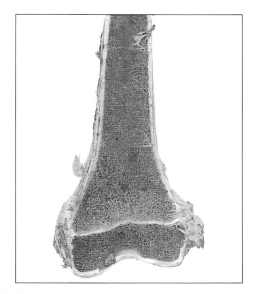

Fig. 9-95. Sickle cell anemia: postmortem longitudinal section of femur showing expansion of red (hematopoietic) marrow down the shaft toward the knee, with thinning of cortical bone. (Courtesy of Dr. J. E. McLaughlin.)

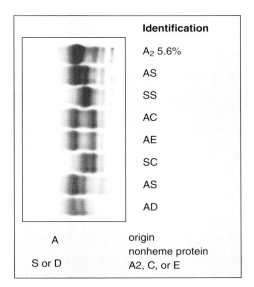

Fig. 9-96. Sickle cell anemia: hemoglobin electrophoresis in cellulose acetate, Ponceau S stain. S and D and A2, C, and E run together. Agar gel separation is usually used to distinguish these. The uppermost lane shows the raised Hb A2 level of β-thalassemia trait. (Courtesy of Gareth Ellis.)

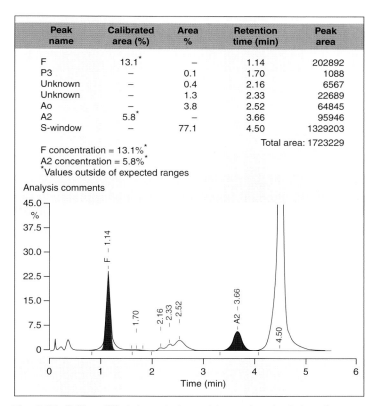

Peak name	Calibrated area (%)	Area %	Retention time (min)	Peak area
F	13.1*	–	1.14	202892
P3	–	0.1	1.70	1088
Unknown	–	0.4	2.16	6567
Unknown	–	1.3	2.33	22689
Ao	–	3.8	2.52	64845
A2	5.8*	–	3.66	95946
S-window	–	77.1	4.50	1329203

Total area: 1723229

F concentration = 13.1%*
A2 concentration = 5.8%*
*Values outside of expected ranges

Analysis comments

Fig. 9-97. Sickle cell/β-thalassemia: hemoglobin analysis by high-performance liquid chromatography (HPLc). HbS 77%, HbF 13.1%, HbA$_2$ 5.8%. (Courtesy of Gareth Ellis.)

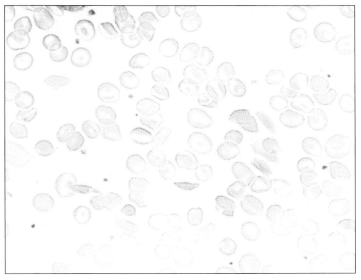

Fig. 9-98. Sickle cell/β-thalassemia: peripheral blood film showing sickle cells, target cells, and microcytic hypochromic cells.

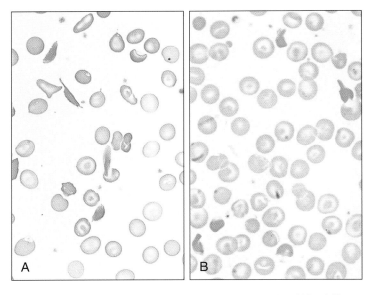

Fig. 9-99. Sickle cell/hemoglobin C disease. **A** and **B,** Peripheral blood films in which sickle cells and target cells are prominent. **B,** Peripheral blood film showing typical irregularly contracted cells. (*B,* Courtesy of Professor B. A. Bain.)

OTHER STRUCTURAL HEMOGLOBIN DEFECTS

Other common hemoglobin abnormalities include hemoglobin C (Fig. 9-100), which may be combined with β^0-thalassemia (Fig. 9-101), hemoglobin D, and hemoglobin E diseases (Figs. 9-102 and 9-103). Rare syndromes produced by hemoglobin abnormalities include hemolytic anemia because of an unstable hemoglobin (Fig. 9-104), hereditary polycythemia, hereditary methemoglobinemia (see Fig. 9-107), and thalassemia syndromes caused by structural variants.

F-CELLS

In normal adults, the synthesis of fetal Hb (Hb F) is reduced to very low levels (<0.6%) and the Hb F is restricted to a subpopulation of erythrocytes termed *F-cells,* which contain, in addition, adult hemoglobin (Hb A $\alpha2\beta2$). Increased levels of Hb F in adult life are characteristic of a heterogeneous group of genetic disorders termed *hereditary persistence of fetal Hb* (HPFH) and $\delta\beta$-thalassemias. The distribution of Hb F could be heterocellular or pancellular, and this has been a criterion for differentiating the $\delta\beta$-thalassemias from the HPFHs (Fig. 9-105).

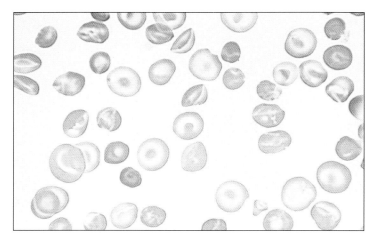

Fig. 9-100. Homozygous hemoglobin C disease: peripheral blood film showing many target cells and irregularly contracted cells. The patient showed a mild hemolytic anemia with low MCV and MCH, splenomegaly, and gallstones.

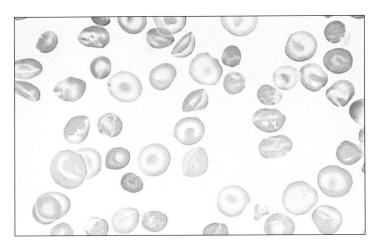

Fig. 9-101. Hemoglobin C/β^0-thalassemia: peripheral blood film showing crystals of hemoglobin C in cells otherwise empty of hemoglobin. (Courtesy of Professor B. A. Bain.)

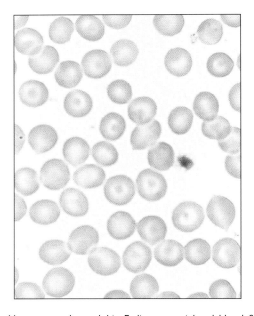

Fig. 9-102. Homozygous hemoglobin E disease: peripheral blood film showing target cells and deeply staining contracted cells. The patient was not anemic. Red cell indices (MCV, MCH) were reduced.

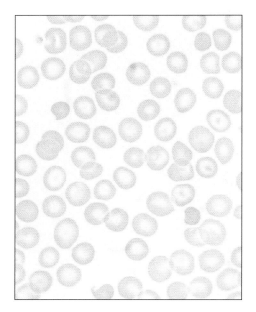

Fig. 9-103. Homozygous hemoglobin E: blood film showing hypochromia, microcytosis, target cells, and irregularly contracted cells. (Hb, 11.9 g/dl; RBC, 6.84 3 109/l; MCV, 54 fl; MCH, 17.4 pg.) (Courtesy of Professor B. A. Bain.)

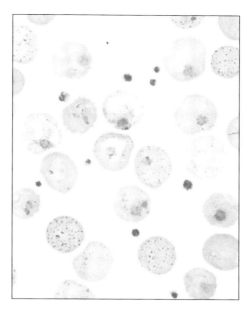

Fig. 9-104. Unstable hemoglobin (Hb-Hammersmith): Postsplenectomy peripheral blood film shows many cells with punctate basophilia or containing single or multiple inclusion bodies composed of precipitated, denatured hemoglobin (seen as Heinz bodies on special staining). The underlying lesion is substitution of the amino acid phenylalanine by serine at position 42 in the β chain.

There is a slight increase of fetal hemoglobin in adult blood in a variety of acquired disorders, such as megaloblastic anemia, acute myeloid leukemia, and paroxysmal nocturnal hemoglobinuria.

Circulating fetal red cells may be found in mothers in the immediate postpartum period, following mixing of fetal and maternal blood at delivery; such cells may be detected by the Kleihauer technique (Fig. 9-106).

METHEMOGLOBINEMIA

The iron atoms in normal hemoglobin are in the ferrous state. Methemoglobin reductase enzymes use NADH or NADPH to reduce methemoglobin, which contains ferric iron, which is formed normally during the life span of the red cell. Methemoglobinemia may arise from an inherited defect in either the α- or β-globin chain of hemoglobin or from deficiency of the enzyme NADH-methemoglobin reductase (Fig. 9-107). In either case, there is an excess of hemoglobin containing ferric iron. Methemoglobin may also be acquired as a result of exposure to drugs or chemicals.

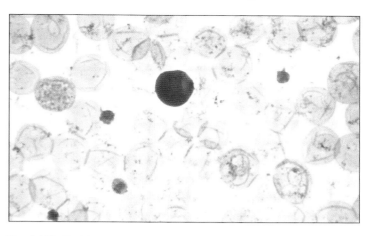

Fig. 9-106. Fetal hemoglobin: acid elution (Kleihauer) technique showing a fetal red cell in maternal blood. The darkly staining fetal cell contains fetal hemoglobin that has resisted elution at low pH. The adult cells appear as "ghosts" because the adult hemoglobin has been leached out of the cells.

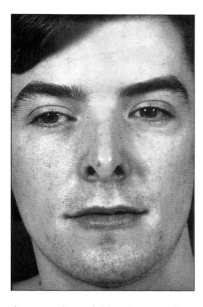

Fig. 9-107. Hereditary methemoglobinemia: cyanosis caused by NADH-methemoglobin reductase deficiency shows a typical slate-gray appearance in this 22-year-old man whose blood count was normal.

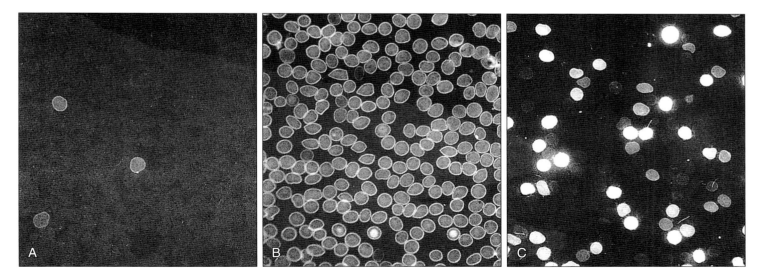

Fig. 9-105. Fetal hemoglobin in peripheral blood anti γ chain immunofluorescence stain. **A,** Normal blood heterocellular distribution (Hb F, 0.4%; F-cells, 2.5%). **B,** Indian hereditary persistence of fetal hemoglobin (HPFH) (Hb F, 22%; F-cells, 100%). **C,** Heterocellular HPFH (Hb F, 2.5%; F-cells, 30%). (Courtesy of Professor S. L. Thein.)

BENIGN DISORDERS OF PHAGOCYTES

Normal white cell appearances and production are discussed in Chapter 4. This chapter is concerned with benign conditions that may be associated with abnormal phagocyte (granulocyte and monocyte) cell morphology or numbers, only some of which are associated with clinical problems.

HEREDITARY VARIATION IN WHITE CELL MORPHOLOGY

PELGER-HUËT ANOMALY

In the Pelger-Huët anomaly, characteristic bilobed neutrophils are found in the peripheral blood. Occasional unsegmented neutrophils with round nuclei are also seen, particularly during infection (Fig. 10-1). The inheritance is dominant. The condition appears to be of no clinical significance, and the affected cells have not been shown to be functionally abnormal. "Pseudo-Pelger" cells occur in acute myeloid leukemia and the myelodysplastic syndromes.

MAY-HEGGLIN ANOMALY

In the May-Hegglin anomaly, a rare condition that has a dominant inheritance pattern, abnormal condensations of RNA appear as mildly basophilic inclusions in the neutrophil cytoplasm (Fig. 10-2). The majority of patients also have thrombocytopenia and giant platelets. Although most affected individuals have no clinical abnormality, in some there are hemorrhagic manifestations. Similar cytoplasmic inclusions, which are termed *Döhle bodies,* may be seen in neutrophils during severe infections (see Fig. 10-13) and occasionally in normal pregnancy.

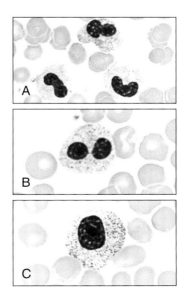

Fig. 10-1. Pelger-Huët anomaly: coarse clumping of the chromatin in **(A)** neutrophils and **(B)** "pince-nez" configurations; **(C)** a single rounded nucleus seen mostly in rare homozygous patients. "Pseudo-Pelger" neutrophils can be seen in myeloid leukemias and the myelodysplastic syndromes.

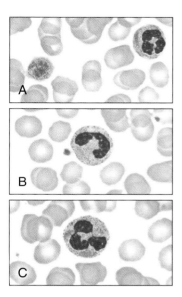

Fig. 10-2. May-Hegglin anomaly: **(A–C)** the neutrophils contain basophilic inclusions 2 to 5 mm in diameter. These inclusions are similar to Döhle bodies (see Fig. 10-13), but are not related to infection. There is an associated mild thrombocytopenia with giant platelets **(A)**.

The gene MYH9 encodes myosin-11A, a protein that enables morphogenesis in various cell types. Defective myosin-11A complexes are due to MYH9 mutations that underlie various macrothrombocytopenias including the May-Hegglin anomaly.

CHÉDIAK-HIGASHI SYNDROME

Chédiak-Higashi syndrome is a severe anomaly associated with giant neutrophil granules. A similar granular abnormality is seen in granulopoietic cells in the marrow and in eosinophils, monocytes, and lymphocytes (Fig. 10-3). The inheritance is autosomal recessive. Affected children usually have neutropenia and thrombocytopenia, and suffer from recurrent severe infections. Clinical examination frequently reveals partial albinism and marked hepatosplenomegaly. The majority die in childhood from infection or hemorrhage.

ALDER'S (ALDER-REILLY) ANOMALY

Alder's (Alder-Reilly) anomaly gives rise to deep purple granules in neutrophils (Fig. 10-4). Similar abnormal granules are found in other granulocytes, monocytes, and lymphocytes. The inheritance is autosomal recessive, and the majority of affected individuals have no clinical problems. Similar leukocyte abnormalities are seen in patients with mucopolysaccharide storage disorders, such as Hurler's and Maroteaux-Lamy syndromes, and occasionally in amaurotic family idiocy (e.g., Spielmeyer-Vogt syndrome; see below).

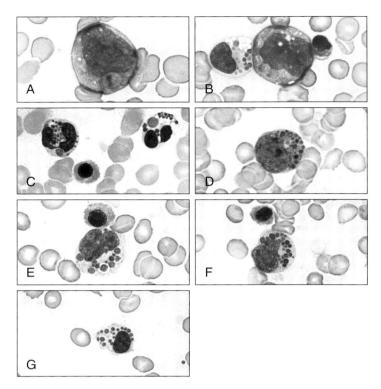

Fig. 10-3. Chédiak-Higashi syndrome: bizarre giant granules are found in the cytoplasm of all types of leukocytes and their precursors: **(A)** promyelocyte; **(B)** promonocyte and lymphocyte; **(C)** neutrophils; **(D)** early eosinophil; **(E, F)** monocytes; and **(G)** lymphocyte.

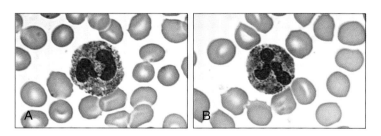

Fig. 10-4. Alder's anomaly: **(A, B)** coarse red-violet granules in neutrophils. In this case there was no associated clinical abnormality.

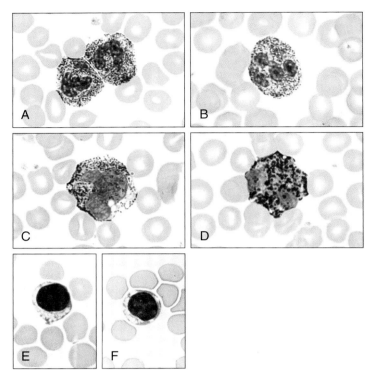

Fig. 10-5. Maroteaux-Lamy syndrome: **(A, B)** coarse red-violet granules in neutrophils, **(C)** monocyte and **(D)** basophil, and **(E, F)** prominent vacuolation of lymphocytes. In this variant of Hurler's syndrome, there are severe skeletal abnormalities and clouding of the cornea.

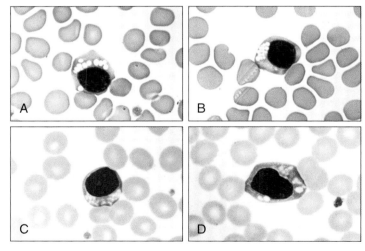

Fig. 10-6. Lymphocyte vacuolation: further examples of prominent cytoplasmic vacuolation in lymphocytes in **(A, B)** mannosidosis and in **(C, D)** the Spielmeyer-Vogt syndrome (juvenile-onset amaurotic idiocy).

MUCOPOLYSACCHARIDOSES VI AND VII

Abnormal granulation of blood granulocytes and monocytes, together with lymphocyte vacuolation, is found in the Maroteaux-Lamy syndrome, which is also known as mucopolysaccharidosis VI (Fig. 10-5). The striking white cell abnormality may also be seen in patients with mucopolysaccharidosis VII. These lysosomal storage disorders are caused by an inherited deficiency of enzymes concerned in the breakdown of acid mucopolysaccharides. Storage-related abnormalities of connective tissue, the heart, the bony skeleton, and the central nervous system (CNS) produce clinical disabilities similar to, but milder than, those found in classic Hurler's syndrome (mucopolysaccharidosis I).

Similar lymphocyte vacuoles may be found (rarely) in patients with inherited defects of enzymes that are involved in the catabolism of oligosaccharide components of glycoproteins (e.g., mannosidosis), and in the rare Spielmeyer-Vogt syndrome (Fig. 10-6).

DORFMAN-CHANARIN SYNDROME

Lipid vacuoles in granulocytes occur in this rare autosomal recessive syndrome in which there is also ichthyosiform erythroderma with variable involvement of the liver, muscles, and CNS (Fig. 10-7). There are genetic faults in triacylglycerol metabolism.

LYSINURIC PROTEIN INTOLERANCE

Lysinuric protein intolerance is a rare autosomal recessive, multisystem disorder characterized by failure to thrive, protein intolerance, pulmonary alveolar proteinosis, osteoporosis, and hemophagocytic-lymphohistiocytosis (Fig. 10-8). There are inherited mutations of the LP1 gene (SLC7A7) on chromosome 14, causing transport defects for lysine, cystine, or ornithine and arginine.

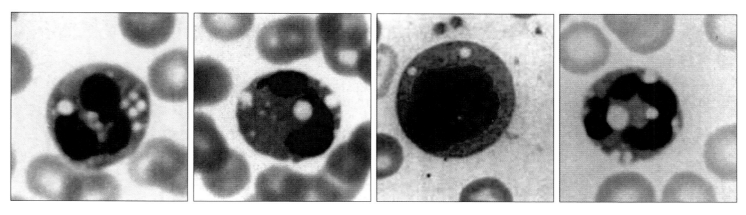

Fig. 10-7. Dorfman-Chanarin syndrome. Lipid-filled clear vacuoles are in netrophils, eosinophils, and monocytes. (Courtesy of Dr. S. Akarsu. By permission *Acta Haemotologica* 117:16–19, 2007.)

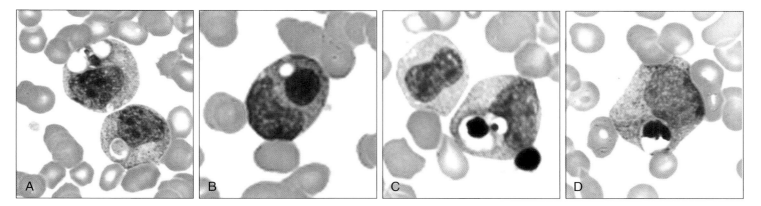

Fig. 10-8. Lysinuric protein intolerance. Hemophagocytosis by myeloid precursors. (Courtesy of Dr. W. C. Gordon, by permission *British Journal Haemotology* 138:1, 2007.)

DISORDERS OF PHAGOCYTIC FUNCTION

Disorders of phagocytic function may be inherited or acquired. Inherited disorders involve adherence, mobility and migration (e.g., leukocyte adhesion deficiency), or phagocytosis and killing. Chronic granulomatous disease (CGD) is a rare disease of killing; 60% of cases are X-linked, and the rest are autosomal recessive (Fig. 10-9). Neutrophils, eosinophils, and monocytes are affected. The patient has recurrent infections, usually with catalase-positive organisms (Fig. 10-10), gram-negative bacilli, or *Aspergillus* species, often in the first year of life. Inability of the neutrophils to reduce nitroblue tetrazolium dye suggests the diagnosis.

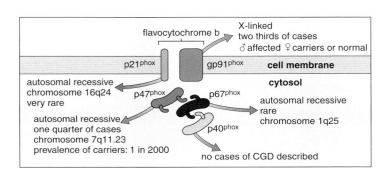

Fig. 10-9. Chronic granulomatous disease: NADPH oxidase components shown to be defective in CGD. The NADPH oxidase is composed of a flavocytochrome b in the membrane of the phagocytic vacuole. This is made up of a protein, gp-91phox, which is the flavocytochrome itself and has the NADPH FAD and two heme binding sites. Its gene, located on the X chromosome, is abnormal in about two thirds of cases of CGD. The gene of the other subunit (p21phox) of this molecule is located on chromosome 16; very occasional defects of this can cause CGD. The genes of the cytosolic proteins p47phox and p67phox are located on chromosome 7 and 1, respectively. Activation of the oxidase is associated with translocation of these two proteins from the cytosol to the membrane, where they bind to the flavocytochrome b. Autosomal recessive CGD is normally associated with the lesion p47phox in about one quarter of cases, and occasionally with p67phox. (Courtesy of Professor A. W. Segal.)

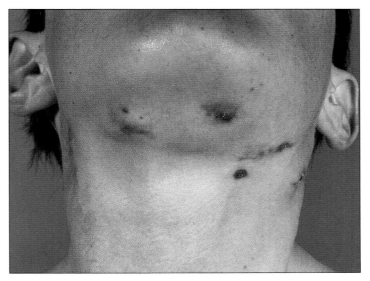

Fig. 10-10. Chronic granulomatous disease: young man with large submental and cervical nodes with poorly healed sinuses as a result of staphylococcal infection. Cervical lymphadenitis, poor healing, and sinus formation are characteristic and can be confused with tuberculosis because of the granulomatous tissue reaction. (Courtesy of Professor A. W. Segal.)

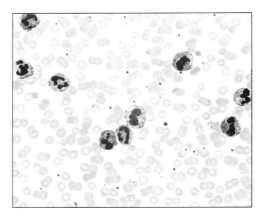

Fig. 10-11. Neutrophil leukocytosis: large numbers of band-form and segmented neutrophils in the peripheral blood. The patient had abdominal sepsis. (WBC, 45 × 10⁹/L; neutrophils, 41 × 10⁹/L.)

TABLE 10-1.	NEUTROPHIL LEUKOCYTOSIS: CAUSES
Bacterial infections Pyogenic – localized or generalized	**Corticosteroid therapy**
	Acute hemorrhage and hemolysis
Inflammation, necrosis Cardiac infarct, ischemia, trauma, vasculitis	**Myeloproliferative disorders** Polycythemia vera, myelofibrosis, chronic myeloid leukemia
Metabolic disorders Uremia, acidosis, gout, poisoning, eclampsia	**Chronic myelomonocytic leukemia**
	Malignant neoplasms

LEUKOCYTOSIS

The term *leukocytosis* refers to an increase in white blood cells (usually to above 12 × 10⁹/L). The most frequent cause is an increase in blood neutrophils. Other leukocytoses involve a predominance of one of the other white cell types found in the blood.

NEUTROPHIL LEUKOCYTOSIS (NEUTROPHILIA)

An increase in neutrophils in the blood of more than 7.5 × 10⁹/L is one of the most frequent abnormalities found in blood counts and blood films (Fig. 10-11). Clinically, fever often results from the release of leukocyte pyrogens. In most neutrophilias the number of band forms increases; occasionally, more primitive cells such as metamyelocytes and myelocytes appear in the peripheral blood (the so-called left shift). In most causes of reactive neutrophil leukocytosis (Table 10-1), toxic changes appear in the neutrophil cytoplasm and on occasion Döhle bodies are present (Figs. 10-12 and 10-13). The neutrophil alkaline phosphatase score (Fig. 10-14) is characteristically elevated.

In some cases of bacterial septicemia, the bacteria ingested by neutrophils may be seen (Fig. 10-15).

HYPERTHERMIA

Body temperatures above 41.1°C (106°F)—most commonly due to heat stroke—are associated with a change in neutrophil (and lymphocyte and monocyte) morphology. The neutrophil change has been termed *botryoid* (Fig. 10-16).

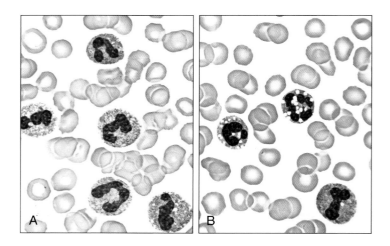

Fig. 10-13. Neutrophil leukocytosis: **(A, B)** Döhle bodies, basophilic inclusions of denatured RNA, can be seen in the cytoplasm of these neutrophils.

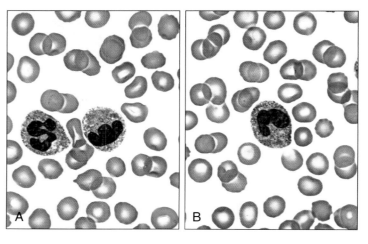

Fig. 10-12. Neutrophil leukocytosis: toxic changes in neutrophils include **(A)** the presence of red-purple granules in the band-form neutrophils and **(B)** cytoplasmic vacuolation.

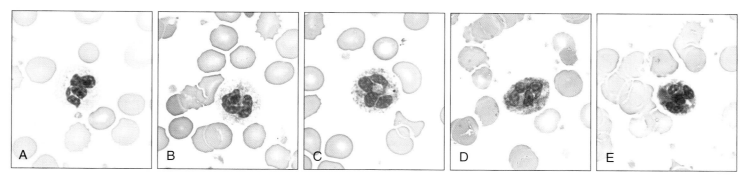

Fig. 10-14. Neutrophil alkaline phosphatase score: after cytochemical staining for alkaline phosphatase activity, 100 neutrophils are assessed for intensity of staining. From **(A)** to **(E)**, the cells score 0, 1, 2, 3, and 4, respectively. High scores are found typically in reactive neutrophil leukocytoses, polycythemia vera, and myelofibrosis. Very low scores are found in chronic myeloid leukemia.

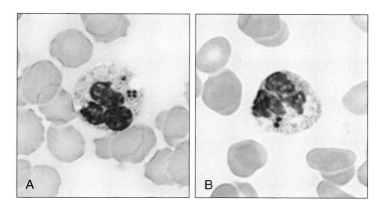

Fig. 10-15. Neutrophil leukocytosis. Neutrophils ingesting bacteria: **(A)** meningococci, **(B)** staphylococci.

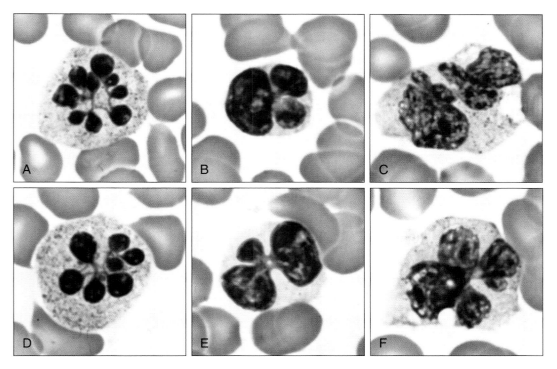

Fig. 10-16. Hyperthermia. Neutrophils with "botryoid" or grape-like nuclei each into six or more lobes (left panels); lymphocytes show nuclear lobation or budding (center panels); monocytes appear binucleate or hyperlobed (right panels). (Courtesy of Dr. P. C. J. Ward, *British Journal of Haemotology* 138:130, 2007.)

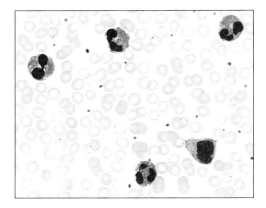

Fig. 10-17. Eosinophilia: four eosinophils and a monocyte in dermatitis herpetiformis. (Total WBC, 20 × 10⁹/L.)

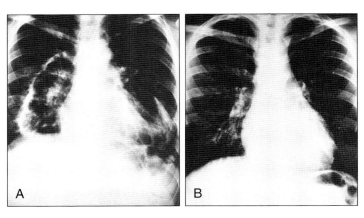

Fig. 10-18. Pulmonary eosinophilia: chest radiographs showing **(A)** diffuse infiltrates in the right middle and lower, and left lower zones. Prominent band shadows suggest areas of collapse. The patient had been taking sulfasalazine for ulcerative colitis. This drug was stopped and prednisolone commenced. **B,** The radiograph shows the same patient 3 weeks later; there is almost complete resolution of the pulmonary changes.

EOSINOPHIL LEUKOCYTOSIS (EOSINOPHILIA)

Eosinophilia is the term applied to an increase in blood eosinophils above 0.4×10^9/L (Fig. 10-17); the causes of eosinophilia are listed in Table 10-2.

There are a number of pulmonary eosinophilic syndromes of varying severity; they are characterized by transient pulmonary infiltrates (Fig. 10-18, *A*), cough, fever, and peripheral eosinophilia. Corticosteroid treatment usually results in the resolution of symptoms and the prompt clearance of infiltrates (Fig. 10-18, *B*). Similar changes may occur in some parasitic infestations when migrating parasites lodge in the lungs.

MONOCYTOSIS AND BASOPHIL LEUKOCYTOSIS

Conditions associated with monocytosis (Fig. 10-19) are listed in Table 10-3. A basophil leukocytosis is seen most frequently in patients with chronic myeloid leukemia (Fig. 10-20) or polycythemia vera. Moderate increases in blood basophils also occur in myxedema, chickenpox, smallpox, and ulcerative colitis.

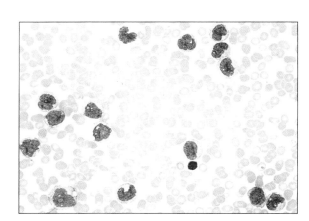

Fig. 10-19. Monocytosis: in this peripheral blood film of chronic myelomonocytic leukemia, with the exception of a single lymphocyte (center), all the nucleated cells shown are monocytes. (Total WBC, 36 × 10⁹/L; monocytes, 30 × 10⁹/L.)

TABLE 10-2.   EOSINOPHILIA: CAUSES

Secondary

Infections (mostly helminthic)
Drugs (anticonvulsants, antibiotics, sulfa drugs, antirheumatics, allopurinol, food allergy)
Pulmonary eosinophilia
Miscellaneous other causes of autoimmune/inflammatory/toxic origin:
  Eosinophilia–myalgia syndrome, toxic oil syndrome
  Eosinophilic fasciitis (Schulman syndrome), Kimura disease, Wells syndrome, Omenn syndrome
  Connective tissue diseases (scleroderma, polyarteritis nodosa, etc.)
  Sarcoidosis, inflammatory bowel disease, chronic pancreatitis
Malignancy (metastatic cancer, Hodgkin lymphoma)
Endocrinopathies (Addison disease, growth factor deficiency, etc.)

Clonal

Acute leukemia (both myeloid and lymphoblastic)
Chronic myeloid disorder
  Molecularly defined
    BCR/ABL-1⁺ chronic myeloid leukemia
    PDGFRA-rearranged eosinophilic disorder (SM-CEL)
    PDGFRB-rearranged eosinophilic disorder
    KIT-mutated systemic mastocytosis
    8p11 syndrome
  Clinicopathologically assigned
    Myelodysplastic syndrome
    Myeloproliferative disorder
      Classic myeloproliferative disorder (polycythemia vera, etc.)
      Atypical myeloproliferative disorder
        Chronic eosinophilic leukemia
        Systemic mastocytosis
        Chronic myelomonocytic leukemia
        Unclassified myeloproliferative disorder

Idiopathic including hypereosinophilic syndrome

TABLE 10-3.   MONOCYTOSIS: CAUSES

Infections
Tuberculosis, brucellosis, bacterial endocarditis, malaria, kala-azar, trypanosomiasis, typhus

Other inflammatory diseases
Sarcoidosis, ulcerative colitis, Crohn's disease, rheumatoid arthritis, systemic lupus erythematosus

Hodgkin's disease and other malignant neoplasms

Acute myelomonocytic and monocytic leukemias

Chronic myelomonocytic leukemia

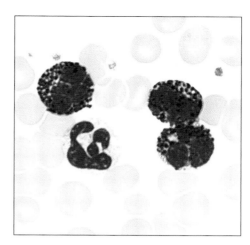

Fig. 10-20. Basophilia: high-power view of three basophils and a neutrophil in a peripheral blood film of chronic myeloid leukemia. (Total WBC, 73 × 10⁹/L; basophils, 7.3 × 10⁹/L.)

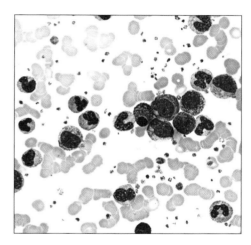

Fig. 10-21. Leukemoid reaction: neutrophils, stab forms, metamyelocytes, myelocytes and a single necrobiotic neutrophil (center) in staphylococcal pneumonia. (WBC, 94 × 10⁹/L.)

LEUKEMOID REACTION

The leukemoid reaction is a benign but excessive leukocytosis that is characterized by the presence of immature cells (myeloblasts, promyelocytes, and myelocytes) in the peripheral blood. Whereas most leukemoid reactions involve blood granulocytes (Fig. 10-21), lymphocytic reactions also occur in some. The majority of these reactions are found in association with severe or chronic infections, and sometimes they are also a feature of widespread metastatic cancer or severe hemolysis. Leukemoid reactions occur more frequently in children.

From the diagnostic point of view, the main problem is to distinguish these reactions from chronic myeloid leukemia. Changes such as toxic granulation, Döhle bodies, and a high neutrophil alkaline phosphatase (NAP) score are characteristically found in leukemoid reactions; large numbers of myelocytes, a low NAP score, and the presence of the Philadelphia chromosome BCR-ABL-1 fusion gene indicate chronic myeloid leukemia.

LEUKOERYTHROBLASTIC REACTION

Another blood cell variation is leukoerythroblastic reaction, in which erythroblasts as well as primitive white cells are found in the peripheral blood (Figs. 10-22 and 10-23). This reaction is most frequently found when a distortion of marrow architecture is present, because of either proliferative disorders of the marrow or marrow infiltrations, or extramedullary erythropoiesis. The principal causes of the leukoerythroblastic reaction are listed in Table 10-4.

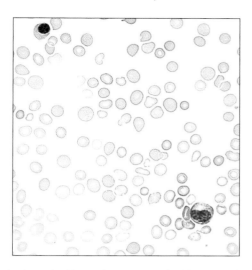

Fig. 10-22. Leukoerythroblastic change: an erythroblast, a myelocyte, red cell polychromasia, anisocytosis, and poikilocytosis, including "teardrop" forms, in myelofibrosis. (Hb, 9.5 g/dL; WBC, 5 × 10⁹/L; 6 erythroblasts per 100 WBCs; platelets, 45 × 10⁹/L.)

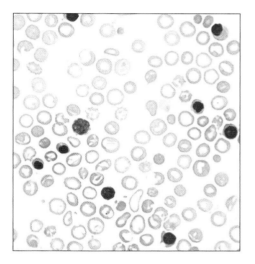

Fig. 10-23. Leukoerythroblastic change: erythroblasts, two lymphocytes, red cell polychromasia, hypochromia, poikilocytosis, acanthocytosis, and spherocytosis. The differential white cell count included metamyelocytes and myelocytes. This is a case of homozygous α-thalassemia (Hb Bart's disease).

TABLE 10-4.	LEUKOERYTHROBLASTIC CHANGE: CAUSES
Metastatic carcinoma in the marrow	
Myelofibrosis	
Myeloid leukemia	
Multiple myeloma	
Hodgkin lymphoma	
Non-Hodgkin lymphoma and histiocytic tumors	
Miliary tuberculosis	
Severe megaloblastic anemia	
Severe hemolysis, particularly in the young	
Osteopetrosis (Albers–Schönberg disease)	

TABLE 10-5.   NEUTROPENIA: CAUSES

Selective

Drug induced:

antiinflammatory – aminopyrine, phenylbutazone

antibacterial – chloramphenicol, co-trimoxazole

anticonvulsants – phenytoin, phenobarbital

antithyroids – carbimazole

phenothiazines – chlorpromazine, promethazine

miscellaneous – tolbutamide, phenindione

Racial or familial:

congenital (Kostmann's syndrome)

Shwachman–Diamond syndrome

Cyclical

Infections:

viral – particularly parvovirus, human immunodeficiency virus, hepatitis

bacterial – typhoid, miliary tuberculosis

protozoal – malaria, kala-azar

Autoimmune:

idiopathic, Felty's syndrome, systemic lupus erythematosus

Bone marrow failure

Aplastic anemia, leukemia, myelodysplasia, myelofibrosis, marrow infiltrations, megaloblastic anemia, drugs, chemotherapy (e.g., alkylating agents, antimetabolites) and radiotherapy

Splenomegaly

NEUTROPENIA

Neutropenia is defined by a blood neutrophil count of less than 2.5 × 10⁹/L. Note, however, that many African and Middle Eastern populations have normal ranges with significantly lower limits than this. Clinical problems related to recurrent infections are associated with absolute levels below 0.5×10^9/L, and neutrophil counts of less than 0.2×10^9/L carry serious risks. Neutropenia may be selective or part of a general pancytopenia (Table 10-5). The majority of neutropenias are caused by reduced granulopoiesis; however, in some patients, the reduced neutrophil counts are caused by increased removal of neutrophils by the reticuloendothelial system or by other tissues. Significant shifts of neutrophils from the circulating population to the marginal pool attached to the vascular endothelium may also be responsible.

SEVERE CONGENITAL NEUTROPENIA (KOSTMANN'S SYNDROME)

A severe congenital neutropenia (SCN), Kostmann's syndrome, is autosomal recessive. It manifests as bacterial infections early in life. The neutrophil count is usually less than 0.2×10^9/L. Bone marrow shows reduced or absent myeloid precursors.

Mutations of ELA2 encoding the neutrophil granule protease, neutrophil elastase (NE) (Fig. 10-24), underlie 50-60% of SCN. Rarely, mutations of the transcriptional repressor Gfil (which regulates ELA2 among other genes) or of enzymes HAX1 (mitochondrial), WAS (cytoskeleton), CSF3R, or G6PC3 (glucose metabolism) underlie such cases. The gene AP3B1, encoding a subunit of a complex involved in subcellular trafficking of vesicular cargo proteins (including NE), is mutated in the Hermansky-Pudlak syndrome type 2 (see p. 441), which is associated with neutropenia. Some mutations of ELA2 underlie cases of congenital cyclical neutropenia.

CLINICAL AND BONE MARROW FINDINGS

In severe neutropenia, painful and intractable infections of the buccal mucosa (Figs. 10-25 and 10-26), throat, skin (Fig. 10-27), and the anal region often occur (see also Chapter 12). Pus is not formed.

Bone marrow examination is essential in all patients with severe neutropenia. Evidence of leukemia or other infiltrations is found in many. In patients with selective depression of granulopoiesis, a reduction in all granulocyte precursors occurs (Fig. 10-28). In some cases, granulopoietic cells are absent (Fig. 10-29), but in others promyelocytes and myelocytes are present with no evidence of mature neutrophils.

MYELOKATHEXIS

A rare syndrome, myelokathexis may be related to myelodysplasia, but it occurs in young patients and is associated with chronic neutropenia and repeated infections. Marrow aspirates show many cells of the neutrophil series with hypersegmentation and longer than normal chromatin strands separating nuclear lobes (Fig. 10-30). Binucleate myelocytes, metamyelocytes, and band forms are a feature. The mature neutrophils are functionally defective.

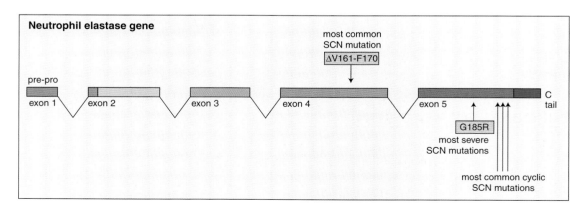

Fig. 10-24. Severe congenital neutropenia (SCN; Kostmann's syndrome). (Adapted from Horwitz MS et al: Hereditary neutropenia, *Blood* 109:1817-1824, 2007.)

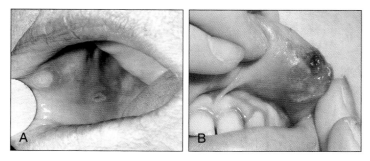

Fig. 10-25. Neutropenia: **(A, B)** ulceration of the buccal mucosa and upper lip in two patients with severe neutropenia.

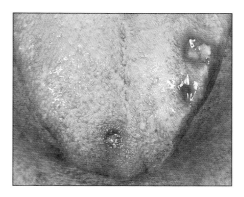

Fig. 10-26. Neutropenia: ulceration of the tongue in severe neutropenia.

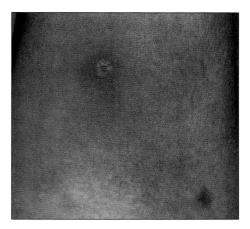

Fig. 10-27. Neutropenia: infected skin lesion with extensive surrounding subcutaneous cellulitis in severe neutropenia. Cultures grew *Staphylococcus aureus* and *Pseudomonas pyocyanea.*

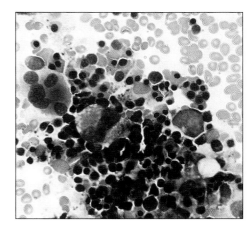

Fig. 10-28. Neutropenia: bone marrow aspirate showing an absence of granulopoietic cells. The small fragment and cell trail contain mainly erythroblasts and megakaryocytes.

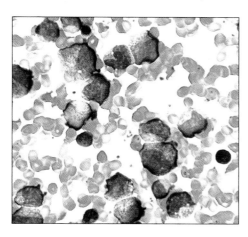

Fig. 10-29. Agranulocytosis: bone marrow aspirate showing numerous promyelocytes and myelocytes with mature neutrophils absent. (Courtesy of Professor R. D. Brunning and the AFIP.)

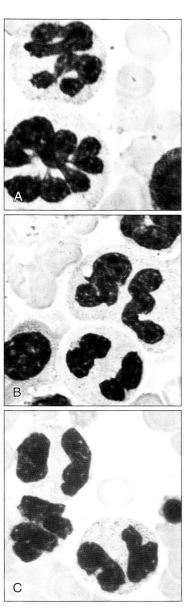

Fig.10-30. Myelokathexis. **A–C,** Bone marrow aspirate showing large band and segmented neutrophils including hyperdiploid forms, with hypersegmentation and abnormal separation of nuclear lobes. Binucleate band forms are apparent.

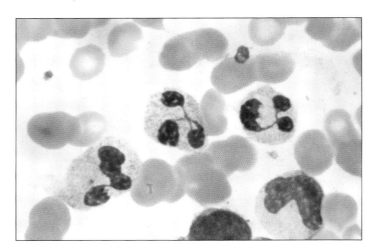

Fig.10-31. Myelokathexis: WHIM syndrome. Neutrophils with abnormal separation of nuclear lobes. The neutrophils may also show cytoplasmic vacuoles and pyknotic nuclei. (Courtesy of Dr. S. Imashuku.)

WHIM SYNDROME

WHIM syndrome consists of Warts, Hypogammaglobulinemia, Infections, and Myelokathexis (Fig. 10-31). It is due to inheritance of a mutation in the gene encoding the receptor CXCR-4 for the stromal factor-1 (SDF-1). The complex SDF-1–CXCR-4 is important in regulating trafficking of leukocytes from marrow to blood and to stromal cells.

LYSOSOMAL STORAGE DISEASES

The lysosomal storage diseases of the reticuloendothelial system (Table 10-6) may result in pancytopenia, vacuolation or abnormal granulation of blood cells, and the accumulation of degenerate foam cells in the bone marrow, liver, and spleen. These lysosomal storage conditions result from defects in lysozymal hydrolytic enzymes (Fig. 10-32). The products of metabolism normally degraded by the specific enzyme that is defective disrupt the lysosomes and damage cell structure.

GAUCHER'S DISEASE

Gaucher's disease is a relatively common familial disorder characterized by the accumulation of glucocerebrosides (especially glucosylce-

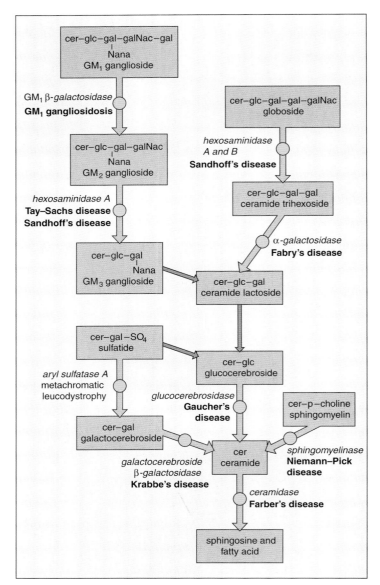

Fig. 10-32. Sphingolipid mechanism: pathways and diseases: the enzymes involved are given in italics, and below each is given the disease (in bold) that results from deficiency of that particular enzyme. cer, Ceramide; glc, glucose; gal, galactose; galNac, acetylgalactosamine; Nana, N-acetylneuraminic acid. (Adapted with permission from Kolodny EH, Tenembaum AL: In Nathan DG, Oski FA, editors: *Hematology of infancy and childhood,* ed 4, Philadelphia, 1992, Saunders, p 1452.)

ramide) in reticuloendothelial cells; it occurs because the enzyme glucocerebrosidase is deficient. Three types occur (Table 10-7):
- Type 1: Chronic adult
- Type 2: Acute infantile neuropathic
- Type 3: Subacute neuropathic with onset in childhood or adolescence

TABLE 10-6. LYSOSOMAL STORAGE DISEASES

Sphingolipidoses	Diseases of complex carbohydrate metabolism
Gaucher's disease	
Niemann–Pick disease	Sialidoses
Farber's disease	Mucolipidoses
GM gangliosidoses	Fucosidosis
	Mannosidosis
Mucopolysaccharidoses	Aspartylglucosaminuria
	Sialic acid storage disease
Hurler's, Scheie's, and Hurler–Scheie disease	
Hunter's disease	**Acid lipase deficiency**
Sanfilippo's disease	
Marquio syndrome	Wolman's disease
Maroteaux–Lamy syndrome	Cholesterol ester storage disease
	Neuronal ceroid lipofuscinoses

TABLE 10-7. CLINICAL MANIFESTATIONS OF GAUCHER'S DISEASE

Manifestation	Type 1	Type 2	Type 3
Onset	1 year	<1 year	2–20 years
Hepatosplenomegaly	++	+/–	+
Bone disease	++	–	+/–
Cardiac valve disease	–	–	+
CNS disease	–	+++	+/–
Oculomotor apraxia	–	+	+/–
Corneal opacities	–	+/–	+/–
Age at death	60–90 years	<5 years	<30 years

Adapted from Hoffbrand AV, Catovsky D, Tuddenham ECD, editors: *Postgraduate haematology,* ed 6, Oxford, 2005, Blackwell Scientific.

The gene is located on chromosome 1 band q21. There is a pseudogene 16 kb downstream from the glucocerebrosidase gene, which is 95% homologous. The disease is caused by gene mutations or deletions or the formation of fusion genes between the functional gene and the pseudogene. The high prevalence in Ashkenazi Jews largely arises from a mutation at cDNA nucleotide 226 (amino acid 370). The chronic adult non-neuropathic form of the disease is accompanied by hepatosplenomegaly (Fig. 10-33) and bone lesions (Fig. 10-34), and sometimes by lymphadenopathy, skin pigmentation, and pingueculae (Fig. 10-35). The most acute neuropathic forms manifest in infancy, and survival beyond the first 3 years of life is rare. A juvenile form may manifest in childhood with features of the chronic adult form, as well as progressive neurologic dysfunction.

A presumptive diagnosis of Gaucher's disease may be made when Gaucher's cells are detected in marrow aspirates (Fig. 10-36, *A* and *C*) and trephine biopsies (Fig. 10-36, *B*). Diagnosis can be confirmed by

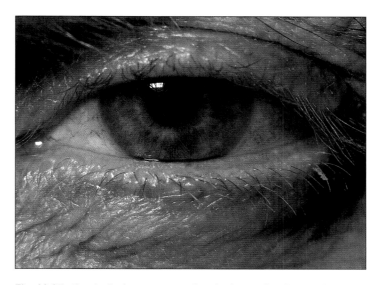

Fig. 10-35. Gaucher's disease: pingueculae, the brownish-yellow wedge-shaped thickenings of the bulbar conjunctiva.

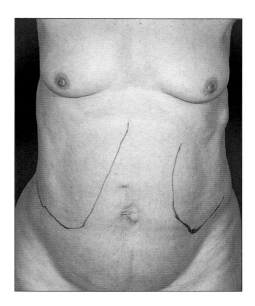

Fig. 10-33. Gaucher's disease: moderate enlargement of both the spleen and liver.

demonstration of absence or severe deficiency of the enzyme glucosylceramide β-glucosidase in fibroblast cultures. Gaucher's cells are also found in the liver and spleen (Fig. 10-36, *D*). Most patients with this condition have elevated plasma acid phosphatase, serum angiotensin-converting enzyme (SACE), ferritin, and transcobalamin II levels.

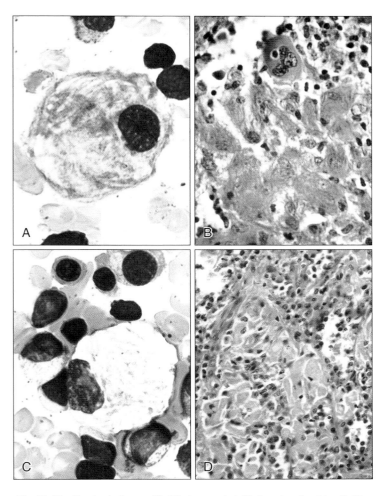

Fig. 10-36. Gaucher's disease: **(A, C)** characteristic histiocytic cells with a fibrillar or "onion-skin" pattern of unstained inclusion material. In biopsy **(B)** these cells are histiocytes with a finely granular cytoplasmic PAS reaction. In the spleen **(D)** the histiocytic cells appear as pale clusters in the reticuloendothelial cords between the venous sinuses.

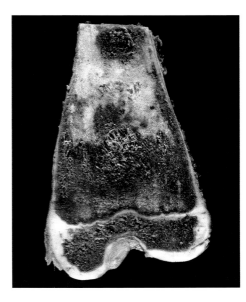

Fig. 10-34. Gaucher's disease: lower end of femur showing expansion of marrow cavity with thinning of cortical bone and multiple infarcted areas (white) giving typical Erlenmeyer flask deformity. There is subchondral bony collapse with osteonecrosis. (Courtesy of Professor R. Brady.)

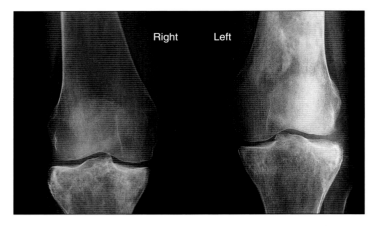

Fig. 10-37. Gaucher's disease: radiograph of the knee joints in a 45-year-old woman shows failure of correct modeling with expansion of the lower ends of the femurs. Bone thinning and loss of trabecular pattern are particularly apparent in the right femur. The sclerosis in the left femur and right tibia is caused by bone infarcts.

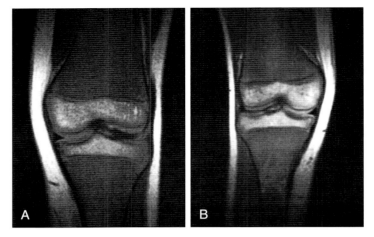

Fig. 10-39. Gaucher's disease: MRI scan of the left knee of an 11-year-old girl, **(A)** before treatment showing Erlenmeyer flask deformity with expansion of the marrow and thinning of the cortical bone—the bone marrow images have uniformly low intensity; **(B)** following 1 year of aglucerase therapy the bone marrow intensity is brighter, and remodeling of the bone is occurring (accompanying a growth spurt). (A, B, Courtesy of Dr. L. Berger.)

Serum chitotriosidase is markedly raised and can be used to monitor efficacy of enzyme therapy. Over 50% of adult patients usually have asymptomatic radiographic changes, such as cortical expansion of the lower end of the femur, which produces a characteristic radiolucent area (Fig. 10-37).

It is now possible to replace the missing enzyme with aglucerase (Ceredase), an enzyme preparation prepared from human placenta. Enzyme made using recombinant DNA techniques, such as imiglucerase (Cerezyme), is now usually preferred. Following therapy there is improvement in blood counts, reduction in liver and spleen size, and remodeling of the bones with reduction of osteoporosis (Fig. 10-38), which can be demonstrated by magnetic resonance imaging (MRI) scan (Fig. 10-39). Substrate reduction therapy with oral agents (e.g., Miglustat and Zavesca) is also being developed.

NIEMANN-PICK DISEASE

Niemann-Pick disease is a sphingomyelin lipidosis, is rarer than Gaucher's disease, and is characterized by extensive tissue storage of sphingomyelin, hepatic and splenic enlargement, and large lipid-filled macrophages in the bone marrow. In its best-defined forms there is an inherited deficiency of the enzyme sphingomyelinase, and sphingomyelin concentration in the tissues is up to 100 times higher than normal. As in Gaucher's disease, acute neuropathic and chronic non-neuropathic forms occur.

The disease is suspected in young children with hepatosplenomegaly when bone marrow aspirates show the presence of foam cells (Fig. 10-40). Confirmation is by showing low levels of sphingomyelinase in fibroblasts cultured from skin or bone marrow. In less severe adult forms of the disease, large numbers of sea-blue histiocytes may be found in bone marrow aspirates, in addition to the classic foam cells (Fig. 10-41).

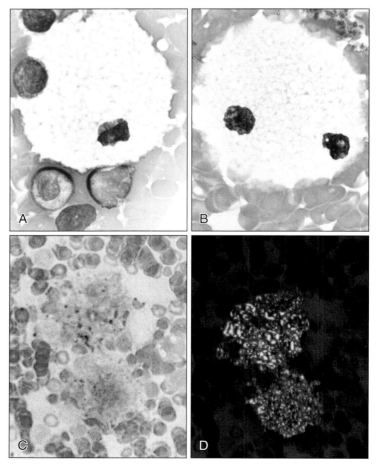

Fig. 10-40. Niemann-Pick disease (infantile): bone marrow showing **(A, C)** typical histiocytic cells with foamy deposits in the cytoplasm; **(B)** the histiocytic cells stain weakly with Sudan black stain for lipid; **(D)** in polarized light, strong red birefringence is present in the Sudan stain. (C, D, Reproduced with permission from Hann IM, Lake BD, Pritchard J, Lilleyman J: *Color atlas of paediatric hematology*, ed 2, Oxford, 1990, Oxford University Press.)

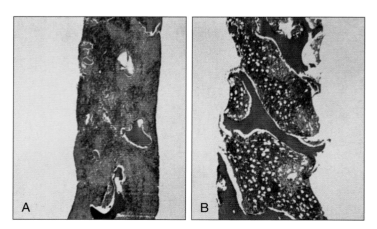

Fig. 10-38. Gaucher's disease: appearances of bone biopsy **(A)** before aglucerase therapy and **(B)** after 12 months of aglucerase therapy. (A, B, Courtesy of Professor R. Brady.)

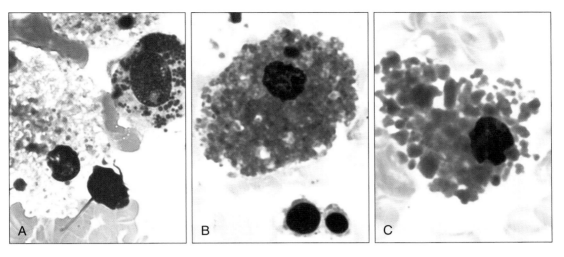

Fig. 10-41. Niemann-Pick disease (adult): bone marrow showing **(A)** typical foam cells, and **(B, C)** prominent histiocytes with sea-blue cytoplasm.

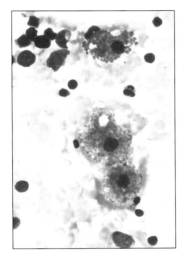

Fig. 10-42. Sea-blue histiocyte syndrome: bone marrow showing typical cells in the cell trails.

TABLE 10-8.   SEA-BLUE HISTIOCYTES IN THE BONE MARROW OR SPLEEN: CAUSES

Frequent, in marrow
Sea-blue histiocyte syndrome
Niemann–Pick disease
Occasional, in marrow
Hyperlipoproteinemia
Hereditary acetyltransferase deficiency
Wolman's disease
Other lipid storage disorders
Chronic myeloid leukemia
Polycythemia vera
Chronic immune thrombocytopenia
Thalassemia
Sickle cell disease
Sarcoidosis
Chronic granulomatous disease

SEA-BLUE HISTIOCYTE SYNDROME

Patients with the rare sea-blue histiocyte syndrome usually have splenomegaly and thrombocytopenic purpura, in some cases with associated hepatic cirrhosis. The inheritance pattern is autosomal recessive.

Bone marrow aspirates contain large numbers of "sea-blue" histiocytes (Fig. 10-42). Phospholipids and sphingomyelin accumulate in tissue, and reduced levels of cellular sphingomyelinase activity have been reported. The syndrome is a variant of Niemann-Pick disease.

Other causes of sea-blue histiocytes in the bone marrow or spleen are listed in Table 10-8.

BENIGN DISORDERS OF LYMPHOCYTES

LYMPHOCYTOSIS

The main causes of an increase in the absolute lymphocyte count are listed in Table 11-1. The count is usually 5-50x10^9/L. Greatly raised levels (>100x10^9/L) may be seen in adults with chronic lymphocytic leukemia. Infants with pertussis and children with acute infectious lymphocytosis, an unusual viral disease, may also have very high lymphocyte counts (Fig. 11-1). Lymphocytoses with large numbers of atypical or "reactive" cells are most often seen in infectious mononucleosis, in other viral illnesses (including infectious hepatitis), and in toxoplasmosis. Unusually heavy smoking is probably, although this is unclear, associated with a benign polyclonal lymphocytosis (Fig. 11-2).

INFECTIOUS MONONUCLEOSIS

Infectious mononucleosis is a disorder characterized by sore throat, fever, lymphadenopathy, and atypical lymphocytes in the blood. The disease appears to be the result of infection with the Epstein-Barr (EB) virus. In affected patients, heterophile antibodies against sheep red cells are found in the serum at high titres (Paul-Bunnell test).

Most patients have lethargy, malaise, and fever. On examination the majority show lymphadenopathy (Fig. 11-3).

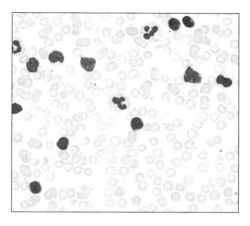

Fig. 11-1. Benign lymphocytes: bordetella pertussis infection. Girl aged 4 presenting with a limp. White cell count 130x10^9/l; normal hemoglobin and platelet count. Immunophenotyping showed the lymphocytes to be T cells, CD4 or CD8 positive. Serology was positive for B pertussis. (Courtesy of Dr. W. Erber).

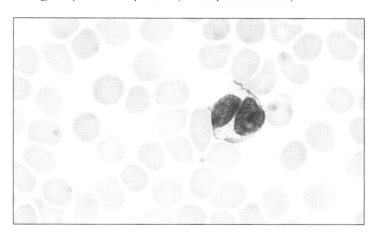

Fig. 11-2. Benign lymphocytosis: representative binucleate lymphocyte in the peripheral blood of a heavy smoker with polyclonal lymphocytosis. (Courtesy of Professor B.A. Bain.)

TABLE 11-1. LYMPHOCYTOSIS: CAUSES

Reactive Lymphocytosis	Stress
Acute infections	Trauma
	Major surgery
Bacterial	Myocardial infarction
Bordetella	Status epilepticus
Pertussis	Septic shock
	Sickle cell crisis
Viral	
Mononucleosis syndrome	**Hypersensitivity reactions**
Epstein–Barr	
Cytomegalovirus	Insect bites
HIV	Drugs
Rubella	
Herpes simplex	**Chronic polyclonal**
Adenovirus	
Viral hepatitis	Cigarette smoking
Dengue fever	Cancer
Human herpes virus type 6	Hyposplenism
(HHV-6)	Thymoma
HHV-8	
Varicella zoster	
	NK Lymphocytosis
Toxoplasma gondii	
	Primary
Acute infectious lymphocytosis	
(unexplained)	Acute lymphoblastic leukemia
	Chronic lymphocytic, prolymphocytic,
Chronic infections	hairy cell, adult T-cell leukemia-lymphoma
	Non-Hodgkin's lymphoma
Tuberculosis, brucellosis,	Monoclonal B-cell lymphocytosis
syphilis, leprosy, leishmaniasis,	Persistent polyclonal B-cell lymphocytosis
stronygloidiasis	Large granular lymphocytic leukemia,
	CD8$^+$, CD4$^+$, α/β or γ/δ T cell types

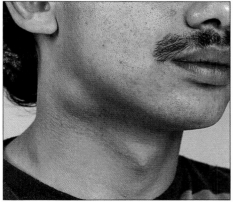

Fig. 11-3. Infectious mononucleosis: cervical lymphadenopathy in a 19-year-old man who had fever and pharyngitis.

Generalized inflammation of the oral and pharyngeal surfaces with follicular tonsillitis (Fig. 11-4) is usual, and some patients show palatal petechiae (Fig. 11-5). Periorbital and facial edema (Fig. 11-6) or a morbilliform rash (Fig. 11-7) may be present.

Palpable splenomegaly occurs in over half the patients. Occasionally, subcapsular hematomas of the spleen (Fig. 11-8) are present and have a tendency to rupture.

The diagnosis is suspected by finding a moderate lymphocytosis (10 to 20 $\times$ 10^9/L) and large numbers of atypical lymphocytes in the peripheral blood film (Fig. 11-9). Fine needle aspiration of a lymph node shows a mixed cell population dominated by reactive lymphocytes (Fig 11-10). Lymph node biopsy is not usually performed. The histological appearances are those of a reactive node with proliferating germinal follicles, increased numbers of T-cells, especially CD8+ve,

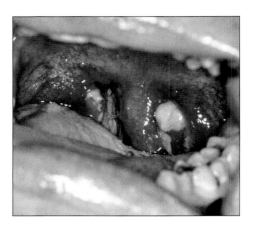

Fig. 11-4. Infectious mononucleosis: gross swelling and hemorrhagic erythema of the oropharynx. The tonsils are covered by a purulent exudate.

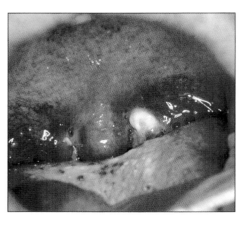

Fig. 11-5. Infectious mononucleosis: oropharynx (same case as shown in Fig. 11-4) showing marked swelling of the uvula and tonsils, and palatal petechial hemorrhage.

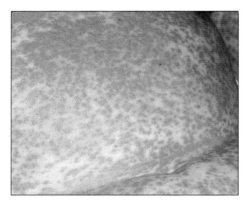

Fig. 11-7. Infectious mononucleosis: morbilliform erythematous skin eruption. There was generalized lymphadenopathy and the spleen was enlarged to 3 cm below the left costal margin.

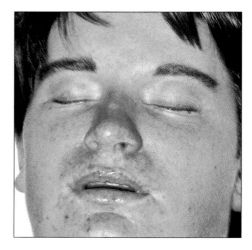

Fig. 11-6. Infectious mononucleosis: marked facial and periorbital edema.

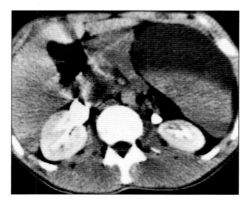

Fig. 11-8. Infectious mononucleosis: abdominal computed tomography (CT) scan showing massive enlargement of the spleen with a large anterior subcapsular hematoma (area of decreased density).

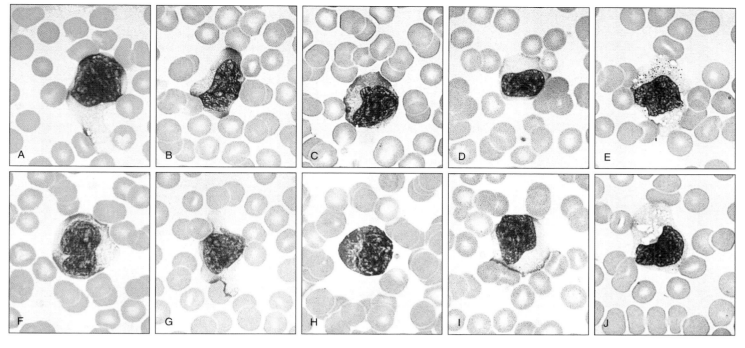

Fig. 11-9. Infectious mononucleosis. **A–J,** Representative "reactive" lymphocytes in the peripheral blood film of a 21-year-old man. These are T lymphocytes reacting to B cells infected by the Epstein-Barr virus. The cells are large with abundant vacuolated cytoplasm; the nuclei often show a fine blast-like chromatin pattern. The edges of the lymphocytes are often indented by adjacent red cells.

Fig. 11-10. Infectious mononucleosis: fine-needle aspirate of cervical lymph node showing a pleomorphic lymphoid population including immunoblasts, centroblasts, centrocytes and small lymphocytes.

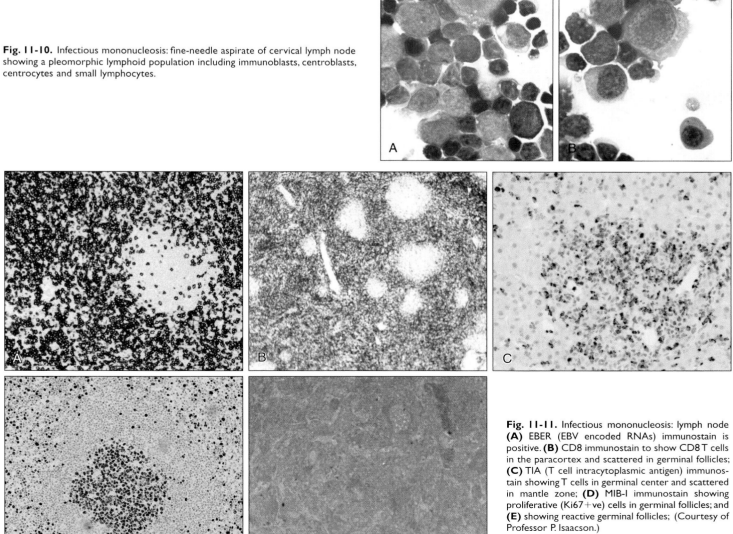

Fig. 11-11. Infectious mononucleosis: lymph node **(A)** EBER (EBV encoded RNAs) immunostain is positive. **(B)** CD8 immunostain to show CD8 T cells in the paracortex and scattered in germinal follicles; **(C)** TIA (T cell intracytoplasmic antigen) immunostain showing T cells in germinal center and scattered in mantle zone; **(D)** MIB-I immunostain showing proliferative (Ki67+ve) cells in germinal follicles; and **(E)** showing reactive germinal follicles; (Courtesy of Professor P. Isaacson.)

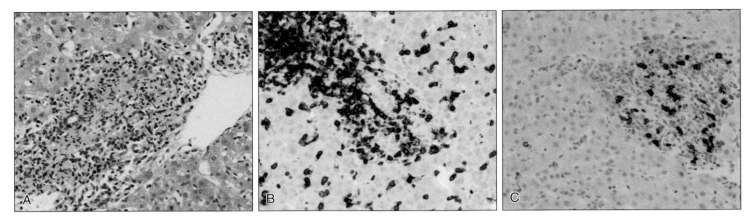

Fig. 11-12. Infectious mononucleosis (same case as Fig 11-10); liver biopsy showing **(A)** Mixed inflammatory cells in portal tract and scattered in sinusoids; **(B)** CD8 immunostain showing CD8 T cells in portal tracts and sinusoids; and **(C)** CD20 immunostain showing B cells in portal tracts and sinusoids. (Courtesy of Professor P. Isaacson.)

and positive staining for the EB virus antigens (Fig 11-11). Jaundice and abnormal liver function occurs in a minority of patients. Liver histology shows mixed inflammatory cells in the portal tracts and sinusoids with a predominance of CD8 +ve T cells (Fig 11-12).

LYMPHADENOPATHY

Infectious mononucleosis is one cause of generalized lymphadenopathy (Table 11-2). A number of conditions including acute leukemia,

toxoplasmosis, infectious hepatitis, human immunodeficiency virus (HIV) infection and follicular tonsillitis are likely to create initial problems in diagnosis. Lymph node biopsy or fine-needle aspiration cytology of the affected nodes may be helpful in differential diagnosis. Reactive lymph nodes are characterized by an overall retention of normal node structure with expansion of follicle cells which show the presence of mixed inflammatory cells, tingible body macrophages, polyclonal T cells and expansion of B cells (centroblasts) at the edge of the germinal centers (Fig 11-13). T cells may infiltrate the germinal center and are a mixture of CD4 and CD8 cells (Fig 11-14).

TABLE 11-2.   LYMPHADENOPATHY: CAUSES

Localized	Generalized
Local infection	**Infections**
Pyogenic infection (e.g., pharyngitis, dental abscess, otitis media), actinomyces	Viral (e.g., infectious mononucleosis, measles, rubella, viral hepatitis), human immunodeficiency virus
Viral infection (e.g., cat scratch fever, lymphogranuloma venereum)	Bacterial (e.g., brucellosis, syphilis, tuberculosis, salmonella, bacterial endocarditis)
Tuberculosis	Fungal (e.g., histoplasmosis)
Lymphoma	Protozoal (e.g., toxoplasmosis)
Hodgkin lymphoma	**Noninfectious inflammatory diseases**
Non-Hodgkin lymphoma	For example, sarcoidosis, rheumatoid arthritis, systemic lupus erythematosus, other connective tissue diseases, Kikuchi's disease, serum sickness
Metastatic tumors	**Leukemia, especially CLL, ALL**
Carcinoma	**Lymphoma**
Malignant melanoma	Non-Hodgkin lymphoma
	Hodgkin lymphoma
	Waldenström's macroglobulinemia
	Rarely, metastatic tumors
	Angioimmunoblastic lymphadenopathy
	Sinus histiocytosis with massive lymphadenopathy (Rosai-Dorfman)
	Autoimmune lymphoproliferative disease
	Reaction to drugs and chemicals
	For example, hydantoins and related chemicals, beryllium
	Hyperthyroidism

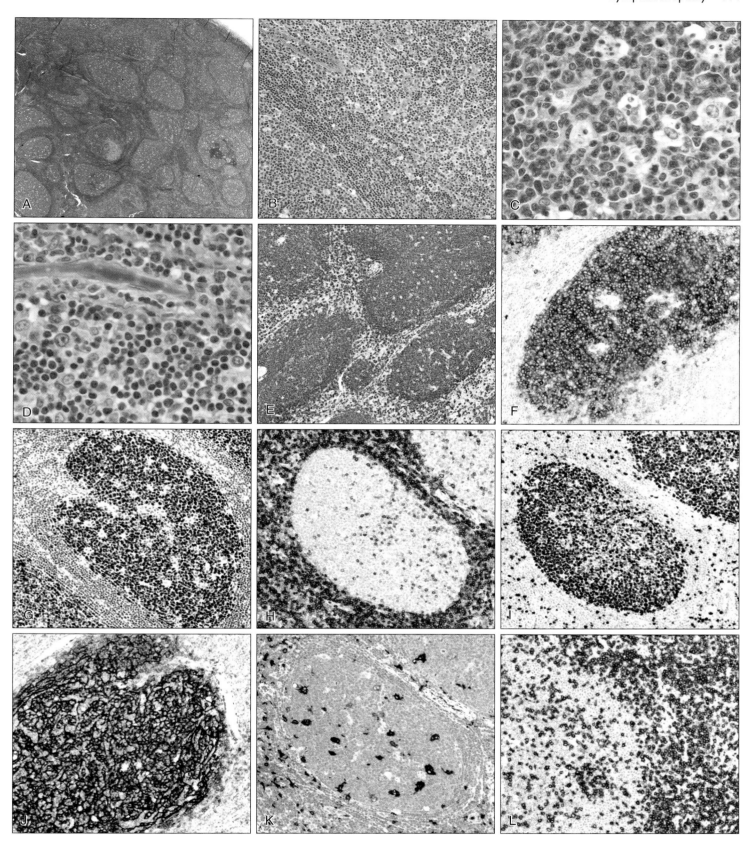

Fig. 11-13. Reactive lymphadenopathy: lymph node histologic findings **(A)** low power showing expanded follicles with mixture of lymphocytes, macrophages, infiltrating cells with surrounding mantle zone intact. **(B)** Higher power showing germinal center with tingible body macrophages, centrocytes, and centroblasts. High endothelial blood vessel and lymphocyte trafficking. **(C)** High power centrocytes and centroblasts. **(D)** Paracortex showing mixed inflammatory cells and blood vessels. **(E)** CD20 immunostain showing germinal center and mantle zone B cells. **(F)** CD10 immunostain showing germinal center B cells. **(G)** BCL-6 immunostain showing nuclear staining of germinal B cells. **(H)** BCL-2 immunostain; mantle zone B cells and scattered T cells are positive. **(I)** MIB-1 immunostain. This is a proliferation marker detecting the Ki67 antigen. The cells in the germinal follicle are positive with a darker zone at the edge. **(J)** CD21 immunostain: follicular dendritic cells are positive and show a network of cell processes. **(K)** CD163 immunostain: tingible body macrophages are positive in the germinal center. **(L)** CD3 immunostain: T cells in the paracortex and a few scattered T cells in the germinal center are positive. (Courtesy of Dr. A. Ramsay.)

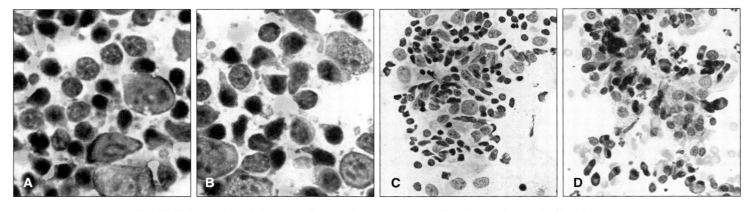

Fig. 11-14. Reactive lymphadenopathy. T cells (red rhodamine labeling) occupy the paracortical area surrounding the mainly B lymphocyte corona that expresses IgM (green fluorescein labeling). A number of T cells are scattered within the germinal center, where immune complexes are also stained strongly by the IgM antisera. **B,** The T cells within the paracortical area are a mixture of CD4+ helper (red) and CD8+ suppressor/cytotoxic (green) cells. **C,** At the edge of a germinal center is a mixture of B lymphocytes expressing κ (red) or λ (green) light chains. (A to C courtesy of Professor M. Chilosi, Professor G. Janossy, and Professor G. Pizzolo.)

Fine needle aspirates show the node to contain a pleomorphic lymphoid population (Fig 11-15) which by flow cytometry can be shown to be polyclonal, expressing kappa and lambda light chains. In toxoplasmosis characteristic small groups of histiocytes may be found (Fig. 11-20). Also, computed tomography (CT) scans may be helpful in distinguishing benign lymphadenopathy from lymphoma (Fig. 11-17).

Lymph node biopsy may be needed to distinguish benign conditions (e.g. infectious, immune reactions, vasculitides) from malignant conditions (Figs 11.18-11.23).

Fig. 11-15. Reactive lymphadenopathy. Fine-needle aspirate of cervical lymph node showing **(A, B)** a pleomorphic lymphoid population with large immunoblasts, centroblasts, paler centrocytes, and small lymphocytes; **(C)** small and medium-sized lymphoid cells and histiocytes; **(D)** plasma cells, histiocytes, and lymphocytes.

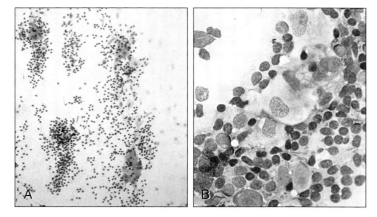

Fig. 11-16. Toxoplasmosis: fine-needle aspirate of cervical lymph node showing **(A)** groups of histiocytic cells in the cell trails; **(B)** at higher magnification predominantly small lymphocytes that surround these histiocytes are seen. (A, Papanicolaou's stain; B, May-Grünwald/Giemsa stain.)

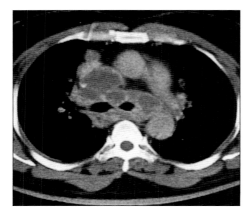

Fig. 11-17. Tuberculosis: CT scan showing tuberculous lymph nodes in the mediastinum. This is typical of tuberculosis. Lymphoma can occasionally produce this appearance. (Courtesy of Dr. L. Berger.)

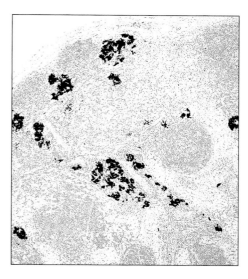

Fig. 11-18. Tattoo pigment in the sinus areas of a lymph node. (Courtesy of Dr. J. E. McLaughlin.)

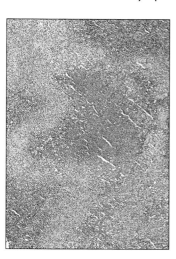

Fig. 11-21. Cat scratch disease: a geographic area of necrosis within a granuloma is visible. (Courtesy of Dr. J. E. McLaughlin.)

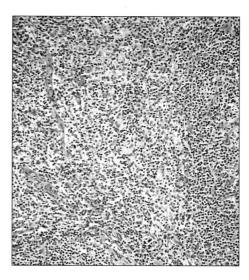

Fig. 11-19. Dermatopathic lymphadenopathy: clear cytoplasm of interdigitating reticulum cells gives an area of pallor above a follicle. Occasional phagocytic cells that contain melanin are visible. (Courtesy of Dr. J. E. McLaughlin.)

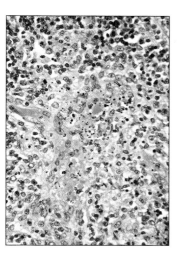

Fig. 11-22. Kawasaki's disease: vasculitic reaction in a lymph node. (Courtesy of Dr. J. E. McLaughlin.)

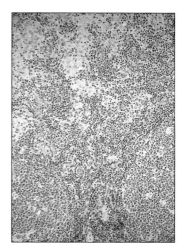

Fig. 11-20. Toxoplasmosis: small clusters of epithelial histiocytes above two hyperplastic follicles. (Courtesy of Dr. J. E. McLaughlin.)

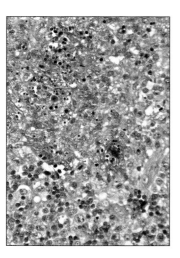

Fig. 11-23. Kawasaki's disease: fibrin (red) deposition in the wall of a small blood vessel. (Courtesy of Dr. J. E. McLaughlin.)

KIKUCHI'S DISEASE

Kikuchi's disease (also called Kikuchi-Fujimoto and histiocytic necrotizing lymphadenitis) was first recognized in Japan, but is now known to have worldwide distribution. It is more common in young women, manifesting with persistent tender or nontender lymphadenopathy; fever and a viral-like prodromal syndrome are frequent, and mild leukopenia may be present. Cervical nodes are involved most often, but any group of nodes may be affected. No associated virus has been found, and systemic lupus erythematosus (SLE) is suggested by the histopathology, but Kikuchi patients rarely develop SLE (Fig. 11-24 through 11-26).

SINUS HISTIOCYTOSIS WITH MASSIVE LYMPHADENOPATHY (ROSAI-DORFMAN DISEASE) (SEE CHAPTER 16)

Sinus histiocytosis with massive lymphadenopathy is a rare condition seen most frequently in young blacks and is characterized by lymphadenopathy, fever, leukocytosis, and hypergammaglobulinemia (see page 287).

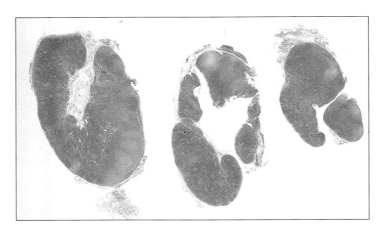

Fig 11-24. Kikuchi disease: Whole mount of lymph node "bread-sliced" into three parts showing pale circumscribed areas of necrosis. (Courtesy of Dr. T. Levine.)

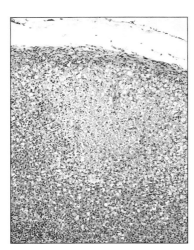

Fig 11-25. Kikuchi disease: Low-power view of cortical area of necrosis. (Courtesy of Dr. T. Levine)

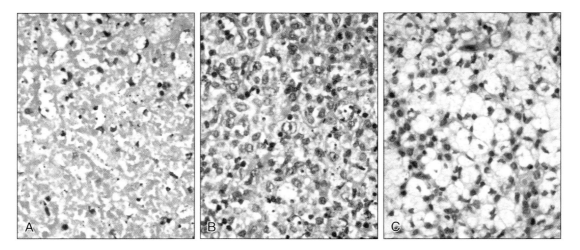

Fig 11-26. Kikuchi disease: **A,** High-power view of necrosis with karyorrhectic debris (note the absence of neutrophils). **B,** Adjacent "cuff" of lymphoblasts, including T-cell blasts and macrophages. **C,** Characteristic "crescentic" or "signet cell" macrophages adjacent to areas of necrosis. (Courtesy of Dr. T. Levine.)

PRIMARY IMMUNODEFICIENCY DISORDERS

The main types of primary and secondary immunodeficiency disease are listed in Table 11-3. A detailed map of the sites of the defects in the congenital immune deficiencies is given in Fig. 11-27. In severe combined immunodeficiency disease, the T- and B-lymphocyte systems fail to develop. There is severe lymphopenia and hypogammaglobulinemia. Affected infants fail to thrive (Fig. 11-28) and die early in life from recurrent infections, such as by *Pneumocystis*

carinii, cytomegalovirus, other viruses, fungi, and bacteria. Atrophy of the thymus occurs (Fig. 11-29); the lymph nodes and spleen are small and devoid of lymphoid cells. The most common cause is deficiency of the enzyme adenosine deaminase (ADA) (Fig. 11-30). Deficiency of another enzyme, purine nucleoside phosphorylase, causes a more selective lack of T cells. Deficiency of ADA has been treated successfully by stem cell transplantation and most recently by "gene therapy" in which the ADA gene is introduced into the patient's lymphocytes in vitro, and the lymphocytes are then reinfused.

TABLE 11-3. IMMUNODEFICIENCY DISORDERS

B-cell disorders	**Primary T-cell deficiency**

X-linked agammaglobulinemia (defect of Bruton's tyrosine kinase, btk)
Autosomal agammaglobulinemia
  Recessive λ5, Igα, BLNK
  Human inducible co-stimulator (ICOS)
Selective IgA or IgM deficiency
IgG subclass deficiencies
Hyper IgM
  Activation-induced cytidine deaminase (AICD) deficiency
  Uracil DNA glycosylase (UNG) deficiency
  CD40 ligand deficiency
  CD40 deficiency
B-cell activation factor from tumor necrosis factor (Baff-R) deficiency
TAC1 deficiency
Common variable immune deficiency
	Congenital thymic aplasia (DiGeorge Syndrome)
	MHC class II deficiency
	Transporter associated with antigen presentation (TAP-1 or TAP-2) MHC class 1 deficiency
	THI deficiency
	  Interferon γ and interferon γ receptor deficiency ⎤ affect T cell/
	  IL- 12 and IL-12 receptor deficiency ⎦ macrophage interaction

	Disorders of cytotoxic T cell/NK function with acute organ damage after viral infection
	X-linked lymphoproliferative (Duncan Syndrome) Chediak–Higashi (see page 159) Griscelli syndrome Familial hemophagocytic syndrome (perforin gene defect) (see page 283)
Severe combined immune deficiency	**Multisystem disorders**
X-Linked Interleukin (IL) receptor γ chain defects in receptors for IL-2, IL-4, IL-7, IL15; α chain defect for IL-7 JAK-3 deficiency ZAP-70 deficiency Adenosine deaminase (ADA), purine nucleoside phosphorylase deficiencies Recombination activating gene (RAG-1 or RAG-2) deficiencies Reticular dysgenesis	Wiskott–Aldrich syndrome (X-linked) Immune dysregulation polyendocrinopathy enteropathy, X-linked (IPEX) WHIM (warts, hypogammaglobulinemia, infections, and myelokathexis) Autoimmune polyendocrinopathy and ectodermal dysplasia Hyper IgE – eczema, hypermobility of joints, lung abnormalities
	Defects of DNA repair with chromosome instability and sensitivity to X-radiation
	Ataxia telangiectasia (immunodeficiency) Nijmegen breakage syndrome

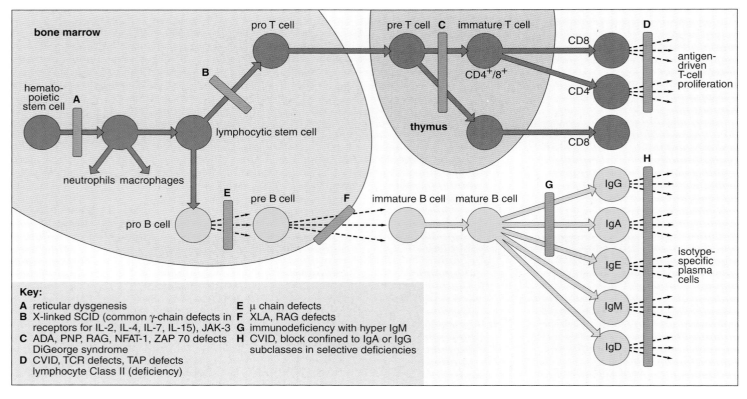

Fig. 11-27. Immunodeficiency disorders: sites of the defects in B- and T-cell development in different types of congenital immune deficiency. *ADA*, adenosine deaminase; *CVID*, common variable immunodeficiency; *JAK-3*, Janus-associated kinase; *NFAT-1*, nuclear factor of activated T cells; *PNP*, purine nucleoside phosphorylase; *RAG*, recombination activation genes; *SCID*, severe combined immunodeficiency; *TAP*, transporter associated with antigen presentation; *XLA*, X-linked agammaglobulinemia; *ZAP-70*, zeta-associated protein. (Courtesy of Dr. A. D. B. Webster.)

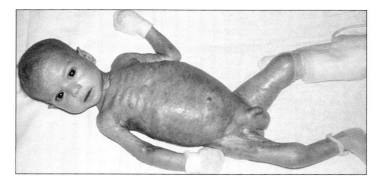

Fig. 11-28. Severe combined immunodeficiency disease caused by adenosine deaminase (ADA) deficiency: severely wasted infant with distended abdomen. There was widespread candidal infection of the mouth and chronic diarrhea. (Courtesy of Professor R. I. Levinsky.)

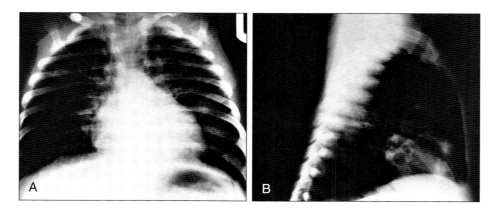

Fig. 11-29. Severe combined immunodeficiency disease: chest radiographs of the infant in Fig. 11-25. **A,** The posteroanterior view shows absence of thymic shadow in the superior mediastinum. **B,** The lateral view confirms the lack of thymus tissue deep in the sternum. (A, B, Courtesy of Professor R. I. Levinsky.)

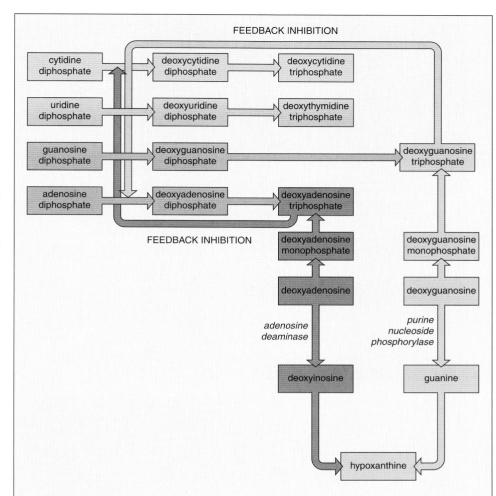

Fig. 11-30. Role of adenosine deaminase (ADA) and purine nucleoside phosphorylase (PNP) in purine degradation. ADA deficiency causes death of cortical thymocytes by accumulation of deoxyadenosine triphosphate (which inhibits DNA synthesis). PNP deficiency produces toxicity to T cells by accumulation of deoxyguanosine triphosphate. ADA and PNP are also involved in adenosine and guanosine degradation, respectively. In both types of deficiency, other biochemical mechanisms of toxicity to proliferating and nonproliferating lymphoid cells may occur.

In the very rare syndrome of lymphoreticular dysgenesis, development of both the reticuloendothelial and lymphoid systems fails. Affected infants die soon after birth from overwhelming infection. Lymphopenia is marked, and stigmata of splenic atrophy may be found in the peripheral blood (Fig. 11-31).

ACQUIRED IMMUNODEFICIENCY SYNDROME

Acquired immunodeficiency syndrome (AIDS) is caused by infection with HIV, a retrovirus of the lentivirus subgroup.

The predominant effects of HIV are produced through infection of T helper (CD4+) cells (Fig. 11-32). Some CD4+ cells are lysed directly by replicating HIV, but the virus remains latent in most host cells, unrecognized by the patient's immune system. When such latently infected T cells are activated, the virus replicates and cell death follows. The CD4 antigen appears to be the main receptor for HIV, and CD4+ antigen-presenting cells are also an important site for viral replication. A chemokine receptor, CCR-5 or CCR-4, is also required for cell entry.

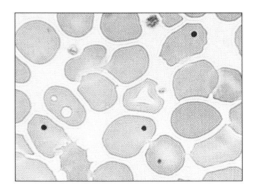

Fig. 11-31. Lymphoreticular dysgenesis: peripheral blood film of a 1-week-old infant. The large numbers of Howell-Jolly bodies (small granular remnants of DNA) are the result of splenic agenesis. There was severe lymphopenia. (Absolute lymphocyte count, 0.1×10^9/L.)

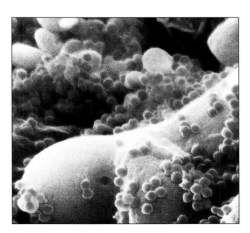

Fig. 11-32. AIDS: scanning electron micrograph of a T lymphocyte infected by HIV. This close-up view shows the hexagonal outline of the virus particles. The virus subgroups (clades) differ in viral sequence. (Courtesy of Lennart Nilsson; © Boehringer Ingelheim International GmbH.)

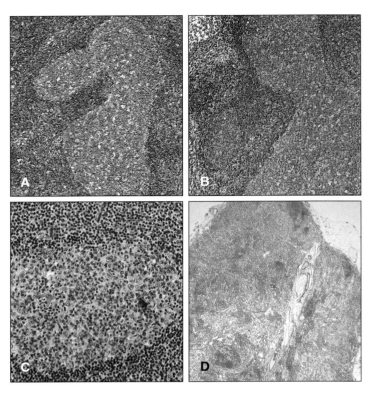

Fig. 11-33. AIDS: sections of lymph nodes infected by HIV show a spectrum of histologic changes. **A, B,** Type I includes follicular and paracortical hyperplasia. Mitotically active germinal centers are numerous in the medulla, as well as the cortex, and present a "geographic outline." Mitotic figures are abundant, and there is extensive cytolyis and phagocytosis of cell remnants by tingible body histiocytes. The mantle zones are attenuated and (in places) absent, and the follicles appear confluent. The interfollicular tissue shows an increase in small vessels. **C,** In the Type II pattern, there is loss of germinal centers but diffuse lymphoid hyperplasia. **D,** In Type III, an end-stage in fatal cases, lymphocyte depletion predominates. (*A, B,* Courtesy of Dr. J. E. McLaughlin. *C,* Reproduced with permission from Ioachim HL: *Pathology of AIDS,* New York, 1989, Gower Medical Publishing.)

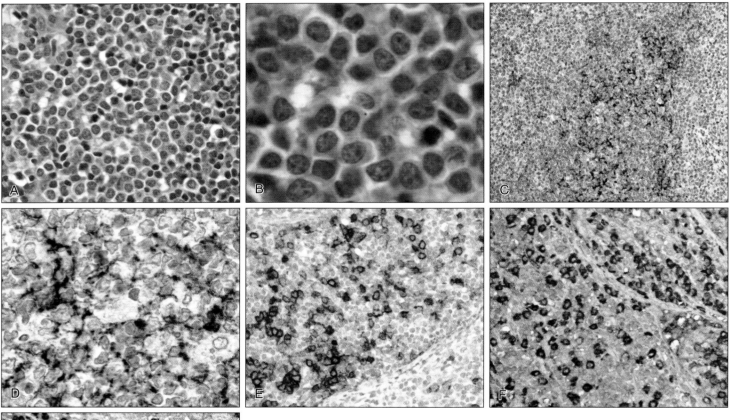

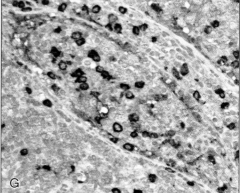

Fig. 11-34. HIV Infection. **A,** Monocytoid B cells with monomorphic B cells with cytoplasm resembling histiocytes, typical of HIV infection but also seen in toxoplasmosis and other conditons. **B,** Monocytoid B cells as a) at higher power. **C,** P24 immunostain; follicle dendritic cells are positive. **D,** P24 immunostain as c) at higher power. **E,** CD138 immunostain showing plasma cells increased in germinal centre and paracortex. **F,** Kappa light chain: the B cells are polytypic. **G,** Lambda light chain: the B cells polytypic (Courtesy of Dr. A. Ramsay).

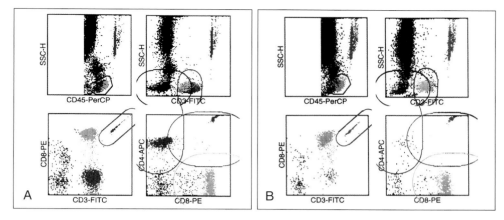

Fig. 11-35. HIV Infection: four color flow cytometry measurement of peripheral blood lymphocyte subpopulations. **A,** normal; **B,** HIV infection. The pink dots represent a known number of beads which are counted in order to quantify the CD4 and CD8 populations. Brown dots = CD4 cells. Green dots = CD8 cells (Courtesy, Department of Immunology, Royal Free Hospital)

Fig. 11-36. HIV infection: the sequence of expression of HIV antigens and different antibodies following primary infection. (Courtesy of Professor M. C. Contreras and the North London Blood Transfusion Center.)

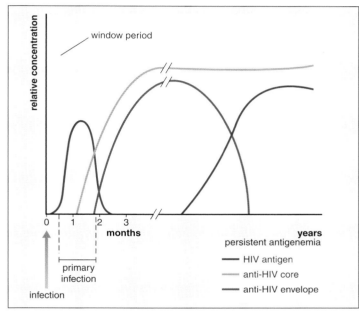

TABLE 11-4.   HUMAN IMMUNODEFICIENCY VIRUS INFECTION: HEMATOLOGIC MANIFESTATIONS

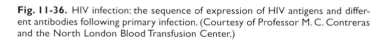

Fall in CD4 lymphocyte count and lymphopenia

Anemia, neutropenia, thrombocytopenia – either singly or combined

Bone marrow changes	Hypercellular (increased plasma cells, lymphocytes)
	Normocellular
	Hypocellular
	Dysplastic changes:
	normoblasts
	granulocytic (giant metamyelocytes, Pelger forms, detached nuclear fragments)
	megakaryocytes
	Increased fibrosis,
	Granulomas (AFB, cryptococcal, uncertain etiology)
	Other infections [e.g., histoplasma, leishmania, pneumocystis (may need culture to demonstrate)]
	Benign nodules
	Gelatinous degeneration
	Infiltration by lymphoma
Low serum vitamin B$_{12}$ and folate levels	
Toxic change as a result of drugs	For example, megaloblastosis caused by azidothymidine, pentamidine
Plasma protein changes	Polyclonal rise in IgG
	Paraprotein

Transmission of the virus is usually by sexual contact, or by blood or blood products, or by breast milk. Particularly common in homosexual men, AIDS is also seen frequently in intravenous drug abusers, hemophiliacs, and other patients who require multiple blood transfusions, as well as in heterosexual contacts of AIDS cases.

The viral load may be as high as 10^7 ribonucleic acid (RNA) copies/ml during acute infection. A prodromal period of about 6 weeks follows the initial infection, after which symptoms that resemble infectious mononucleosis may occur. A proportion of patients pass through the asymptomatic and persistent lymphadenopathy stages to the AIDS-related complex (ARC) and fully developed AIDS.

Examination of involved lymph nodes reveals characteristic abnormalities (Figs. 11-33 and 11-34). Depletion of CD4 cells is progressive, and the peripheral blood shows lymphopenia and an alteration in the T-lymphocyte subsets, with a fall in the CD4+:CD8+ (helper:suppressor) ratio from the normal value of 1.5 to 2.5:1 to less than 1:1 (Fig. 11-35). A polyclonal rise in serum immunoglobulins is often found, in some cases with a paraprotein present. The diagnosis is confirmed by detection of antibodies to one or more HIV surface antigens, or by detection of the antigens themselves (Fig. 11-36). Hematologic abnormalities may include anemia, neutropenia, or thrombocytopenia (Table 11-4); these are often autoimmune

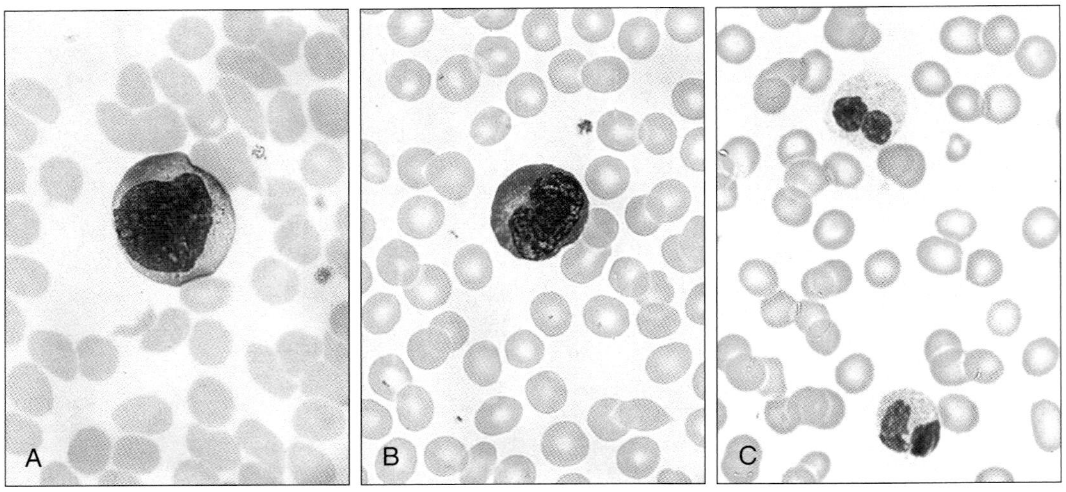

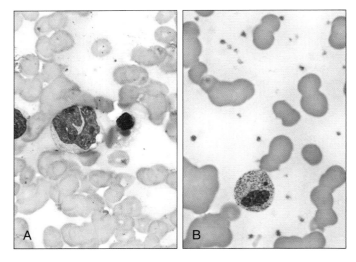

Fig. 11-37. HIV infection: peripheral blood showing **(A, B)** immunoblasts and **(C)** pseudo-Pelger cells. (*C*, Courtesy of Dr. D. Swirsky.)

in origin, but sometimes result from direct infection of hematopoietic stem and progenitor cells in the bone marrow. The cytopenias may also be caused by dysplastic changes (Figs. 11-37 to 11-40), fibrosis (Fig. 11-41), or lymphoma in the marrow.

A wide spectrum of opportunistic organisms cause infections in AIDS patients, including atypical mycobacteria (Fig. 11-42), *Pneumocystis carinii* (Fig. 11-43), cytomegalovirus (Fig. 11-44) and *Cryptococcus, Histoplasma* (Fig. 11-45), and *Leishmania* (Fig. 11-46).

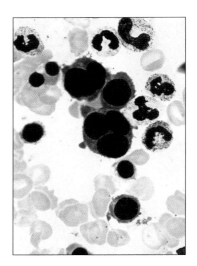

Fig. 11-38. HIV infection: bone marrow aspirate showing dyserythropoietic changes.

Fig. 11-39. HIV infection: dysmyelopoiesis with **(A)** giant metamyelocyte and **(B)** detached nuclear fragment. (*B*, Courtesy of Professor. B. A. Bain.)

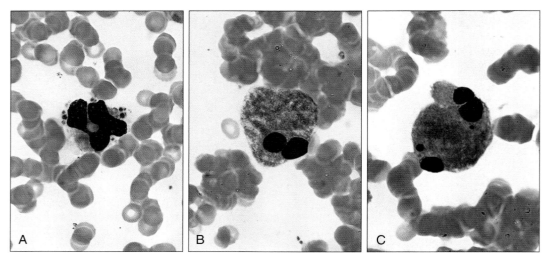

Fig. 11-40. HIV infection. **A–C,** Bone marrow aspirate showing dysplastic megakaryoctes.

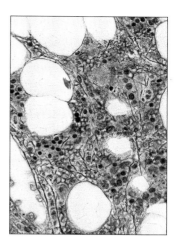

Fig. 11-41. HIV infection: bone marrow trephine biopsy showing dense reticulin network. (Silver stain.) (Courtesy of Dr. C. Costello.)

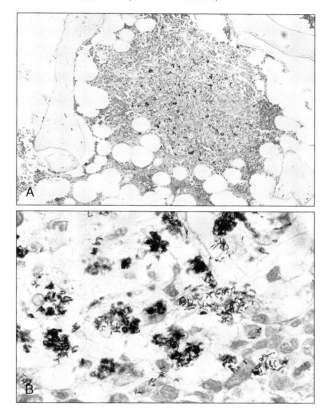

Fig. 11-42. AIDS: bone marrow trephine biopsy. **A,** Granuloma showing strong positivity with Ziehl-Nielsen stain. **B,** Higher power shows large numbers of acid-fast bacilli. (A, B, Courtesy of Dr. B. W. Baker and Dr. E. B. Knottenbelt.)

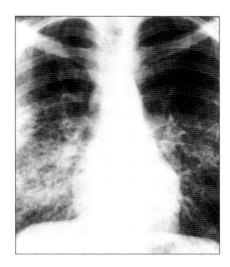

Fig. 11-43. AIDS: chest radiograph in *Pneumocystis carinii* infection, showing extensive, predominantly central interstitial opacities.

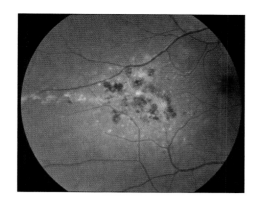

Fig. 11-44. AIDS: cytomegalovirus retinitis. (Courtesy of Dr. S. Imashuku.)

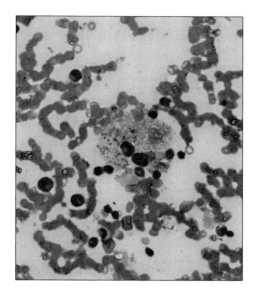

Fig. 11-45. AIDS: bone marrow aspirate showing histoplasmosis, visible as faintly staining fine fungal organisms in macrophages. (Courtesy of Dr. C. Costello.)

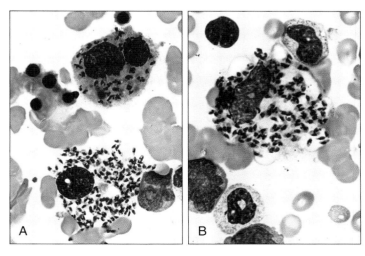

Fig. 11-46. AIDS: bone marrow aspirate showing Leishman-Donovan bodies.

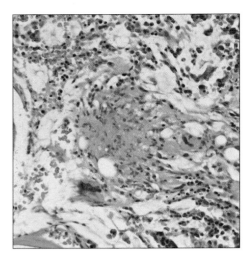

Fig. 11-47. AIDS: bone marrow trephine biopsy showing granuloma of uncertain etiology. (Courtesy of Dr. C. Costello.)

Often non-specific granuloma are found (Fig. 11-47). A proportion of the patients develop Kaposi's sarcoma, a vascular skin tumor of endothelial cell origin associated with Kaposi's sarcoma herpesvirus (KSHV) or human herpesvirus 8 (HHV8) (Figs. 11-48 and 11-49); other patients may develop non-Hodgkin lymphoma, which is likely to be high grade, and they have a 20% incidence of lymphoma in the central nervous system (Figs. 11-50 to 11-53). Primary effusion lymphoma is an unusual B cell lymphoma associated with HHV8 viral infection (see Fig 19-78).

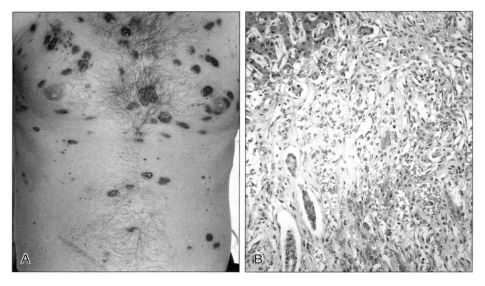

Fig. 11-48. AIDS, Kaposi's sarcoma: **A,** Multiple vascular tumors of endothelial origin on the chest of an HIV antigen–positive homosexual male. **B,** infiltration of the portal areas of the liver. (A, Courtesy of Dr. I. V. D. Weller.)

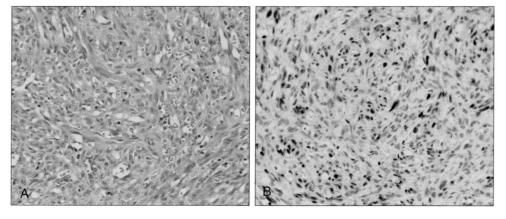

Fig. 11-49. A, AIDS, Kaposi's sarcoma: vascular endothelial cells with blood lakes. **B,** AIDS Kaposi sarcoma: p24 immunostain is positive.

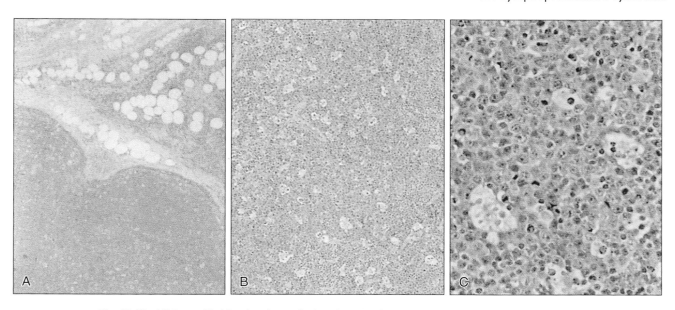

Fig. 11-50. AIDS, non-Hodgkin lymphoma. **A,** Lymph node showing replacement of normal architecture by tumor, which is extending into surrounding fat. **B, C,** Higher magnifications show the tumor to comprise lymphoblasts and "starry sky" tingible body macrophages.

Fig. 11-51. AIDS, non-Hodgkin lymphoma: fine-needle aspirate of cervical lymph node showing lymphoblasts with cytoplasm that is strongly basophilic. Some of the cells show prominent cytoplasmic vacuoles (same case as shown in Fig. 11-50).

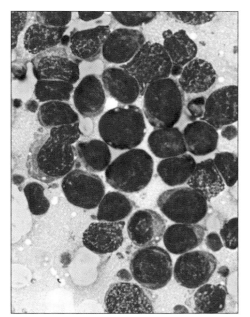

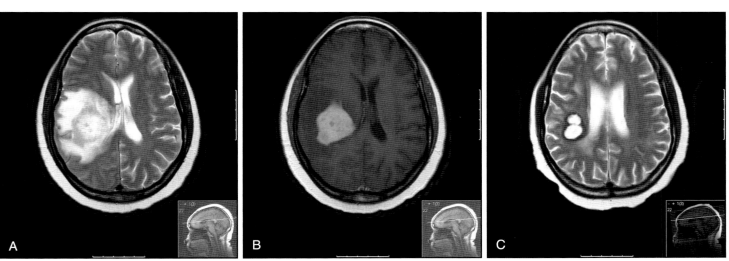

Fig. 11-52. AIDS, Cerebral lymphoma MRI. A, T2W MR brain scan showing heterogeneous mass and adjacent edema in right inferior frontoparietal region. There is compression of the right lateral ventricle and displacement of midline structures. Biopsy showed diffuse large B cell lymphoma. B, The mass enhances after intravenous gadolinium injection. C, Enhanced image after chemotherapy showing regression of the mass. (Courtesy of the Department of Radiology, the Royal Free Hospital.)

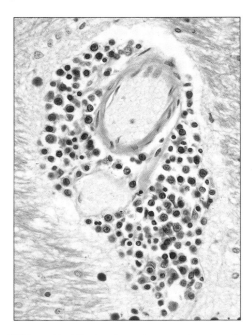

Fig. 11-53. AIDS, non-Hodgkin lymphoma: invasion of perivascular space of the brain by a high-grade systemic lymphoma. (Courtesy of Dr. J. E. McLaughlin.)

AUTOIMMUNE LYMPHOPROLIFERATIVE SYNDROME

Autoimmune lymphoproliferative syndrome is characterized by lymphadenopathy (Fig. 11-54), hepatosplenomegaly, autoimmune hemolytic anemia, neutropenia, thrombocytopenia, and hypergam-

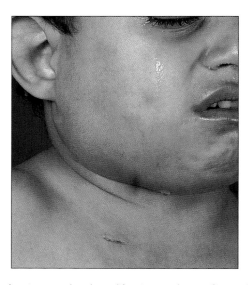

Fig. 11-54. Autoimmune lymphoproliferative syndrome: 8-year-old girl with marked generalized lymphadenopathy and hepatosplenomegaly. Her brother had similar clinical findings. (Courtesy of Professor H. G. Prentice.)

maglobulinemia with a high proportion of circulating CD3+, CD4–, and CD8+ T cells. The lymph nodes show loss of normal architecture with reduction of B cells (Fig. 11-55). The disease is associated with mutations in the FAS gene with defective apoptosis in response to anti-FAS antibody and presumably failure of normal apoptosis by lymphoid cells in vivo.

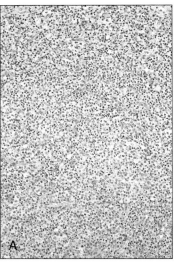

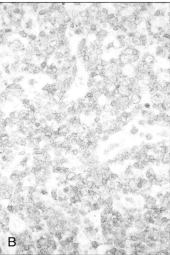

Fig. 11-55. Autoimmune lymphoproliferative syndrome. **A,** Lymph node biopsy at low power showing replacement of normal architecture by a uniform population of T lymphocytes with effacement of cortical structures. **B,** Immunoperoxidase stain at higher power showing that the majority of lymphocytes express CD3 antigens. (A, B, Courtesy of Dr. J. E. McLaughlin and Professor H. G. Prentice.)

ACUTE LEUKEMIAS

The acute leukemias are the result of accumulation of early myeloid or lymphoid precursors in the bone marrow, blood, and other tissues, and are thought to arise by somatic mutation(s) of a single cell within a minor population of stem or early progenitor cells in the bone marrow or thymus (Fig. 12-1). Acute leukemia may arise de novo or be the terminal event in a number of preexisting blood disorders, for example, polycythemia rubra vera, chronic myeloid leukemia, or one of the myelodysplastic syndromes. At presentation at least 20% and usually more than 80% of marrow cells are blasts.

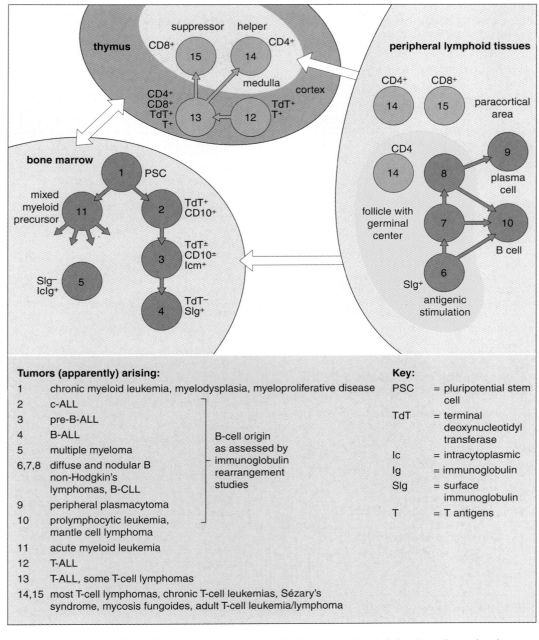

Tumors (apparently) arising:

1   chronic myeloid leukemia, myelodysplasia, myeloproliferative disease
2   c-ALL
3   pre-B-ALL
4   B-ALL
5   multiple myeloma
6,7,8   diffuse and nodular B non-Hodgkin's lymphomas, B-CLL
9   peripheral plasmacytoma
10   prolymphocytic leukemia, mantle cell lymphoma
11   acute myeloid leukemia
12   T-ALL
13   T-ALL, some T-cell lymphomas
14,15   most T-cell lymphomas, chronic T-cell leukemias, Sézary's syndrome, mycosis fungoides, adult T-cell leukemia/lymphoma

(6,7,8,9,10: B-cell origin as assessed by immunoglobulin rearrangement studies)

Key:

PSC   = pluripotential stem cell
TdT   = terminal deoxynucleotidyl transferase
Ic   = intracytoplasmic
Ig   = immunoglobulin
SIg   = surface immunoglobulin
T   = T antigens

Fig. 12-1. Tumor cells: similarities between the tumor cells of acute and chronic leukemias, malignant lymphomas and myeloma, and early bone marrow, thymic, or peripheral lymphoid cells. Although the malignant cells may resemble these progenitor or more mature cells, it is possible that the cell of origin of the hematologic malignancy is an earlier (more primitive) cell. B-ALL, C-ALL, and pre-B-ALL are now classified by WHO (2008) according to cytogenetics (Table 12-1).

TABLE 12-1.   WORLD HEALTH ORGANIZATION (2008) CLASSIFICATION OF TUMORS
OF THE HEMATOPOIETIC AND LYMPHOID TISSUES

MYELOPROLIFERATIVE NEOPLASMS		**AML with myelodysplasia-related changes**	9895/3
Chronic myelogenous leukemia, *BCR-ABL1* positive	9875/3	**Therapy-related myeloid neoplasms**	9920/3
Chronic neutrophilic leukemia	9963/3		
Polycythemia vera	9950/3	**Acute myeloid leukemia, NOS**	9861/3
Primary myelofibrosis	9961/3	AML with minimal differentiation	9872/3
Essential thrombocythemia	9962/3	AML without maturation	9873/3
Chronic eosinophilic leukemia, NOS	9964/3	AML with maturation	9874/3
Mastocytosis		Acute myelomonocytic leukemia	9867/3
Cutaneous mastocytosis	9740/1	Acute monoblastic and monocytic leukemia	9891/3
Systemic mastocytosis	9741/3	Acute erythroid leukemia	9840/3
Mast cell leukemia	9742/3	Acute megakaryoblastic leukemia	9910/3
Mast cell sarcoma	9740/3	Acute basophilic leukemia	9870/3
Extracutaneous mastocytoma	9740/1	Acute panmyelosis with myelofibrosis	9931/3
Myeloproliferative neoplasm, unclassifiable	9975/3		
		Myeloid sarcoma	9930/3
MYELOID AND LYMPHOID NEOPLASMS ASSOCIATED			
WITH EOSINOPHILIA AND ABNORMALITIES OF		**Myeloid proliferations related to Down syndrome**	
PDGFRA, PDGFRB,* OR *FGFR1		Transient abnormal myelopoiesis	9898/1
Myeloid and lymphoid neoplasms with *PDGFRA*		Myeloid leukemia associated with Down syndrome	9898/3
rearrangement	*9965/3*		
Myeloid neoplasms with *PDGFRB* rearrangement	*9966/3*	**Blastic plasmacytoid dendritic cell neoplasm**	9727/3
Myeloid and lymphoid neoplasms with *FGFR1*			
abnormalities	*9967/3*	**ACUTE LEUKEMIAS OF AMBIGUOUS LINEAGE**	
		Acute undifferentiated leukemia	9801/3
MYELODYSPLASTIC/MYELOPROLIFERATIVE		Mixed phenotype acute leukemia with	
NEOPLASMS		t(9;22)(q34;q11.2); *BCR-ABL1*	*9806/3*
Chronic myelomonocytic leukemia	9945/3	Mixed phenotype acute leukemia with t(v;11q23); *MLL*	
Atypical chronic myeloid leukemia, *BCR-ABL1*		rearranged	*9807/3*
negative	9876/3	Mixed phenotype acute leukemia, B/myeloid, NOS	*9808/3*
Juvenile myelomonocytic leukemia	9946/3	Mixed phenotype acute leukemia, T/myeloid; NOS	*9809/3*
Myelodysplastic/myeloproliferative neoplasm,		*Natural killer (NK) cell lymphoblastic*	
unclassifiable	9975/3	*leukemia/lymphoma*	
Refractory anemia with ring sideroblasts			
associated with marked thrombocytosis	9982/3	**PRECURSOR LYMPHOID NEOPLASMS**	
MYELODYSPLASTIC SYNDROMES		**B-lymphoblastic leukemia/lymphoma**	
Refractory cytopenia with unilineage dysplasia		B-lymphoblastic leukemia/lymphoma, NOS	*9811/3*
Refractory anemia	9980/3	B-lymphoblastic leukemia/lymphoma with recurrent	
Refractory neutropenia	*9991/3*	genetic abnormalities	
Refractory thrombocytopenia	*9992/3*	B-lymphoblastic leukemia/lymphoma with t(9:22)	
Refractory anemia with ring sideroblasts	9982/3	(q34;q11.2); *BCR-ABL1*	*9812/3*
Refractory cytopenia with multilineage dysplasia	9985/3	B-lymphoblastic leukemia/lymphoma with t(v;11q23);	
Refractory anemia with excess blasts	9983/3	*MLL* rearranged	*9813/3*
Myelodysplastic syndrome associated with isolated		B-lymphoblastic leukemia/lymphoma with t(12;21)	
del(5q)	9986/3	(p13;q22); *TEL-AML1 (ETV6-RUNX1)*	*9814/3*
Myelodysplastic syndrome, unclassifiable	9989/3	B-lymphoblastic leukemia/lymphoma with	
Childhood myelodysplastic syndrome		hyperdiploidy	*9815/3*
Refractory cytopenia of childhood	9985/3	B-lymphoblastic leukemia/lymphoma with	
		hypodiploidy (hypodiploid ALL)	*9816/3*
		B-lymphoblastic leukemia/lymphoma with	
ACUTE MYELOID LEUKEMIA LEUKEMIA (AML)		t(5;14)(q31;q32) *(IL3-IGH)*	*9817/3*
AND RELATED PRECURSOR NEOPLASMS		B-lymphoblastic leukemia/lymphoma with	
		t(1;19)(q23; p13.3); *E2A-PBX1 (TCF3-PBX1)*	*9818/3*
AML with recurrent genetic abnormalities			
AML with t(8;21)(q22;q22); *RUNX1-RUNX1T1*	9896/3	**T-lymphoblastic leukemia/lymphoma**	*9837/3*
AML with inv(16)(p13.1q22) or t(16;16)(p13.1;q22);			
CBFB-MYH11	9871/3	**MATURE B-CELL NEOPLASMS**	
Acute promyelocytic leukemia with t(15;17)		Chronic lymphocytic leukemia/small lymphocytic	
(q22;q11-12); *PML-RARA*	9866/3	lymphoma	9823/3
AML with t(9;11)(p22;q23); *MLLT3-MLL*	9897/3	B-cell prolymphocytic leukemia	9833/3
AML with t(6;9)(p23;q34); *DEK-NUP214*	*9865/3*	Splenic B-cell marginal zone lymphoma	9689/3
AML with inv(3)(q21q26.2) or t(3;3)(q21;q26.2);		Hairy cell leukemia	9940/3
RPN1-EVI1	*9869/3*	*Splenic B-cell lymphoma/leukemia, unclassifiable*	9591/3
AML (megakaryoblastic) with t(1;22)(p13;q13);		*Splenic diffuse red pulp small B-cell lymphoma*	9591/3
RBM15-MKL1	*9911/3*	*Hairy cell leukemia-variant*	9591/3
AML with mutated NPM1	9861/3		
AML with mutated CEBPA	9861/3		

Modified from Swerdlow SH, Campo E, Harris NL, Jaffe ES, Pileri SA, Stein H, Thiele J, Vardiman JW: *WHO Classification of Tumours of Haematopoietic and Lymphoid Tissues,* ed 4, Lyon, 2008. International Agency for Research on Cancer.

The diseases are divided into two main subgroups: acute myeloid (myeloblastic, myelogenous) leukemia (AML) and acute lymphoblastic leukemia (ALL), and further subdivided on cytogenetic and morphologic grounds into various subcategories (Table 12-1). The previous French-American-British (FAB) scheme based on morphology divided AML into subtypes M0 to M7 and ALL into subtypes L1, L2, and L3 (Table 12-2). The World Health Organization (WHO) (2008) classification is largely based on cytogenetics. Table 12-1 also gives the WHO (2008) classification of all the other tumors of the hematopoietic and lymphoid tissues.

TABLE 12-1. WORLD HEALTH ORGANIZATION (2008) CLASSIFICATION OF TUMORS OF THE HEMATOPOIETIC AND LYMPHOID TISSUES—cont'd

Lymphoplasmacytic lymphoma	9671/3	Adult T-cell leukemia/lymphoma	9827/3
Waldenström macroglobulinemia	9761/3	Extranodal NK/T cell lymphoma, nasal type	9719/3
Heavy chain diseases	9762/3	Enteropathy-associated T-cell lymphoma	9717/3
Alpha heavy chain disease	9762/3	Hepatosplenic T-cell lymphoma	9716/3
Gamma heavy chain disease	9762/3	Subcutaneous panniculitis-like T-cell lymphoma	9708/3
Mu heavy chain disease	9762/3	Mycosis fungoides	9700/3
Plasma cell myeloma	9732/3	Sézary syndrome	9701/3
Solitary plasmacytoma of bone	9731/3	Primary cutaneous CD30 positive T-cell	
Extraosseous plasmacytoma	9734/3	lymphoproliferative disorders	
Extranodal marginal zone lymphoma of mucosa-		Lymphomatoid papulosis	9718/1
associated lymphoid tissue (MALT lymphoma)	9699/3	Primary cutaneous anaplastic large cell lymphoma	9718/3
Nodal marginal zone lymphoma	9699/3	Primary cutaneous gamma-delta T-cell lymphoma	*9726/3*
Pediatric nodal marginal zone lymphoma	9699/3	*Primary cutaneous CD8 positive aggressive*	
Follicular lymphoma	9690/3	*epidermotropic cytotoxic T-cell lymphoma*	9709/3
Pediatric follicular lymphoma	9690/3	*Primary cutaneous CD4 positive small/medium T-cell*	
Primary cutaneous follicle center lymphoma	*9597/3*	*lymphoma*	9709/3
Mantle cell lymphoma	9673/3	Peripheral T-cell lymphoma, NOS	9702/3
Diffuse large B-cell lymphoma(DLBCL), NOS	9680/3	Angioimmunoblastic T-cell lymphoma	9705/3
T cell/histiocyte rich large B-cell lymphoma	9688/3	Anaplastic large cell lymphoma, *ALK* positive	9714/3
Primary DLBCL of the CNS	9680/3	*Anaplastic large cell lymphoma, ALK negative*	9702/3
Primary cutaneous DLBCL, leg type	9680/3		
EBV positive DLBCL of the elderly	9680/3	**HODGKIN LYMPHOMA**	
DLBCL associated with chronic inflammation	9680/3	Nodular lymphocyte predominant Hodgkin lymphoma	9659/3
Lymphomatoid granulomatosis	9766/1	Classical Hodgkin lymphoma	9650/3
Primary mediastinal (thymic) large B-cell lymphoma	9679/3	Nodular sclerosis classical Hodgkin lymphoma	9663/3
Intravascular large B-cell lymphoma	9712/3	Lymphocyte-rich classical Hodgkin lymphoma	9651/3
ALK-positive large B-cell lymphoma	9737/3	Mixed cellularity classical Hodgkin lymphoma	9652/3
Plasmablastic lymphoma	9735/3	Lymphocyte-depleted classical Hodgkin lymphoma	9653/3
Large B-cell lymphoma arising in HHV8-associated			
multicentric Castleman disease	*9738/3*	**HISTIOCYTIC AND DENDRITIC CELL NEOPLASMS**	
Primary effusion lymphoma	9678/3	Histiocytic sarcoma	9755/3
Burkitt lymphoma	9687/3	Langerhans cell histiocytosis	9751/3
B-cell lymphoma, unclassifiable, with features		Langerhans cell sarcoma	9756/3
intermediate between diffuse large B-cell lymphoma		Interdigitating dendritic cell sarcoma	9757/3
and Burkitt lymphoma	9680/3	Follicular dendritic cell sarcoma	9758/3
B-cell lymphoma, unclassifiable, with features		Fibroblastic reticular cell tumor	9759/3
intermediate between diffuse large B-cell lymphoma		Indeterminate dendritic cell tumor	9757/3
and classical Hodgkin lymphoma	9596/3	Disseminated juvenile xanthogranuloma	
MATURE T-CELL AND NK-CELL NEOPLASMS		**POST-TRANSPLANT LYMPHOPROLIFERATIVE**	
T-cell prolymphocytic leukemia	9834/3	**DISORDERS (PTLD)**	
T-cell large granular lymphocytic leukemia	9831/3	Early lesions	
Chronic lymphoproliferative disorder of NK-cells	9831/3	Plasmacytic hyperplasia	9971/1
Aggressive NK cell leukemia	9948/3	Infectious mononucleosis-like PTLD	9971/1
Systemic EBV positive T-cell lymphoproliferative		Polymorphic PTLD	9971/3
disease of childhood	*9724/3*	Monomorphic PTLD (B- and T/NK-cell types)*	
Hydroa vacciniforme-like lymphoma	*9725/3*	Classical Hodgkin lymphoma–type PTLD*	

NOS, not otherwise specified.
The italicized numbers are provisional codes for the 4th edition of ICD-O. While they are expected to be incorporated in the next ICD-O edition, they currently remain subject to changes.
The italicized histologic types are provisional entities, for which the WHO Working Group felt there was insufficient evidence to recognize as distinct diseases at this time.
*These lesions are classifed according to the leukemia or lymphoma to which they correspond, and are assigned the respective ICD-O code.

TABLE 12-2.   FAB (MORPHOLOGIC) CLASSIFICATION
OF ACUTE MYELOID LEUKEMIA

M_0

Large, agranular blasts (resemble ALL L_2, rarely L_1). Myeloperoxidase negative or <3% positive; B-, T-lineage markers negative; CD13 and/or CD33 positive; myeloperoxidase positive by immunochemistry or electron microscopy; TdT may be positive.

M_1

Blast cells, agranular and granular types (Types I and II) >90% of nonerythroid cells. At least 3% of these are peroxidase or Sudan black positive.
Remaining 10% (or less) of cells are maturing granulocytic cells.

M_2

Sum of agranular and granular blasts (Types I and II) is from 30% to 89% of nonerythroid cells.
Monocytic cells, <20%.
Granulocytes from promyelocytes to mature polymorphs, >10%.

M_3

Majority of cells are abnormal promyelocytes with heavy granulation.
Characteristic cells that contain bundles of Auer rods ("faggots") invariably present.
Note: Microgranular variant also occurs (Fig. 12-34).

M_4

In the marrow, blasts >30% of nonerythroid cells.
Sum of myeloblasts, promyelocytes, myelocytes and later granulocytes is between 30% and 80% of nonerythroid cells.
>20% of nonerythroid cells are monocyte lineage.
If monocytic cells exceed 80%, diagnosis is M_5.
Notes: If marrow findings as above and peripheral blood monocytes (all types) are >5.0 × 10^9/L, diagnosis is M_4.
If monocyte count <5.0 × 10^9/L, M_4 can be confirmed on basis of serum lysozyme, combined esterase, etc.
Diagnosis of M_4 confirmed if >20% of marrow precursors are monocytes (confirmed by special stains).

M_4 with eosinophilia

Eosinophils >5% of nonerythroid cells in marrow.
Eosinophils are abnormal.
Eosinophils are chloroacetate and periodic acid–Schiff positive.

M_5

80% of marrow nonerythroid cells are monoblasts, promonocytes, or monocytes.
M_{5a}, 80% of monocytic cells are monoblasts.
M_{5b}, <80% of monocytic cells are monoblasts; remainder are predominantly promonocytes and monocytes.

M_6

The erythroid component of the marrow exceeds 50% of all nucleated cells.
30% of the remaining nonerythroid cells are agranular or granular blasts (Types I and II).
Note: If >50% erythroid cells but <30% blasts, diagnosis becomes myelodysplastic syndrome.

M_7

30% at least of nucleated cells are blasts.
Blasts identified by platelet peroxidase on electron microscopy or by monoclonal antibodies.
Increased reticulin is common.

Modified from Bennett JM, Catovsky D, Daniel MT, et al: Proposed revised criteria for classification of acute myeloid leukemia. A report of the French-American-British Cooperative Group, *Ann Intern Med* 103:620-625, 1985.

CLINICAL FEATURES

Acute leukemia manifests with features of bone marrow failure (anemia, infections, easy bruising or hemorrhage) and may or may not include features of organ infiltration by leukemic cells. The organs usually involved are the lymph nodes, spleen and liver, meninges and central nervous system (CNS), testes (particularly in ALL), and skin (particularly in the M3 type of AML). Rarely, a visible deposit of leukemic blasts is seen in the eye (Fig. 12-26) or in other tissues

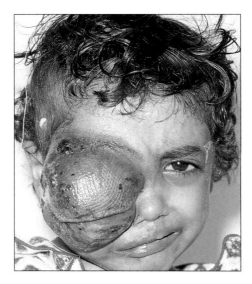

Fig. 12-2. Acute myeloid leukemia: chloroma of the eye in a 12-year-old girl with AML M2.

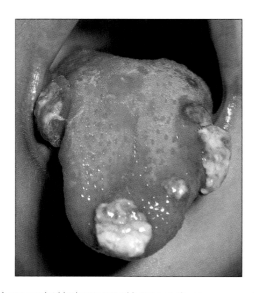

Fig. 12-3. Acute myeloid leukemia: raised lesions on the tongue caused by deposits of leukemic blasts in a 41-year-old man with AML M4.

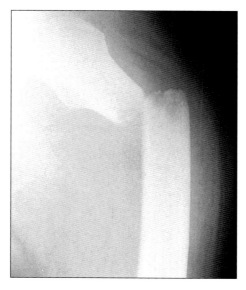

Fig. 12-4. Acute myeloid leukemia: pathologic fracture of left upper femur in an 82-year-old woman.

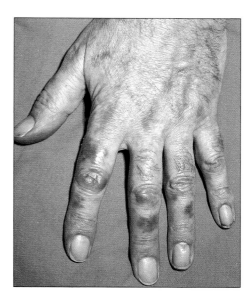

Fig. 12-5. Acute myeloid leukemia: Sweet's syndrome (acute febrile neutrophilic dermatosis) in a 62-year-old man with AML M4: bullous pyoderma. (Courtesy of Professor H. G. Prentice.)

(Figs. 12-3 and 12-4). Occasionally, patients show Sweet's syndrome (acute febrile neutrophilic dermatitis), which occurs in other malignant diseases (Fig. 12-5).

Infections are often bacterial in the early stages and particularly affect the skin (Figs. 12-6 and 12-7), pharynx, and perianal (Fig. 12-8) and perineal (Fig. 12-9) regions. Bacterial infections may lead to the adult respiratory distress syndrome (Fig. 12-10). Fungal infections are particularly common in patients with prolonged periods of neutropenia (Figs. 12-11 and 12-13) who have undergone multiple courses of chemotherapy and antibiotic therapy.

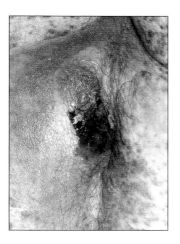

Fig. 12-8. Acute myeloid leukemia: this perianal lesion was found to be the result of a mixed infection by *Escherichia coli* and *Streptococcus fecalis*.

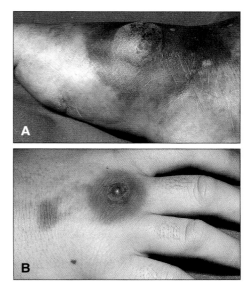

Fig. 12-6. Acute myeloid leukemia. **A,** A purplish black bullous lesion with surrounding erythema caused by infection from *Pseudomonas pyocyanea* on the foot. **B,** Similar but less marked infection on the back of the hand.

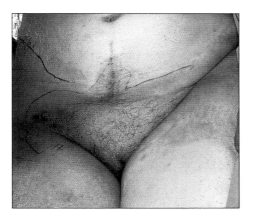

Fig. 12-9. Acute myeloid leukemia: cellulitis of the perineum, lower abdomen, and upper thighs caused by *Pseudomonas pyocyanea*.

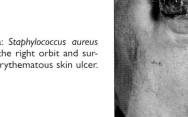

Fig. 12-7. Acute myeloid leukemia: *Staphylococcus aureus* was isolated from **(A)** infection of the right orbit and surrounding tissue and **(B)** a necrotic erythematous skin ulcer.

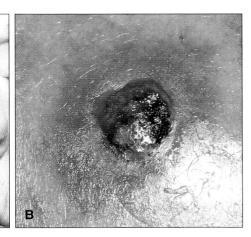

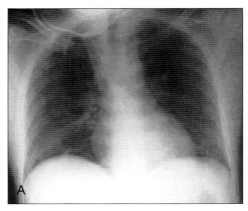
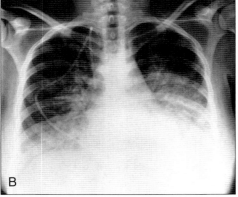

Fig. 12-10. Acute myeloid leukemia. **A,** Chest radiograph of 22-year-old man showing widespread interstitial shadowing resulting from adult acute respiratory distress syndrome associated with *Streptococcus mitis* infection during induction therapy. **B,** Interstitial shadowing in lower and middle zones bilaterally in a 23-year-old woman with septicemia from *Pseudomonas pyocyanea* following chemotherapy. She developed a fatal adult respiratory distress syndrome.

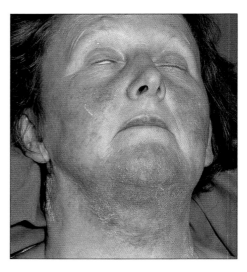

Fig. 12-11. Acute myeloid leukemia: spreading cellulitis of the neck and chin resulting from mixed streptococcal and candidal infection, previous chemotherapy, and prolonged periods of neutropenia.

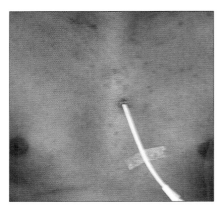

Fig. 12-13. Acute myeloid leukemia: candidal septicemia. Typical skin rash in a 22-year-old Sri Lankan man with severe neutropenia caused by intensive chemotherapy.

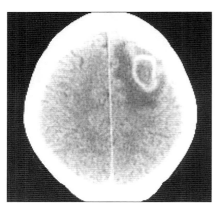

Other viral (especially herpetic), protozoal, or fungal infections are frequent, particularly in the mouth, and may become generalized and life threatening (Figs. 12-14 to 12-17). Hemorrhage of the skin or mucous membranes is usually petechial (Figs. 12-18 and 12-19).

Infiltration of the skin that manifests as a widespread, raised, nonitchy hemorrhagic rash and swelling of the gums (Fig. 12-20) are characteristic of the M5 type of AML; nodular and localized skin infiltrates may also occur (Fig. 12-21).

Fig. 12-14. Acute myeloid leukemia: CT scan showing encapsulated brain lesion in right frontal zone caused by aspergillosis infection with surrounding hypodense area caused by inflammation.

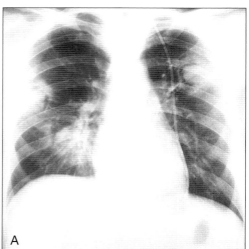
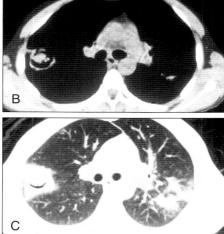

Fig. 12-12. Acute myeloid leukemia: this 32-year-old-man had received repeated chemotherapy for refractory disease. Three pulmonary mycotic cavities are visible: **(A)** radiograph; **(B, C)** computed tomography (CT) scans. (*B, C,* Courtesy of Dr. A. R. Valentine.)

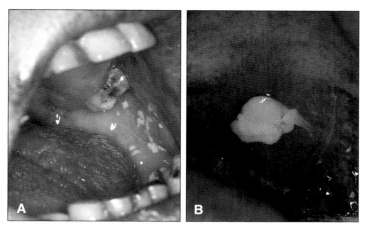

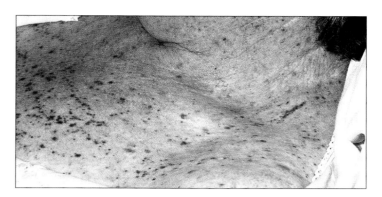

Fig. 12-18. Acute myeloid leukemia: petechial hemorrhages covering the upper chest and face in severe thrombocytopenia.

Fig. 12-15. Acute myeloid leukemia. **(A)** Plaques of *Candida albicans* in the mouth, with a lesion of herpes simplex on the upper lip. **B,** Candidal plaque on the soft palate.

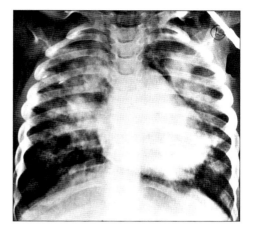

Fig. 12-16. Acute myeloid leukemia: chest radiograph showing patchy consolidation bilaterally caused by measles infection in a child. (Courtesy of Professor J. M. Chessells.)

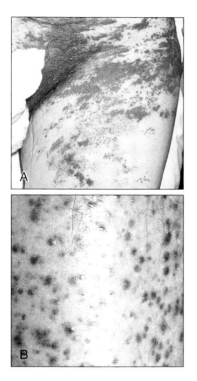

Fig. 12-19. Acute myeloid leukemia. **A,** Marked ecchymoses, petechial hemorrhages, and bruises over the groin and thigh. **B,** Close-up view of petechial hemorrhages over the leg.

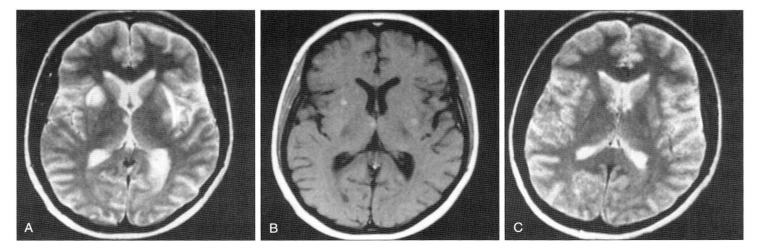

Fig. 12-17. Acute myeloid leukemia. **A, B,** Magnetic resonance imaging (MRI) scans showing multiple small opacities. The patient, a 23-year-old woman, complained of headaches and diplopia. The diagnosis of toxoplasmosis was made, and **(C)** she responded rapidly to antitoxoplasmosis therapy. (*A–C,* Courtesy of Dr. A. R. Valentine.)

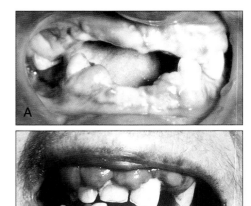

Fig. 12-20. Acute myeloid leukemia, M5 subtype. **A, B,** Leukemic infiltration of the gums results in their expansion and thickening, and partial covering of the teeth.

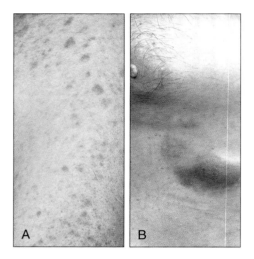

Fig. 12-21. Acute myeloid leukemia, M5 subtype. **A,** Multiple, raised, erythematous skin lesions caused by leukemic infiltration. **B,** Close-up view of nodular skin lesion.

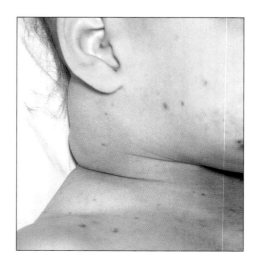

Fig. 12-22. Acute lymphoblastic leukemia: marked cervical lymphadenopathy in a 4-year-old boy. (Courtesy of Professor J. M. Chessells.)

In ALL, lymphadenopathy is more common (Fig. 12-22). In the T-cell variant (T-ALL), there is often upper mediastinal enlargement, caused by a thymic mass, which responds rapidly to therapy (Fig. 12-23). Although meningeal involvement is more frequent in children and younger subjects with ALL, it may occur at all ages, manifesting with nausea, vomiting, headaches, visual disturbances, photophobia,

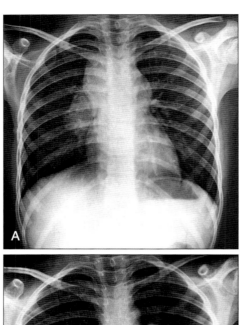

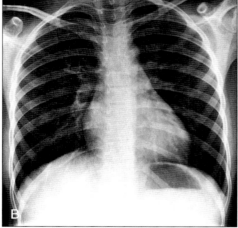

Fig. 12-23. Acute lymphoblastic leukemia, T-cell subtype: chest radiographs of a 4-year-old boy showing **(A)** upper mediastinal widening caused by thymic enlargement; **(B)** disappearance of thymic mass following 1 week of therapy with vincristine and prednisolone.

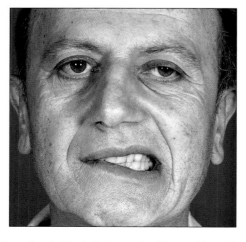

Fig. 12-24. Acute lymphoblastic leukemia: this 59-year-old man has facial asymmetry because of a right lower motor neuron seventh nerve palsy resulting from meningeal leukemic infiltration. (Courtesy of Professor H. G. Prentice.)

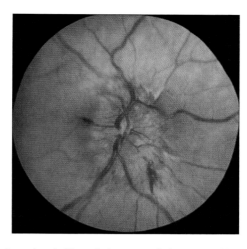

Fig. 12-25. Acute lymphoblastic leukemia: papilledema caused by meningeal disease. There is blurring of the disk margin with venous enlargement and retinal hemorrhages.

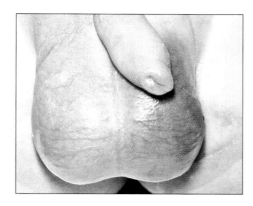

Fig. 12-28. Acute lymphoblastic leukemia: testicular swelling and erythema of the left side of the scrotum caused by testicular infiltration. (Courtesy of Professor J. M. Chessells.)

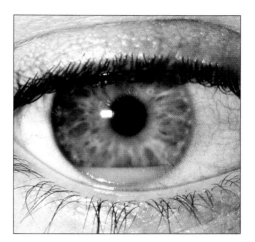

Fig. 12-26. Acute lymphoblastic leukemia: leukemic infiltration in the anterior chamber of the eye obscures the lower rim of the iris. (Courtesy of Professor J. M. Chessells).

and features of the cranial nerve palsies (Fig. 12-24). Papilledema may be found on examination (Fig. 12-25), and infiltration may occur at any site (Figs. 12-26 and 12-27). Testicular relapse is common, although it is only rarely detectable clinically on presentation (Fig. 12-28). Bone involvement may produce characteristic radiographic findings (Fig. 12-29).

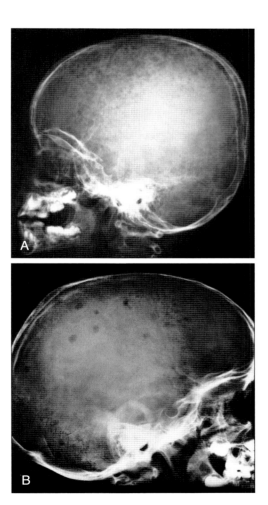

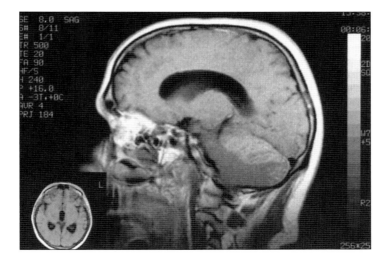

Fig. 12-27. Acute lymphoblastic leukemia: MRI scan showing dilated cerebral ventricles with expansion of the cerebellum and blockage of the viaduct between the third and fourth ventricles. The patient, a 33-year-old man, had headache, diplopia, and blast cells in the cerebrospinal fluid. (Courtesy of Dr. A. R. Valentine.)

Fig. 12-29. Acute lymphoblastic leukemia: radiographs of childrens' skulls showing **(A)** mottled appearance caused by widespread leukemic infiltration of bone and **(B)** multiple punched-out lesions caused by leukemic deposits. (Courtesy of Professor J. M. Chessells.)

MICROSCOPIC APPEARANCES

ACUTE MYELOID LEUKEMIA

The FAB morphologic classification criteria are given in Table 12-2. The WHO recognizes three favorable prognosis cytogenetic sub-groups: t(8;21) differentiated (M2) (Fig. 12-30); Inv (16), a type of myelomonocytic leukemia (M4) with abnormal myelomonocytic

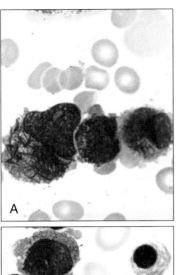

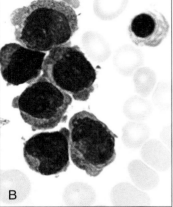

Fig. 12-32. Acute myeloid leukemia, t (15;17) subtype. **A, B,** Promyelocytes containing coarse azurophilic granules, and bundles of Auer rods ("faggots") in **(A).** The nuclei contain one or two nucleoli.

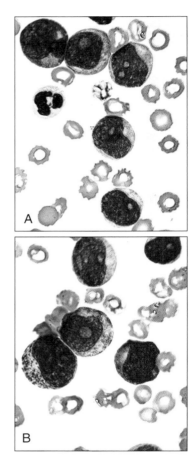

Fig. 12-30. Acute myeloid leukemia,t (8;21) subtype: **(A)** bone marrow aspirates showing myeloblasts with promyelocytes with azurophilic granules also present; **(B)** blast cells with folded nuclei, one or two nucleoli, less than 20 azurophilic granules (type II blasts) or greater than 20 azurophilic granules (type III blasts) per cell, and occasional Auer rods.

cells and eosinophils with basophilic granules (Fig. 12-31); and the t(15;17) promyelocytic subtype (Figs. 12-32 and 12-33). The typical form shows bundles of rodlike structures ("faggots"), which are aggregates of granules and can be seen with special stains (see Fig. 12-75). These cells contain procoagulant material, which, when released into the circulation, causes disseminated intravascular coagulation; this type also has a microgranular variant (Fig. 12-34). In AML M3, treatment with all-trans retinoic acid (ATRA) produces differentiation of the blasts (Fig. 12-35) often with full remission being obtained.

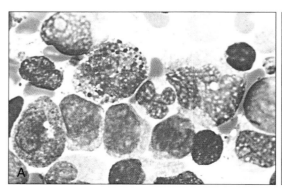

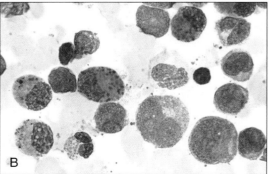

Fig. 12-31. Acute myeloid leukemia, inv (16) subtype. **A, B,** Blast cells, abnormal myelomonocytic cells, and eosinophils with basophilic granules.

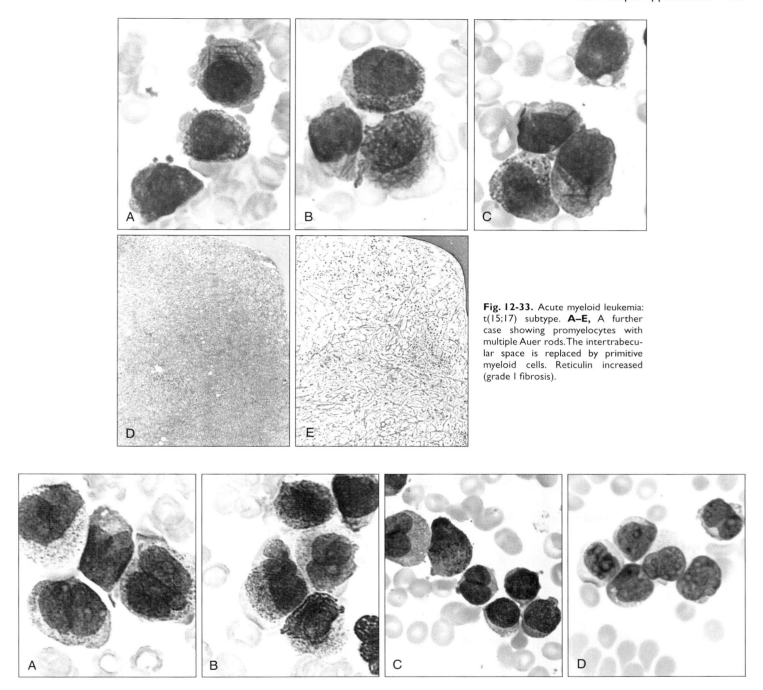

Fig. 12-33. Acute myeloid leukemia: t(15;17) subtype. **A–E,** A further case showing promyelocytes with multiple Auer rods. The intertrabecular space is replaced by primitive myeloid cells. Reticulin increased (grade 1 fibrosis).

Fig. 12-34. Acute myeloid leukemia, t(15;17). **A–D,** Microgranular variant. The usually bilobed cells contain numerous small azurophilic granules. (*C and D,* Courtesy of Professor J. M. Bennett.)

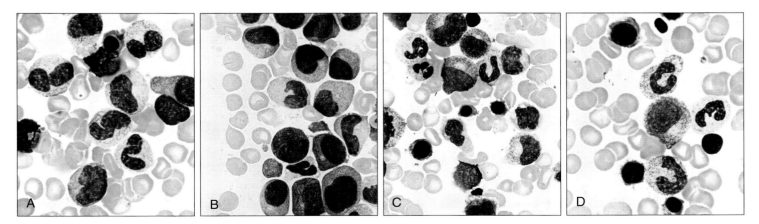

Fig. 12-35. Acute myeloid leukemia,t (15;17). **A–D,** Differentiation of myeloblasts into myelocytes and neutrophils during treatment with ATRA. Abnormal myelocytes and neutrophils containing Auer rods are seen. (*A–D,* Courtesy of Professor M. T. Daniel.)

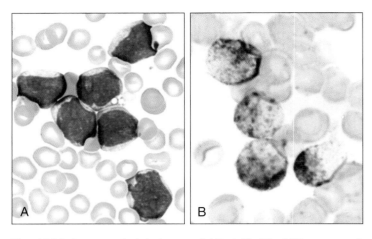

Fig. 12-36. Acute myeloid leukemia: t(9;11) (p22;q23) (MLL rearranged). **A,** Monoblastic (M5a) with over 80% blasts in the marrow. **B,** Nonspecific esterase-positive confirming monocytic lineage. FISH showed disruption of MLL gene in 96% of interphase nuclei analyzed. The patient was a 24-year-old man with no previous chemotherapy or radiotherapy.

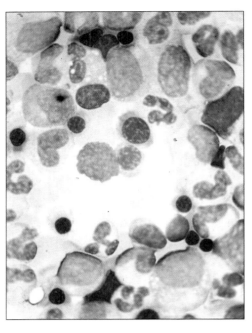

Fig. 12-38. Acute myeloid leukemia t(8;13) after topoisomerase inhibitor therapy. Myeloblasts and abnormal monocytes and neutrophils are present. (Courtesy of Professor B. A. Bain.)

Another myelomonocytic subgroup is characterized by chromosomal rearrangements involving the MLL gene on chromosome 11, for example, AML with t(9;11) (p22;q23); MLL3-MLL (Fig. 12-36). These cases may arise de novo or follow previous chemotherapy or radiotherapy. AML with t(6;9)(p23;q34) (DEK-NUP214); inv (3) q21;q26.2 (RPN1-EVII); t(1;22) p13; q13) (RBM15-MLLI) are listed by WHO. AML with mutated NPM1 and with nucleated CEBPA are described later in this chapter in the section on fluorescent in situ hybridization (FISH).

Acute myeloid leukemia with multilineage dysplasia may also arise de novo (Fig. 12-37) or follow previous chemotherapy. Other cases arise particularly after topisomerase inhibitor therapy, for example, with etoposide (Fig. 12-38).

On May-Grünwald/Giemsa staining the minimally differentiated (M0) subclass is the least differentiated (Fig. 12-39) and can only be diagnosed with certainty after immunophenotyping and immunocytochemistry or electron microscopy (or both). The cases without differentiation (M1) subclass show agranular and granular blasts (Fig. 12-40), the blasts showing zero (type I) or less than 20 granules (type II). The differentiated (M2) subclass shows definite differentiation to promyelocytes (Fig. 12-41). Rare subtypes show abnormal metachromatic granules (Fig. 12-42) with or without basophilic granules (Figs. 12-43 and 12-44).

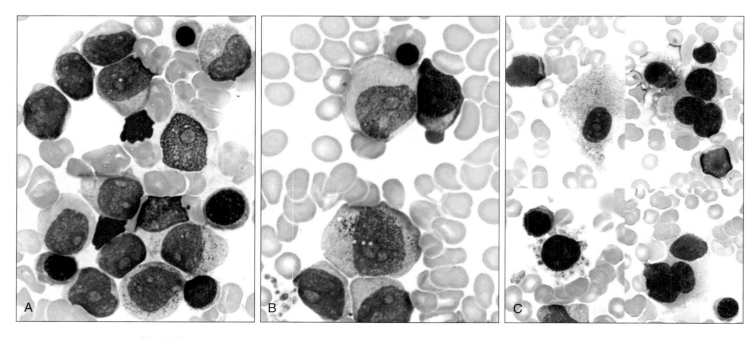

Fig. 12-37. A–C, Acute myeloid leukemia with multilineage dysplasia. **A,** Myeloblasts, many with Auer rods. Dysplastic changes in granulopoiesis erythropoiesis and megakaryocytes. The patient was a 68-year-old woman with no previous history of myelodysplasia.

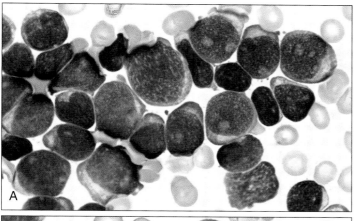

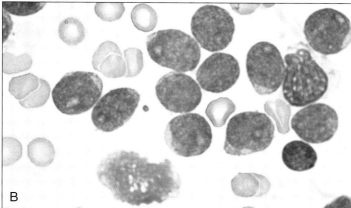

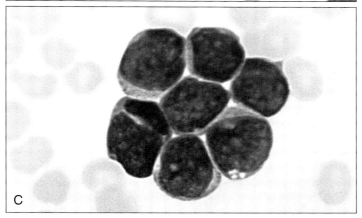

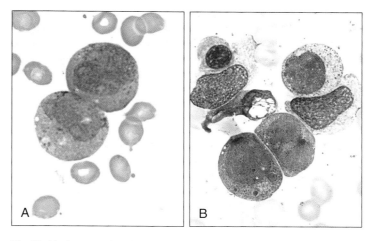

Fig. 12-41. Acute myeloid leukemia with differentiation (M2) subtype. **A, B,** Unusual large, vacuolated inclusions (pseudo–Chédiak-Higashi) are present in blast cells. (Courtesy of Dr. D. Swirsky.)

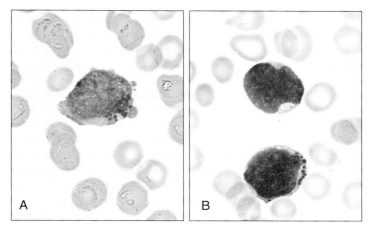

Fig. 12-42. Acute myeloid leukemia with differentiation, (M2) subtype: rare basophilic differentiation (peripheral blood). (Courtesy of Professor D. Catovsky.)

Fig. 12-39. Acute myeloid leukemia minimally differentiated (M0) subtype. **A–C,** Bone marrow aspirates showing large blasts resembling ALL L2 subtype. Granules are absent (Type I blasts), myeloperoxidase and Sudan black staining negative, CD13 and/or CD33 positive; myeloperoxidase is positive by electron microscopy or immunocytochemistry. TdT may be positive. (Courtesy of Dr. M. T. Daniel, Professor J. M. Bennett, and Dr. A. B. Mehta.)

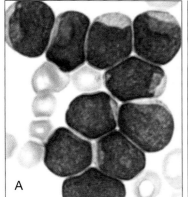
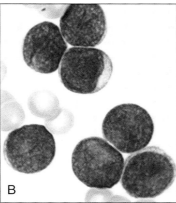
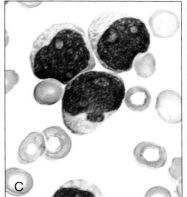
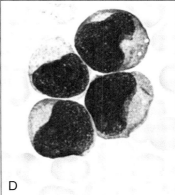

Fig. 12-40. Acute myeloid leukemia without differentiation (M1) subtype. **A,** Bone marrow aspirates showing blasts with large, often irregular, nuclei with one or more nucleoli, and with varying amounts of eccentrically placed cytoplasm. Either no definite granulation (type I blasts) is present or a few azurophilic granules and occasional Auer rods can be seen (type II blasts). At least 3% of cells stain with Sudan black or myeloperoxidase.

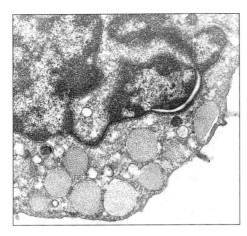

Fig. 12-43. Acute myeloid leukemia, M2 subtype: ultrastructure of the blasts shown in Fig. 12-42. Cytoplasmic granules show stippled pattern. (Courtesy of Professor D. Catovsky.)

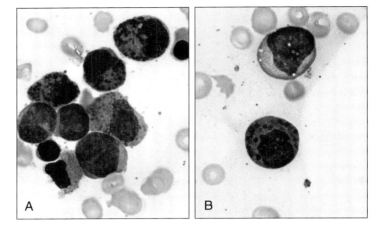

Fig. 12-44. Acute myeloid leukemia with differentiation, rare (M2) subtype: with abnormal eosinophils **(A)**, three myeloblasts, and four abnormal eosinophils with metachromatic granules; **(B)** neoplastic myelocyte with coarse basophilic and eosinophilic granulation. (a, b Courtesy of Dr K van Poucke and Prof. M Peetermans.

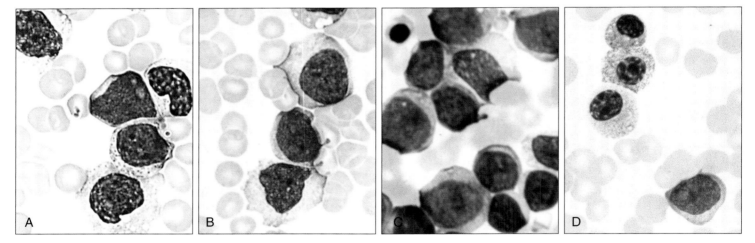

Fig. 12-45. Acute myeloid leukemia, myelomonocytic (M4) subtype. **A–C,** Blast cells contain cytoplasmic granules (myeloblasts and promyelocytes) or pale cytoplasm with occasional vacuoles and granules, and folded or rounded nuclei (monoblasts). **D,** Abnormal pseudo-Pelger forms may occur.

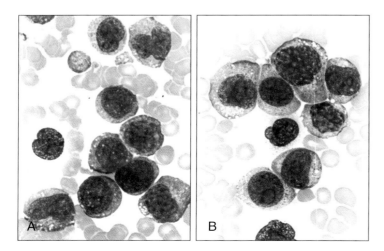

Fig. 12-46. Acute myeloid leukemia, myelomonocytic (M4) subtype: mixture of blast cells with features of primitive myeloid and monocytic cells; CD13 and CD33 were positive.

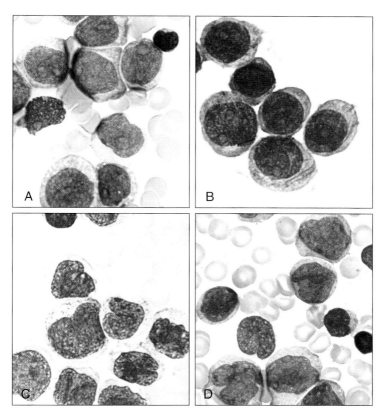

Fig. 12-47. Acute leukemia, monoblastic and monocytic (M5) subtype: blast cells with pale cytoplasm or perinuclear "haloes" and cytoplasmic vacuoles but only occasional granules. Their usually centrally placed nuclei are folded, rounded, or kidney shaped. **A, B,** Monoblastic subtype: 80% of the cells are monoblasts. **C, D,** Monocytic subtype: less than 80% of the cells are monoblasts. The remaining cells are promonocytes and monocytes. The cells in **(B)** show ribosome lamellar complexes. (*B, D,* Courtesy of Professor D. Catovsky.)

Acute myelomonocytic leukemia (M4) shows a mixture of blasts with promyelocytic and monocytic differentiation, the latter consisting of less than 20% of the total (Figs. 12-45 and 12-46).

Acute monoblastic leukemia (M5a) (Fig. 12-47) shows over 80% monoblasts. The monocytic type (M5b) shows more differentiated "promonocytes" or monocytic cells (see Fig. 12-47). Serum and urinary lysozyme are high. An unusual subtype with M4 or M5 features shows erythrophagocytosis (Fig. 12-48). In subclass acute erythroid leukemia (M6) over 50% of cells are erythroid precursors with bizarre dyserythropoietic forms. In the pure erythroid form over 80% of the

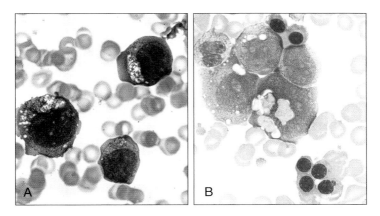

Fig. 12-48. Acute myelomonocytic/monoblastic leukemia (M4/M5) subtype with erythrophagocytosis and t(8;16). **A,** In this case the blasts were M5 subtype; other similar cases are M4 subtype. A bleeding diathesis with features of fibrinolysis (not disseminated intravascular coagulation as in M3) is often present. **B,** Child with M4/M5 subtype with t(8;16) showing erythrophagocytosis. (*A,* Courtesy of Professor D. Catovsky. *B,* Courtesy of Dr. D. Swirsky.)

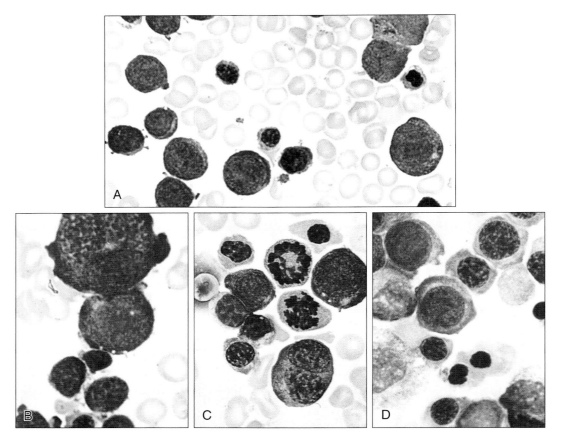

Fig. 12-49. Acute erythroid leukemia (M6) subtype: **A,** there is a preponderance of erythroid cells at all stages of development. **B–D,** High-power views of bone marrow aspirate showing erythroid predominance with many dyserythropoietic features, such as multinucleate cells (gigantoblasts), vacuolated cytoplasm, abnormal mitoses, and megaloblastic nuclei.

cells are erythroid (Fig. 12-49). In the erythroid/myeloid form, the relative proportions are more equal (Fig. 12-50). Features of myelodysplasia may also be present in other cell lines.

Acute megakaryoblastic leukemia (M7) is rare. It is often associated with fibrosis of the marrow (Figs. 12-51 and 12-52) and is recognized by the appearance of the blasts, special staining for platelet peroxidase, electron microscopy, or monoclonal antibodies to cell surface antigens.

RARE TYPES OF ACUTE MYELOID LEUKEMIA

Rare types of AML include acute mast cell leukemia (Fig. 12-53), acute panmyelosis with myelofibrosis (Fig. 12-54), myeloid sarcoma (Fig. 12-55), acute natural killer (NK) cell leukemia (Figs. 12-56 and 12-57), and acute eosinophilic leukemia (Fig. 12-58). A rare appearance of the marrow in AML, partial necrosis is shown in Fig. 12-59. Hemophagocytosis by myeloid blasts is an infrequent finding in several subgroups (Fig. 12-60).

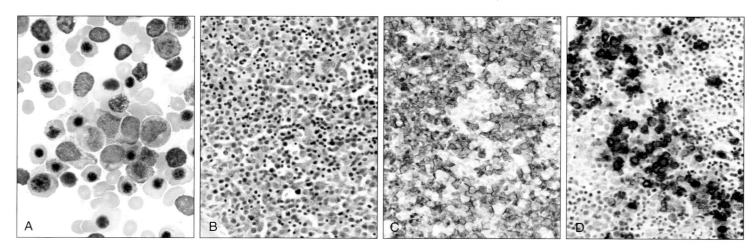

Fig. 12-50. Acute erythroid leukemia, erythroid/myeloid. **A,** Bone marrow aspirate, predominance of erythroid cells, many with dyserythropoietic features: large, paler myeloblasts, one with an Auer rod also present. **B–D,** Bone marrow trephine biopsy; **B,** showing hypercellularity with a mixture of smaller, densely straining erythroblasts and pale, larger myeloblasts; **C,** anti-glycophorin immunostain shows erythroid cells positive, myeloblasts negative; **D,** myeloperoxidase stain shows myeloblasts positive, erythroid cells negative. (Courtesy of Dr. W. Erber.)

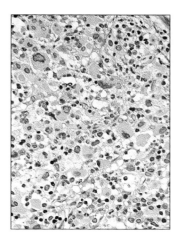

Fig. 12-51. Acute megakaryoblastic leukemia, M7 subtype: bone marrow trephine biopsy showing large blasts with amorphous pink cytoplasm interspersed with residual small hematopoietic cells.

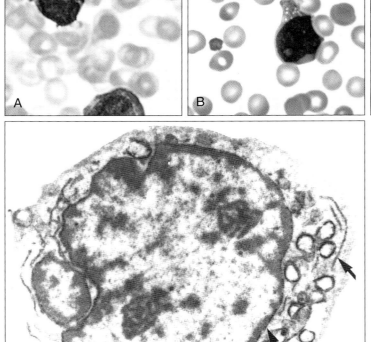

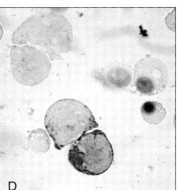

Fig. 12-52. Acute myeloid leukemia, (M7) subtype. **A–D,** The megakaryoblasts are large, primitive cells with basophilic cytoplasm. Some show abortive platelet budding. **D,** The cells are positive for platelet peroxidase; immunoperoxidase stain. **E,** Megakaryoblast: morphologically, this cell resembles a lymphoblast but is identified by the reactivity with the platelet–peroxidase reaction (linear black areas) in the endoplasmic reticulum and nuclear membrane (arrows). Mitochondria are nonspecifically positive. (Courtesy of Dr. E. Matutes and Professor D. Catovsky.)

Fig. 12-53. Acute mast cell leukemia. **A–C,** Bone marrow showing typical blasts with basophilic and vacuolated cytoplasm. In this case the leukemia arose de novo; other cases follow systemic mastocytosis (although usually other forms of AML complicate this disease) or occur as transformation of chronic myeloid leukemia.

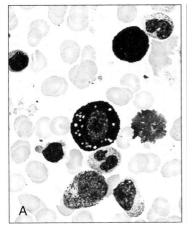

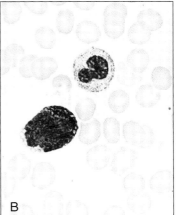

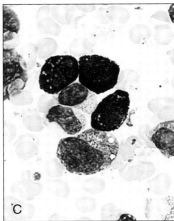

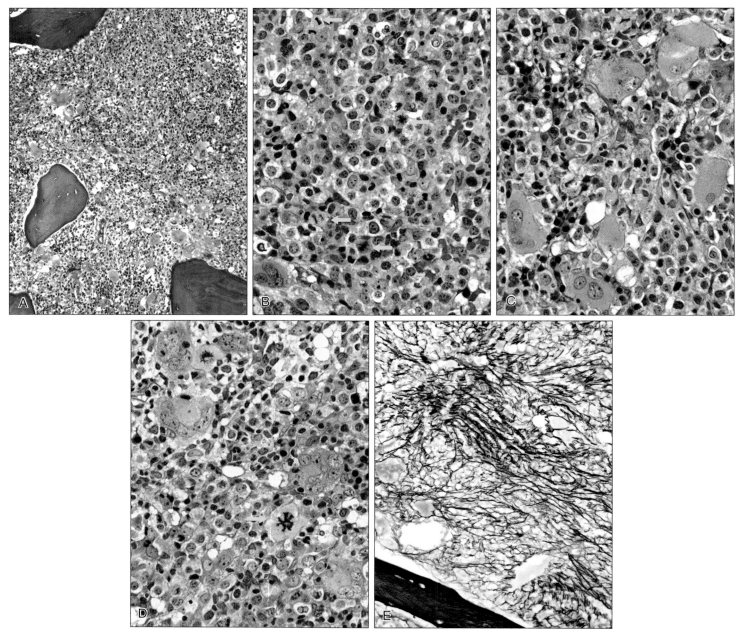

Fig. 12-54. Acute panmyelosis with myelofibrosis: the patient had pancytopenia. (Hb 9.0 g/dl, WBC 2.3 × 10^9/L, neutrophils 0.16 × 10^9/L, blasts 0.9 × 10^9/L, platelets 37 × 10^9/L.) The blood film showed only mild anisocytosis and poikilocytosis with no tear-drop cells. A very occasional erythroblast was present; there was no splenomegaly. Attempts at marrow aspiration failed. **A,** The trephine biopsy shows a hypercellular marrow with replacement of normally developing cells with primitive myeloid and erythroid cells and megakaryocytes. **B,** Myeloid and erythroid blasts at higher magnification. Arrows point to cells in mitosis. **C** and **D,** Abnormal small and large megakaryoblasts and megakaryocytes showing nonlobated and hypolobated nuclei with a dispersed vesicular chromatin pattern. There are two megakaryoblasts in mitosis. **E,** Reticulin staining shows a marked increase in reticulin fiber density and thickness with extensive fiber intersections. (Grade 2 fibrosis.)

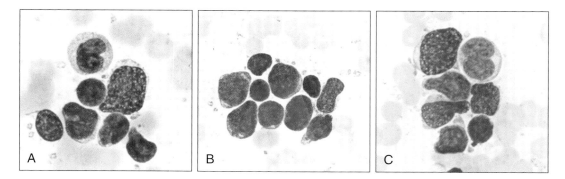

Fig. 12-55. A–C, Myeloid sarcoma; the patient was an 85-year-old man with a 6.5 cm mass in the left axilla. Normal blood count. Smears from a fine-needle aspirate show replacement of normal nodal lymphocytes with primitive myeloid hematopoietic cells. Marker studies showed positivity for CD33, CD34, CD15, CD117, aberrant CD56, and CD7. Bone marrow at presentation was normal. Seven months later he developed typical and fatal AML M4 subtype.

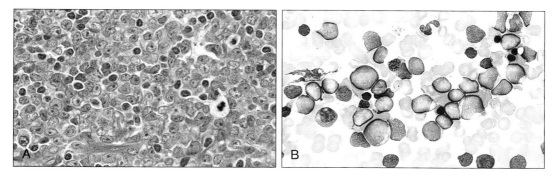

Fig. 12-56. Acute myeloid leukemia, NK cell subtype: 54-year-old man with cervical lymphadenopathy. **A,** Biopsy showed diffusive infiltration of cells with round and irregular small nucleoli and scanty cytoplasm. **B,**The bone marrow shows an infiltrate of immature blasts with of varied morphology. The cells were myeloperoxidase negative but CD2+, CD7+, CD33+, CD56+, and HLA-DR+. (*A, B,* Courtesy of Dr. R. Suzuki.)

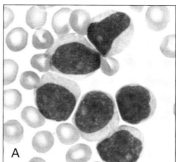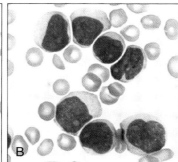

Fig. 12-57. Acute NK cell leukemia. The cells were CD 56+ and CD4+. The large blast cells have a vesicular chromatin pattern, prominent nucleoli, and pale relatively agranular cytoplasm.

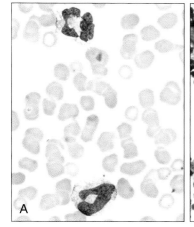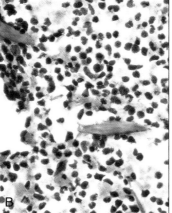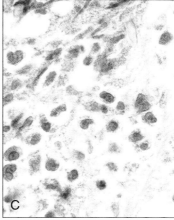

Fig. 12-58. Acute myeloid leukemia, rare eosinophilic subtype: 55-year-old man treated with chemotherapy for carcinoma of the bladder 10 years previously. **A,** Peripheral blood showing abnormal eosinophils. **B,** Bone marrow aspirate showing eosinophilic blasts, necrotic cells, and Charcot-Leyden crystals. **C,** Bone marrow trephine showing necrotic cells and Charcot-Leyden crystals. (Hb, 11.0 g/dl; WBC, 23.2 × 10⁹/L; platelets, 24 × 10⁹/L.) (Courtesy of Dr. A. G. Smith.)

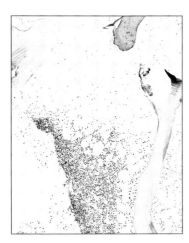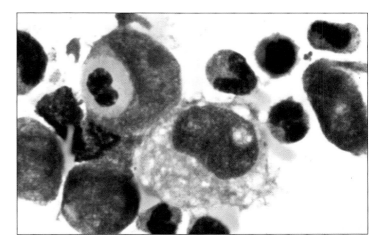

Fig. 12-59. Acute myeloid leukemia: trephine biopsy showing partial necrosis of bone marrow. (Courtesy of Dr. R. Kumar.)

Fig. 12-60. Acute myeloid leukemia t(16; 21). Marked hemophagocytosis by leukemic blasts cells. (Courtesy Dr. S. Imashuku.)

CONGENITAL ACUTE LEUKEMIA

Figure 12-61 illustrates a rare type of acute leukemia, congenital acute leukemia. This is usually myeloid and characterized by extensive extramedullary infiltration, including in the skin.

ACUTE LEUKEMIA AND DOWN SYNDROME

An increased incidence of both ALL and AML occurs in Down syndrome. In the first year of life, AML is the more usual (Fig. 12-62). A transient myeloproliferative syndrome also occurs more frequently in Down syndrome than in normal infants. The blood and bone marrow appearances are morphologically similar to those in AML, usually with over 30% of blasts in the blood (Figs. 12-63 to 12-65). A specific JAK2 mutation (JAK2 R683) and multiple gene deletions occur in about 25% of Down Syndrome ALL cases.

ACUTE LYMPHOBLASTIC LEUKEMIA

Lymphoblasts show little evidence of differentiation and the appearances of the cells are similar whether the case is classified as leukemia or lymphoma, but the cases divide into B- and T-cell varieties. The B-lineage cases are now divided by WHO into subvarieties with recurrent cytogenetic/molecular genetic markers and those not otherwise

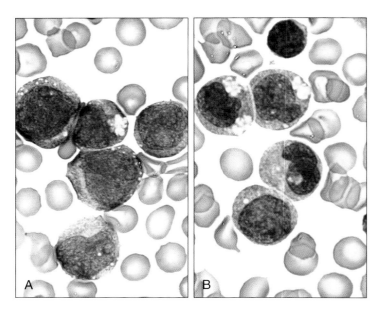

Fig. 12-61. Congenital acute myeloid leukemia. **A, B,** Peripheral blood films of a male infant born with anemia, hepatosplenomegaly, and skin lesions. There are large numbers of myeloblasts with prominent cytoplasmic vacuolation. (Hb, 10.1 g/dl; WBC, 92 × 10⁹/L; blasts, 85%; platelets, 15 × 10⁹/L.) (*A, B,* Courtesy of Professor J. M. Chessels.)

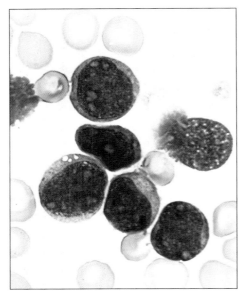

Fig. 12-63. Transient myeloproliferative disorder: Down syndrome. Peripheral blood film from a 3-day-old girl with Down syndrome (Hb, 16.2 g/dl; WBC, 62 × 10⁹/L [blasts, 50% to 55%]; platelets, 28 × 10⁹/L). The blasts have basophilic cytoplasm, dispersed nuclear chromatin, and several nucleoli. Azurophilic granules are present in one of the blasts. The WBC increased to 77 × 10⁹/L on day 5, but then resolved spontaneously by 8 weeks, when the blood film was normal. There was no recurrence within a 5-year follow-up. (Courtesy of Professor R. D. Brunning and the AFIP.)

specified (see Table 12-1). These varieties cannot be distinguished by conventional light microscopy. Cases with smaller, more uniform cells with scanty cytoplasm were classified by FAB as L1 (Fig. 12-66), whereas those with blasts differing widely in size, with prominent nucleoli and greater amounts of cytoplasm, were classified as L2 (Fig. 12-67). L2 tends to include more of the adult cases and also most of those immunologically typed as T-ALL. This morphologic subdivision is now obsolete. Rare subtypes show coarse granules (Fig. 12-68, *A*) or a reactive eosinophilia (Fig. 12-68, *B*).

The Burkitt (L3) variant shows multiple small vacuoles throughout a basophilic cell cytoplasm and often overlying the nucleus (Fig. 12-69). The bone marrow in all variants is hypercellular, with leukemic blasts making up at least 80% of the marrow cell total (Fig. 12-70). In ALL, blasts may be seen in the cerebrospinal fluid (Fig. 12-71) or testes (Fig. 12-72).

In T-ALL, blasts are difficult to distinguish from B-lineage blasts morphologically; special stains, flow cytometry, cytogenetics, and gene rearrangement studies are needed (Fig. 12-73).

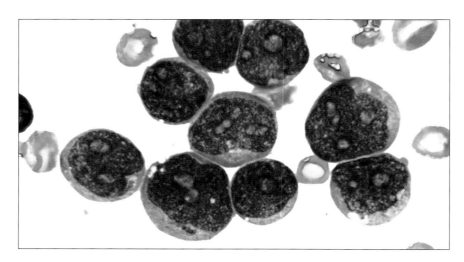

Fig. 12-62. Acute myeloid leukemia: Down syndrome. Peripheral blood showing numerous myeloblasts in a child younger than 1 year old. (Courtesy of Professor R. D. Brunning and the AFIP.)

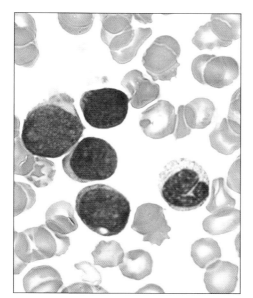

Fig. 12-64. Transient myeloproliferative disorder: Down syndrome. Peripheral blood film from a 20-day-old girl (Hb, 16.4 g/dl; WBC, 54 × 10⁹/L; platelet count normal). Approximately 50% of the white blood cells are blasts. The platelets are large; occasional platelets are poorly granulated. The white cell count returned to normal after 3 weeks, but increased 3 months later following a bacterial infection when blast cells were again numerous. This resolved but relapsed 2 months later, at which time the child was treated for acute leukemia. (Courtesy of Professor R. D. Brunning and the AFIP.)

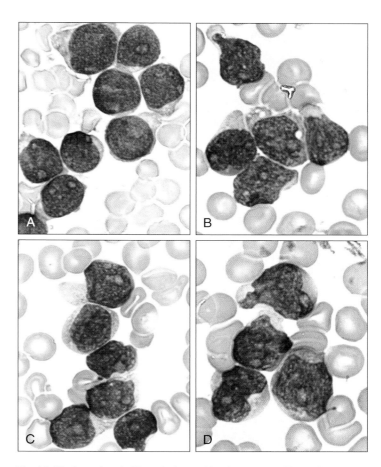

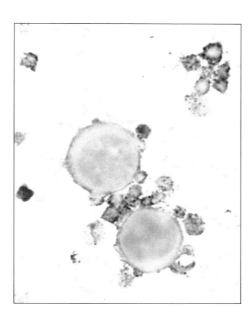

Fig. 12-65. Transient myeloproliferative disorder: Down syndrome. Peripheral blood from the child described in Fig. 12-64 reacted with monoclonal antibody to CD61 (platelet glycoprotein IIIa; AP-AAP technique). The megakaryocytes, pro-megakaryocytes, and platelets are positive; the blasts (not shown) were nonreactive. (Courtesy of Professor R. D. Brunning and the AFIP.)

Fig. 12-67. Acute lymphoblastic leukemia, L2 subtype. **A–D,** Blast cells that vary considerably in size and amount of cytoplasm; the nuclear-to-cytoplasmic ratio is rarely as high as in L1. The nuclei are variable in shape and often contain many nucleoli.

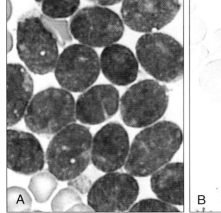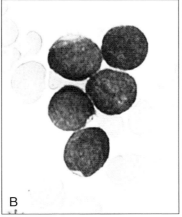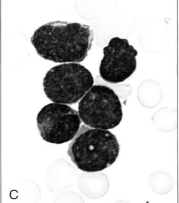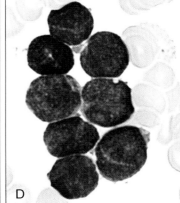

Fig. 12-66. Acute lymphoblastic leukemia, small cell (L1) subtype. **A–D,** Rather small, uniform blast cells with scanty cytoplasm, and rounded or cleft nuclei with usually a single nucleolus.

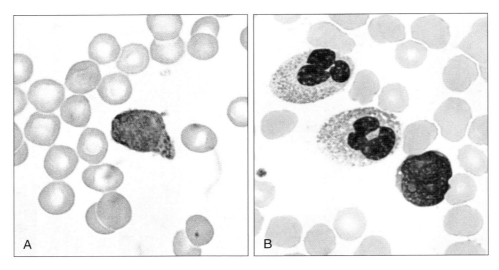

Fig. 12-68. Acute lymphoblastic leukemia. **A,** Rare subtype with granules. **B,** Rare subtype with eosinophilia—peripheral blood film showing a lymphoblast and two eosinophils. (WBC, 36 × 10⁹/L; lymphoblasts, 14 × 10⁹/L; eosinophils, 20 × 10⁹/L.) (*A*, Courtesy of Dr. A. Cantu-Reynoldi; see also Cantu-Reynoldi A, Invenizzi R, Biondi A, et al: Biological and clinical features of acute lymphoblastic leukemia with cytoplasmic granules or inclusions: description of eight cases, *Br J Haematol* 73:309-314, 1989.)

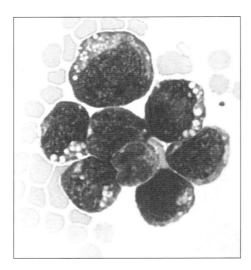

Fig. 12-69. Acute lymphoblastic leukemia, Burkitt lymphoma (L3) subtype: blast cells with deeply staining blue cytoplasm containing numerous small perinuclear vacuoles. This appearance is typical of B-ALL.

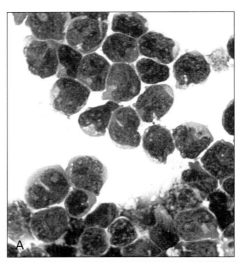

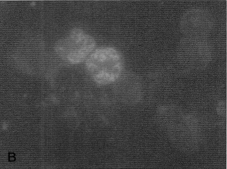

Fig. 12-71. Acute lymphoblastic leukemia. **A,** High-power view of cytospin of cerebrospinal fluid, showing a deposit of blast cells of varying morphology. The patient had the features of meningeal leukemia. **B,** Indirect immunofluorescent staining of cerebrospinal fluid for terminal deoxynucleotidyl transferase (TdT). These few cells, difficult to recognize morphologically, show nuclear TdT staining typical of lymphoblasts. (Courtesy of Professor K. F. Bradstock.)

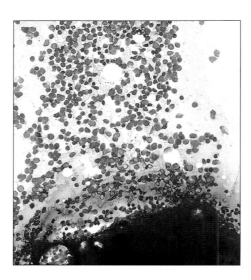

Fig. 12-70. Acute lymphoblastic leukemia: low-power view of bone marrow fragment showing hypercellularity of cellular trails, of which over 80% are blast cells.

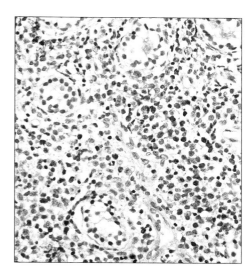

Fig. 12-72. Acute lymphoblastic leukemia: low-power view of testicular infiltrate, showing leukemic blast cells in the interstitial tissues and in the seminiferous tubular epithelium.

TABLE 12-3. SCORING SYSTEM FOR MARKERS PROPOSED BY THE EUROPEAN GROUP FOR IMMUNOLOGY CLASSIFICATION OF LEUKEMIA (EGIL)

Score	B lymphoid	T lymphoid	Myeloid
2	CytCD79a* Cyt IgM CytCD22	CD3(m/cyt) anti-TCR (αβ or γδ)	MPO
1	CD19 CD20 CD10	CD2 CD5 CD8 CD10	CD17 CD13 CD33 CD65
0.5	TdT CD24	TdT CD7 CD1a	CD14 CD15 CD64

*CD79a may also be expressed in some cases of precursor T-lymphoblastic leukemia/lymphoma

If >2 points is scored for myeloid and for one of the lymphoid lineages, the case is classified as biphenotypic.

ACUTE MIXED CELL LEUKEMIA

Blast cells may show features of both myeloid and lymphoid cells. These may be due to aberrant expression of markers or to the presence of two populations (Fig. 12-74). The criteria for diagnosis of biphenotypic leukemia with two or more blast cell populations of different lineages are given in Table 12-3.

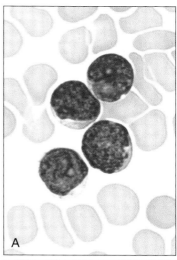
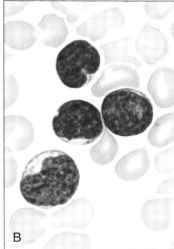

Fig. 12-73. Acute T-lymphoblastic leukemia. The majority of the blasts cells in the peripheral blood are small with sparse cytoplasm, condensed chromatin, and inconspicuous nucleoli. Some of the cells have a nuclear cleft. The patient was a 24-year-old man with hemoglobin 12.0 g/dl, WBC 115 × 10⁹/L, and platelets 15 × 10⁹/L. The cells were CD1a+, CD2+, cCD3+, CD5+, CD4/CD8+, CD7+, and TdT+.

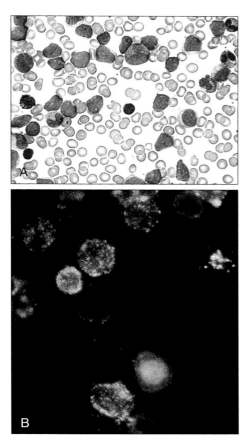

Fig. 12-74. Acute leukemia, mixed cell (myeloid/lymphoblastic) type. **A,** Bone marrow aspirate showing blasts of varying size and morphology. Some have scanty cytoplasm without granules, whereas others, usually larger, have eccentric nuclei, substantial cytoplasm, and granules. **B,** Bone marrow aspirate seen by indirect immunofluorescence shows one population of cells (lymphoblastic) to have nuclear TdT (green) whereas another population (myeloid) has myeloid (CD33) surface antigen (yellow/orange). (Courtesy of Professor G. Janossy.)

CYTOCHEMISTRY

Cytochemical stains may aid the identification of the different sub-types of acute leukemia (Table 12-4). In AML, special stains such as myeloperoxidase or Sudan black are used to confirm the presence of granules in the myeloid cells. The dual esterase stain may also be used (Fig. 12-75). Monocytic differentiation is demonstrated by nonspe-cific esterase staining, which may be combined with chloracetate staining to differentiate monoblasts and myeloblasts in the same case (Fig. 12-76). The periodic acid-Schiff (PAS) reagent may show block positivity in the erythroid variant (Fig. 12-77).

In ALL, the special stains of value are as follows:
- •PAS, which shows block positivity in precursor B-ALL, usually showing the (CD10) antigen (Fig. 12-78)
- •Acid phosphatase, which shows eccentric Golgi body staining in T-ALL (Fig. 12-79)
- •Oil red O, which stains lipid material in Burkitt ALL (Fig. 12-80) that appears as vacuoles on conventional May-Grünwald/Giemsa staining

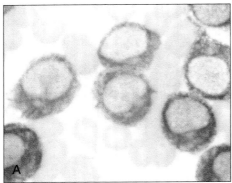
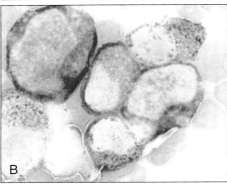

Fig. 12-76. Acute myeloid leukemia: bone marrow aspirates of (A) monoblastic subtype shows deep orange staining by nonspecific esterase, and of (B) myelo-monocytic subtype shows deep orange staining of the monoblast cytoplasm by nonspecific esterase and blue staining of myeloblast cytoplasm by chloracetate.

TABLE 12-4. ACUTE LEUKEMIA: CYTOCHEMISTRY

	Precursor B-ALL	T-ALL	AML		
			M₁–M₃	M₄–M₅	M₆–M₇
Myeloperoxidase	–	–	+/++	+	–
Sudan black	–	–	+/++	+	–
Nonspecific esterase	–	–	–	++	+ (focal)
Periodic acid–Schiff	+ (coarse)	–	–	+	+ (fine)
Acid phosphatase	–	+ (focal)	–	+ (diffuse)	+ (focal)

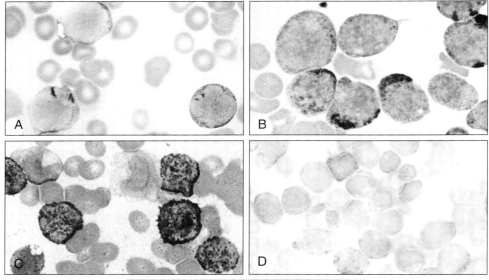
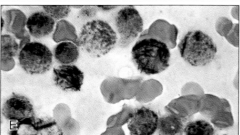

Fig. 12-75. Acute myeloid leukemia: bone marrow aspirates of (A, B) M2 subtypes show black-staining cytoplasmic granules and Auer rods; (C) myelomonocytic subtype myeloblasts with black cytoplasmic granules (the monoblasts show only background staining); (D) t(8;21) subtype shows multiple, blue-staining cytoplasmic granules; (E) t(15;17) subtype shows multi-ple Auer rods ("faggots"). (A–C, Sudan black; D, myeloperoxidase; E, dual esterase stains.) (E, Courtesy of Professor J. M. Bennett.)

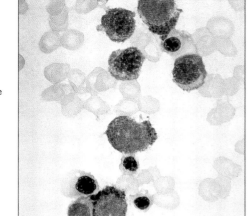

Fig. 12-77. Acute myeloid leukemia, M6 subtype: bone marrow aspirate in which the cytoplasm of some of the erythroblasts shows block positive red staining by PAS.

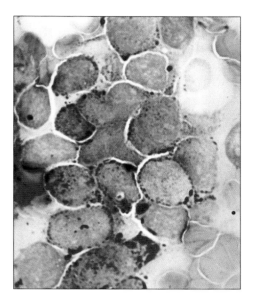

Fig. 12-78. Acute lymphoblastic leukemia, precursor B: bone marrow aspirate showing cells with one or more coarse granules in the cytoplasm. PAS stain.

Fig. 12-79. Acute lymphoblastic leukemia, T-cell subtype: bone marrow aspirate shows red cytoplasmic staining with marked coloration of the Golgi zone adjacent to or indented into the nucleus. Acid phosphatase stain.

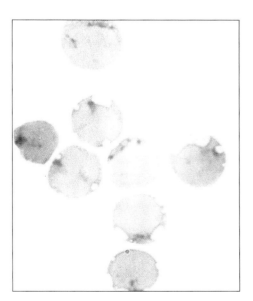

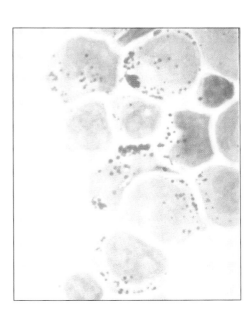

Fig. 12-80. Acute lymphoblastic leukemia, Burkitt (L3) subtype: bone marrow aspirate stained with oil red O shows prominent cytoplasmic lipid collections corresponding to some of the vacuoles shown by Romanowsky staining (see Fig. 12-69).

TABLE 12-5A. ACUTE LEUKEMIA: PANELS OF MONOCLONAL (OR POLYCLONAL) ANTIBODIES RECOMMENDED BY THE BRITISH COMMITTEE FOR STANDARDS IN HAEMATOLOGY AND BY THE U.S. CANADIAN CONSENSUS GROUP FOR THE DIAGNOSIS AND CLASSIFICATION OF ACUTE LEUKEMIA

		BCSH	Consensus group
Primary panel	B lymphoid	CD19, cCD22, cCD79a, CD10	CD10, CD19, anti-κ, anti-λ
	T lymphoid	cCD3, CD2	CD2, CD5, CD7
	Myeloid	CD13, CD117, anti-cMPO	CD13, CD14, CD33
	Not lineage specific	Nuclear TdT	CD34, HLA-DR
Secondary panel	B lymphoid	μ, SmIg (anti-κ and anti-λ), CD138	CD20, Sm/cCD22
	T lymphoid	CD7	CD1a, Sm/cCD3, CD4, CD8
	Myeloid	CD33, CD41, CD42, CD61, anti-glycophorin A	CD15, CD16, CD41, CD42b, CD61, CD64, CD71, CD117, anti-cMPO, anti-glycophorin A
	Not lineage specific	CD45	CD38, nuclear TdT
	Nonheatmopoietic	MAb for the detection of small round cell tumors of childhood	
Optional	B lymphoid	CD15 (a myeloid marker often expressed on *MLL*-rearranged B lymphoblasts) and 7.1/NG2 (also for *MLL*-rearranged ALL)	
	T lymphoid	Anti-TCRαβ, anti-TCRγδ	
	Myeloid	Anti-lysozyme, CD14, CD36, anti-PML (MAb PL1-M3, HLA-DR for negativity in M3 AML)	

c, cytoplasmic; CD, cluster of differentiation; MAb, monoclonal antibody; MPO, myeloperoxidase; Sm, surface membrane; TCR, T-cell receptor; TdT, terminal deoxynucleotidyl transferase

IMMUNOLOGY

Immunologic characterization of leukemic cells is now carried out using fluorescent-labeled antibodies to surface, cytoplasmic, and nuclear antigens of leukemia cells and counting these using flow cytometry using fluorescence-activated cell sorting (FACS) analysis. Panels of antibodies have been established for initial screening and for subsequent more detailed analysis (Table 12-5AB). The pattern of antigen expression varies according to the cytogenetic and morphologic features of the leukemic cells. Figure 12-81, *A*, shows typical findings in AML, and Fig. 12-81, *B*, illustrates a case with an aberrant phenotype. This may subsequently be useful in detection in minimal residual disease. Typical findings in B-lineage ALL and T-cell ALL are shown in Figs. 12-82 and 12-83. Cytoplasmic

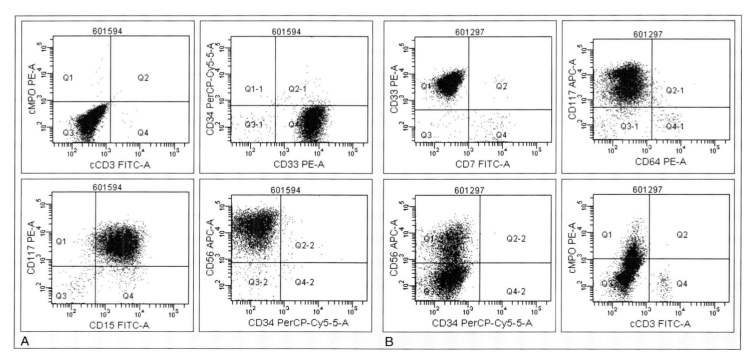

Fig. 12-81. Acute myeloid leukemia: flow cytometry. **A,** The blast cells are positive for CD15, CD33, CD117, cMPO, and HLA; CD34 and CD64 negative. **B,** The blast cells show an aberrant phenotype, being CD33, CMPO, and CD117 positive but also CD56 positive. (Courtesy of Immunophenotyping Laboratory, Royal Free Hospital.)

TABLE 12-5B. FLOW CYTOMETRIC IMMUNOPHENOTYPING FOR HEMATOLOGIC NEOPLASMS

Reagents of clinical utility in the evaluation of maturing myeloid and monocytic neoplasms			Adapted from F.E. Craig and K.A. Foon Blood III: 3941-3967
Reagent	Normal distribution	Clinical utility in myeloid and monocytic neoplasms	Comments
CD1[1]b	Maturing neutrophilic and monocytic cells, some lymphoid cells.	May be aberrantly expressed in AML, MDS, and MPD.	—
CD13	Neutrophillic and monocytic cells.	Indicator of neutrophillc and monocytic lineage in acute leukemia. May be aberrantly expressed in AML, MDS, and MPD.	
CD14	Monocytes.	Indicator of monocytic differentiation.	Not a sensitive marker of immature monocytes.
CD15	Maturing neutrophillic cells and monocytes and NK cells.	May be aberrantly expressed in AML, MDS, and MPD.	—
CD16	Maturing neutrophilic cells, monocytes, and NK cells.	May be aberrantly expressed in AML, MDS, and MPD.	—
CD33	Neutrophillic and monocytic cells.	May be aberrantly expressed in AML, MDS, and MPD.	Some normal variability in intensity of expression.
CD34	B-cell and T-cell precursors and myeloblasts.	Indentification and enumeration of blasts.	Not all blasts are CD34.
CD45	All B cells (weaker intensity on precursors and plasma cells), all T cells (weaker intensity on precursors).	Identification of blasts (CD45 gaining often with low orthogonal (side) light scatter).	—
CD56	NK cells and NK-like T cells.	May be aberrantly expressed in AML, MDS, and MPD.	Low level of expression on regenerating normal neutrophillic and monocytic cells and with growth factor simulation.
CD117	Immature neutrophillic cells and most cells.	Identification myeloblasts and mast cells.	May be present in myeloma and some T-cell neoplasms.
HLA-DR	Myeloblasts, monocytes, all B cells, activated T cells.	Identification of promyelocytae, such as APL. May be aberrantly expressed in AML, MDS, and MPD.	Non-APL AML may also be negative.
CD2*	Tcells, NK cells	May be aberrantly expressed in AML; some association with inv16. May be aberrantly expressed in systemic mastocytosis.	—
CD4*	T-cell subset, monocytic	Often positive in AML, particularly with monocytic differentiation.	Also mature T-cell neoplasms and HDN.
CD7*	Tcells and NK cells.	May be aberrantly expressed in AML, MDS, and MPD.	
CD25*	Activated B cells and T cells	May be aberrantly expressed in systemic mastocytosis.	Reported association with BCR/ABL-ALL.
CD36*	Monocytes, erythroid cells, mogakaryocytes and platelets.	When used in combination with CD64 is a more sensitive marker of monocytic differentiation than CD14	—
CD38*	Precursor B cells (hematogones), normal follicle center B cells, immature and activated T cells, plasma cells (bright intensity), myeloid and monocytic cells, and erythroid precursors.	Identification of early bone marrow progenitor cell populations for further evaluation of phenotypic abnormalities.	—
CD41*	Megakaryocytes and platelets.	Megakaryocytic differentiation.	May detect nonspecific binding of platelet proteins to other cells such as monocytes.
CD 61*	Megakaryocytes and platelets.	Megakaryocytic differentiation.	May detect nonspecific adherence of platelet proteins to other cells such as monocytes. Sometimes combined with CD42b to distinguish platelets from blasts.
CD 61	Megakaryocytes and platelets.	Megakaryoctyic differentiation.	May demonstrate fewer problems with adherence of platelet proteins.
CD64*	Monocytes and intermediate neutrophilic precursors.	Identification of monocytic differentiation. May be aberrantly expressed in AML, MDS, and MPD.	Gained on mature neutrophils with sepsis.
CD71*	Erythroid precursors (bright), myeloid, activated lymphoid, proliferating cells.	Identification of immature erythroid cells. Possibly expressed in MDS.	—
cMPO*	Neutrophillic and monocytic cells.	Indicator of myeloid differentiation.	In contrast to cytochemical stain, measures the presence of antigen, not enzyme activity.
CD117*	Immature neutrophillic cells and mast cells.	Identification of myeloblasts.	May be expressed by cells more mature cells than blasts.
CD123*	Monocytes, neutrophils, basophils, megakaryocytes, and plasma cytoid dendritic cells (bright).	Identification HDN. Positive some AML, especially with monocytic differentiation	Plasmacytoid dendritic cells may be increased in some reactive conditions such as Castleman disease and Kikuchi lymphadentitis and in association with MPD.
CD163*	Monocytes, macrophage.	Indicator of monocytic differentiation.	—
CD235a*	Erythroid precursors	Indicator of erythroid maturation.	Not present on some immature erythroid precursors.

Reagents included in this table were recommended in the consensus guidelines.
— indicates no entry.
* Those reagents may be considered for secondary evaluation after other reagents listed have been used in the initial evaluation.

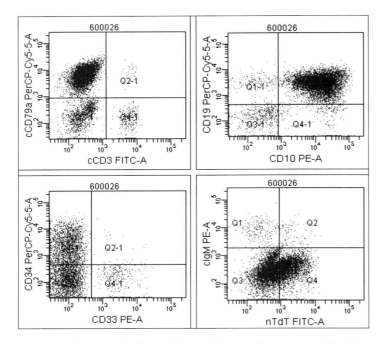

Fig. 12-82. Acute lymphoblastic leukemia: B-lineage flow cytometry. The blast cells are CD10, CD19, CD34, CD79a, and TdT positive; cCD3 and IgM negative. (Courtesy of Immunophenotyping Laboratory, Royal Free Hospital.)

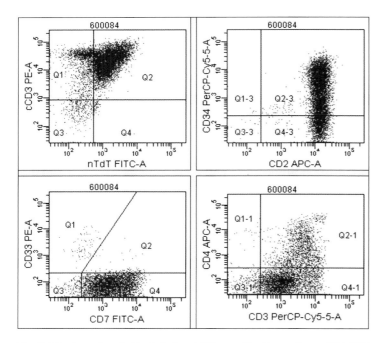

Fig. 12-83. Acute lymphoblastic leukemia; T-lineage. The blast cells are CD4, CD7, cCD3, CD34, and TdT positive. (Courtesy of Immunophenotyping Laboratory, Royal Free Hospital.)

(c) immunoglobulin (cIg) and cCD3 are relatively specific markers for B-lineage and T-lineage ALL, respectively. Nuclear terminal deoxynucleotide transferase–like surface antigens (TdT-like surface antigens) can be detected by FACS but also by immunoperoxidase staining of blood or bone marrow (Fig. 12-84). The criteria for diagnosis of biphenotypic leukemias have been given (Table 12-3), and the value of TdT detection in identifying extramedullary ALL cells is shown in Fig. 12-71.

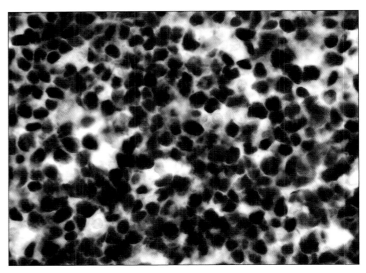

Fig. 12-84. Acute lymphoblastic leukemia: bone marrow cells staining positive for TdT by immunoperoxidase. (Courtesy of Dr. A. Ramsay.)

CYTOGENETICS

Cytogenetic analysis is now essential for the exact characterization of the acute leukemias, decisions on management, and prognosis.

The human somatic cell contains 23 pairs of chromosomes. These are numbered 1 to 22 in descending order of size plus one pair, the sex chromosomes, being XX in females and XY in males. The term *karyotype* is used to describe the chromosomal makeup of a cell. The letters p and q refer to the short and long chromosomes, respectively. The dark or lighter staining bands are detected by Giemsa (G) or quinacrine (Q) techniques and numbered from the centromere outward. Groups of bands are regions, also numbered outward from the centromere. Translocations are denoted by t,

TABLE 12-6. ACUTE LEUKEMIA: CYTOGENETIC ABNORMALITIES (see also Table 12-1)

Acute myeloid leukemia		Acute lymphoblastic leukemia
Relatively specific		**Precursor B-ALL**
M_1 t(3;v)*		t(12;21) (p13;q22)¶
M_2 t(8;21) (q22;q22)		t(9;22) (q34;q11)
M_3 t(15;17) (q22;q21)		t(4;11) (q21;q23)
M_4 inv(16) (p13;q22) or del(16) (q22)†		t(1;19) (q23;p13)
$M_4(M_5)$ t(8;16) (p11;p13)		del(6q)
M_{5a} t(11;v) (q23;v)		t(11;14) (q13;q32)
M_{5b} t(8;16)(p11;p13)		t or del 12p12
M_6 del(20)(q11)		6q–
		9p–
Others		+21
t(9;22) (q34;q11)	M_1, biphenotypic	Hyperdiploidy 50–65 chromosomes
t(6;9) (p23;q34)‡	M_2, M_4	Near haploidy 26–34 chromosomes
t(3;3) (q21;q29) inv(3) (q21;q26)§		
+9	M_6	**B-ALL**
+11, +13	M_0, M_1	t(8;14) (q24;q32)
+22	M_4 Eo	t(8;22) (q24;q11)
+4	M_2, M_4 with MDS	t(2;8) (p11–13;q24)
+8	M_1, M_4, M_5	
+21		**T-ALL**
5q–/–5	secondary AML, MDS	t or del 14q11
7q–/–7	secondary AML, MDS	t(11;14) (p13;q11)
t or del	secondary AML	t(10;14) (q24;q11)
12p11–p13‡		t(1;14) (p34;q11)
		6q–
		9p–

*v = various other chromosomes §associated with thrombocytosis
†associated with abnormal eosinophils ¶detectable only by molecular methods
‡with increased basophils

M_0–M_6 refers to previous FAB morphological classification

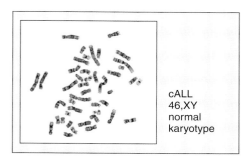

Fig. 12-85. Acute lymphoblastic leukemia: a representative bone marrow cell with normal karyotype (46, XY). (Courtesy of Dr. E. Nacheva.)

followed by the chromosome numbers (lower number first) in brackets and then the bands included in subsequent brackets. The abbreviation *inv* indicates an inversion, *ins* indicates an insertion, *del* indicates a deletion, and *der* indicates the derivative chromosome resulting from a translocation. Gain or loss of a whole chromosome is shown by + or − in front of the number, gain or loss of part of a chromosome by + or − after the number.

Table 12-6 shows the more common cytogenetic findings in the acute leukemias, and Fig. 12-85 shows a normal karyotype, albeit in a case of B-lineage ALL.

The frequencies of more common cytogenetic changes in adult and childhood AML are shown in Fig. 12-86 and the analysis of karyotype of a sample of blood or bone marrow for cytogenetic changes in Fig. 12-87. The various chromosomes can be

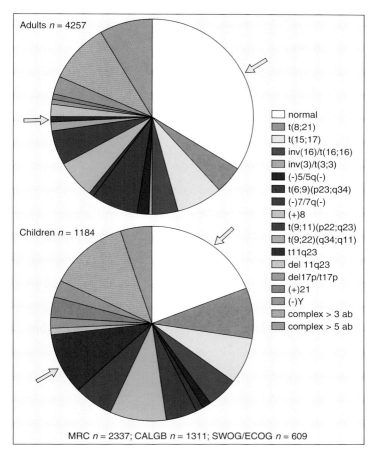

Fig. 12-86. Acute myeloid leukemia: distribution of the most common chromosome abnormalities in adults and children. (Adapted from Mrozek K. et al: *Blood Reviews* 18:115-136, 2004.)

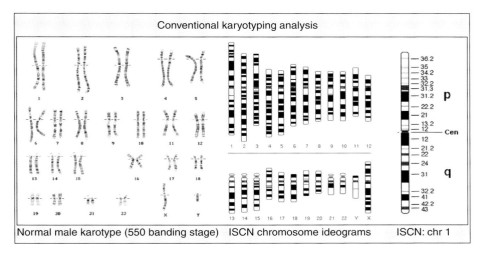

Fig. 12-87. Conventional karyotyping analysis: international system for chromosome nomenclature (ISCN), p (short arm), and q (long arm) with numbers assigned to each band. (Courtesy of Dr. E. Nacheva.)

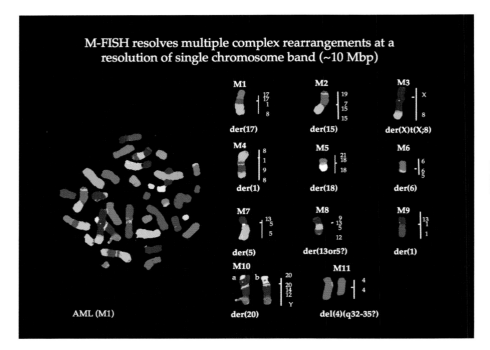

Fig. 12-88. Acute myeloid leukemia: identification of complex chromosome changes by color karyotyping using M-FISH. (Courtesy of Dr. E. Nacheva.) (See Fig. 12-98.)

distinguished using "whole chromosome paints" (Fig. 12-88). The structural chromosome abnormalities in three favorable prognosis AML groups, t(8;21), t(15;17), inv(16) and also t(6;9) as an example of a translocation found in therapy related AML are illustrated in Figs. 12-89 to 12-91. The translocations t(8;21) (RUNXI-ETO) and inv(16) (SMMHC-CBFB) in AML and t(12;21) (TEL-RUX1) in childhood ALL cause disruption of the core binding factor complex CBF made up of RUNXI (also known as AML1) and CBFβ (Fig 12-92). The normal CBF dimer recognizes and binds specific deoxyribonucleic acid (DNA) sequences through RUNX1 and regulates many genes important in the differentiation of hematopoietic cells, for example, IL-3 and GM-CSF. Mice lacking RUNXI fail to develop normal hematopoiesis.

In ALL hyperdiploidy carries a favorable prognosis (Fig. 12-93). The frequencies of the various translocations in childhood ALL are shown in Fig. 12-94. The incidence is different in adults; for example, t(9;22) occurs in up to 25% of cases over age 40 years.

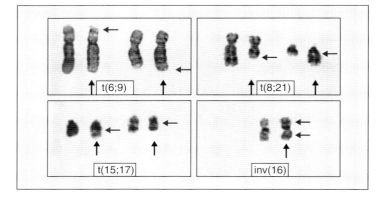

Fig. 12-90. Acute myeloid leukemia: partial karyograms showing common rearrangements in AML. In each karyogram, the translocated chromosome is on the right (arrowed) in each pair; red arrows mark the regions of chromosome breakage and rejoining: t(6;9) (p22;q34); t(8;21) (q22;q22); t(15;17) (q22;q12); inv(16) (p13;q22). (Courtesy of Professor L. M. Secker-Walker.)

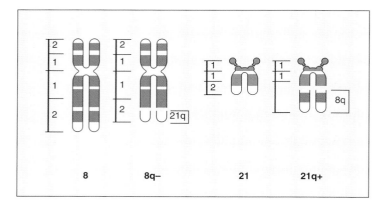

Fig. 12-89. Acute myeloid leukemia, t(8;21) subtype: diagrammatic systematized description of the structural aberration t(8;21). (Courtesy of Professor L. M. Secker-Walker.)

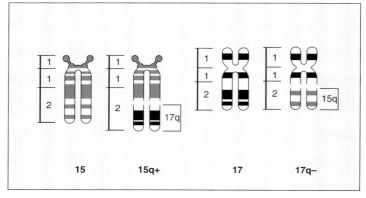

Fig. 12-91. Acute myeloid leukemia, t(15;17) subtype (acute promyelocytic leukemia, APL): systematized description of the structural aberration t(15;17). (Courtesy of Professor L. M. Secker-Walker.)

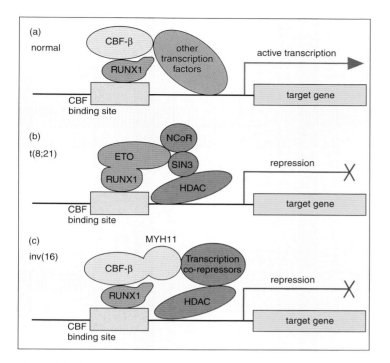

Fig. 12-92. The genes encoding components of the CBF transcription factor complex are frequent targets in AML. **A,** RUNX1 binds a specific DNA sequence motif, and recruits CBF-β to form a heterodimeric complex. This then acts as a transcriptional organizer, attracting other specific transcription factors and promoting target gene transcription. **B,** The t(8;21) translocation results in fusion of RUNX1 to the ETO protein, which recruits a series of transcriptional repressors, including histone deacetylases, leading to target gene inactivation. **C,** In cells carrying the inv (16) rearrangement, the CBF-β-MYH11 fusion protein binds to RUNX1 and then recruits transcriptional repressors.

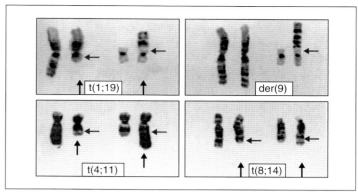

Fig. 12-95. Acute lymphoblastic leukemia: partial karyograms showing common translocations in patients with ALL. The translocated chromosomes are on the right (arrowed) of each pair; the red arrows mark the regions of chromosome breakage and rejoining: t(1;19) (q21;p13); der(19) t(1;19) (q23;p13); t(4;11) (q21;q23); t(8;14) (q24;q32). (Courtesy of Professor L. M. Secker-Walker.)

Cytogenetic analysis of acute leukemia cells may help confirm the diagnosis and indicate the subtype in which characteristic abnormalities may occur.

The translocations shown in Fig. 12-95 with the exception of der(19) are associated with a poor prognosis. Translocations (9;22), t(1;19) and the variant der (19) and t(4;11) are characteristic for early B-lineage ALL and t(8;14) for B-ALL (see Figs. 12-95 and 12-96).

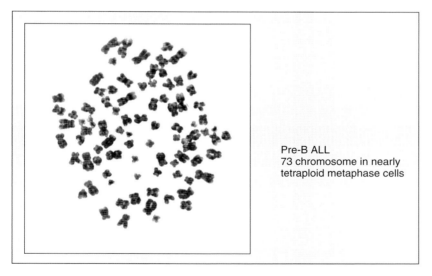

Pre-B ALL
73 chromosome in nearly
tetraploid metaphase cells

Fig. 12-93. Acute lymphoblastic leukemia: a representative hyperdiploid bone marrow cell pre-B-ALL with 73 chromosomes. (Courtesy of Dr. E. Nacheva.)

Fig. 12-94. Acute lymphoblastic leukemia: cytogenetic abnormalities. Distribution of translocation-generated oncogenes. (Modified from Look AT: Oncogenic transcription factors in the human acute leukemias, *Science* 278:1059-1064, 1997.)

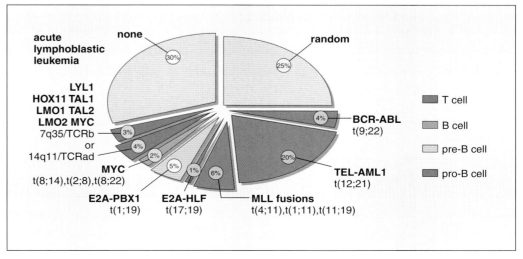

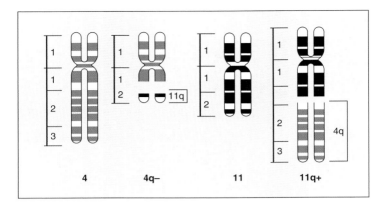

Fig. 12-96. Acute lymphoblastic leukemia, t(4;11): from a patient with blasts of null phenotype (TdT+, CD10−). Systematized description of the structural aberration. The translocated chromosomes are on the right in each pair. (Courtesy of Professor L. M. Secker-Walker.)

FLUORESCENT IN SITU HYBRIDIZATION

Fluorescent in situ hybridization (FISH) can be used to examine interphase as well as dividing cells (Figs. 12-97 and 12-98). It is able to detect gain or loss of all or part of a chromosome or a translocation, in some cases where the translocated or lost material is not visible by light microscopy (Figs. 12-98 and 12-99). A cryptic translocation t(12;21) (p13;q22) occurs in 30% of B-lineage ALL (Fig. 12-100, *A*). Using the MLL probe, FISH can show rearrangements within the gene (Fig. 12-100, *B*).

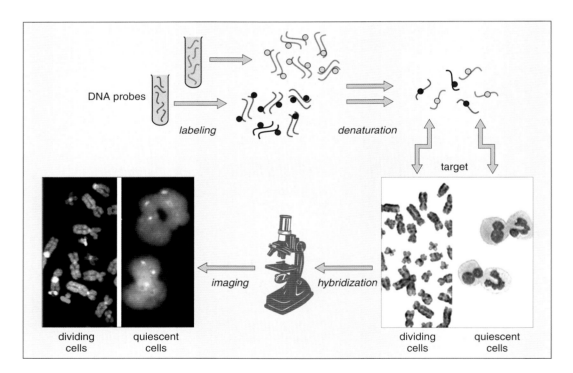

Fig. 12-97. Principle of fluorescence in situ hybridization (FISH). (Courtesy of Dr. E. Nacheva.)

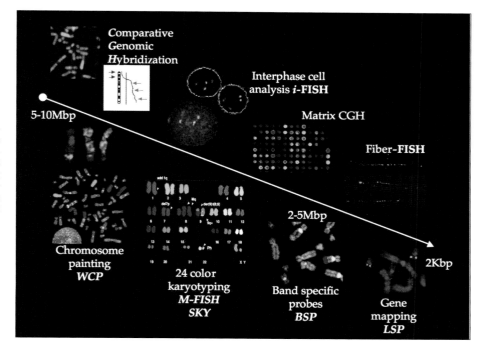

Fig. 12-98. Summary of fluorescence in situ hybridization (FISH) techniques. Below the diagonal line methods for analysis of dividing cells are illustrated: whole chromosome painting (WCP), color karyotyping (SKY and M-FISH), band-specific paints (BSP), and locus-specific probes (LSP). Above the diagonal line methods for analysis of interphase cells are illustrated: comparative genomic hybridization (CGH), i-FISH, matrix CGH, and fiber FISH. (Courtesy of Dr. E. Nacheva.)

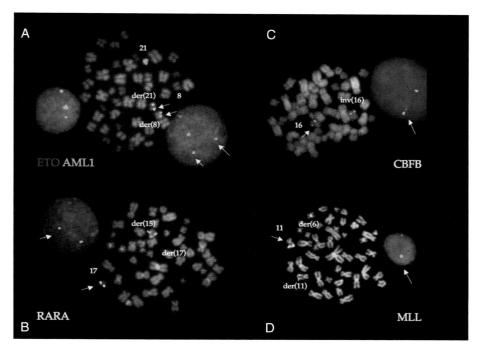

Fig. 12-99. Acute myeloid leukemia: identification of typical chromosome rearrangements by FISH in both metaphase and nondividing cells. **A,** Using dual color, dual-fusion FISH probe to detect ETO/AML fusion resulting from t(8;21). **B–D,** Using break-apart dual-color FISH probes to detect RARA gene rearrangements associated with t(15;17) and variants of thereof, CBFA rearrangement associated with inv(16) and MLL gene rearrangement associated with t(6;11). (Courtesy of Dr. E. Nacheva.)

Fig. 12-100. Acute lymphoblastic leukemia: FISH analysis. **A,** Metaphase from a childhood patient with ALL showing the translocation t(12;21) by chromosome "painting." Chromosomes 12 are painted red and chromosomes 21 green. This chromosome abnormality is not visible by conventional cytogenetic analysis. FISH elegantly reveals the exchange of material on the derived chromosomes 12 and 21. **B,** FISH using probes for the centromere of chromosome 11 (green) and the MLL gene (red), normally on chromosome 11, reveals a reciprocal translocation between chromosomes 6 and 11 that results in the rearrangement of MLL, which is detected as a splitting of the MLL signal between the derived chromosomes 6 and 11. (A, B, Courtesy of Dr. C. J. Harrison.)

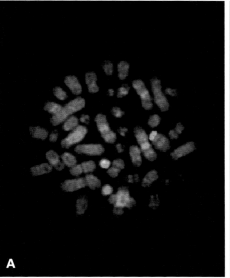
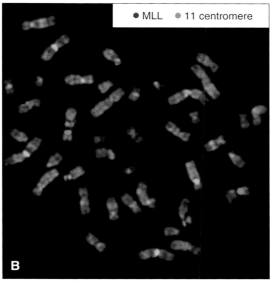

MOLECULAR STUDIES

Between 40% and 50% of adult AML cases have normal cytogenetics (NC) by light microscopy and have been placed in an intermediate prognostic group between the favorable group with, for example,

TABLE 12-7.   ACUTE MYELOID LEUKEMIA: GENE MUTATIONS AND GENE-EXPRESSION CHANGES IN PATIENTS WITH NORMAL CYTOGENETICS

Gene mutation	Gene location
FMS-related tyrosine kinase 3 (FLT3) gene	13q12
Nucleophosmin, member 1 (NPM1) gene	5q35
Partial tandem duplication (PTD) of the myeloid/lymphoid or mixed lineage leukemia (MLL) gene	11q23
Overexpression of the brain and acute leukemia (BAALC) gene	8q22.3
Mutations of the CC AAT/enhanced-binding protein α (CEBPA) gene	1q13.1
Overexpression of the ETS-related gene ERG	21q22.3

Adapted from Mrozek L et al: *Blood* 109:431-438, 2007. Also, see text for TET2.

t(8;21), inv(16), or t(15;17) and the unfavorable group with, for example, -7, inv(3), balanced translocations including 11q23 other than t(9;11), or with a complex karyotype (see Fig. 12-86). The NC group, however, shows submicroscopic alterations that may be detected by molecular tests or special staining and that strongly influence outcomes (Table 12-7 and Fig. 12-101). The most frequent are internal tandem duplication (ITD) of the FLT3 gene (Fig. 12-102). This occurs particularly in NC patients and those with t(15;17). In the NC patients the white cell and blast counts tend to be higher than those without FLT3 ITD. It carries an unfavorable prognosis. On the other hand, point mutations usually within the activation loop of the FLT3 tyrosine kinase, found in 5% to 14% of the NC patients, do not affect prognosis.

Mutations in the nucleophosmin member1 (NPM1) gene are found in 46% to 62% of AML NC patients. The protein has several functions, including prevention of nucleolar aggregation, regulation of ribosomal protein assembly and transport. The protein is normally localized to the nucleus but if mutated is usually aberrantly expressed in the cell cytoplasm (Figs. 12-103 to 12-105). Both FLT3 and NPM1 mutations may be detected using molecular techniques (Fig. 12-106).

Acquired mutations of TET2, a tumor suppressor gene at 4q24, occur in 10% to 20% of patients with myeloid neoplasms including AML, MDS, myeloproliferative diseases, CML, CMML, and systemic mastocytosis. TET2 mutations may precede other clonal genetic lesions, e.g. JAK-2 or chromosome translocations. The other mutational changes in gene expression seen in NC AML cases, including mutated CEBPA, are listed in Table 12-7 and are less frequent.

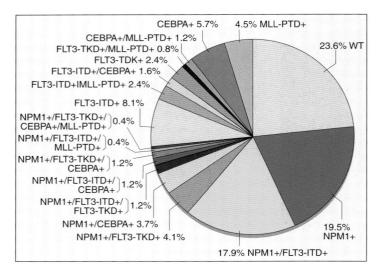

Fig. 12-101. Acute myeloid leukemia: pie chart based on 246 patients analyzed for the presence or absence of mutations in NPM1 and CEBPA genes, FLT3-ITD, FLT3-TDK, and MLLPTD. (Adapted from Mrozek L et al: *Blood* 109:431-438, 2007.)

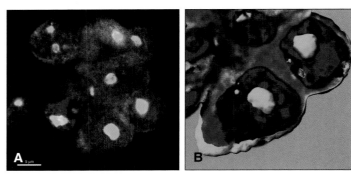

Fig. 12-103. Subcellular distribution of nucleophosmin (NPM) in the human acute myeloid leukemia cell line OCI-AML3, which carries a mutation of the NPM1 gene. **A,** Cells show the expected nucleolar positivity and the aberrant cytoplasmic expression of NPM (immunofluorescence and confocal microscope analysis; nuclei are stained red with propidium iodide). **B,** Three-dimensional reconstruction of two OCI-AML3 cells. An electronic cut of the image sparing nucleoli was performed to better visualize nuclear and aberrant cytoplasmic distribution of NPM. (Courtesy of Professor I. Nicoletti and Professor B. Falini.)

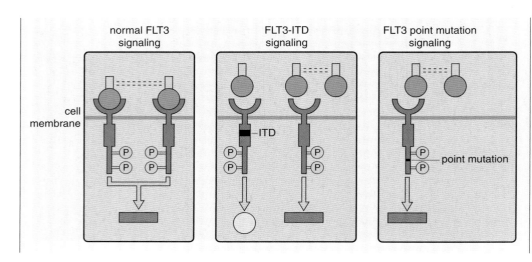

Fig. 12-102. Normal FLT3 signaling and disruption that may occur because of two major classes of mutations: internal tandem duplications (ITD) of 3 to 400 base pairs in exons 14 or 15 (15% to 35% of cases of AML) or missense point mutations in exon 20 in the intracellular domain (5% to 10% of cases of AML). Modified from Emanuel P (2007) The Hematologist ASH News and Reports, p. 10.

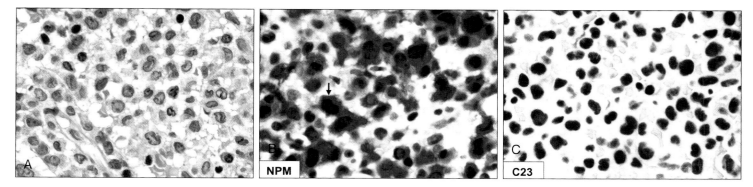

Fig. 12-104. Bone marrow biopsy from AML with mutated NPM1. **A,** Diffuse infiltration by leukemic cells with monoblastic appearance. **B,** Most leukemic cells show the expected nuclear positivity and the aberrant cytoplasmic expression of NPM (arrow). **C,** The leukemic cells from the same case show nucleus-restricted expression of C23/nucleolin. Immunostaining of paraffin sections with monoclonal antibodies recognizing both wild-type and mutated NPM **(B)** or C23/nucleolin **(C).** Immuno–alkaline phosphatase anti–alkaline phosphatase (AP-AAP) technique hematoxylin counterstaining. (Courtesy of Professor B. Falini.)

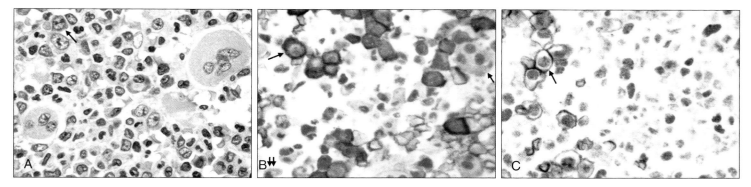

Fig. 12-105. Multilineage involvement in AML with mutated NPM1 (bone marrow biopsy, paraffin sections). **A,** The marrow is infiltrated by myeloid blasts, abnormal immature erythroid cells (long arrow), and dysplastic megakaryocytes. **B,** Double AP-AAP/immunoperoxidase staining for NPM (blue) and glycophorin (brown). All leukemic cells of the erythroid lineage (long arrow), and dysplastic megakaryocytes (short arrow). **C,** Double AP-AAP/immunoperoxidase staining for all C23/nucleolin (blue) and glycophorin (brown). All leukemic cells of different lineages (the long arrow indicates an immature erythroid cell) show nucleus-restricted expression of C23/nucleolin. (Courtesy of Professor B. Falini.)

Fig. 12-106. Gene scan fragment analysis. Identification of FLT3 internal tandem duplication and nucleophosmin 4bp insertion in AML patients. PCR is performed using fluorescently labeled primers; products are run on the ABI 3130 genetic analyzer. Nucleophosmin wild-type patients show only one peak; patients heterozygous for the mutation show a second peak 4bp larger (B—blue peaks) (lower panel). Similarly, the FLT3 internal tandem deletion (ITD) patients who are wild type show a single peak (upper panel). Patients who have an ITD have a large peak; the size of the peak will be determined by the length of the ITD (green peaks). Wild-type nucleophosmin (blue) and wild-type FLT3 (green); orange peaks are the size standards. (Courtesy of V. Duke and Dr. L. Foroni.)

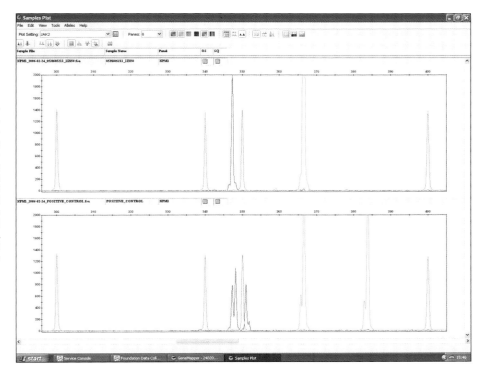

GENE ARRAYS

Quantification of the expression of thousands of genes using microarray technology can be used to molecularly classify leukemias, including subgroups of AML and ALL (Figs. 12-107 to 12-111).

These techniques are not widely available but may in the future define biological and clinically relevant subgroups of AML and ALL (see Figs. 12-107 to 12-111). These techniques are not applicable to the detection of minimal residual disease.

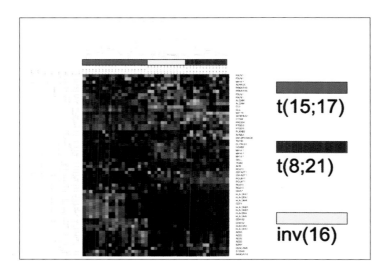

Fig. 12-107. Hierarchic cluster analysis of the gene expression pattern of the set of 13 predictor genes as identified according to adapted class prediction methodology. The three distinct cytogenetic AML subgroups can clearly be separated based on their gene expression profiles. Each row represents a leukemia sample and each column a gene. GenBank accession numbers are shown on the top. Varying expression levels are shown on a scale from black (no gene expression) to bright red (highest expression). The subgroups are colored according to their chromosomal aberrations. (Courtesy of Professor T. Haferlach and *Proceedings of the National Academy of Sciences* 99:10012, 2002.)

Fig. 12-108. Principle component analysis (PCA) based on U133A expression data of WHO-classified AML subtypes with recurrent chromosome aberrations and normal bone marrow mononuclear cells from healthy volunteers. Sixty AML samples comprising the color-coded subgroups t(15;17) (n = 20), t(8;21) (n = 13), inv(16) (n = 12), and t(11q34)/MLL gene rearrangement positive samples (n = 15) can accurately be discriminated and are different from normal bone marrow (n = 9). (Courtesy of Professor T. Haferlach. From *Seminars in Hematology* 40:281-295, 2003.)

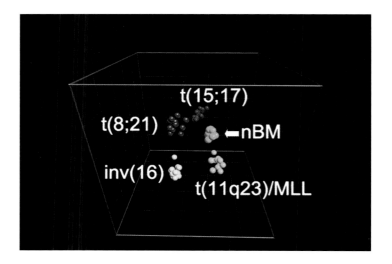

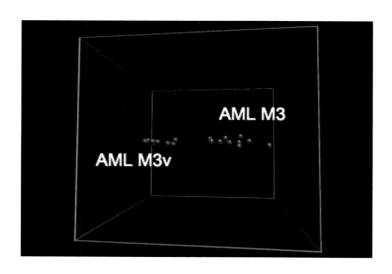

Fig. 12-109. Visualization of genes differentially expressed in M3 and M3v. In the hierarchic cluster analysis and the PCA, the feature space consisted of measured expression data on genes differentially expressed between FAB M3 and M3v. In the hierarchic clustering, the normalized expression value for each gene was coded by color (standard deviation from mean). Red indicates high expression and green low expression in a cell. (Courtesy of Professor T. Haferlach.)

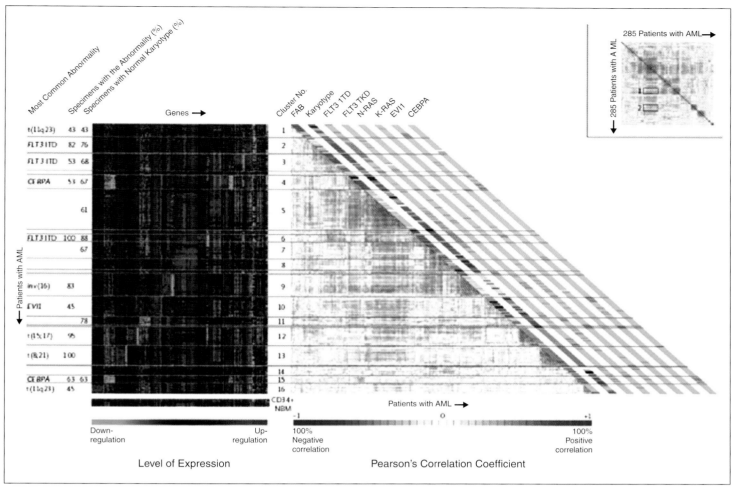

Fig. 12-110. In panel (A), the correlation visualization tool displays pairwise correlations between the samples. The colors of the cells relate to Pearson's correlation coefficient values, with deeper colors indicating higher positive (red) or negative (blue) correlations. One hundred percent negative correlation would indicate that genes with a high level of expression in one sample would always have a low level of expression in the other sample, and vice versa. Box 1 indicates a positive correlation between clusters 5 and 9 and box 2 a negative correlation between clusters 5 and 12. The red diagonal line displays the intraindividual comparison of results for a patient with AML (i.e., 100% correlation). To reveal the patterns of correlation, we applied a matrix-ordering method to rearrange the samples. The ordering algorithm starts with the most highly correlated pair of samples and, through an interactive process, sorts all the samples into correlated blocks. Each sample is joined to a block in an ordered manner so that a correlation trend is formed within a block, with the most correlated samples at the center. The blocks are then positioned along the diagonal of the plot in a similar ordered manner. Panel (B) shows all 16 clusters identified on the basis of the correlation view. The French-American-British (FAB) classification and karyotype based in cytogenetic analyses are depicted in the columns along the original diagonal of the correlation view; FAB subtype M0 is usually indicated in black, subtype M1 in green, subtype M3 in purple, subtype M3 in orange, subtype M4 in yellow, subtype M5 in blue, and subtype M6 in gray; normal karyotypes are indicated in green, inv(16) abnormalities in yellow, t(8;21) abnormalities in purple, t(15;17) abnormalities in orange, 11q23 abnormalities in blue, 7(q) abnormalities in red, +8 aberations in pink, complex karyotypes (those involving more than three chromosomal abnormalities) in black, and other abnormalities in gray. FLT3 internal tandem duplication (ITD) mutations; FLT3 mutations in the tyrosine kinase domain (TKD); N-RAS, K-RAS, and CEBPA mutations; and the overexpression of EVI1 are depicted in the same set of columns: red indicates the presence of a given abnormality and green its absence. The levels of expression of the top 40 genes identified by the significance analysis of microarrays of each of the 16 clusters, as well as in normal bone marrow (NBM) and CD34+ cells, are shown on the left-hand side. The scale bar indicates an increase (red) or a decrease (green) in the level of expression by a factor of at least 4 relative to the geometric mean of all samples. The percentages of the most common abnormalities (those present in more than 40% of specimens) and the percentages of specimens in each cluster with a normal karyotype are indicated. (Courtesy of Professor T. Haferlach and Valk et al: *New England Journal of Medicine* 350:1622, 2004.)

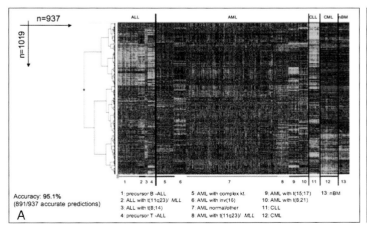
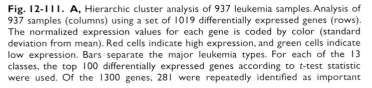
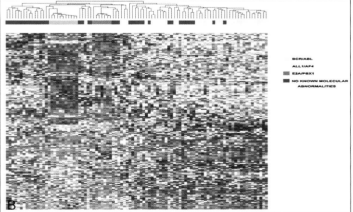

Fig. 12-111. A, Hierarchic cluster analysis of 937 leukemia samples. Analysis of 937 samples (columns) using a set of 1019 differentially expressed genes (rows). The normalized expression values for each gene is coded by color (standard deviation from mean). Red cells indicate high expression, and green cells indicate low expression. Bars separate the major leukemia types. For each of the 13 classes, the top 100 differentially expressed genes according to t-test statistic were used. Of the 1300 genes, 281 were repeatedly identified as important diagnostic markers and overlapped among the lists of the top 100 genes, resulting in 1019 nonoverlapping genes. B, Gene expression profiles of adult B-lineage acute lymphoblastic leukemia (ALL) samples. Supervised clustering reveals distinct gene expression profiles for samples with ALL/AF4, E2A/PBX1 and less distinct profiles for samples with BCR/ABL or no molecular abnormalities. (A, Courtesy of Professor T. Haferlach and *Blood* 106:1193, 2005. B, Courtesy of Professor R. Foa and Dr. S. Chiaretti.)

MINIMAL RESIDUAL DISEASE

Detection of residual leukemia cells in the peripheral blood or bone marrow of patients in complete remission clinically, by blood count and by examination of blood or bone marrow by light microscopy using normal staining, can be performed immunologically by flow cytometry (Table 12-8), in which residual cells of an aberrant leukemic phenotype are sought (Fig. 12-112) or by molecular methods. These are applicable to B-lineage or T-lineage ALL in which the exact clonal rearrangement of immunoglobulin or T-cell receptor genes is first analyzed (Figs. 12-113 to 12-118) and the remission blood or bone marrow sample is then tested quantitatively for this clone, most frequently using real-time polymerase chain reaction (RT-PCR). Alternatively, if the patient has a chromosomal translocation (Table 12-9), this can also be used as a marker for MRD (Fig. 12-119), using either DNA analysis or more frequently when the breakpoint is large, using reverse transcriptase PCR (Figs. 12-120;12-121).

TABLE 12-8. LEUKEMIA-ASSOCIATED IMMUNOPHENOTYPES THAT CAN BE IDENTIFIED AT DIAGNOSIS OF ACUTE LEUKEMIA AND SUBSEQUENTLY BE USED TO MONITOR MINIMAL RESIDUAL DISEASE

Type of abnormality	Example
Adherent expression of an antigen more appropriate to another lineage	Lymphoid-associated antigens, such as CD2, CD4, CD5, CD7, CD19, or CD20, on myeloid cells Myeloid-associated antigens, such as CD13, CD15, CD33, CD65, or CD66c, on lymphoid cells Natural killer or T-lineage-associated antigens, such as CD56, expressed on B lymphoblasts
Asynchronous expression of antigens or failure to express expected antigens synchronously	Co-expression of terminal deoxynucleotidyl transferase, CD10 and strong CD34 with cytoplasmic μ chain or strong CD19, CD20, CD21, or CD22 Co-expression of CD34 or terminal deoxynucleotidyl transferase with CD11b, CD14, CD15, strong CD33, or CD65 Failure to express CD13 and CD33 synchronously
Abnormally weak or abnormally strong antigen expression	Increased expression of CD10 Increased expression of CD33
Expression of antigens that are not usually expressed in cells being examined	Presence in the bone marrow of cells (i) expressing CD1a or (ii) expressing both cytoplasmic CD3 and either terminal deoxynucleotidyl transferase or CD34 or (iii) co-expressing CD4 and CD8

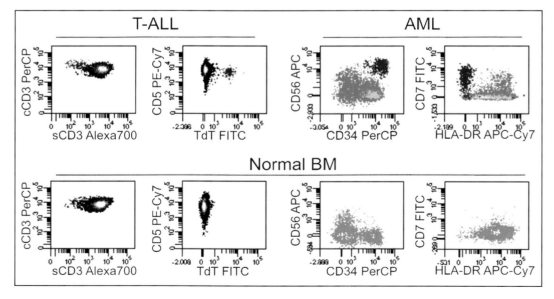

Fig. 12-112. Immunophenotypes: detection of minimal residual disease (MRD) in acute leukemia by flow cytometry. *Top,* Bone marrow (BM) samples from a patient with T-lineage acute lymphoblastic leukemia (T-ALL) and from one with acute myeloid leukemia (AML), both in morphologic remission, were labeled with combinations of 8 to 10 monoclonal antibodies simultaneously. Red dots in the density plots are the result of the combined immunophenotypic profile of the cell population and indicate MRD; they correspond to 0.02% of mononuclear cells in the T-ALL sample and 0.3% in the AML sample. *Bottom,* Results of a BM sample obtained from a healthy individual and stained with the same antibodies is shown. (Courtesy of Professor D. Campana.)

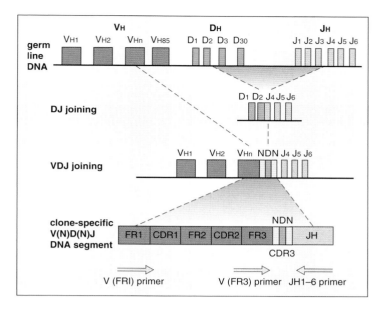

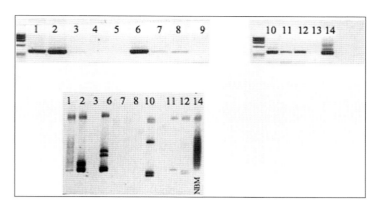

Fig. 12-113. IgH locus: the partial germ line locus is shown on top, followed by a hypothetical rearrangement event. Positions of primers that can be used for PCR gene amplification of the resulting rearrangement are shown by orange arrows. V, variable regions; D, diversity regions; J, joining regions; N, random regions inserted by TdT during gene rearrangement. (Courtesy of Dr. L. Foroni.)

Fig. 12-116. Heteroduplex analysis. Leukemia analysis using heteroduplex gel electrophoresis. Gene screening using primers for TCR gamma genes was performed and amplification verified by running an aliquot on an agarose gel electrophoresis, as illustrated in Fig. 12-115. An aliquot of the visible bands was then denatured for 5 minutes at 94° C and cooled to 5° C for 1 hour before loading onto an acrylamide nondenaturing vertical gel. The gel was run for 2 hours at 100 V and bands visualized by Sybersafe staining. Lane numbers on the upper gel correspond to lane numbers on the bottom gel. The presence of a monclonal (lane 11), biclonal (lanes 2,6,10,12), and polyclonal (lane 14) is clearly shown by this approach. This is a more powerful technique to distinguish clonal versus polyclonal rearrangements for antigen-receptor gene analysis compared with agarose gel resolution. (Courtesy of Dr. L. Foroni.)

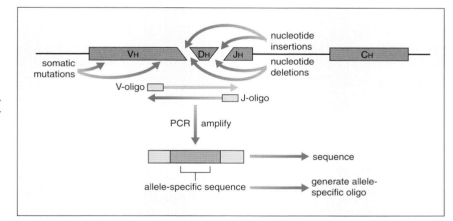

Fig. 12-114. Minimal residual disease: detection in precursor B-ALL using PCR amplification with clone-specific primers or probe.

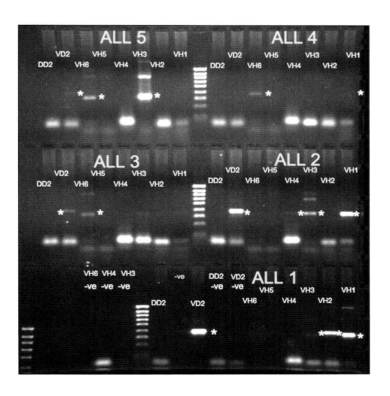

Fig. 12-115. Leukemia analysis. Representative ethidium bromide agarose gel of five different newly diagnosed leukemias. Approximately 200 ng of DNA was tested per lane with a combination of immunoglobulin VH (VH-JH primer combinations for the six major Ig V (VH1 to VH6) gene families), and by TCR delta (DH-JH primer combination). Approximately one third of the PCR product was then run on a 1.5% agarose gel and bands visualized by Sybersafe staining. In this image the positive VH amplification for each combination of primers is marked by an asterisk. A 100bp ladder is used for the correct sizing of each PCR fragment. Primer dimmer combinations are visible in the low part of each set of run. Negative controls are also marked. The negative TCR delta tests are not shown. (Courtesy of Dr. L. Foroni.)

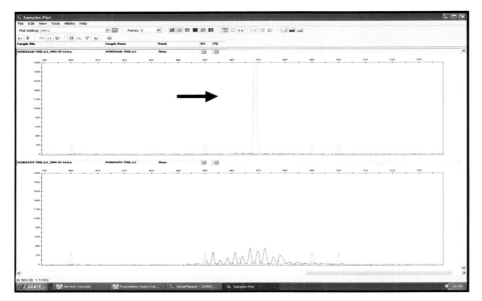

Fig. 12-117. Gene scan fragment analysis. Detection of IgVH clone in patients with B-precursor acute lymphoblastic leukemia. PCR is performed using one fluorescently labeled primer and one nonlabeled primer. PCR products are then run together with formamide on the ABI 3130. Each VH gene primer is labeled with a different fluorescent label, allowing for the PCR reactions to be pooled before running on the fragment collector. Size standard appears orange. *Top,* Clone identified as a single peak on fragment analysis. *Bottom,* Polyclonal IgVH trace seen when there is no individual clone present. (Courtesy of V. Duke and Dr. L. Foroni.)

Fig. 12-118. Gene scan fragment analysis. T-cell receptor gamma clone identification. PCR performed using fluorescently labeled forward primers for TCRγ 1 to 8, 9, 10, and 11 together with nonlabeled Jγ reverse primer. PCR products are then run on the ABI 3130 fragment analyzer. This patient has a TCRγ 1 to 8 clone, which will need to be sequenced to identify the clone and the CDR3 region. (Courtesy of V. Duke and Dr. L. Foroni.)

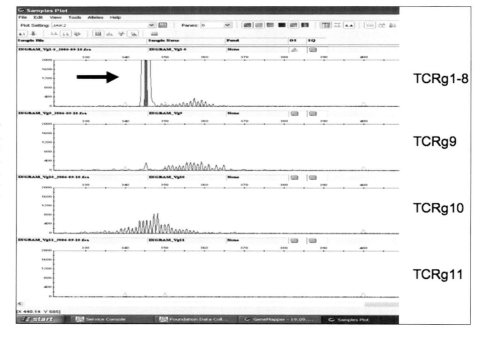

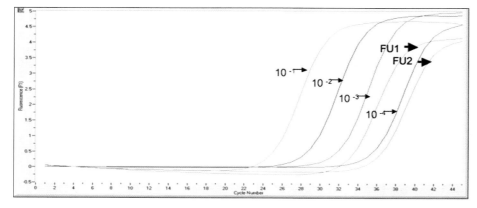

Fig. 12-119. Real-time (RT)-PCR quantification of minimal residual disease (MRD) using immunoglobulin gene analysis of peripheral blood. This image illustrates RT-PCR for antigen-receptor gene analysis. Dilution of presentation material from 10^1 to 10^4 of DNA from the leukemic sample into normal mononuclear cells (obtained from six normal donor buffy-coats) is shown, and each dilution is marked by an arrow and the individual dilution amount. Two follow-up samples (FU1 and FU2) measurements are given. FU1 is quantified between 10^4 and 10^3 whereas FU2, though positive, is outside the quantitative range (POQR) of the presentation standard curve. (Courtesy of Dr. L. Foroni.)

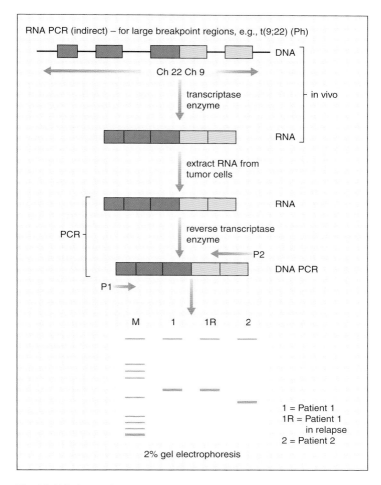

RNA PCR (indirect) – for large breakpoint regions, e.g., t(9;22) (Ph)

M   1   1R   2

1 = Patient 1
1R = Patient 1
     in relapse
2 = Patient 2

2% gel electrophoresis

Fig. 12-120. Molecular cytogenetics: RNA PCR [indirect—for large breakpoint regions, e.g., t(9;22) (Ph)].

TABLE 12-9   TRANSLOCATIONS SUITABLE FOR PCR ANALYSIS: (UPPER) ALL, B LINEAGE; (MIDDLE) ALL, T LINEAGE; (LOWER) AML

Acute lymphoblastic leukemia: B lineage

	Chromosomal translocation	Molecular target	DNA or RNA
Precursor B	t(9;22)	BCR-ABL	RNA
	t(1;19)	E2A-PBX1	RNA
	t(17;19)	HLF-E2A	RNA
	t(4;11)	AF4-MLL	RNA
	t(12;21)	TEL-AML1	RNA
	11q23 translocations	MLL-AF	RNA
B-ALL	t(8;14)	MYC-Sμ	DNA

Acute lymphoblastic leukemia: T lineage

	Chromosomal translocation	Molecular target	DNA or RNA
T-ALL	TAL interstitial deletion	TAL-SIL	DNA
	t(1;14)	TAL-1-TCRδ	DNA
	t(10;14)	HOX11-TCRδ	DNA
	t(11;14)	11p13-TCRδ	DNA

Acute myeloid leukemia

FAB subtype	Chromosomal translocation	Molecular target	DNA or RNA
M₂	t(8;21)	CBFα-/MTGA*	RNA
M₂ or M₄	t(6;9)	DEK-CAN	RNA
M₃	t(15;17)	PML-RARα	RNA
M₄	inv 16	CBFβ-MCHII	RNA
Non-specific	t(9;22)	BCR-ABL	RNA
	t(9;11)	MLL-AF9	RNA

*CBFα = AML1; MTGA = ETO

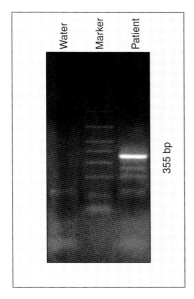

Fig. 12-121. Reverse transcriptase (RT): PCR analysis of an APL patient at diagnosis. The PML-RARA fusion product (cDNA) has been amplified using nested oligonucleotides from the PML and RARA genes. Lane 1, water control; Lane 2, low-molecular-weight (Cambio) DNA marker; Lane 3, patient sample. All APL patients with a t(15;17) translocation express either the 5′ (a single 355 bp fusion message) or the 3′ (a series of various fusion messages caused by alternate splicing) PML breakpoint. (Courtesy of Dr. P. Devaraj.)

CHRONIC MYELOID LEUKEMIAS AND MYELOMONOCYTIC/ MYELOPROLIFERATIVE DISORDERS

The major disease is Philadelphia (Ph) chromosome–positive chronic myeloid leukemia (CML) (Table 13-1). Rare types of CMLs include Ph-negative, BCR-ABL–negative CML and chronic neutrophilic, eosinophilic, and monocytic leukemias. The myelodysplastic/ myeloproliferative diseases chronic myelomonocytic leukemia (CMML), juvenile myelomonocytic leukemia (JMML), and refractory anemia with ringed sideroblasts associated with marked thrombocytosis are also discussed in this chapter.

CHRONIC MYELOID LEUKEMIA (BCR REARRANGEMENT POSITIVE)

CML is most frequently seen in the middle-aged but occurs at all ages. In most patients there is replacement of normal marrow by cells with an abnormal G-group chromosome, the Ph chromosome (Fig. 13-1). This abnormality is a result of reciprocal translocation involving chromosome 9 band q34 and chromosome 22 band q11. The cellular oncogene ABL (now termed ABL1), which codes for a tyrosine protein kinase (TPK), is translocated to a specific breakpoint cluster region (BCR) of chromosome 22. Part of the BCR (the 5′ end) remains on chromosome 22, and the 3′ end moves to chromosome 9 together with the oncogene *SIS* (which codes for a protein with close homology to one of the two subunits of platelet-derived growth factor). As a result of the translocation onto chromosome 22, a chimeric BCR/ABL messenger ribonucleic acid (mRNA) is produced (Fig. 13-2), which results in the synthesis of a 210 kDa protein with considerably enhanced TPK activity compared with the normal 145 kDa *ABL* oncogene product (Table 13-2). The fusion gene may be detected by the fluorescent in situ hybridization (FISH) technique (Fig. 13-3).

Cases of Ph-positive acute lymphoblastic leukemia (ALL) may show a similar molecular abnormality to that in typical Ph-positive CML, but some show a breakpoint on chromosome 22 outside the major BCR region but in the first intron of the gene (minor BCR, or m-BCR breakpoint). In these, the product of the translocated ABL gene is a 190 kDa protein also of enhanced TPK activity (see Table 13-2).

TABLE 13-1. CHRONIC MYELOID AND MYELOMONOCYTIC LEUKEMIAS: CLASSIFICATION

Type	Molecular genetics
BCR-rearrangement positive CML	>95% BCR-ABL1 p210 <5% p190 or p230
BCR-rearrangement negative CML	Various cytogenetic abnormalities
Chronic neutrophilic leukemia	Deletions of chromosome 20q and trisomy 21 or 9 in some
Chronic eosinophilic leukemia	FIPILI-PDGFR-α (in those who respond to Imatinib) generated by interstitial deletion on chromosome 4q12
Chronic monocytic leukemia	Very rare
Chronic myelomonocytic leukemia	PDGFR-β rearrangement in a minority who respond to Imatinib
Juvenile myelomonocytic leukemia	30% PTPN11 (encodes SHP-2) mutations 20% K-RAS or N-RAS mutations 10% NF1 mutation
Refractory anemia with ringed sideroblasts associated with marked thrombocytosis	Somatic mutations of JAK2 and MPL

BCR, breakpoint cluster region; CML, chronic myeloid leukemia

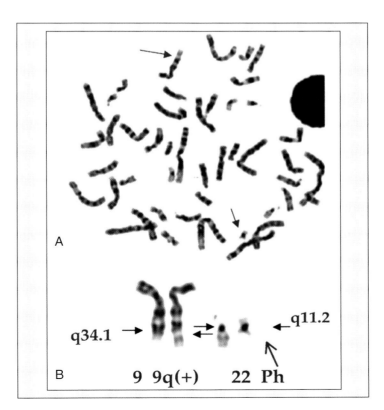

Fig. 13-1. Chronic myeloid leukemia. **A,** G-banded metaphase cell with *arrows* pointing to the Ph and der(9) chromosomes. **B,** Partial karyotype showing the reciprocal translocation t(9;22)(q34;q11). The *arrows* indicate the breakpoints. (Courtesy of Dr. E. Nacheva.)

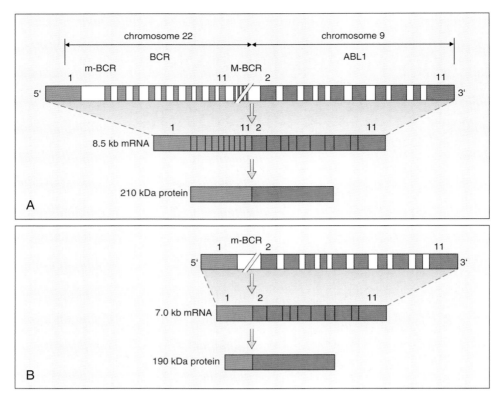

Fig. 13-2. Chronic myeloid leukemia. **A,** Chimeric BCR/ABL mRNA encoded for partly by the breakpoint cluster region (BCR) of chromosome 22 and partly by the ABL1 oncogene translocated from chromosome 9 to 22. The breakpoint is almost always in the major BCR (M-BCR) region, a 5 to 6 kb region 3′ to exon 11. Small exons numbered b1, b2, b3, and so on occur in the M-BCR region, and the breakpoint is usually between b3 and b4 or b2 and b3, giving rise to fusion genes b3a2 or b2a2, respectively. The resultant 85 kb mRNA is expressed as a 210 kDa protein (p210). **B,** In Ph-positive acute lymphoblastic leukemia (ALL) the breakpoint may be in the M-BCR region, but may also occur in the first intron, the minor BCR (m-BCR) region. The fusion gene is termed e1a2. A 7.0 kb mRNA is formed that codes for a 190 kDa protein (p190).

CLINICAL FEATURES

The symptoms are related to hypermetabolism and include anorexia, lassitude, weight loss, and night sweats. Splenomegaly is usual and frequently massive (Fig. 13-4). Features of anemia, a bleeding disorder, visual disturbance because of retinal disease (Figs. 13-5 and 13-6), neurologic symptoms, and occasionally gout (Fig. 13-7) may occur. As in chronic lymphocytic leukemia (CLL), this condition is only discovered in some patients during routine blood counting. The white cell count is usually between 50×10^9/L and 500×10^9/L (but may be over 500×10^9/L; Fig. 13-8), and a complete spectrum of granulocytic cells is seen in the blood film (Figs. 13-9 to 13-11). Basophils are often prominent, and the levels of myelocytes, metamyelocytes, and neutrophils exceed those of the more primitive blast cells and promyelocytes. The bone marrow is hypercellular with a granulocytic predominance (Figs. 13-12 to 13-15).

TABLE 13-2. CHRONIC MYELOID LEUKEMIA: PATTERNS OF INVOLVEMENT OF THE Ph CHROMOSOME, THE BCR (5.8 KB) REGION, AND THE ABL TPK IN CML AND ALL

Condition	Pattern
Normal	Ph−, BCR− → 145 kDa TPK
Chronic myeloid leukemia	Ph+, BCR+ → 210 kDa TPK
	Ph−, BCR+ → 210 kDa TPK
	Ph−, BCR− → 145 kDa TPK (atypical cases; ?myelodysplasia)
Acute lymphoblastic leukemia	Ph+, BCR+ → 210 kDa TPK (?blast transformation of CML)
	Ph+, BCR− → 190 kDa TPK (?de novo ALL)
	Ph−, BCR− → 145 kDa TPK (de novo ALL)

ALL, Acute lymphoblastic leukemia; *BCR1,* rearrangement within the 5.8 KB BCR region; *CML,* chronic myeloid leukemia.

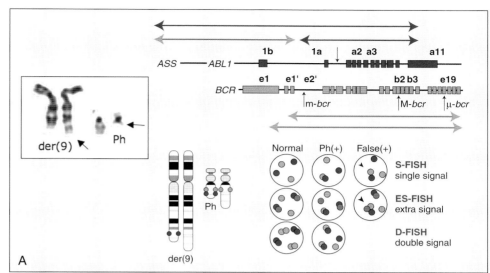

Fig. 13-3. Chronic myeloid leukemia. **A,** Different types of fluorescent in situ hybridization (FISH) probes to detect the BCR/ABL1 fusion. The top part shows the sequence of the BCR *(green)* and ABL1 *(red)* covered by the FISH probes. S-FISH detects the fusion signal only on the Ph chromosome. Extra signal FISH (ES-FISH, *blue*) detects the der(9) chromosome, and a *blue-red-green* cluster identifies the BCR/ABL1 fusion. Double FISH (D-FISH) uses probes to specify BCR and ABL1 breakpoints, and both products, Ph and der(9), give a fusion signal. **B,** D-FISH BCR/ABL1 probe image showing a typical Ph-positive cell with FISH signals *(top)* and diagram *(bottom)* showing a one G *(green)*, one R *(red)*, and two Y *(yellow)* signal pattern. **C,** A cell with typical deletions of der(9) chromosome with only one fusion signal on the Ph chromosome as seen in 10% to 15% of patients with chronic myeloid leukemia. (Courtesy of Dr. E. Nacheva.)

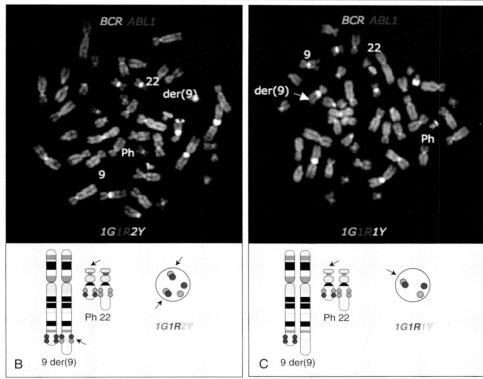

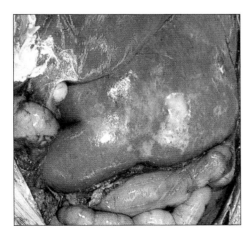

Fig. 13-4. Chronic myeloid leukemia: abdominal contents at autopsy of a 54-year-old man. The grossly enlarged spleen extends toward the right iliac fossa. The central pale area covered by fibrinous exudate overlays an extensive splenic infarct. The liver is moderately enlarged.

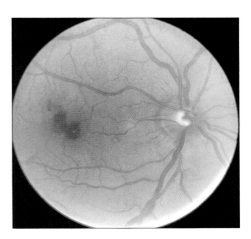

Fig. 13-5. Chronic myeloid leukemia: ocular fundus in the hyperviscosity syndrome showing distended retinal veins and deep retinal hemorrhages at the macula. (Hb, 14 g/dl; white blood cell count [WBC], 590 $\times$ 10^9/L; platelets, 1050 $\times$ 10^9/L.)

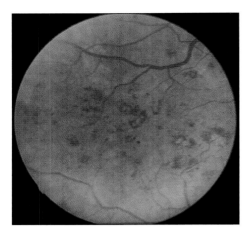

Fig. 13-6. Chronic myeloid leukemia: ocular fundus (same case as shown in Fig. 13-5) showing prominent leukemic infiltrates fringed by areas of retinal hemorrhage.

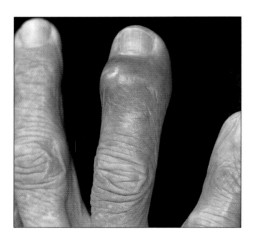

Fig. 13-7. Chronic myeloid leukemia: acute inflammation and swelling of the fourth finger because of uric acid deposition. (Hb, 8.6 g/dl; WBC, 540 × 10⁹/L; platelets, 850 × 10⁹/L; serum uric acid, 0.85 mmol/L.)

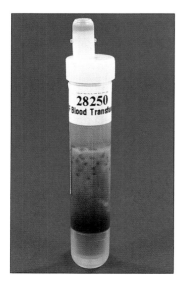

Fig. 13-8. Chronic myeloid leukemia: peripheral blood, from a 22-year-old woman, showing vast increase in buffy coat. (Hb, 6.1 g/dl; WBC, 532 × 10⁹/L; platelets, 676 × 10⁹/L.)

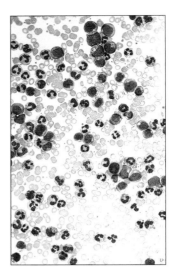

Fig. 13-9. Chronic myeloid leukemia: peripheral blood film showing cells in all stages of granulocytic development. (Hb, 16.8 g/dl; WBC, 260 × 10⁹/L; platelets, 140 × 10⁹/L.)

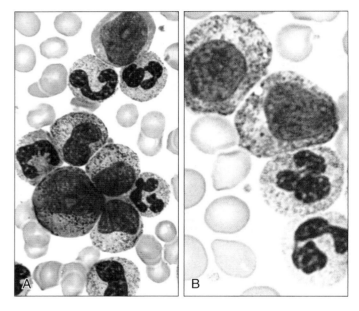

Fig. 13-10. Chronic myeloid leukemia. **A** and **B,** Peripheral blood films showing a myeloblast, promyelocytes, myelocytes, metamyelocytes, and band and segmented neutrophils.

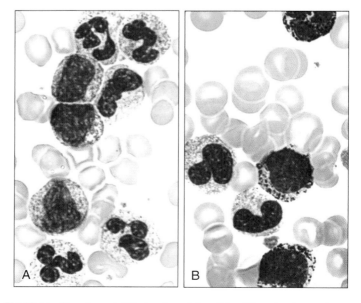

Fig. 13-11. Chronic myeloid leukemia: peripheral blood films showing myelocytes, a metamyelocyte, and band and segmented neutrophils **(A)** and basophils and metamyelocytes **(B).**

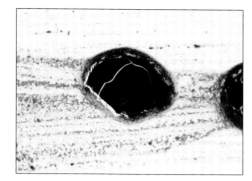

Fig. 13-12. Chronic myeloid leukemia: bone marrow aspirate showing hypercellular fragment and trails.

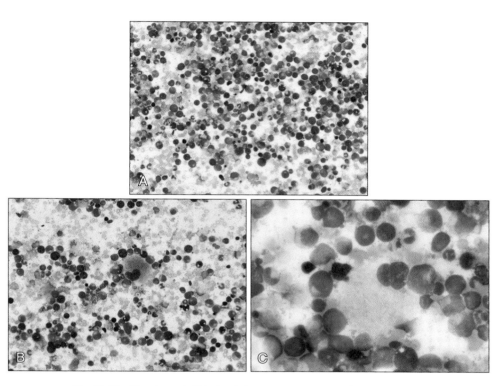

Fig. 13-13. Chronic myeloid leukemia bone marrow aspirate showing increased granulocytes and precursors with blasts <5% **(A)**, small megakaryocyte **(B)**, and pseudo-Gaucher cell **(C).**

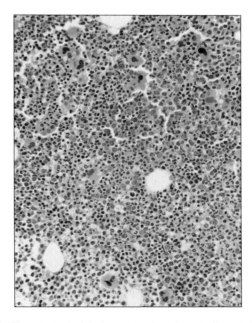

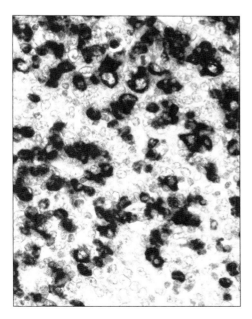

Fig. 13-14. Chronic myeloid leukemia: trephine biopsy showing hypercellular hematopoiesis with increased granulopoiesis and small megakaryocytes.

Fig. 13-15. Chronic myeloid leukemia: trephine bone marrow biopsy stained for neutrophil elastase (a myeloid-specific marker) with immunophosphatase. (Courtesy of Professor D.Y. Mason.)

ACCELERATED PHASE

This is characterized by anemia, increasing white cell count and spleen size not responding to therapy, peripheral blood basophils to >20% of circulating white cells (Fig. 13-16), persistent thrombocytopenia (<100 × 10^9/L), or thrombocytosis (>1000 × 10^9/L) not responding to therapy, with increased blasts in the blood or marrow to 10% to 19% (Figs. 13-16 to 13-18). There may be proliferation of dysplastic cells in the granulocytic lineage (Figs. 13-19 and 13-20) with small dysplastic megakaryocytes in sheets (Fig. 13-21, *A*) in the marrow with increased fibrosis (Fig. 13-21, *B*). Cytogenetic analysis often shows clonal evolution, e.g., +8, +Ph, iso-17q or +19.

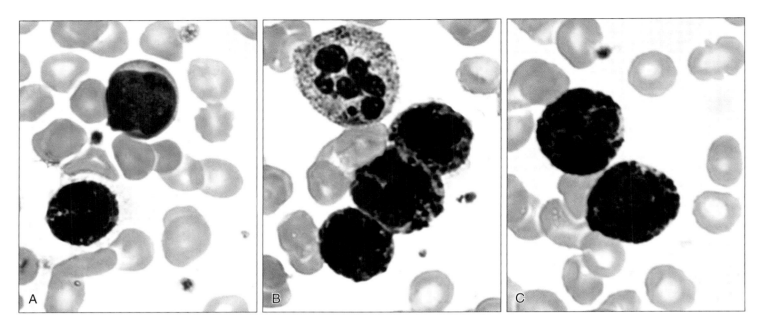

Fig. 13-16. Chronic myeloid leukemia: accelerated phase. Peripheral blood films showing marked basophilia and presence of a myeloblast.

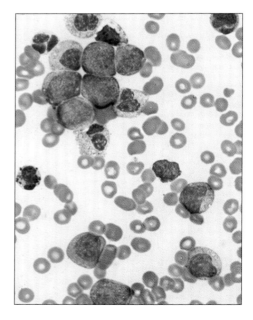

Fig. 13-17. Chronic myeloid leukemia: accelerated phase. Peripheral blood film showing basophils, myeloblasts, and thrombocytopenia. (Courtesy of Dr. W. Erber.)

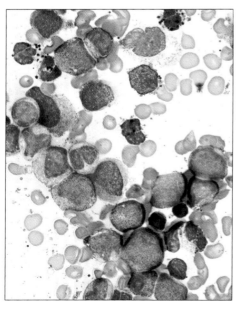

Fig. 13-18. Chronic myeloid leukemia: accelerated phase. Bone marrow aspirate showing basophilia, myeloblasts 10%, and increased promyelocytes. (Courtesy of Dr. W. Erber.)

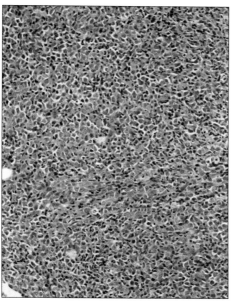

Fig. 13-19. Chronic myeloid leukemia; accelerated phase. Trephine biopsy showing myeloid hyperplasia with increased population of early cells. (Courtesy of Dr. W. Erber.)

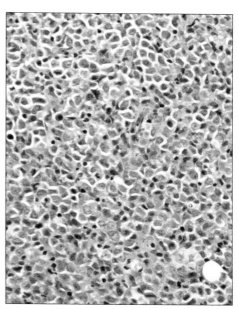

Fig. 13-20. Chronic myeloid leukemia: accelerated phase. Higher power to show myeloid hyperplasia with increased early granulocyte precursors. (Courtesy of Dr. W. Erber.)

Fig. 13-21. Chronic myeloid leukemia: accelerated phase. **A,** Trephine biopsy showing clustering of abnormal small megakaryocytes. **B,** Trephine biopsy showing increase in reticulum fiber density and thickness with some cross-linking of fibers—Thiele scale grade 2 fibrosis (silver stain).

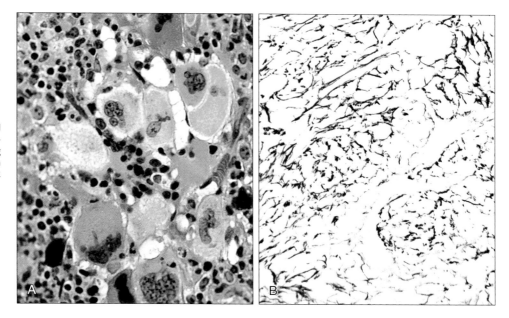

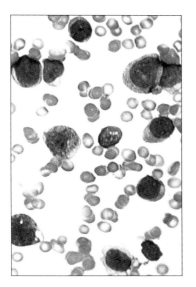

Fig. 13-22. Chronic myeloid leukemia: peripheral blood film showing blast cell transformation. Over half the white cells seen are primitive blast forms. (Hb, 8.5 g/dl; WBC, 110 × 10⁹/L [blasts, 65 × 10⁹/L]; platelets, 45 × 109/L.)

BLAST TRANSFORMATION

Before the introduction of Imatinib, in about 70% of patients there was a terminal metamorphosis to an acute malignant form of leukemia (Figs. 13-22 to 13-25), which is associated with rapid deterioration of the patient and progressive bone marrow failure. Splenic enlargement and infiltration of the skin (Figs. 13-26 and 13-27), CNS, and other non-hematopoietic tissues may occur. The transformation may be myeloblastic, lymphoblastic (see Fig. 13-25), mixed, or (rarely) megakaryoblastic (Figs. 13-28 and 13-29). At least 30% of the marrow cells are blasts.

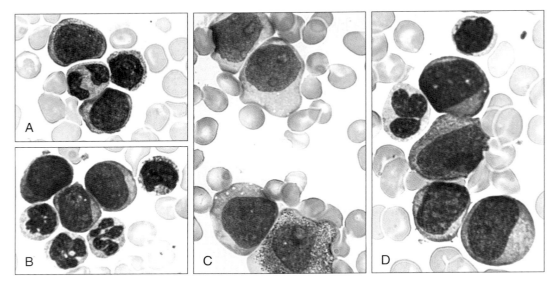

Fig. 13-23. Chronic myeloid leukemia. **A–D,** Peripheral blood films at high magnification showing myeloblastic transformation. Numerous myeloblasts, atypical neutrophils, and abnormal promyelocytes are seen.

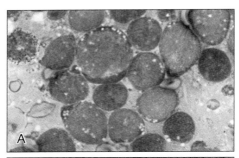

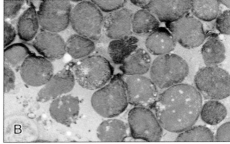

Fig. 13-24. Chronic myeloid leukemia. **A** and **B,** Bone marrow aspirates showing lymphoblastic transformation. There are vacuolated lymphoblasts and residual basophil granulocytes or precursors. (*A,* Courtesy of Dr. K. van Pouche and Professor Z. Berneman.)

Fig. 13-25. Chronic myeloid leukemia (CML): common features in the genome profile of CML samples at lymphoid blast transformation revealed by one Mb bacterial artificial chromosome (BAC) array comparative genomic hybridization (CGH) analysis (SGI2600 chip) as seen in four cases, including **(A)** gain of the 1q31–q44 region, **(B)** loss of about 300 kbp at 6q21, **(C)** loss of the BAC clones at 9p, **(D)** loss of 13q31, and **(E)** gain at 16p12. Colored dots represent the fluorescent ratio (FR) of the BAC clones along a chromosome, and each color represents a different sample. (Courtesy of Dr. E. Necheva.)

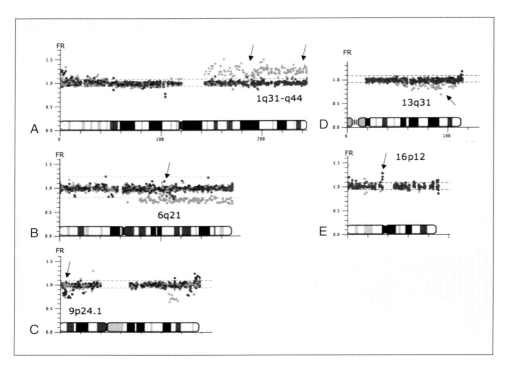

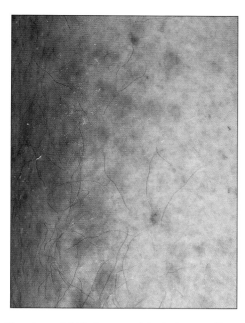

Fig. 13-26. Chronic myeloid leukemia: nodular leukemic infiltrates in the skin over the anterior surface of the tibia in a 48-year-old woman with blast cell transformation.

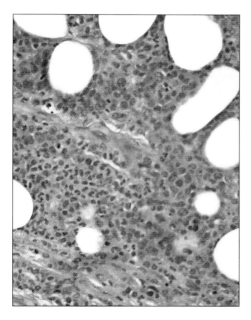

Fig. 13-27. Chronic myeloid leukemia: histologic section of the skin lesion shown in Fig. 13-26, illustrating extensive perivascular infiltration with mononuclear cells and polymorphs in the deeper layers of the dermis.

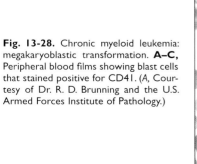

Fig. 13-28. Chronic myeloid leukemia: megakaryoblastic transformation. **A–C,** Peripheral blood films showing blast cells that stained positive for CD41. (A, Courtesy of Dr. R. D. Brunning and the U.S. Armed Forces Institute of Pathology.)

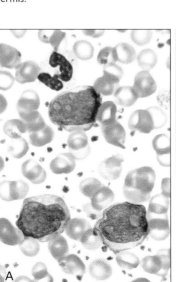
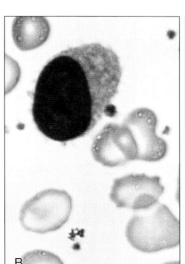
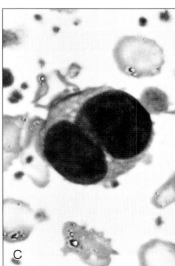

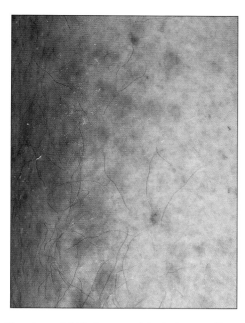

Fig. 13-29. Chronic myeloid leukemia: megakaryoblastic transformation. Bone marrow showing atypical megakaryocytes and megakaryoblasts. (Courtesy of Dr. R. D. Brunning and the U.S. Armed Forces Institute of Pathology.)

TREATMENT

Initial chemotherapy is with imatinib, which blocks the adenosine triphosphate (ATP) binding site of the BCR-ABL kinase (Fig. 13-30). Over 80% of patients respond hematologically with complete remission and become Ph negative, although the presence of the BCR-ABL mRNA can usually be detected by RT-PCR in the peripheral blood. Patients may become resistant to imatinib through a variety of mechanisms, most often because of acquisition of point mutations in the ABL kinase domain. Second-generation drugs dasatinib and nilotinib are now in clinical use.

Hydroxyurea, alpha-interferon, busulfan, and allogeneic stem cell transplantation, which have been the mainstays of treatment in the past, are now used in a minority of patients.

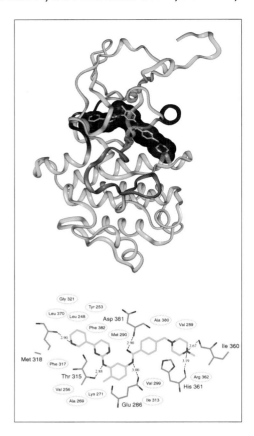

Fig. 13-30. Chronic myeloid leukemia. Crystal structure of the kinase domain of ABL in complex with imatinib. (Courtesy of Dr. J. Kuriyan and Dr. M. Seeliger. From Kuriyan J, Seeliger M: *Cancer Res* 62:4236–4243, 2002.)

PHILADELPHIA-NEGATIVE CHRONIC MYELOID LEUKEMIA

Some patients with typical disease are Ph negative but are found to have the BCR-ABL rearrangement on molecular analysis. Other patients with Ph-negative and BCR-ABL rearrangement–negative disease have a variant or an atypical CML that is usually associated with fewer myelocytes, more monocytoid cells, and atypical neutrophils in the peripheral blood. Severe anemia and thrombocytopenia are more frequent than in classic CML (Fig. 13-31). The prognosis for Ph-negative, BCR-ABL–negative CML is generally worse than that for Ph-positive, BCR-ABL–positive or Ph-negative, BCR-ABL–positive CML.

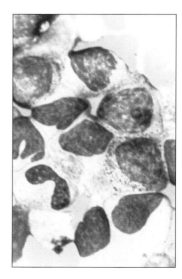

Fig. 13-31. Chronic myeloid leukemia: Ph chromosome negative, BCR-ABL rearrangement negative. Bone marrow aspirate showing myelocytes, metamyelocytes, and "paramyeloid" cells, features of myelodysplasia.

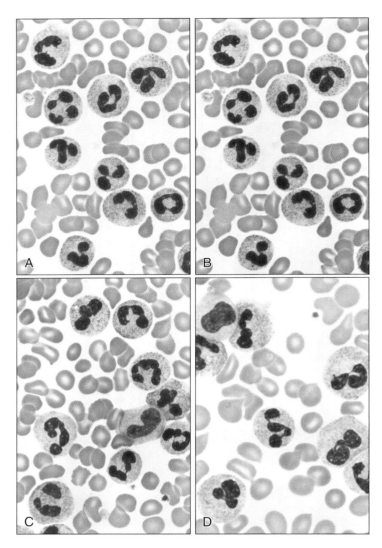

Fig. 13-32. Chronic neutrophilic leukemia: 83-year-old man, slight splenomegaly. Peripheral blood film showed increased neutrophils with less than 5% myelocytes and promyelocytes and occasional blasts. (Hemoglobin, 6.5 g/dl; white cells, 160×10^9/L; platelets, 350×10^9/L. Cytogenetics normal, BCR-ABL and JAK-2 negative.)

CHRONIC NEUTROPHILIC LEUKEMIA

Chronic neutrophilic leukemia (CNL) is a rare myeloproliferative disease characterized by sustained peripheral blood neutrophilia, bone marrow hypercellularity caused by neutrophil proliferation, and hepatosplenomegaly (Fig. 13-32). The Ph chromosome and *BCR-ABL* fusion gene are absent, and cytogenetics are usually normal. In up to 20% of cases, another neoplasm is present, most frequently multiple myeloma.

CHRONIC EOSINOPHILIC LEUKEMIA

Chronic eosinophilic leukemia (CEL) is characterized by a clonal proliferation of eosinophil precursors in the marrow with a persistent peripheral blood eosinophilia often with eosinophil precursors (Fig. 13-33). There is organ damage caused by eosinophil infiltration. There is activation of a protein kinase caused by formation of fusion genes in four distinct recurrent breakpoint clusters that code for the following: (1) platelet-derived growth factor α *(PDGFRA)* at 4q12; (2) platelet-derived growth factor receptor β *(PDGFRB)* at 5q31-33;

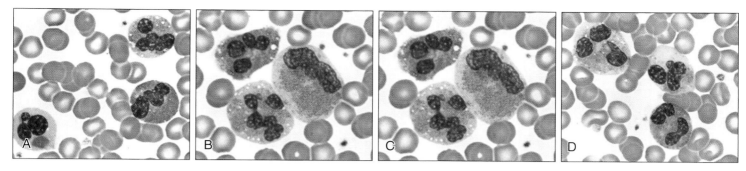

Fig. 13-33. Chronic eosinophilic leukemia: peripheral blood film. FIPILI-PDGFRA positive, BCR-ABL negative, cytogenetics normal. (Hemoglobin, 11.0 g/dl; white cells 45.0 × 10⁹/L; eosinophils, 37.4 × 10⁹/L; eosinophil myelocytes and promyelocytes, 2.7 × 10⁹/L; platelets, 190 × 10⁹/L.) Complete remission was achieved by treatment with imatinib.

(3) fibroblastic growth factor receptor 1 *(FGFR1)* at 8p11; and (4) Janus kinase 2 *(JAK2)* at 9p24. More than 35 different fusion genes have been associated with CEL or an eosinophil myeloproliferative disease. The most common is *FIPILI-PDGFRA,* generated by an 800 kb interstitial deletion on chromosome 4q12 that is not visible cytogenetically.

CEL has a male preponderance. The disease may be associated with marrow fibrosis and terminate as acute myeloid leukemia. The FIPILI-PDGFRA–positive patients respond to imatinib.

Eosinophilia–myeloproliferative disease "8p11" is associated with rearrangement of FGFRI caused by 8p11 translocations. The patients show a myeloproliferative/myelodysplastic disease with usually marked eosinophilia in the blood. There is a high incidence of associated non-Hodgkin's lymphoma or lymphoblastic leukemia. The disease often rapidly transforms into acute myeloid leukemia.

CHRONIC MYELOMONOCYTIC LEUKEMIA

Chronic myelomonocytic leukemia (CMML) is a myeloproliferative/myelodysplastic syndrome characterized by a persistent monocytosis of >1.0 × 10⁹/L in the peripheral blood, the absence of the *BCR-ABL* fusion gene, <20% blasts in the marrow, and dysplasia in one or more myeloid lineage. The proportion of monocytes is nearly always >10% of the white blood cells (Fig. 13-34). The blood monocytes may appear normal or show abnormal granulation, unusual nuclear lobe formation, or finely dispersed chromatin (Figs. 13-35 and 13-36). Dysgranulopoiesis is usually present. There may be anemia and thrombocytopenia, both mild at presentation. The bone marrow is usually hypercellular with granulocytic hyperplasia with increased monocytes, dyserythropoiesis often with ringed sideroblasts, and micromegakaryocytes. CMML has

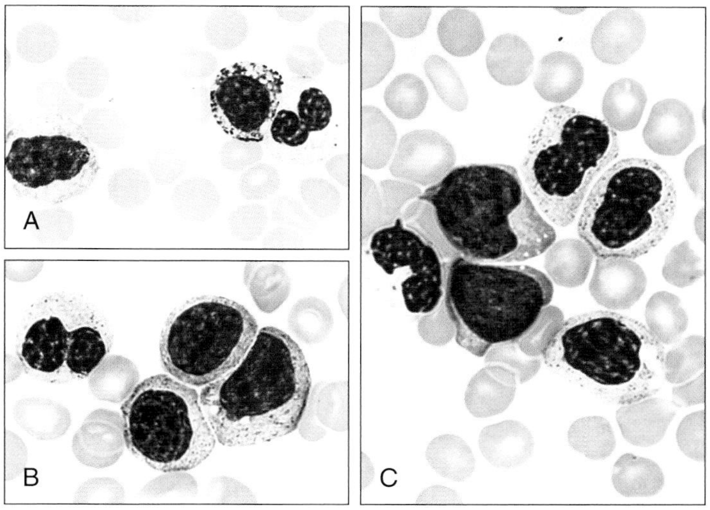

Fig. 13-35. Chronic myelomonocytic leukemia (CMML): myelodysplastic syndrome. **A** and **B,** Peripheral blood films showing white cells in CMML. Most cells are more monocytoid than those in Fig. 13-36, and the neutrophil shown is agranular.

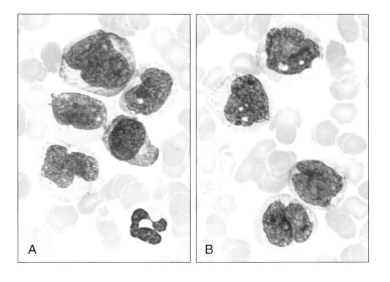

Fig. 13-34. Chronic myelomonocytic leukemia (CMML). **A–C,** Peripheral blood films showing white cells in CMML. Many atypical myelomonocytic cells and pseudo-Pelger neutrophils, some agranular, are shown.

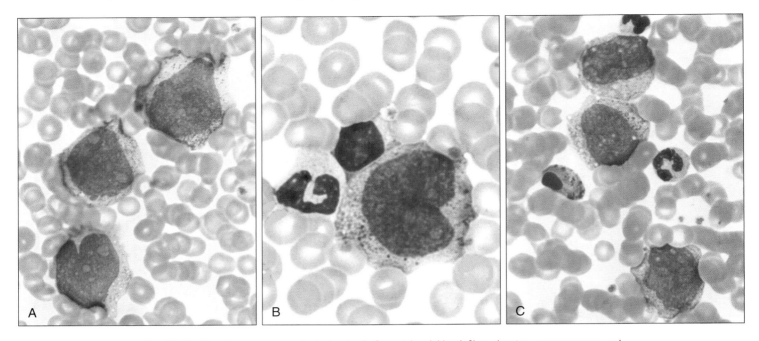

Fig. 13-36. Chronic myelomonocytic leukemia: **A-C,** peripheral blood films showing promonocytyes and a monoblast.

been divided into two groups: *1* is with <5% blasts in the blood and <10% in the marrow and *2* is with 5% to 19% blasts in the blood and 10% to 19% in the marrow. Cytogenetic changes are frequent but not specific and include +8, −7/del (7q), and abnormalities of 12.

JUVENILE MYELOMONOCYTIC LEUKEMIA

This disease of children is characterized by overproduction of myeloid cells that infiltrate the bone marrow and systemic tissues. There is often marked lymphadenopathy and eczematoid rash (Fig. 13-37). The blood film shows myelomonocytoid cells usually with anemia and thrombocytopenia (Figs. 13-38 and 13-39). Up to 30% of patients progress to AML. A characteristic in vitro feature of the disease

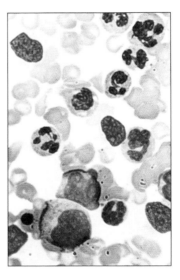

Fig. 13-38. Juvenile chronic myeloid leukemia: peripheral blood film from the infant in Fig. 13-37 shows a predominance of myelomonocytoid cells.

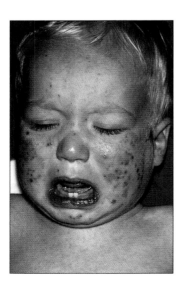

Fig. 13-37. Juvenile chronic myeloid leukemia: eczematoid facial rash and lip bleeding in an 8-month-old infant. There was moderate splenomegaly. Cytogenetic studies failed to demonstrate the presence of the Ph chromosome. (Hb, 10.5 g/dl; WBC, 120 × 10⁹/L; platelets, 85 × 10⁹/L.) (Courtesy of Professor J. M. Chessells.)

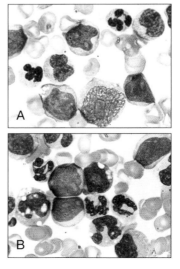

Fig. 13-39. Juvenile chronic myeloid leukemia. **A** and **B,** Peripheral blood films showing occasional blast forms, myelomonocytic cells, and atypical agranular band and segmented neutrophils.

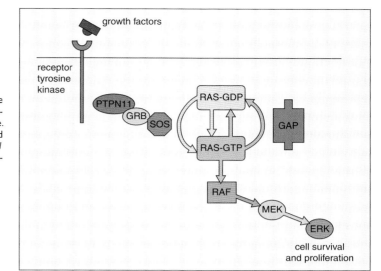

Fig. 13-40. Noonan syndrome. The *PTPN11* gene encodes a protein, tyrosine phosphatase, involved in the RAS-MAPK pathway for cell signaling. *PTPN11* accounts for approximately 50% of the gene mutations found in Noonan syndrome. Since its discovery, mutations in other genes in the pathway have been implicated in Noonan syndrome (e.g., *SOS1, KRAS,* and *RAF1*). Somatic mutations in *PTPN11* are also found in juvenile myelomonocytic leukemia (JMML). (Courtesy of Professor M. A. Patton.)

is that the cells are exquisitely sensitive to the growth factor granulocyte-macrophage colony-stimulating factor (GM-CSF) and form abnormal numbers of colonies in culture. Children with two genetic disorders, Noonan syndrome (NS) and neurofibromatosis 1 (NF1), are at increased risk of developing JMML, as well as, more rarely, monocytosis or transient myelomonocytic disorders. Mutations in the bone marrow in the genes NF1 or PTPNII are present in cases of JMML not associated with NS or NF1. The protein products of both genes are involved in the RAS signaling pathway (Fig. 13-40). RAS activation to the guanosine triphosphate (GTP) state is necessary for its intracellular signaling in pathways from external stimuli such as growth factors, including GM-CSF (see Fig. 13-40).

In addition to mutations of PTPNII and NF1, mutations of NRAS and KRAS2 have been found in about 25% of cases of JMML. These mutations introduce amino acid substitutions that result in proteins that remain in the GTP-bound active conformation because of resistance to GTPase-activating protein, as well as lack of intrinsic GTPase activity.

NOONAN SYNDROME

This dominant developmental disorder is a characterized by short stature; facial abnormalities, including hypertelorism, low-set ears, and ptosis (Figs. 13-41 and 13-42); cardiac defects;

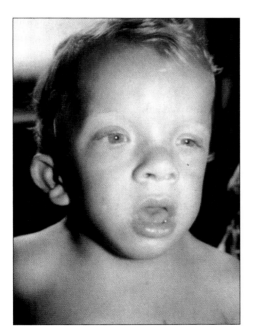

Fig. 13-41. Noonan syndrome. Young child showing facial features of Noonan syndrome, including hypertelorism, ptosis, and low-set ears. (Courtesy of Professor M. A. Patton.)

Fig. 13-42. Noonan syndrome. Older child showing neck webbing and pectus excavatum. (Courtesy of Professor M. A. Patton.)

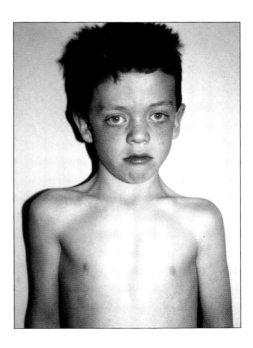

skeletal abnormalities; mental retardation; genitourinary defects; and factor XI deficiency. About half of these patients have germline missense mutations of the gene PTPNII, encoding the tyrosine phosphatase SHP-2 (see Fig. 13-40) involved in the RAS signaling pathway. Mutations in SOS1, KRAS, and RAF1 have also been described in NS. Approximately one third of patients with NS develop JMML.

NEUROFIBROMATOSIS I

Individuals with NF1 are at increased risk of benign and malignant diseases that arise in the embryonic neural crest. Children (but not adults) with NF1 are also predisposed to JMML and, less frequently, other myeloid malignancies. The NF1 gene codes for neurofibromin, which acts as a GTPase-activating protein. This appears to act as a tumor suppressor gene for JMML.

REFRACTORY ANEMIA WITH RINGED SIDEROBLASTS ASSOCIATED WITH MARKED THROMBOCYTOSIS (RARS-T)

This disorder usually shows 15% or more ringed sideroblasts in the marrow, erythroid and megakaryocytic dysplasia, and platelet counts greater than $1000 \times 10^9/L$ (Fig. 13-43). The JAK-2-V617F mutation is present in about half the patients and cells homozygous for the mutation may be present. MPL-W515 mutations are present in a minority of the JAK-2-V617F negative patients.

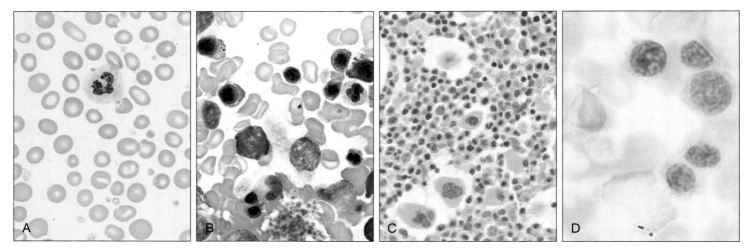

Fig. 13-43. Refractory anemia with ring sideroblasts (RARS) associated with marked thrombocytosis. **A,** Peripheral blood film shows marked red cell anisocytosis with increased platelets. **B,** Bone marrow aspirate shows dyserythropoesis with bi- and tri-nucleated erythroblasts. **C,** Trephine biopsy shows increased megakaryocytes with mononuclear forms. **D,** Perls' stain shows ring sideroblasts. (Courtesy of Dr. W. Erber.)

MYELODYSPLASTIC SYNDROMES

The myelodysplastic syndromes are a group of clonal hematopoetic stem cell diseases with cytopenia(s) and dysplastic features in one or more myeloid lineage. There is ineffective hematopoiesis. The proportion of blasts in the marrow may be normal or increased but below 20%; otherwise the disease is classified as acute myeloid leukemia. Myelodysplasia usually occurs in elderly subjects who have an anemia, persistent neutropenia and thrombocytopenia, or various combinations of these. Typically, the anemia is macrocytic and there is no enlargement of the liver, spleen, and lymph nodes.

The myelodysplastic syndromes are classified by the World Health Organization (WHO) into seven subgroups (Table 14-1). The hematologic findings combined with cytogenetic findings can be used to obtain a prognostic score (Table 14-2). The higher the score, the worse the prognosis.

Cytogenetic abnormalities are common, occurring in about 50% of primary and 90% of secondary myelodysplastic syndromes (Fig. 14-1). They are more common in refractory anemia with excess blasts (RAEB) than in refractory anemia (RA), neutropenia (RN) or thrombocytopenia (RT), or RA with ring sideroblasts (RARS). Abnormalities include the following:

- Chromosome deletion or loss (e.g., del 5q/monosomy 5 [see Fig. 14-8], del 7q/monosomy 7, del 11q, del 12p, del 13q, del 17p, del 20q, monosomy 7 [see Fig. 14-23], loss of Y)
- Chromosome gain (e.g., trisomy 8, trisomy 11)

TABLE 14-1.   MYELODYSPLASTIC SYNDROMES: FAB AND WORLD HEALTH ORGANIZATION (WHO 2008) CLASSIFICATION

Disease	Blood findings	Bone marrow findings
Refractory cytopenias with unilineage dysplasia (RCUD) Refractory anemia (RA); Refractory neutropenia (RN); Refractory thrombocytopenia (RT)	Unicytopenia or bicytopenia[1] No or rare blasts	Unilineage dysplasia ≥ 10% of the cells in one myeloid linease < 5% blasts < 15% of erythroid precursos are ringed sideroblasts
Refractory anemia with ringed sideroblasts (RARS)	Anemia No blasts	Erythroid dysplasia *only* ≥ 15% of erythroid precursos are ringed sideroblasts < 5% blasts
Refractory cytopenia with multilineage dysplasia (RCMD)	Cytopenias (bicytopenia or pancytopenia) No or rare blasts No Auer rods < 1 × 10⁹/L monocytes	Dysplasia in ≥ 10% of cells in ≥ 2 myeloid lineages (neutrophil and/or erythroid precursos and/or megakaryocytes) < 5% blasts in marrow No Auer rods ± 15% ringed sideroblasts
Refractory anemia with excess blasts-1 (RAEB-1)	Cytopenias < 5% blasts[2] No Auer rods < 1 × 10⁹/L monocytes	Unilineage or multilineage dysplasia 5% to 9% blasts No Auer rods
Refractory anaemia with excess blasts-2 (RAEB-2)	Cytopenia(s) 5% to 19% blasts Auer rods ±[3] < 1 × 10⁹/L monocytes	Unilineage or multilineage dysplasia 10% to 19% blasts Auer rods ±[3]
MDS associated with isolated del(5q)	Anemia Usually normal or increased platelet count No or rare blasts (< 1%)	Normal to increased megakaryocytes with hypolobated nuclei < 5% blasts No Auer rods Isolated del(5q) cytogenetic abnormality
Myelodysplastic syndrome, unclassified (MDS-U)	Cytopenias ≤ 1% blasts[2]	Unequivocal dysplasia in < 10% of cells in one more myeloid cell lines when accompanies by a cytogenetic abnormality considered as presumptive evidence for a diagnosis of MDS < 5% blasts No Auer rods

RARS is also known as primary acquired sideroblastic anemia (see page 85).
[1]Bicytopenia may occasionally be observed. Cases with pancytopenia should be classified as MDS-U.
[2]If the marrow myeloblast percentage is <5% but there are 2-4% myeloblasts in the blood, the diagnostic classification is RAEB 1. Cases of RCUD and RCMD with 1% myeloblasts in the blood should be classified as MDS, U.
[3]Cases with Auer rods <5% myeloblasts in the blood and <10% in the marrow should be classified as RAEB 2.

TABLE 14-2. MYELODYSPLASTIC SYNDROMES: PROGNOSTIC SCORES BASED ON WORLD HEALTH ORGANIZATION (WHO 2002) CLASSIFICATION

	+0	+1	+2	+3
WHO category	RA, RARS, del 5q	RCMD, RCMDS	RAEB-1	RAEB-2
Karyotype*	Good	Intermediate	Poor	–
Transfusion requirement (1 or more unit every 8 weeks)	Nil	Regular	–	–

*Good = normal karyotype or isolated – Y, del 5q, del 20q;
Intermediate = other abnormality;
Poor = complex karyotype ≥ 3 abnormalities or chromosome 7 abnormalities

RA, Refractory anemia; *RAEB*, RA with excess blasts; *RARS*, RA with ring sideroblasts; *RCMDS*, refractory cytopenia with multilineage dysplasia and ring sideroblasts. RAEB-1 = 5%–9% marrow blasts; RAEB-2 = 10%–19% marrow blasts.

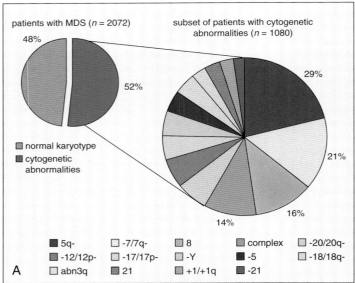

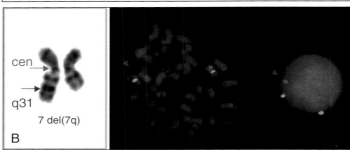

Fig. 14-1. Myelodysplastic syndromes. **A,** Frequency of cytogenetic abnormalities. **B,** Deletion or loss of the long arm of chromosome 7 by FISH. G-banded partial karyotype with *arrows* pointing to the location of the FISH probes. Metaphase and nondividing cells display typical loss of the signal from the long arm of chromosome 7. (*A,* Adapted with permission from Giagounidis A: *Haematological Reports* 2(14):5–10, 2006. *B,* Courtesy of Dr. E. Nacheva.)

- Chromosome rearrangement (e.g., t3q26, t[1;7], t11q23)
- Complex (three or more abnormalities) karyotypes; these and chromosome abnormalities give a poor prognosis.

Clinically, these patients have symptoms related to bone marrow failure with frequent infective episodes (Figs. 14-2 and 14-3) and bleeding abnormalities (Fig. 14-4). As a consequence of these complications, many patients die of severe neutropenia or thrombocytopenia,

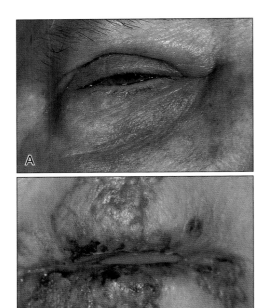

Fig. 14-2. Myelodysplastic syndrome. **A,** Skin infection spreading from the eyelids. **B,** Extensive herpes simplex eruptions spreading from the lip margins to adjacent skin. Both patients had refractory anemia with excess blasts (RAEB).

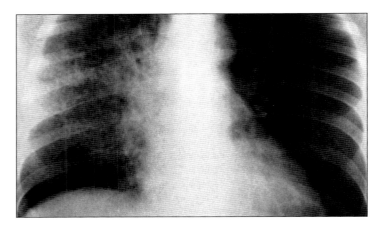

Fig. 14-3. Myelodysplastic syndrome: chest radiograph (portable film) of a 62-year-old man with Legionnaires' disease. There is widespread patchy consolidation throughout the right lung.

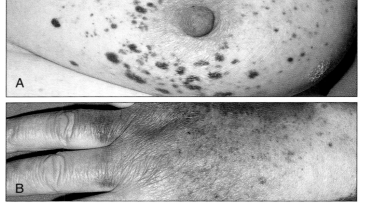

Fig. 14-4. Myelodysplastic syndrome. **A,** Extensive purpura of the skin of the breast in a 35-year-old woman with refractory anemia (RA). **B,** Extensive ecchymoses and purpura of the skin over the back of the hand (same patient). (Hb, 8 g/dl; white blood cell count [WBC], 4 × 10⁹/L; platelets, 20 × 10⁹/L.)

but in others the disease progresses to frank acute myeloid leukemia (AML). In the past, these syndromes, particularly those with normal numbers of blasts (<5%) in the marrow, have been referred to as *preleukemia.*

The blood film abnormalities in each subgroup are highly variable. General features include macrocytic red cells, qualitative

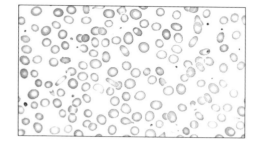

Fig. 14-5. Myelodysplastic syndrome: peripheral blood film in refractory anemia (RA) shows marked anisocytosis and poikilocytosis. (Hb, 7.9 g/dl; white blood cell count [WBC], 5.4 × 10⁹/L [neutrophils, 1.8 × 10⁹/L]; platelets, 120 × 10⁹/L.)

granulocytic and monocytic changes (see following text), and giant platelets. In patients with RA, RN, or RT gross morphologic changes may not occur (Fig. 14-5). In RARS, a dimorphic red cell population frequently occurs (Fig. 14-6). Agranular neutrophils, pseudo-Pelger cells, and cells difficult to diagnose as monocytic or granulocytic are seen in peripheral blood (Fig. 14-7). Patients with RAEB often show leucoerythroblastic changes. Thrombocytosis occurs typically in the 5q- (an interstitial deletion, usually 5q11 or 5q13 to 5q33) syndrome variant of RA (Fig. 14-8). The deleted gene is RPS14 encoding a ribosomal protein. In this syndrome, bone marrow megakaryocytes have a characteristic hypolobulated appearance (Fig. 14-9).

The bone marrow in the myelodysplastic syndromes is typically hypercellular and shows morphologic abnormalities, often in all three series of hematopoietic cells. There is usually evidence of dyserythropoiesis, with nuclear atypia (budding, bridging, karyorrhexis, multinuclearity, hyperlobation), some megaloblastosis, and ring sideroblasts (Figs. 14-10 to 14-15). In about 20% of cases in all seven subgroups, an increase in reticulin occurs (Fig. 14-16), and in occasional cases, the marrow is hypocellular.

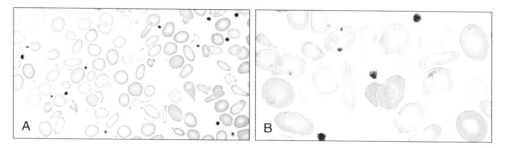

Fig. 14-6. Myelodysplastic syndrome: peripheral blood films in refractory anemia with ring sideroblasts (RARS) showing marked red cell anisocytosis and poikilocytosis (**A**). Although the majority of cells are markedly hypochromic, there is a second population of normochromic cells. At higher magnification a red cell shows two small basophilic inclusions (Pappenheimer bodies) (**B**). Perls' staining demonstrated that similar inclusions were Prussian blue positive (siderotic granules). These granules were far more numerous after splenectomy.

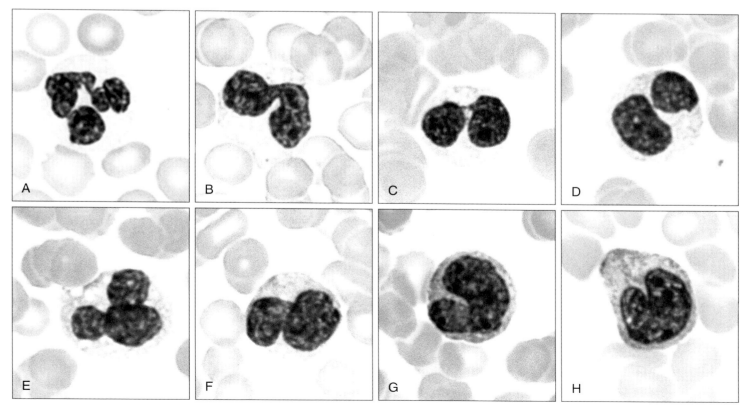

Fig. 14-7. Myelodysplastic syndrome: refractory cytopenia with multilineage dysplasia peripheral blood films showing white cells. Agranular neutrophils, atypical myelomonocytic cells, and pseudo-Pelger neutrophils, some also agranular, are shown.

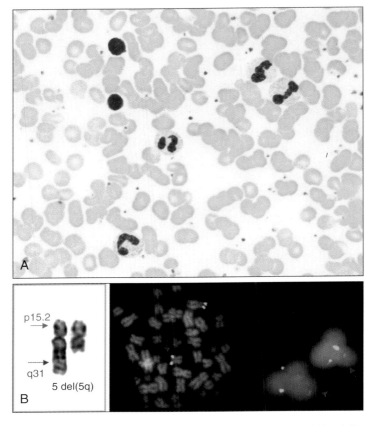

Fig. 14-8. Myelodysplastic syndrome. **A,** 5q- syndrome: peripheral blood film from a 75-year-old woman showing macrocytes, hyposegmented neutrophils, and thrombocytosis. **B,** 5q- syndrome: FISH analysis showing loss of long (q) arm of chromosome 5. G-banded partial karyotype with arrows pointing to the location of the FISH probes. (Courtesy of Dr. E. Nacheva.)

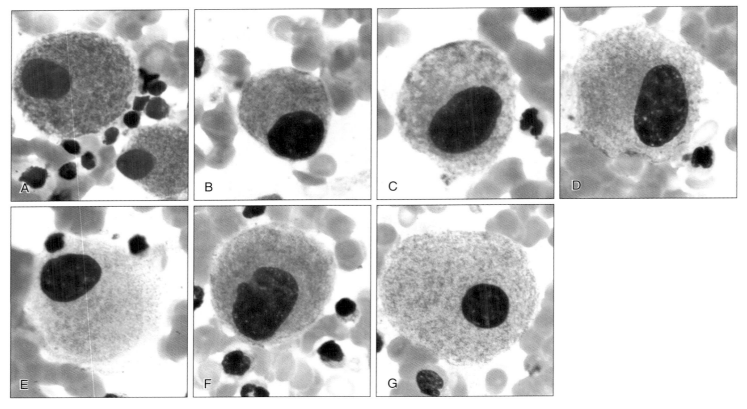

Fig. 14-9. Myelodysplastic syndrome: 5q-syndrome. Bone marrow aspirates show abnormal hypolobulated megakaryocytes.

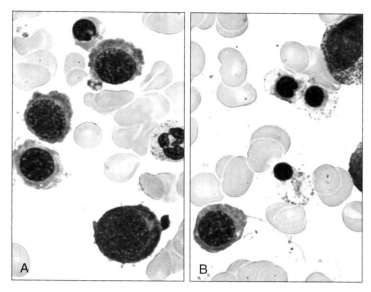

Fig. 14-10. Myelodysplastic syndrome. **A** and **B,** Bone marrow cell trails in refractory anemia with ring sideroblasts (RARS) showing marked defective hemoglobinization and vacuolation in later-stage polychromatic and pyknotic erythroblasts.

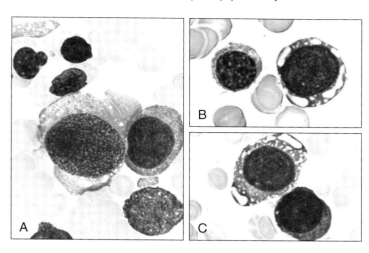

Fig. 14-13. Myelodysplastic syndrome: bone marrow aspirates in refractory anemia with excess blasts (RAEB)—I showing abnormal proerythroblasts and megaloblast-like changes **(A)** and prominent cytoplasmic vacuolation in the basophilic erythroblasts **(B** and **C),** evidence of dyserythropoiesis.

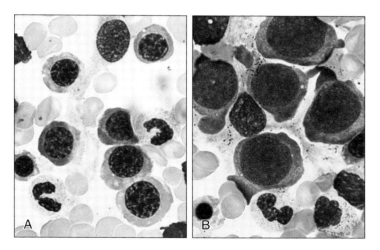

Fig. 14-11. Myelodysplastic syndrome: bone marrow cell trails in refractory anemia with ring sideroblasts (RARS) showing erythroblasts with vacuolation of cytoplasm in later cells and mild megaloblastic features **(A)** and a prominent group of proerythroblasts **(B).**

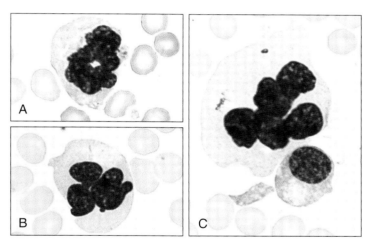

Fig. 14-14. Myelodysplastic syndrome. **A–C,** Bone marrow aspirates in refractory anemia with excess blasts (RAEB)—I showing three examples of polyploid multinucleate polychromatic erythroblasts, further evidence of gross dyserythropoiesis.

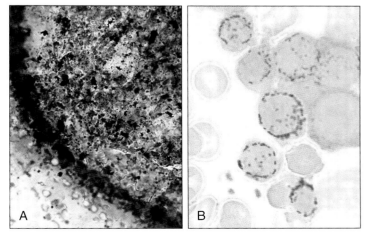

Fig. 14-12. Myelodysplastic syndrome: bone marrow fragment in refractory anemia with ring sideroblasts (RARS) showing increased iron stores **(A)** and pathologic ring sideroblasts at higher magnification **(B).** (Perls' stain.)

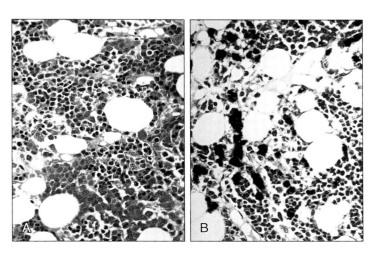

Fig. 14-15. Myelodysplastic syndrome: trephine biopsies in refractory anemia with excess blasts (RAEB)—I showing clusters of blast forms and prominent hemosiderin-laden macrophages **(A).** Gross increase in reticuloendothelial iron stores is confirmed by Perls' staining **(B).**

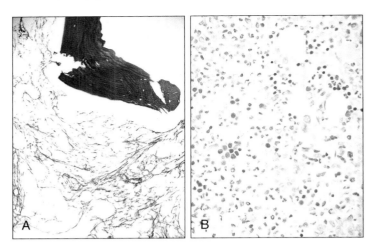

Fig. 14-16. Myelodysplastic syndrome: refractory cytopenia with multilineage displasia. Trephine biopsy showing increased reticulin fiber density **(A)**. (Silver impregnation stain.) **B,** Foci of immature myeloid cells in intertrabecular area (ALIP).

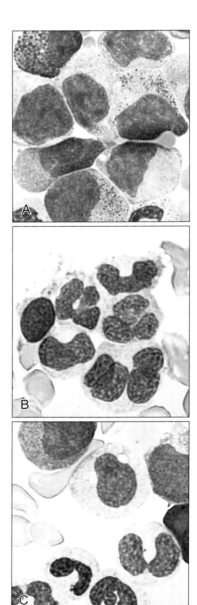

Fig. 14-17. Myelodysplastic syndrome: bone marrow aspirates in refractory anemia with excess blasts (RAEB)–1 showing disturbed granulopoiesis with agranular promyelocytes **(A)** and agranular neutrophils and abnormal myelomonocytic cells **(B and C)**; some cells ("paramyeloid" cells) are difficult to classify as monocytic or granulocytic.

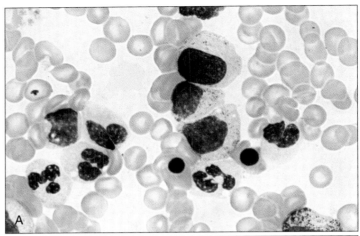

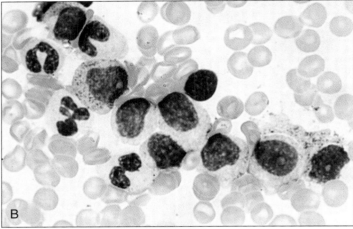

Fig. 14-18. Myelodysplastic syndrome. **A** and **B,** Bone marrow aspirate in refractory cytopenia with multilineage dysplasia showing abnormal agranular neutrophils, myelocytes, promyelocytes, and abnormal myelomonocytic cells.

Granulocytic abnormalities include hypogranular or agranular myelocytes, metamyelocytes and neutrophils, pseudo-Pelger cells (Figs. 14-17 and 14-18), pseudo-Chediak Higashi granules, and hypersegmented or polyploid neutrophils and Auer rods. Megakaryocytic abnormalities include small mononuclear or binucleate forms (see Figs. 14-9 and 14-19) or large megakaryocytes with multiple round nuclei and large granules in the cytoplasm.

In the more advanced myelodysplastic syndromes, there is also an increase in the blast cell population, but by definition, these cells remain <20% of the marrow cell total. When the level of blast cells exceeds this figure, evolution to AML has occurred (Fig. 14-20). Abnormal localization of immature precursors (ALIP) in the bone marrow in patients without excess blasts has been found to be an independent prognostic factor (see Figs. 14-16 and 14-21).

Copper deficiency has been reported in a few cases to mimic myelodysplasia in the blood and bone marrow (Fig. 14-22). In patients with comorbidities likely to result in nutritional deficiency (e.g., intestinal malabsorption), copper deficiency should be excluded.

The management of myelodysplastic syndromes is unsatisfactory. In the elderly, treatment is often with supportive therapy alone or with mild chemotherapy (e.g., low-dose subcutaneous cytosine arabinoside). Lenalidomide (Revlimid), a thalidomide derivate, is helpful in some cases, particularly those with the 5q- syndrome. Azacitidine and decitabine are demethylating agents with favorable responses in a minority of cases of RAEB. Erythropoietin is used either alone or in combination with granulocyte colony-stimulating factor (G-CSF) for patients with RA requiring transfusion. Chemotherapy, as for AML, is given in younger patients with RAEB, with or without stem cell transplantation, and this approach offers a possible cure.

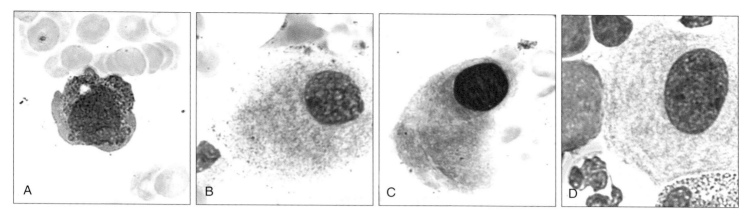

Fig. 14-19. Myelodysplastic syndrome. **A–D,** Bone marrow aspirates showing an atypical megakaryoblast and three atypical mononuclear megakaryocytes, all of which show evidence of cytoplasmic maturation and granulation.

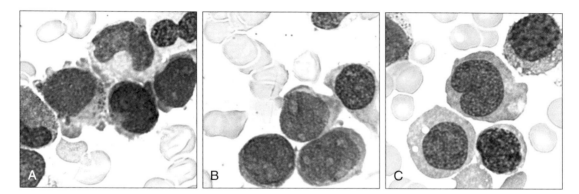

Fig. 14-20. Myelodysplastic syndrome transformed to acute myeloid leukemia. **A–C,** Bone marrow aspirates in refractory anemia with excess blasts (RAEB), which has progressed to acute myeloid leukemia after a period of observation, showing increased numbers of blast cells, some of which have atypical features. The blast cells make up 23% of the marrow cell total. Agranular neutrophils and myelomonocytic cells are also evident.

Fig. 14-21. Myelodysplastic syndrome. **A** and **B,** Trephine biopsy. Both views show abnormal intertrabecular localization of nests of immature myeloid cells (ALIPs).

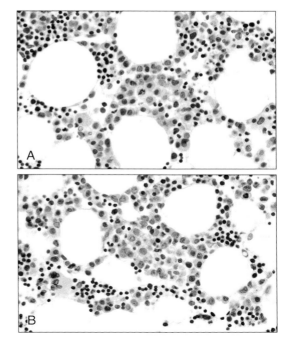

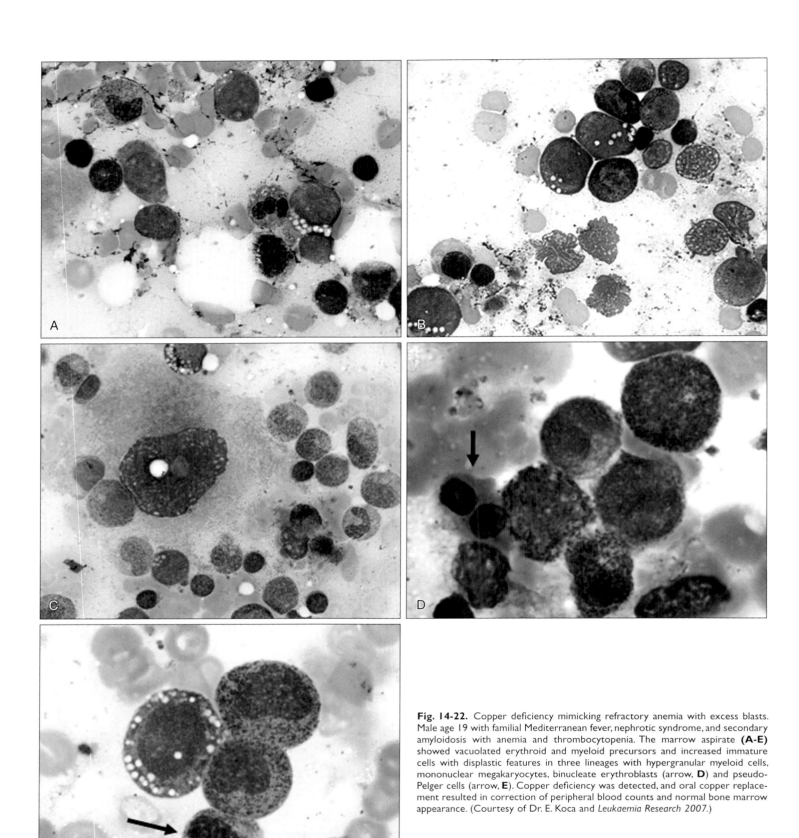

Fig. 14-22. Copper deficiency mimicking refractory anemia with excess blasts. Male age 19 with familial Mediterranean fever, nephrotic syndrome, and secondary amyloidosis with anemia and thrombocytopenia. The marrow aspirate **(A-E)** showed vacuolated erythroid and myeloid precursors and increased immature cells with displastic features in three lineages with hypergranular myeloid cells, mononuclear megakaryocytes, binucleate erythroblasts (arrow, **D**) and pseudo-Pelger cells (arrow, **E**). Copper deficiency was detected, and oral copper replacement resulted in correction of peripheral blood counts and normal bone marrow appearance. (Courtesy of Dr. E. Koca and *Leukaemia Research 2007.*)

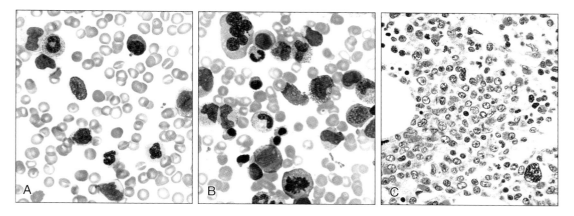

Fig. 14-23. Myelodysplastic syndrome, monosomy 7 of childhood. **A,** Peripheral blood film showing mature monocytes, neutrophils, occasional immature cells, and a plasma cell. **B,** Bone marrow aspirate showing increased numbers of monocytes and promonocytes and a large multinucleated polychromatic erythroblast. **C,** Trephine biopsy showing increased cellularity, centrally placed immature myeloid cells (ALIP), and reduced megakaryocytes. (*A* and *B,* Courtesy of Dr. R. D. Brunning and the U.S. Armed Forces Institute of Pathology.)

MONOSOMY 7 SYNDROME OF CHILDHOOD

Monosomy 7 syndrome of childhood is a form of myelodysplasia that occurs in children, usually boys, between ages 6 months and 8 years. Hepatosplenomegaly is normally marked. There is usually monocytosis and anemia, as well as dysplastic changes in the marrow (Fig. 14-23). Transformation to AML is frequent.

MYELOPROLIFERATIVE DISORDERS

Polycythemia vera or poycythemia rubra vera, essential thrombocythemia, and myelofibrosis make up the nonleukemic myeloproliferative disorders. A clonal proliferation is responsible for the overlapping expansion of erythropoietic, granulopoietic, and megakaryocytic components in the marrow and, in advanced disease, of the liver and spleen. In the World Health Organization (WHO) classification, these conditions are listed with chronic myeloid leukemias (discussed in Chapter 13) and proliferative disorders of mast cells.

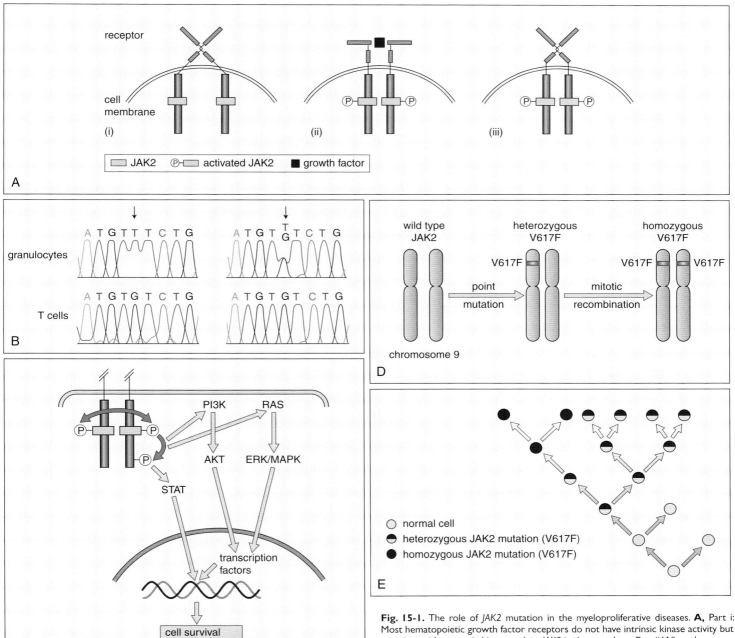

Fig. 15-1. The role of *JAK2* mutation in the myeloproliferative diseases. **A,** Part i: Most hematopoietic growth factor receptors do not have intrinsic kinase activity but associate with a protein kinase such as *JAK2* in the cytoplasm. Part ii: When the receptor binds a growth factor the cytoplasmic domains move closer together and the *JAK2* molecules can activate each other by phosphorylation. Part iii: The *V617F JAK2* mutation allows the *JAK* protein to become activated even when no growth factor is bound. **B,** DNA sequencing shows homozygous G to T mutation in *JAK2* in granulocytes but not in T lymphocytes *(left)* and heterozygous mutation *(right)*. **C,** *JAK2* activation leads to cell survival and proliferation through activation of three major pathways: the *STAT* transcription factors, the *PI3K* pathway acting through *Akt*, and *Ras* activation, which subsequently activate *ERK* and *MAPK*. **D,** The development of homozygosity for the *V617F* mutation is a two-step process, with the initial point mutation followed by mitotic recombination of chromosome 9p between the *JAK2* locus and the centromere. (This results in loss of heterozygosity but a diploid DNA copy.) **E,** A model for the development of myeloproliferative disease following *JAK2 (V617F)*. This leads to a survival advantage of the neoplastic cells. (*B,* After Kralovic R et al: *N Eng J Med* 352:1779–1790, 2005.)

TABLE 15-1.   MOLECULAR LESIONS ASSOCIATED WITH MYELOPROLIFERATIVE DISORDERS

Abnormality	Association
Recurrent genetic lesions	
BCR-ABL	Chronic myeloid leukemia (100%)
JAK2 V617F	Polycythemia vera (95%), essential thrombocythemia (50%–60%), idiopathic myelofibrosis (50%–60%), and other myeloid disorders (1%–5%)
JAK2 exon12	Polycythemia vera or idiopathic erythrocytosis
MPL W515K/L	Idiopathic myelofibrosis (5%) and essential thrombocythemia (1%)
KIT mutations	Systemic mastocytosis
F1P1L1–PDGFRA	Chronic eosinophilic leukemia
PDGFRB fusion genes	Chronic myelomonocytic leukemia (rare)
FGFR fusion genes	Chronic myelomonocytic leukemia (rare)
Other cytogenetic lesions	
Trisomy 9	Amplifies JAK2 gene and associated with JAK2 V617F mutation
Trisomy 8	Found in myeloproliferative disorders, myelodysplasia, and acute myeloid leukemias: target genes not identified
Trisomy 1q	Caused by duplication, trisomy, or unbalanced translocations
20q deletion	Found in myeloproliferative disorders and myelodysplasia; associated with JAK2 V617F mutation and precedes it in some cases; target genes not identified
5q and 7q deletions	Thought to reflect changes secondary to cytotoxic therapy; target genes not identified
13q deletion	Associated with idiopathic myelofibrosis; overlap of commonly deleted region and the region for chronic lymphocytic leukemia
Dysregulated genes and proteins	
BCR-XL	Overexpressed in polycythemia vera as a result of constitutive JAK–STAT signaling; antiapoptopic effects in erythroid cells
NFE2	Upregulated in JAK2-positive myeloproliferative diseases; may affect erythroid differentiation
PRV1	RNA levels increased in polycythemia vera but unlikely to play a direct role in disease pathogenesis because protein levels are not increased
MPL	Surface levels of proteins decreased and aberrantly glycosylated in myeloproliferative disorders; role in disease pathogenesis unclear

After Campbell PJ, Green AR: *N Eng J Med* 355:2452–2466, 2006.

A single acquired point mutation of the cytoplasmic Janus-associated tyrosine kinase *JAK2 (V617F)* occurs (heterozygous or homozygous) in the marrow and blood of almost all patients with polycythemia vera and approximately half of those with essential thrombocythemia and myelofibrosis (Fig. 15-1). The mutation occurs in a highly conserved region of the pseudokinase domain that is believed to negatively regulate *JAK2* signaling. *JAK2* is involved in transducing signals from cytokines and growth factors, including erythropoietin, granulocyte-macrophage colony-stimulating factor, and thrombopoietin. The mutation is responsible for uncontrolled myeloproliferation associated with these disorders. In polycythemia vera the presence of homozygosity increases with time. Other genetic lesions associated with myeloproliferative disorders are listed in Table 15-1. Recent studies have suggested that aberrant microRNA may contribute to the molecular pathogenesis of polycythemia vera.

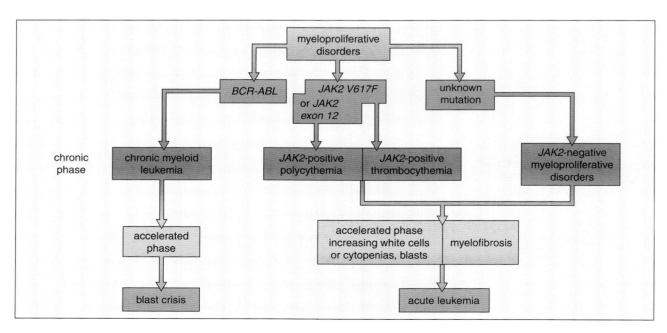

Fig. 15-2. Molecular pathogenesis of the myeloproliferative disorders.

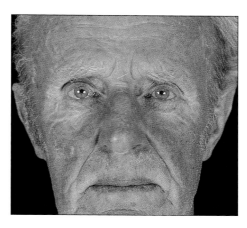

Fig. 15-3. Polycythemia vera: facial plethora in a 65-year-old man. (Hb, 22 g/dl; WBC, 17 × 10⁹/L; platelets, 550 × 10⁹/L; total RCV, 65 ml/kg.)

Many patients with polycythemia vera and essential thrombocythemia have features of both, and as with Ph-positive chronic myeloid leukemia, there is a natural evolution or acceleration of the proliferation, which may be associated with further genetic lesions. In polycythemia vera and essential thrombocythemia, an increase in fibrosis results in findings indistinguishable from idiopathic myelofibrosis (Fig. 15-2). The accelerated phase may be associated not only with myelofibrosis, but also with either increasing white cell counts or neutropenia or thrombocytopenia. The transformation to acute leukemia in a minority of patients probably reflects the acquisition of further mutations.

POLYCYTHEMIA VERA

Polycythemia vera is predominantly a disease of the middle-aged and elderly. Clinical problems are related to the increase in blood volume and viscosity and to the hypermetabolism associated with the myeloproliferation. The clinical features include plethora (Figs. 15-3 and 15-4), headaches, lethargy, dyspnea, fluid retention, bleeding symptoms, weight loss, night sweats, and general pruritus made worse by hot baths, acne rosacea (Fig. 15-5), and other forms of dermatitis. There is often suffusion of the conjunctiva (Fig. 15-6) and marked engorgement of retinal vessels (Figs. 15-7 and 15-8).

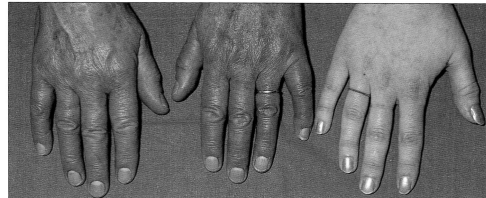

Fig. 15-4. Polycythemia vera: the hands of a 50-year-old woman (on the *left*) appear congested and plethoric. (Hb, 20 g/dl; WBC, 15 × 10⁹/L; platelets, 490 × 10⁹/L.) The hand on the *right* is of a healthy 35-year-old woman. (Hb, 14.5 g/dl.)

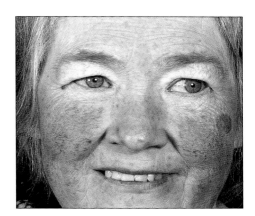

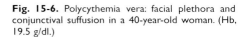

Fig. 15-5. Polycythemia vera: acne rosacea in a middle-aged woman after treatment by venesection.

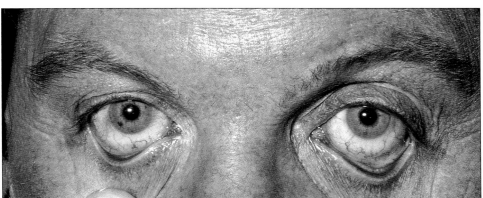

Fig. 15-6. Polycythemia vera: facial plethora and conjunctival suffusion in a 40-year-old woman. (Hb, 19.5 g/dl.)

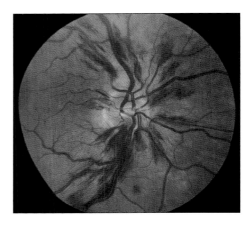

Fig. 15-7. Polycythemia vera: gross distention of retinal vessels with conspicuous hemorrhage and mild swelling of the optic disc in hyperviscosity syndrome. The patient had headaches, lassitude, confusion, and blurred vision. (Hb, 23.5 g/dl; WBC, 35 × 10⁹/L; platelets, 950 × 10⁹/L.) (Courtesy of Professor J. C. Parr.)

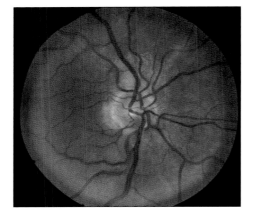

Fig. 15-8. Polycythemia vera: same retina as shown in Fig. 15-7 following venesection. The vessels and disc have returned to normal, and the areas of hemorrhage have resolved. (Courtesy of Professor J. C. Parr.)

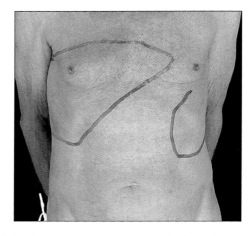

Fig. 15-9. Polycythemia vera: enlarged liver and spleen of the patient shown in Fig. 15-1.

Mild to moderate splenomegaly (Fig. 15-9) is found in 70% of patients, and the liver is palpable in 50%. High blood uric acid levels are accompanied by gout (Fig.15-10) in about 15% of cases. Major thrombosis and hemorrhage dominate the course of untreated polycythemia. Portal or hepatic venous thrombosis is a serious complication.

The blood count reveals erythrocytosis and often a neutrophil leukocytosis and thrombocytosis; no primitive cells are seen in the peripheral blood film. There may be an increase in basophils.

The *JAK2* mutation (Fig. 15-11) is present in blood granulocytes and marrow in over 95% of patients.

Bone marrow aspirates typically show hyperplastic, normoblastic erythropoiesis and granulopoiesis with increased numbers of megakaryocytes (Figs. 15-12 and 15-13). Trephine biopsies confirm the hyperplastic hematopoiesis, and clusters of megakaryocytes are often prominent (Figs. 15-14 and 15-15). In most patients hematopoietic tissue makes up 90% or more of the intertrabecular space. Silver impregnation techniques often show some increase in reticulin fiber density (Fig. 15-16). Studies with radioactive iron (not now performed) usually demonstrated that erythropoiesis is confined to central skeletal sites without extramedullary activity (Fig. 15-17).

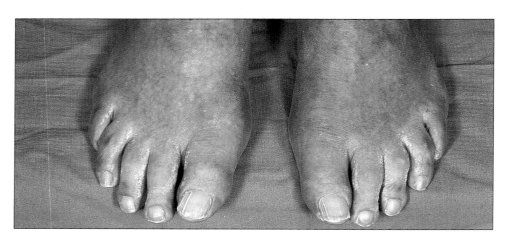

Fig. 15-10. Polycythemia vera: acute gout with inflammation and swelling of the metatarsal and interphalangeal joints of the right great toe. The skin also shows a dusky plethora. (Hb, 21.5 g/dl; total RCV, 53 ml/kg; serum uric acid, 0.9 mmol/L.)

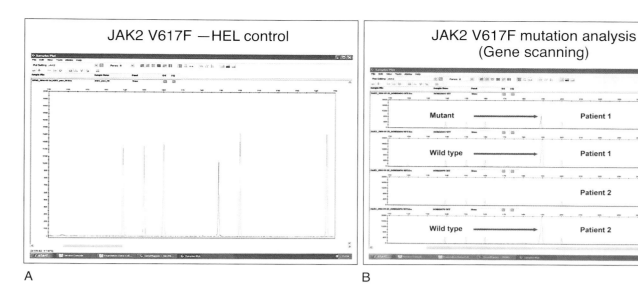

Fig. 15-11. Identification of *JAK2 V617F* mutations using fluorescently labeled primers. The sequence of the primers is specific either for the Wild type (WT) or for the *V617F* mutation; the reverse primer for both reactions is the same. **A,** HEL cell line positive for the point mutation (size standard appears as orange peaks). **B,** Patient 1 is heterozygous for *V617F* because both WT and mutant fragments amplified. Patient 2, however, is WT for *JAK2*. (Courtesy Dr. Foroni)

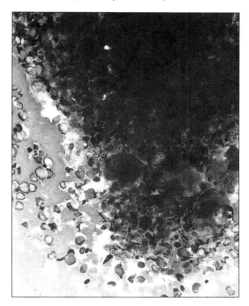

Fig. 15-12. Polycythemia vera: bone marrow aspirate showing the edge of a hypercellular fragment. Marrow fat cells are absent.

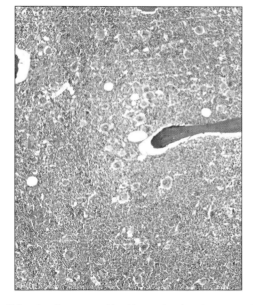

Fig. 15-14. Polycythemia vera: trephine biopsy showing almost complete filling of the intertrabecular space with hyperplastic hematopoietic tissue.

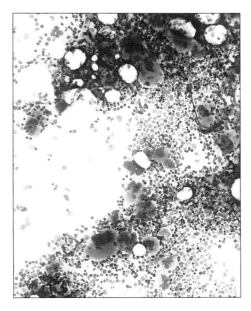

Fig. 15-13. Polycythemia vera: bone marrow aspirate with hypercellular cell trails and bone marrow fragments but incomplete replacement of marrow fat spaces. Megakaryocytes are especially prominent in the cell trails.

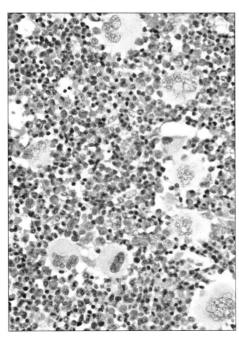

Fig. 15-15. Polycythemia vera: higher-power view of Fig. 15-14 showing hyperplasia of erythropoiesis, granulopoiesis, and megakaryocytes.

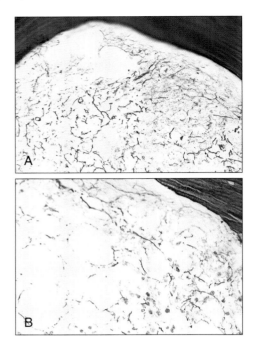

Fig. 15-16. Polycythemia vera: silver impregnation staining shows a moderate increase in the density of reticulin fibers **(A)** compared with normal bone marrow **(B)**.

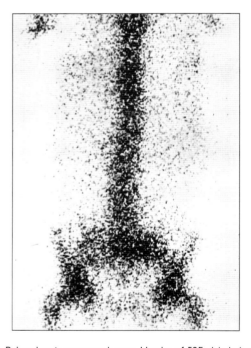

Fig. 15-17. Polycythemia vera: trunk scan. Uptake of 52Fe-labeled transferrin in the axial skeleton indicates that erythropoiesis is confined to the bone marrow.

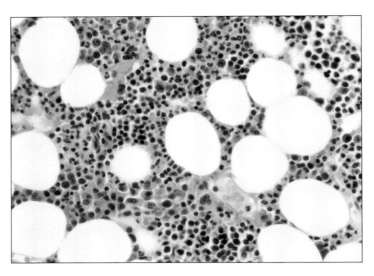

Fig. 15-18. Polycythemia and idiopathic erythrocytosis in *JAK2 exon 12* mutation. Trephine biopsy in a patient with *K539L JAK2* mutation. There is only mild hyper-cellularity and isolated erythroid hyperplasia. Megakaryocytes show normal morphology and no clustering. (Courtesy of Dr. Wendy Erber.)

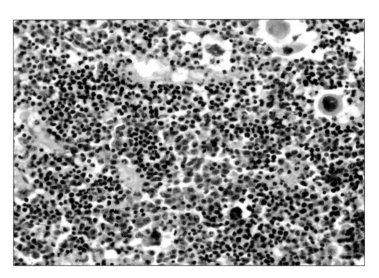

Fig. 15-19. Polycythemia and idiopathic erythropoiesis in *JAK2 exon 12* mutation. Trephine biopsy in a patient with 12del 542,543 *JAK2* mutation. There is marked hypercellularity with dominant erythropoiesis and normal megakaryocytes. (Courtesy of Dr. Wendy Erber.)

TABLE 15-2. PROPOSED DIAGNOSTIC CRITERIA FOR POLYCYTHEMIA VERA

***JAK2*-positive polycythemia**

(diagnosis requires the presence of both criteria)

A1	High hematocrit (>52% in men or >48% in women) or an increased red-cell mass (>25% above predicted value)
A2	Mutation in *JAK2*

***JAK2*-negative polycythemia vera**

(diagnosis requires the presence of A1, A2, and A3, plus either another A criterion or two B criteria)

A1	Increased red-cell mass (>25% above predicted value) or a hematocrit ≥60% in men or >56% in women
A2	Absence of mutation in *JAK2*
A3	No causes of secondary erythrocytosis (normal arterial oxygen saturation and no elevation of serum erythropoietin)
A4	Palpable splenomegaly
A5	Presence of acquired genetic abnormality (excluding *BCR-ABL*) in hematopoietic cells
B1	Thrombocytosis (platelets >450 × 10⁹/L)
B2	Neutrophilia (neutrophils >10 × 10⁹/L; >12.5 × 10⁹/L in smokers)
B3	Splenomegaly on radiography
B4	Endogenous erythroid colonies or low serum erythropoietin

Modified from Campbell PJ, Green AR: *N Eng J Med* 355:2452–2466, 2006.

Recently a group of *V617F*-negative patients with polycythemia vera or idiopathic erythrocytosis have been identified with gain in function mutations involving the exon 12 region of the *JAK2* gene. These patients had isolated erythrocytosis, low erythropoietin levels, and bone marrows showing erythroid hyperplasia without abnormalities of granulopoiesis or megakaryocytes (Figs. 15-18 and 15-19). Unlike cultured erythroid colonies in patients with *V617F*-positive polycythemia vera, those with exon 12 mutations are not homozygous for the *JAK2* mutation.

Proposed diagnostic criteria for polycythemia vera are shown in Table 15-2. In the presence of the *JAK2* mutation, the traditional measurement of red cell mass is now only performed occasionally.

TABLE 15-3.   CAUSES OF POLYCYTHEMIA

Primary (increased red cell volume)	Secondary (increased red cell volume)	Relative (normal red cell volume)

Polycythemia vera
Familial (congenital)
	As a result of compensatory erythropoietin increase in:
	  high altitudes
	  heavy smoking
	  cardiovascular disease
	  pulmonary disease and alveolar hypoventilation
	  increased affinity hemoglobins (familial polycythemia)
	  methemoglobinemia (rarely)
	
	As a result of inappropriate erythropoietin increase in:
	  renal disease – hydronephrosis, vascular impairment,
	    cysts, carcinoma
	  massive uterine fibromyomata
	  hepatocellular carcinoma
	  cerebellar hemangioblastoma
		"Stress" or "spurious" polycythemia
		
		Dehydration:
		  water deprivation
		  vomiting
		  diuretic therapy
		
		Plasma loss:
		  burns
		  enteropathy

JAK2-negative polycythemia vera may be differentiated from other causes of polycythemia (Table 15-3) by identifying a low serum erythropoietin and a normal arterial oxygen saturation. In polycythemia vera circulating erythroid progenitors BFU-E and CFU-E are increased and grow in vitro independently of added erythropoietin. Relative polycythemia is excluded by blood volume studies.

Treatment of polycythemia vera is aimed at maintaining a normal hematocrit. Patients are managed with venesection or treated with cytotoxic drugs, usually hydroxyurea, or with radioactive phosphorus. Trials of *JAK2* inhibitors are in progress.

Typically there is a median survival of 10 to 15 years. Transition to the accelerated phase with myelofibrosis occurs in about 30% of cases, and death from acute myeloid leukemia occurs in less than 10% of patients.

PRIMARY CONGENITAL POLYCYTHEMIA

In this rare condition mutations in the genes coding for factors involved in the hypoxia sensing pathway have been found to be associated with increased erythropoietin production. A homozygous mutation in the von Hippel-Lindau (*VHL*) gene is present in familial erythrocytosis found in the Chuvash population. In other isolated cases there have been mutations in the gene for the propyl hydroxlase domain containing proteins (*PHD2*) or the hypoxia inducible factor (*HIF2A*) gene.

Mutations in the erythropoietin receptor gene (*EPOR*) have been found in a few patients.

ESSENTIAL THROMBOCYTHEMIA

A diagnosis of essential thrombocythemia is considered when a sustained rise in platelet count occurs, in some cases in excess of $1000 \times 10^9/L$, with no other underlying cause. There are usually abnormalities of platelet function, and in severe cases the clinical course may be dominated by recurrent hemorrhage and thrombosis. In many patients the raised platelet count is found on routine testing and there are no symptoms for many years, particularly in younger patients. In some patients this disorder is not easily distinguished from myelofibrosis and particularly polycythemia vera, of which many consider thrombocythemia to be merely a variant.

The *JAK2 V617F* mutation is found in 50% to 60% of patients. Unlike polycythemia vera, homozygosity for the mutation is not a feature. Other genetic mutations are possibly responsible for most *JAK2 V617F*–negative cases, for example, activation mutations in the thrombopoietin receptor gene *MPL* in less than 5%, but in some patients, the disease appears to have a polyclonal origin.

The dominant clinical problem is bleeding from the gastrointestinal tract and, less frequently, epistaxis, menorrhagia, hematuria, or hemoptysis. Spontaneous bruising often appears (Fig. 15-20), and cerebrovascular accidents may occur in the elderly. Blockage of peripheral blood vessels may result in erythromelalgia (Fig. 15-21), ischemia, and gangrene (Fig. 15-22).

The peripheral blood film shows a distinctive increase in platelet count, and the platelets are often of abnormal morphology with many giant forms. Howell-Jolly bodies and other stigmata of splenic atrophy are found in a third of severe cases, and careful search may reveal the presence of megakaryocyte fragments (Figs. 15-23 to 15-26).

Splenic atrophy (Fig. 15-27) often increases the severity of platelet elevation in the peripheral blood as obliteration of the splenic red pulp areas, in which platelet pooling normally occurs, results in the entire marrow platelet production being accommodated in the general circulation.

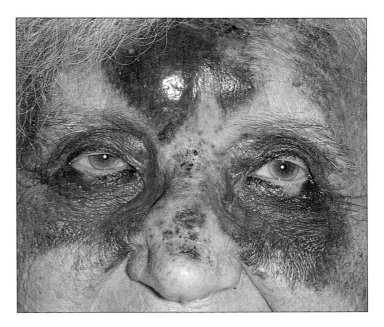

Fig. 15-20. Essential thrombocythemia: hemorrhage into subcutaneous tissues following minor trauma. Gross defects of platelet aggregation with adenosine diphosphate, adrenaline, and thrombin were found. (Platelets, 2300 $\times$ 10^9/L.)

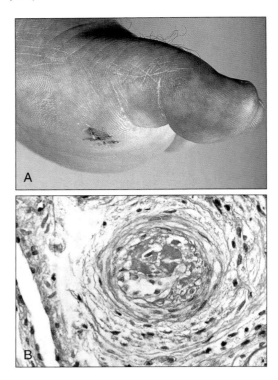

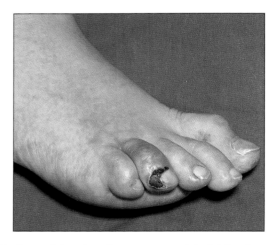

Fig. 15-21. Essential thrombocythemia: erythromelalgia. **A,** Severe burning pain and hot, red congestion of the forefoot and toes in a 39-year-old man. (Platelet count, 875 × 10⁹/L.) **B,** Section of a skin biopsy showing thrombotic occlusion of an arteriole with proliferative changes in the peripheral wall. (*A* and *B,* Courtesy of Professor J. J. Michiels.)

Fig. 15-22. Essential thrombocythemia: gangrene of the left fourth toe. (Platelets, 1900 × 10⁹/L.)

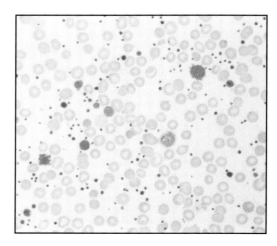

Fig. 15-23. Essential thrombocythemia: peripheral blood film showing a gross increase in platelet numbers.

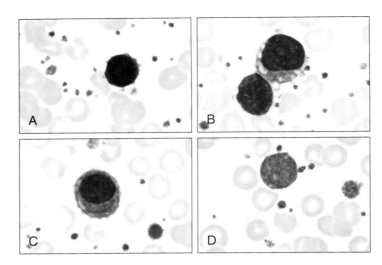

Fig. 15-24. Essential thrombocythemia. **A–D,** Peripheral blood films showing circulating megakaryocyte fragments.

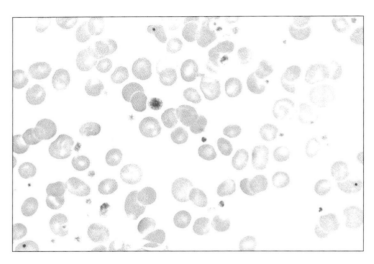

Fig. 15-25. Essential thrombocythemia: blood film showing features of splenic atrophy. The red cells show anisocytosis and mild polychromasia and three contain Howell-Jolly bodies. There is an increase in both platelet number and size.

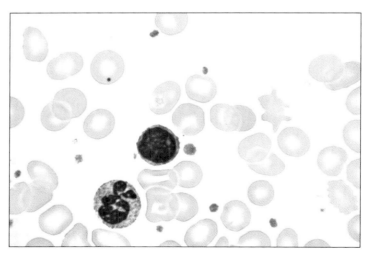

Fig. 15-26. Essential thrombocythemia: peripheral blood film at high magnification showing features of splenic atrophy, including a Howell-Jolly body, red cell targeting, crenation, and acanthocytosis.

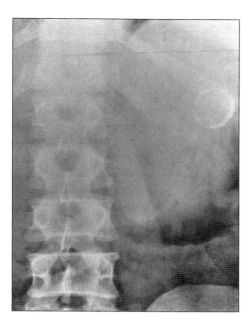

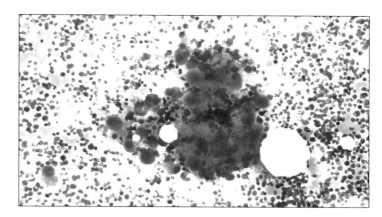

Fig. 15-29. Essential thrombocythemia: bone marrow aspirate cell trail showing a prominent cluster of megakaryocytes.

Fig. 15-27. Essential thrombocythemia: abdominal radiograph showing a small spherical calcified mass (at *upper right*). The blood film showed features of splenic atrophy. At autopsy the fibrotic remnant of spleen weighed only 30 g and had extensive areas of dystrophic calcification.

Aspiration of bone marrow may be difficult. There is usually a general hyperplasia of hematopoietic cells with a striking increase in the number of megakaryocytes (Fig. 15-28), which are often found in cohesive clusters (Fig. 15-29). The megakaryocytes tend to show many nuclear lobes and their average cell volume is above normal (Figs. 15-30 and 15-31). In many patients the dominant feature is masses of adherent platelets that may be confused with marrow fragments (Fig. 15-32). Trephine biopsy preparations reflect the dramatic increase in the megakaryocyte population; large numbers of abnormal megakaryocytes are seen at all stages of development (Figs. 15-33 to 15-35). Silver impregnation techniques demonstrate an increase in reticulin patterns intermediate between those of polycythemia vera and myelofibrosis. Compared with myelofibrosis (see the following section), radiologic scanning shows only modest expansion of hematopoietic tissue (Fig. 15-36).

Proposed diagnostic criteria for essential thrombocythemia are shown in Table 15-4, and the condition must be differentiated from other causes of a high platelet count (Table 15-5).

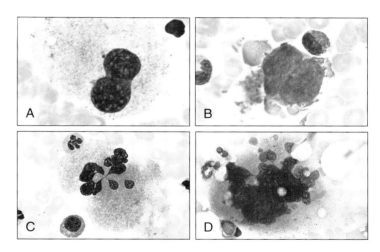

Fig. 15-30. Essential thrombocythemia: bone marrow aspirate showing binucleate megakaryocyte **(A)**; binucleate megakaryoblast with cytoplasmic differentiation **(B)**; and relatively low **(C)** and high **(D)** nuclear ploidy in hypersegmented megakaryocytes.

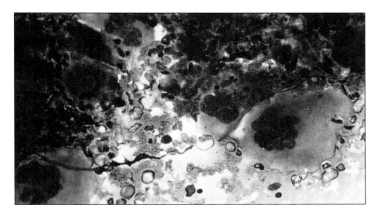

Fig. 15-28. Essential thrombocythemia: bone marrow aspirate fragment showing a marked increase in the number of megakaryocytes.

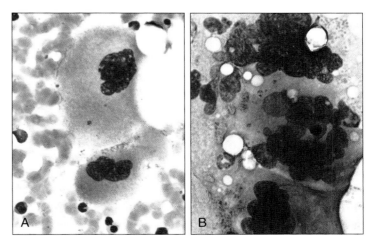

Fig. 15-31. Essential thrombocythemia: bone marrow aspirates showing clumping of megakaryocytes with definite cell borders **(A)** and lack of cytoplasmic separation **(B)**.

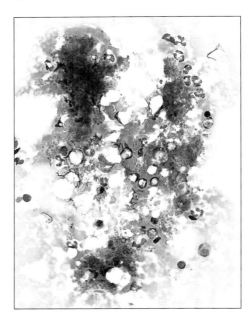

Fig. 15-32. Essential thrombocythemia: bone marrow aspirate cell trail showing large masses of aggregated platelets.

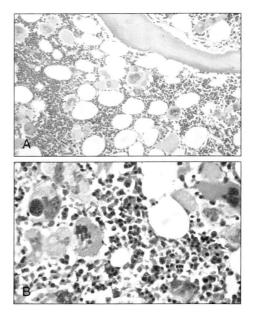

Fig. 15-33. Essential thrombocythemia: trephine biopsy showing that the overall cellularity of hematopoietic tissue is not greatly increased (**A**) but also showing large numbers of megakaryocytes (**B**), seen particularly well at higher magnification.

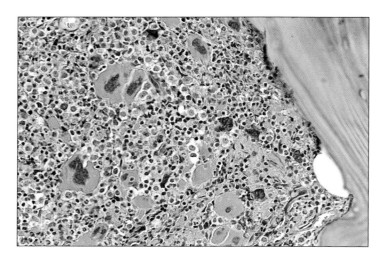

Fig. 15-34. Essential thrombocythemia: trephine biopsy. There is a marked increase in cellularity with prominent megakaryocytes.

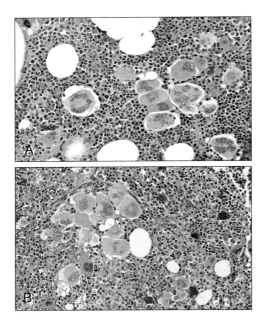

Fig. 15-35. Essential thrombocythemia: trephine biopsy. In two different patients (**A** and **B**) there is clustering of large megakaryocytes of high nuclear ploidy.

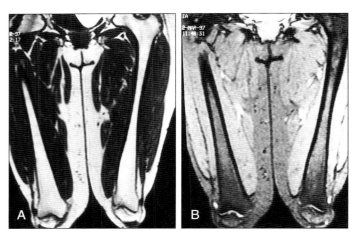

Fig. 15-36. Magnetic resonance imaging: essential thrombocythemia. **A,** T1 sequence. **B,** T2 sequence. The femoral marrow is fatty (grade 0). (*A* and *B,* Courtesy of Professor C. Rozman.)

TABLE 15-4.   PROPOSED DIAGNOSTIC CRITERIA FOR ESSENTIAL THROMBOCYTHEMIA

***JAK2*-positive thrombocythemia**

(diagnosis requires the presence of all three criteria)

A1   Platelets >450 × 10⁹/L
A2   Mutation in *JAK2*
A3   No other myeloid cancer, especially *JAK2*-positive polycythemia, myelofibrosis, or myelodysplasia

***JAK2*-negative essential thrombocythemia**

(diagnosis requires the presence of all five criteria)

A1   Platelets >600 × 10⁹/L on two occasions at least 1 month apart
A2   Absence of mutation in *JAK2*
A3   No reactive causes for thrombocythemia
A4   Normal ferritin (>20 µg/L)
A5   No other myeloid disorder, especially chronic myeloid leukemia, myelofibrosis, polycythemia vera, or myelodysplasia

Modified from Campbell PJ, Green AR: *N Eng J Med* 355:2452–2466, 2006.

TABLE 15-5.	CAUSES OF A HIGH PLATELET COUNT
Reactive	**Endogenous**
Hemorrhage	Essential thrombocythemia
Trauma	Some cases of polycythemia vera, myelofibrosis, and chronic myeloid leukemia
Postoperative	
Chronic iron deficiency	
Malignancy	
Chronic infections	
Connective tissue diseases	
Postsplenectomy with continuing anemia and active marrow	

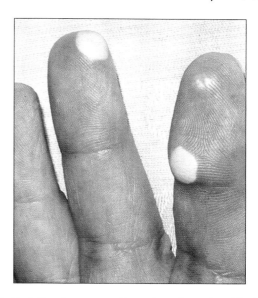

Fig. 15-38. Myelofibrosis: gouty tophi on the index and middle fingers of a 55-year-old man.

Hydroxyurea, busulfan (now largely obsolete), α_2-interferon, and ^{32}P have been used to reduce platelet production. Anagrelide is a newer drug with no leukemogenic action compared with ^{32}P but with side effects on the cardiovascular system and gut in some patients. Low-dose aspirin therapy is used to reduce the risk of thrombosis in asymptomatic patients who show no evidence of excess bruising or hemorrhage.

MYELOFIBROSIS

In myelofibrosis—a myeloproliferative disease that is also known as myelosclerosis, agnogenic myeloid metaplasia, or idiopathic myelofibrosis—the hematopoietic cell proliferation is more generalized, with splenic and hepatic involvement. There is often extension of hematopoietic marrow from central skeletal sites into the long bones of the leg and arm.

This disorder is related closely to polycythemia vera, and over 30% of patients have a previous history of that disease. The associated increase in marrow fiber production is marked and the effectiveness of hematopoiesis is decreased.

The *V617F* mutation is present in over 50% of patients. In *JAK2*-negative patients other mutations may be responsible for the myeloproliferation; for example, an activating mutation in the thrombopoietic receptor *(MPL)* gene is found in 10%. Idiopathic myelofibrosis is indistinguishable from myelofibrosis secondary to polycythemia vera or essential thrombocythemia, and the diagnostic criteria for these conditions are the same. Some patients diagnosed with idiopathic myelofibrosis probably are in the accelerated phase of previously undiagnosed polycythemia vera or essential thrombocythemia. The fibrosis, angiogenesis, and new bone formation in myelofibrosis are the result of a polyclonal response to cytokines and growth factors (e.g., transforming growth factor β [TGF-β], basic fibroblast growth factor [bFGF], and vascular endothelial growth factor [VEGF]) produced by megakaryocytes and monocytes from the myeloproliferative clone.

Myelofibrosis usually occurs in middle-aged and elderly patients. Most patients initially have symptoms caused by anemia, splenic enlargement (Fig. 15-37), or hypermetabolism, such as night sweats, anorexia, and weight loss. Some may complain of bone pain and gout (Fig. 15-38).

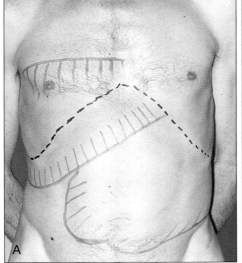 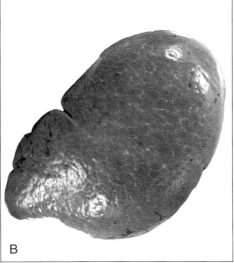

Fig. 15-37. Myelofibrosis. **A,** Splenohepatomegaly; **B,** the patient's spleen shows a well-defined notch in the superior border. The prominent indent in the inferior border was palpable during clinical examination.

Radiologic imaging (Figs. 15-39 and 15-40) is able to provide evidence of the expansion of skeletal myeloproliferative activity. A minority of cases shows generalized osteosclerosis (Fig. 15-41).

As a result of a hyperkinetic portal circulation, in some cases of long standing, the patient develops portal hypertension and may have bleeding esophageal varices or ascites (Figs. 15-42 and 15-43).

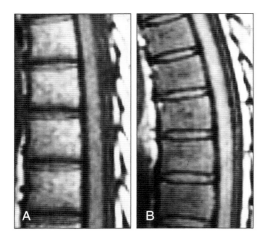

Fig. 15-39. Magnetic resonance imaging: T1 sequence. Dorsal vertebrae in essential thrombocythemia **(A)** and myelofibrosis **(B).** By comparison with the spinal cord, it can be seen that in **A** the vertebral signal is not decreased, whereas in **B** there is a marked decrease. (*A* and *B*, Courtesy of Professor C. Rozman.)

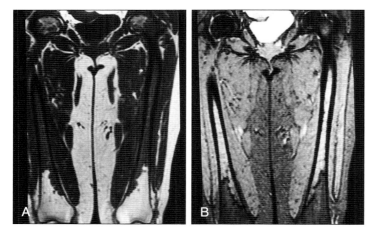

Fig. 15-40. Magnetic resonance imaging: myelofibrosis. Both femurs (except distal diaphyses) display a decreased signal in the T1 sequence **(A)** and a corresponding increase in the T2 sequence **(B)** indicating expansion of hematopoietic tissue. (*A* and *B*, Courtesy of Professor C. Rozman.)

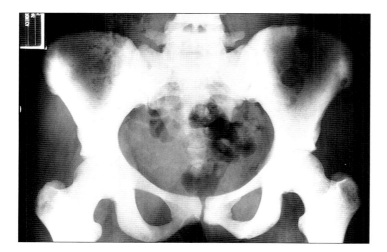

Fig. 15-41. Myelofibrosis: pelvic radiograph showing a generalized increase in bone density from osteosclerosis.

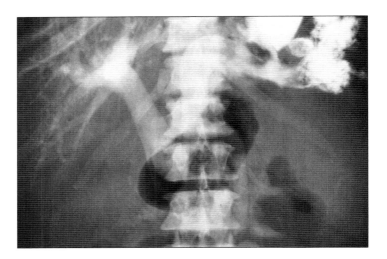

Fig. 15-42. Myelofibrosis: transsplenic portal venogram showing gross dilation of the splenic, inferior mesenteric, and portal veins and increased bone density in the vertebral bodies. A great increase in splenic blood flow results in a hyperkinetic portal circulation, which, together with the obstructive effects of extramedullary hematopoiesis, may be important in the pathogenesis of portal hypertension.

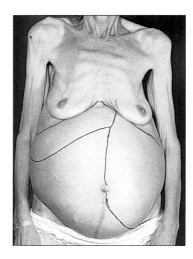

Fig. 15-43. Myelofibrosis: gross wasting and abdominal distention from massive splenomegaly, hepatomegaly, and ascites.

Most patients have a normochromic anemia of moderate or marked severity. It may be macrocytic in those who are folate deficient or microcytic with associated iron deficiency. The peripheral blood usually shows florid leukoerythroblastic change, and the number of nucleated red cells often exceeds the number of leukocytes. Marked polychromasia, anisocytosis, and poikilocytosis with "teardrop" red cells are typical changes (Fig. 15-44). In occasional patients with extensive osteosclerosis, the blood film shows marked leukoerythroblastic change with circulating megakaryocyte fragments (Fig. 15-45). Occasionally these fragments dominate the blood film (Fig. 15-46).

Attempts at bone marrow aspiration are usually unsuccessful, but trephine biopsy reveals a variable degree of hematopoietic cell activity and marrow fibrosis (Figs. 15-47 to 15-50). Silver impregnation techniques show an increase in reticulin fiber density and thickness (Fig. 15-51); only in advanced disease is there collagen deposition and, in 10% of cases, osteosclerosis (Figs. 15-52 and 15-53). Recently, the severity of marrow fibrosis was graded on a scale of 0 to 3 by a European Consensus Committee (Fig. 15-54).

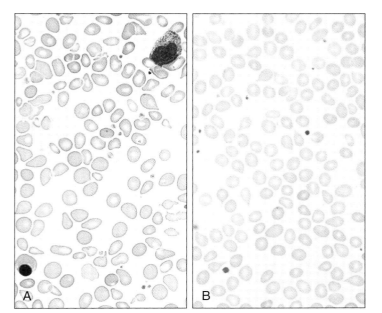

Fig. 15-44. Myelofibrosis: peripheral blood films showing leukoerythroblastic changes with red cell polychromasia, anisocytosis, and poikilocytosis, including "teardrop" forms (the nucleated cells are an erythroblast and a late myelocyte) **(A)**; red cell anisocytosis and poikilocytosis with "teardrop" forms in early disease **(B)**.

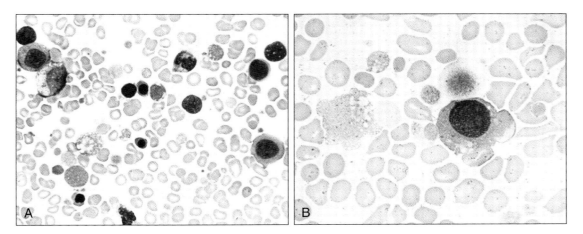

Fig. 15-45. Myelofibrosis/osteomyelofibrosis: peripheral blood films showing myelocytes, erythroblasts, and megakaryocyte fragments **(A)**; at higher magnification, megakaryocyte fragments **(B)**.

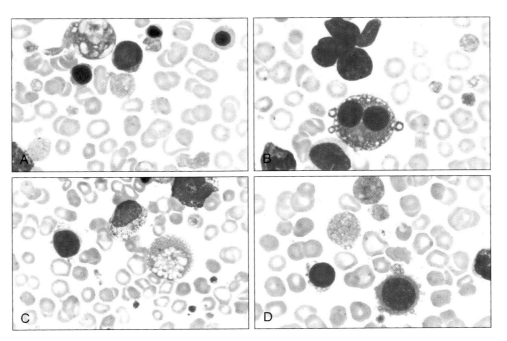

Fig. 15-46. Myelofibrosis: blood film. The images show bizarre giant platelets and megakaryocyte fragments.

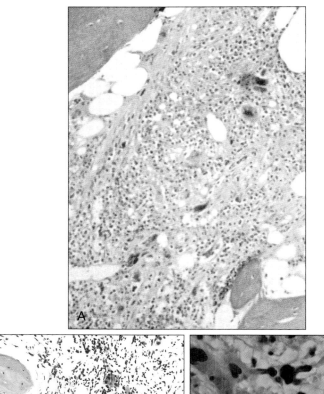

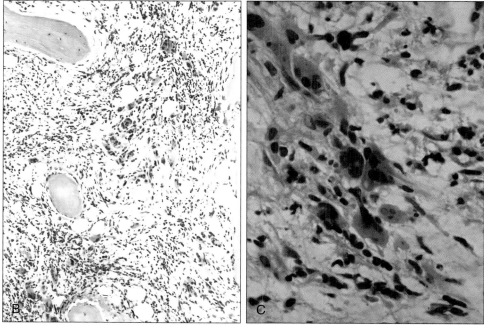

Fig. 15-47. Myelofibrosis: trephine biopsies showing most of the intertrabecular space occupied by cellular loose connective tissue contains scattered hematopoietic cells, including prominent megakaryocytes, fat cells making up less than 15% of the intertrabecular space, and extensive deposition of loose connective tissue around hematopoietic cells **(A** and **B)**; the prominence of megakaryocytes in the myelofibrotic tissue at higher magnification **(C)**.

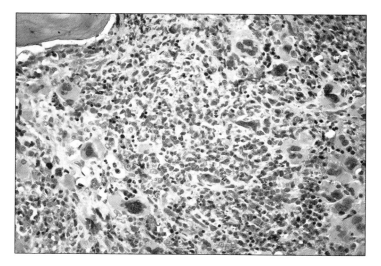

Fig. 15-48. Transitional or accelerated phase myeloproliferative disease: trephine biopsy showing complete filling of intertrabecular space by hyperplastic hematopoietic tissue with large numbers of megakaryocytes and increased stromal connective tissue between hematopoietic cells. This patient has clinical features of both polycythemia vera and myelofibrosis. The blood film showed leukoerythroblastic features and splenic enlargement extending 20 cm below the left costal margin. (Hb, 18.5 g/dl; WBC, 120 $\times$ 10^9/L; platelets, 450 $\times$ 10^9/L; total RCV, 49 ml/kg.)

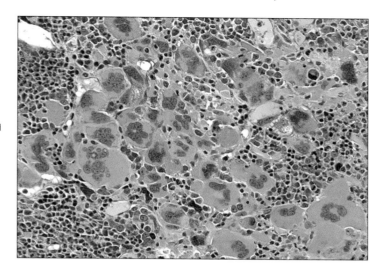

Fig. 15-49. Myelofibrosis: trephine biopsy showing a large cluster of adherent and aggregated megakaryocytes with high nuclear ploidy.

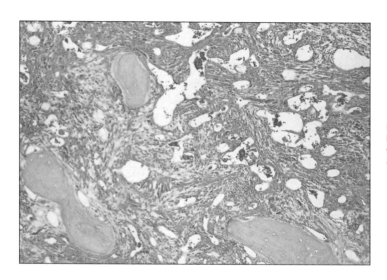

Fig. 15-50. Transitional or accelerated phase myeloproliferative disease: trephine biopsy showing prominent dilated venous sinuses surrounded by hyperplastic and fibrotic hematopoietic tissue. The blood film showed leukoerythroblastic change. (Hb, 19.5 g/dl; WBC, 38 × 10⁹/L; platelets, 850 × 10⁹/L; total RCV, 44 ml/kg.)

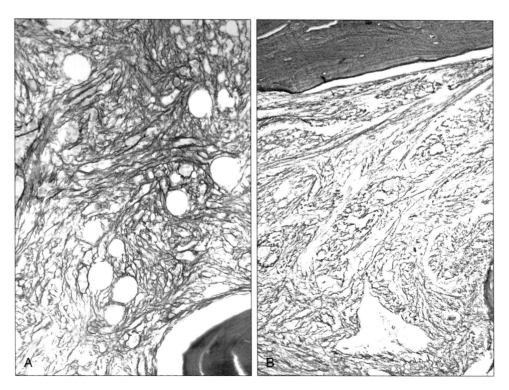

Fig. 15-51. Myelofibrosis: silver impregnation stains of same cases as Fig. 15-50 **(A)** and Fig. 15-47, *B* **(B).** In both biopsies there is a marked diffuse increase in reticulin fiber density and thickness with many intersections (Thiele scale—grade 2).

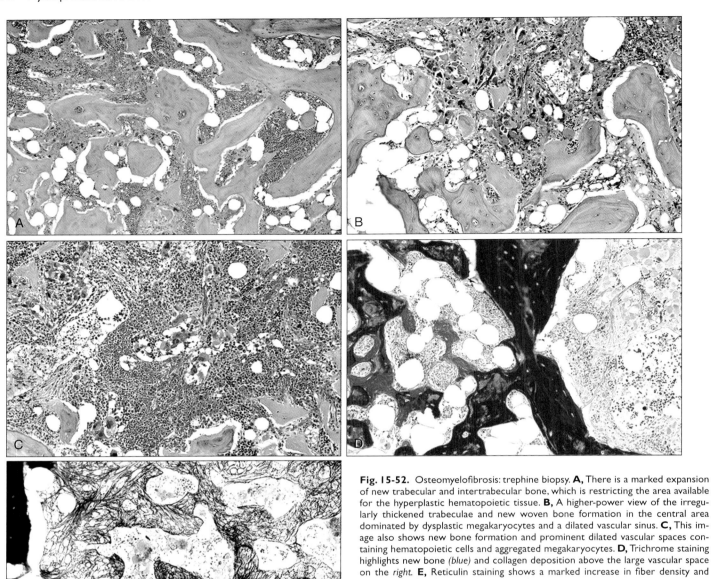

Fig. 15-52. Osteomyelofibrosis: trephine biopsy. **A,** There is a marked expansion of new trabecular and intertrabecular bone, which is restricting the area available for the hyperplastic hematopoietic tissue. **B,** A higher-power view of the irregularly thickened trabeculae and new woven bone formation in the central area dominated by dysplastic megakaryocytes and a dilated vascular sinus. **C,** This image also shows new bone formation and prominent dilated vascular spaces containing hematopoietic cells and aggregated megakaryocytes. **D,** Trichrome staining highlights new bone *(blue)* and collagen deposition above the large vascular space on the *right.* **E,** Reticulin staining shows a marked increase in fiber density and thickness and outlines numerous vascular sinuses.

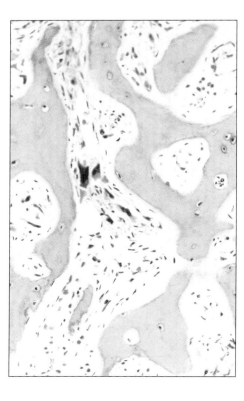

Fig. 15-53. Osteomyelofibrosis: trephine biopsy showing replacement of normal intertrabecular tissue by a fibrous connective tissue containing only isolated hematopoietic cells (the larger central cells are megakaryocytes). There is an increased amount of trabecular bone with an irregular lamellar pattern.

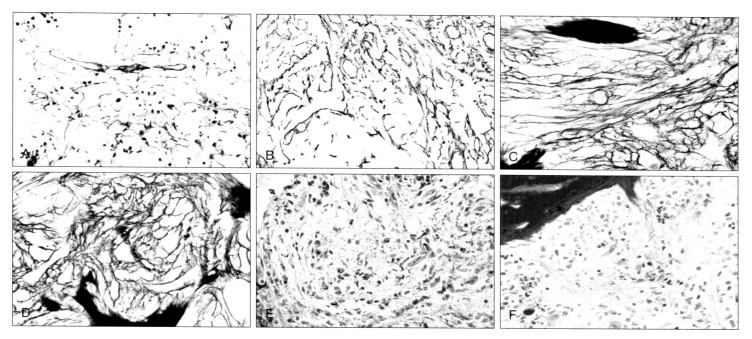

Fig. 15-54. European Consensus Committee grades of marrow fibrosis—Thiele scale. **A,** Grade 0: scattered linear reticulin with no crossovers corresponding to normal marrow. The reticulin aggregation in the center is a small blood vessel. **B,** Grade 1: loose network of reticulin with many intersections. **C,** Grade 2: diffuse and dense increase in reticulin with extensive intersections, occasionally with focal bundles of collagen and/or osteosclerosis. **D,** Grade 3: diffuse and dense increase in reticulin with extensive intersections with coarse bundles of collagen often with extensive osteosclerosis. **E,** Grade 2: same case as **C** showing a few focal collagen fibers staining *blue*. (Masson trichrome stain.) **F,** Grade 3: same case as **D** and Fig. 15-52 showing coarse bundles of collagen and associated osteosclerosis. (Masson trichrome stain.) (Thiele J et al: *Hematologica* 90:1128–1132, 2005.)

Radioisotope investigations were used to determine the severity of the disease. Whole-body scanning techniques used cyclotron-produced ^{52}Fe to assess the distribution of the injected radioiron in the body (Figs. 15-55 and 15-56). These tests are now obsolete. Extramedullary hematopoiesis may also be confirmed from a liver biopsy or after splenectomy (Figs. 15-57 and 15-58).

Proposed diagnostic criteria for myelofibrosis are listed in Table 15-6. Myelofibrosis must be differentiated from causes of reactive marrow fibrosis (Table 15-7).

Treatment of myelofibrosis is unsatisfactory. Supportive red cell transfusions are required in severely anemic patients. Alkylating agents, hydroxyurea, thalidomide with or without steroids, and splenectomy may help in selected patients. Folic acid may be given to prevent deficiency.

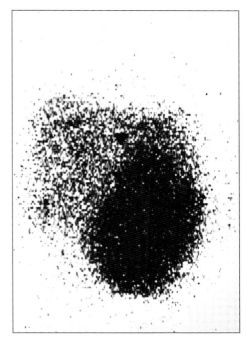

Fig. 15-55. Myelofibrosis: trunk scan showing dominant uptake of 52Fe-labeled transferrin into the enlarged spleen and liver with no evidence of skeletal concentration, a pattern consistent with predominant extramedullary hematopoiesis.

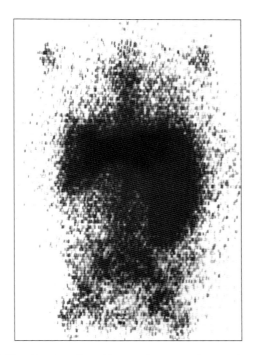

Fig. 15-56. Transitional myeloproliferative disease: trunk scan showing obvious uptake of 52Fe-labeled transferrin in the liver and spleen, as well as in the central skeleton.

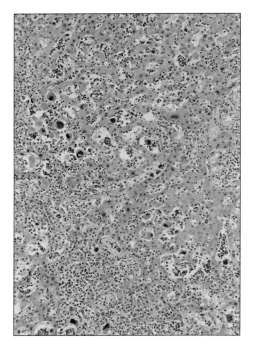

Fig. 15-57. Myelofibrosis: extramedullary hematopoiesis. Liver biopsy shows groups of erythroblasts, granulopoietic cells, and multinucleate megakaryocytes in the sinuses.

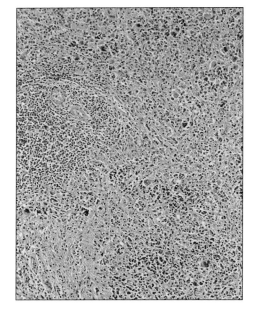

Fig. 15-58. Myelofibrosis: extramedullary hematopoiesis. Section of spleen following splenectomy shows similar groups of hematopoietic cells in the reticuloendothelial cords and sinuses.

TABLE 15-6.   PROPOSED DIAGNOSTIC CRITERIA FOR IDIOPATHIC MYELOFIBROSIS

JAK2-positive myelofibrosis

(diagnosis requires the presence of A1 and A2 and any two B criteria)

A1   Reticulin grade 2 or 3 (on a scale of 0–3)
A2   Mutation in *JAK2*
B1   Palpable splenomegaly
B2   Otherwise unexplained anemia (hemoglobin <11.5 g/L for men; <10.0 g/L for women)
B3   Teardrop red cells on peripheral blood film
B4   Leukoerythroblastic blood film (presence of at least two nucleated red cells or immature myeloid cells in peripheral blood film)
B5   Systemic symptoms (drenching night sweats, weight loss >10% over 6 months, or diffuse bone pain)
B6   Histologic evidence of extramedullary hematopoiesis

JAK2-negative idiopathic myelofibrosis

(diagnosis requires the presence of A1, A2, A3, and any two B criteria)

A1   Reticulin grade 2 or 3 (on a scale of 0–3)
A2   Absence of mutation in *JAK2*
A3   Absence of *BCR-ABL* fusion gene
B1   Palpable splenomegaly
B2   Otherwise unexplained anemia (hemoglobin <11.5 g/L for men; <10.0 g/L for women)
B3   Teardrop red cells on peripheral blood film
B4   Leukoerythroblastic blood film (presence of at least two nucleated red cells or immature myeloid cells in peripheral blood film)
B5   Systemic symptoms (drenching night sweats, weight loss >10% over 6 months, or diffuse bone pain)
B6   Histologic evidence of extramedullary hematopoiesis

Modified from Campbell PJ, Green AR: *N Eng J Med* 355:2452–2466, 2006; and Barosi G et al: *Br J Hematol* 104:730–737, 1999.

TABLE 15-7.   CAUSES OF MARROW FIBROSIS

Myelofibrosis

Infections: tuberculosis (see Chapter 27); osteomyelitis (focal fibrosis)

Malignant lymphoma, including Hodgkin lymphoma (see Chapters 19-21)

Occasionally, chronic myeloid leukemia (see Chapter 13) and other leukemias, especially AML M$_7$ (see Chapter 12)

Metastatic carcinoma, especially breast and prostate (see Chapter 27)

Excess irradiation

Benzene poisoning

Excess fluorine

Paget's disease (focal fibrosis; see Chapter 27)

Osteopetrosis (see Chapter 27)

LEUKEMIC TRANSFORMATION OF POLYCYTHEMIA VERA AND MYELOFIBROSIS

It is generally accepted that transformation is part of the natural history of the myeloproliferative syndrome and probably reflects the acquisition of further mutations. Transition to myelofibrosis from polycythemia vera occurs in approximately 30% of cases and to acute leukemia in less than 10%. The latter is usually acute myeloid leukemia (AML), but the occurrence of acute lymphoblastic leukemia has been described. The incidence of leukemia is similar in those treated with either radioactive phosphorus or alkylating agents. Hydroxyurea is now used in preference to either because it is considered not to predispose to leukemic transformation. Of patients with myelofibrosis, 10% develop a terminal leukemia (Figs. 15-59 to 15-62). Survival beyond leukemic transformation in either condition is brief.

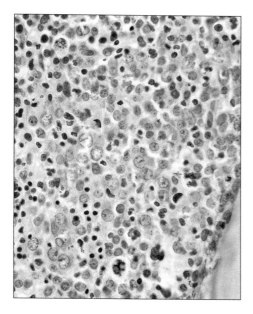

Fig. 15-61. Myelofibrosis transformed into acute myeloid leukemia. Higher-power view of the right field in Fig. 15-43 shows predominantly primitive myeloid blast cells and promyelocytes. Following a 9-year history of myelofibrosis, the patient sought treatment for a fever and bronchopneumonia. (Hb, 7.1 g/dl; WBC, 6 × 10^9/L; blasts, 4.5 × 10^9/L; neutrophils, 0.6 × 10^9/L; platelets, 40 × 10^9/L.)

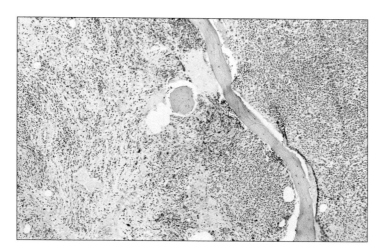

Fig. 15-59. Myelofibrosis transformed into acute leukemia. Trephine biopsy shows areas *(left field)* that are consistent with myelofibrosis, but the intertrabecular space *(right field)* contains sheets of closely packed mononuclear cells with no obvious stromal connective tissue.

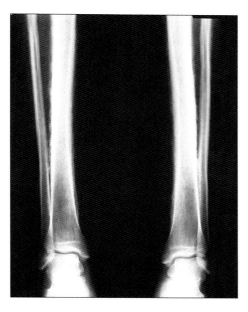

Fig. 15-62. Myelofibrosis transformed into acute myeloid leukemia: radiograph of the lower legs of a middle-aged man showing extensive periosteal elevation caused by infiltration of myeloid blast cells from underlying medullary bone. Although the medullary cavities of these bones in adults usually contain only fat, hematopoietic tissue may extend to distal skeletal tissue in long-standing myeloproliferative disease.

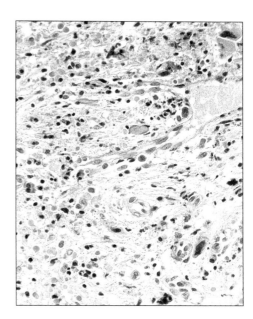

Fig. 15-60. Myelofibrosis transformed into acute leukemia. Higher-power view of the left field in Fig. 15-59 shows isolated hematopoietic cells surrounded by a loose fibrous connective tissue.

MYELOPROLIFERATIVE DISORDER UNCLASSIFIABLE

This designation is applied to cases with clinical and laboratory features of a myeloproliferative disease (Fig. 15-63) but who fail to satisfy the diagnostic criteria for any specific entity or features that overlap two or more categories. Some cases represent an early stage of development, and others may be at an advanced accelerated phase of myeloproliferation that obscures the earlier disorder.

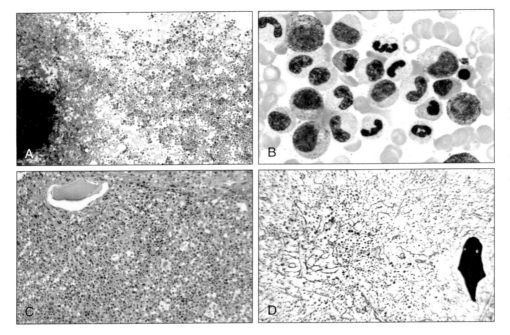

Fig. 15-63. Myeloproliferative disease unclassifiable. Bone marrow images from a 78-year-old man with mild splenomegaly, Hb 15.1 g/dl, neutrophils 32 × 10⁹/L, myelocytes 4.0 × 10⁹/L, promyelocytes 1.2 × 10⁹/L, platelets 530 × 10⁹/L, and mild red cell anisocytosis. **A,** Marrow aspirate showing hypercellular fragment and cell trail. **B,** At higher power the aspirate shows a dominance of granulopoiesis. **C,** Trephine biopsy showing complete replacement of fat by predominantly myelopoietic cells. Megakaryocytes are of low nuclear ploidy and are not seen in clusters. **D,** The reticulin stain shows a minimal increase in fiber density and thickness.

MAST CELL DISEASE

Mast cells are derived from hematopoietic stem cells. In mast cell disease (mastocytosis) there is an abnormal proliferation in the skin or other organs. In many variants of mastocytosis, particularly those with systemic involvement, there is a somatic mutation of *c-KIT,* the proto-oncogene that encodes a receptor tyrosine kinase for stem cell factor (SCF). The most common mutation is the point mutation Asp816Val, which results in spontaneous activation of the KIT protein and a consequent clonal expansion of mast cells.

Other activating mutations affecting the same codon have been identified in a minority of adult cases of cutaneous mastocytosis (Asp816Tyr, Asp816Phe). The WHO classification of mastocytosis is shown in Table 15-8.

CUTANEOUS MASTOCYTOSIS

Cutaneous mastocytosis is the most frequently found form, accounting for 80% of all cases of mastocytosis. The mastocytosis is confined to the skin. The lesions show urticaria when stroked and are pigmented. Urticaria pigmentosa, or macular papular mastocytosis (Figs. 15-64 and 15-65), is the most common form and occurs in both children and adults. Diffuse cutaneous mastocytosis, another variant, is less common and is seen only in children. Cutaneous mastocytoma (Fig. 15-66) occurs as a solitary, benign-appearing tumor usually in infants. In all of these conditions there is no systemic involvement and no elevation of the serum tryptase.

Fig. 15-64. Urticaria pigmentosa. **A,** Mast cells fill the papillary dermis. **B,** A higher-power view of the mast cells. (H & E.) (Courtesy of Dr. David Weedon. From Weedon D: *Skin pathology,* ed 2, Churchill Livingstone, 2002.)

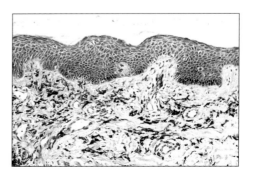

Fig. 15-65. Urticaria pigmentosa. Numerous mast cells are present in the upper dermis. There is also mild hyperpigmentation of the basal layer. (Toluidine blue.) (Courtesy of Dr. David Weedon. From Weedon D: *Skin pathology,* ed 2, Elsevier Science.)

TABLE 15-8.	MASTOCYTOSIS: WORLD HEALTH ORGANIZATION (2008) CLASSIFICATION

Cutaneous mastocytosis
Indolent systemic mastocytosis
Systemic mastocytosis with associated clonal, hematologic non–mast cell lineage disease
Aggressive systemic mastocytosis
Mast cell leukemia
Mast cell sarcoma
Extracutaneous mastocytoma

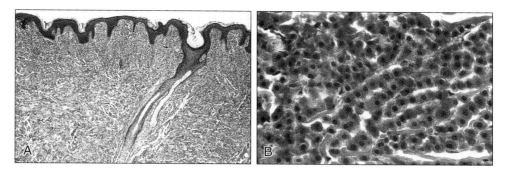

Fig. 15-66. Cutaneous mastocytoma: low power **(A)** high power **(B).** The tumor cells have abundant eosinophilic cytoplasm and uniform darkly staining nuclei. (Courtesy of Dr. Phillip H. McKee. From McKee PH, Calonje E, Granter SR: *Pathology of the skin,* ed 3, Elsevier Mosby, 2005.)

SYSTEMIC MASTOCYTOSIS

In systemic mastocytosis patients may have weight loss, fatigue, or fever. Persistent and progressive eruptive cutaneous lesions (Fig. 15-67) may be associated with pruritus and urticaria. Symptoms such as abdominal pain, diarrhea, flushing, syncope, headaches, tachycardia, or dyspnea result from release of mediators (e.g., histamine, proteases, eicosanoids, or heparin). Occasionally bone pain, fractures, or arthralgia may occur. There may be splenomegaly and, less frequently, hepatomegaly or lymphadenopathy. Radiography may reveal osteosclerosis or multiple irregular lytic skeletal lesions.

In many patients there is anemia, leukocytosis, eosinophilia, or leukopenia. In patients with aggressive forms of the disease, bone marrow failure may occur. In approximately 30% of patients, there is an associated clonal hematopoietic non–mast cell disorder (AHNMD), and the blood count and film may show abnormality related to these conditions. Significant numbers of mast cells are seen in blood films only in very rare cases classified as mast cell leukemia (see the following section). Serum tryptase levels are elevated in most patients.

Although bone marrow involvement by systemic mastocytosis is usually established in trephine biopsies, the diagnosis may also be evident in marrow aspirates (Fig. 15-68). Because most mast cells tend to adhere to the marrow fragments, squash preparations often produce the greatest number of mast cells (Fig. 15-69). The aspirate may show findings consistent with a coexisting hematopoietic clonal disorder (e.g., myelodysplastic syndrome [Figs. 15-70 and 15-71], acute myeloid leukemia, or myeloproliferative or lymphoproliferative disease [Fig. 15-72]).

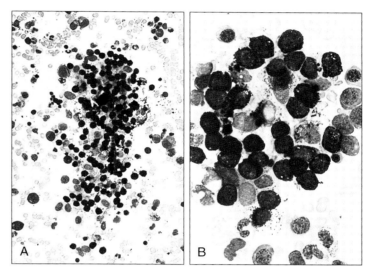

Fig. 15-68. Systemic mastocytosis: bone marrow aspirate showing an extensive accumulation of mast cells at low **(A)** and higher **(B)** power.

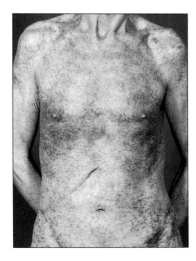

Fig. 15-67. Systemic mastocytosis: generalized pigmented and nodular cutaneous eruption seen after splenectomy and psoralen and ultraviolet A (PUVA) therapy.

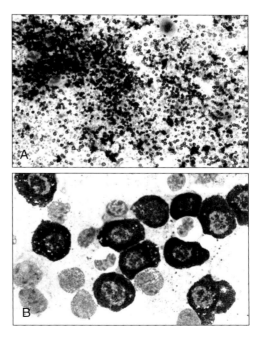

Fig.15-69. Systemic mastocytosis: bone marrow aspirate. **A,** Large numbers of mast cells are seen in the squashed fragment and cell trails. **B,** Typical mast cells at higher magnification.

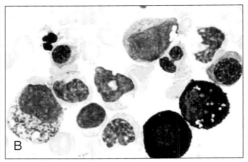
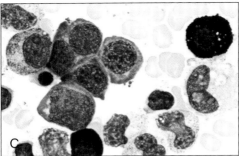

Fig. 15-70. Systemic mastocytosis and myelodysplastic syndrome (refractory anemia with ring sideroblasts): bone marrow aspirate. **A,** The fragment and cell trail are hypercellular with hematopoietic cells and large numbers of mast cells. **B,** At higher magnification, two mast cells and a dysplastic late erythroblast are shown. **C,** Macronormoblastic basophilic erythroblasts and mast cells.

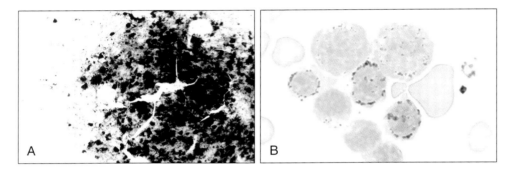

Fig. 15-71. Systemic mastocytosis and myelodysplastic syndrome (refractory anemia with ring sideroblasts): bone marrow aspirate in patient shown in Fig. 15-70. **A,** Fragmental iron stores are markedly increased. **B,** "Ring" sideroblasts.

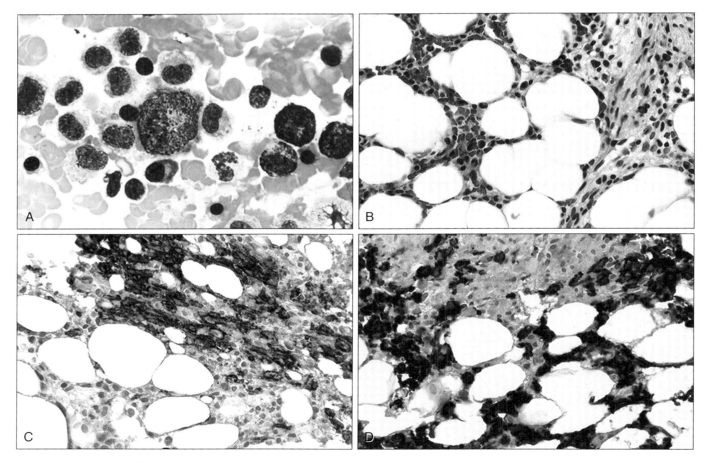

Fig. 15-72. Systemic mastocytosis and hairy cell leukemia. **A,** Bone marrow aspirate showing typical hairy cells and atypical mast cells. **B,** Bone marrow trephine biopsy shows spindle-shaped mast cells adjacent to marrow containing many hairy cells. **C,** Immunohistologic staining for mast cell tryptase shows strong positivity in the spindle-shaped mast cells. **D,** Immunohistologic staining for CD20 identifies the hairy cell population. (All images courtesy of Dr. James W. Vardiman.)

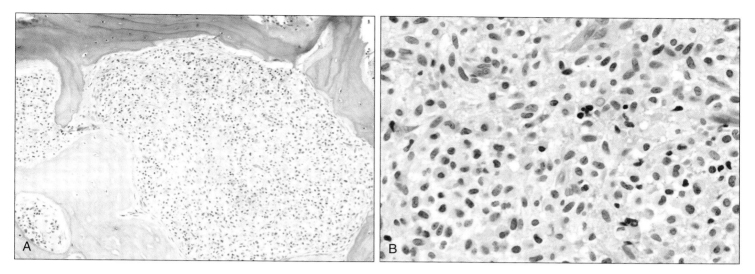

Fig. 15-73. Systemic mastocytosis: trephine biopsy. **A,** In the intertrabecular spaces there is almost complete replacement of normal hematopoietic cells by sheets of neoplastic mast cells. The bony trabeculae are thickened and show changes of early osteosclerosis. **B,** At higher magnification the densely packed mast cells include spindled forms with oval nuclei. (Courtesy of Dr. Christopher McNamara.)

In trephine biopsies the distribution of the neoplastic mast cells may be focal, peritrabecular, perivascular, or random. There may be associated lymphocytes, eosinophils, or fibroblasts. In patients with aggressive disease, the involvement is more extensive, with widespread replacement of normal hematopoietic cells (Figs. 15-73 and 15-74). Thickening of bony trabeculae and osteosclerosis may be evident. Osteolytic lesions are less common.

Although mast cell metachromatic granules may be seen with Giemsa or toluidine blue stains (see Fig. 15-73), immunostaining for mast cell tryptase is the most reliable method of identification (Fig. 15-75, *A*). CD117 is also a positive marker for mast cells (Fig. 15-75, *B*) but is not specific. Neoplastic mast cells, unlike normal mast cells, express both CD25 (Fig. 15-75, *C*) and CD2 on their surface.

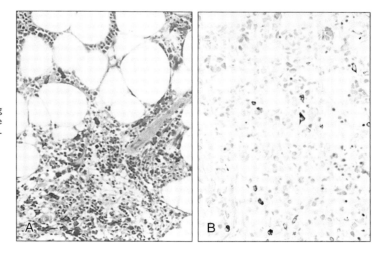

Fig. 15-74. Systemic mastocytosis: trephine biopsy. **A,** Low power view showing perivascular accumulation of mast cells. Mast cells are also present around the edge of a lymphoid follicle. **B,** Characteristic metachromatic staining reaction in the cytoplasm of mast cells with toluidine blue.

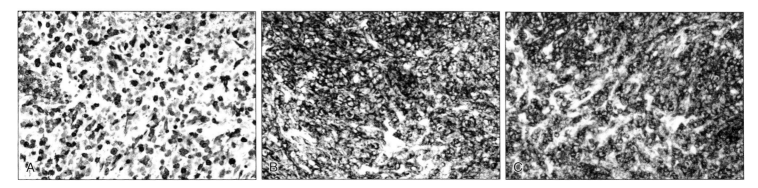

Fig.15-75. Systemic mastocytosis: trephine biopsy. Immunohistologic staining reveals strong positivity for mast cell tryptase **(A),** CD117 **(B),** and CD25 **(C).** (Courtesy of Dr. Christopher McNamara.)

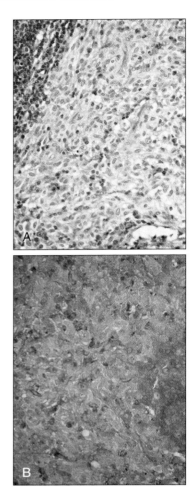

Fig. 15-76. Systemic mastocytosis: sections of spleen showing mononuclear histocyte-like cells on staining with hematoxylin and eosin **(A)** and toluidine blue **(B)** to demonstrate the cytoplasmic metachromasia. (*A* and *B*, Courtesy of Dr. J. E. McLaughlin.)

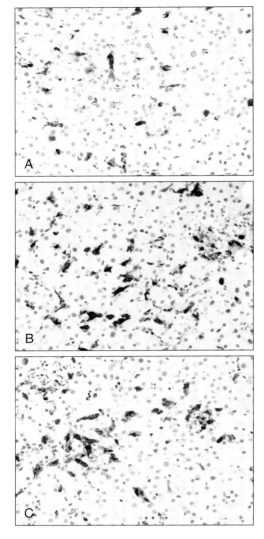

Fig. 15-78. Systemic mastocytosis: liver biopsy. Immunohistologic staining shows strong positivity in mast cells with mast cell tryptase **(A)**, CD117 **(B)**, and CD25 **(C)**. (Courtesy of Dr. Christopher McNamara.)

Splenectomy may show extensive splenic disease (Fig. 15-76), and liver biopsy may identify periportal and sinus mast cell infiltration with associated fibrosis (Figs. 15-77 and 15-78) or even cirrhosis.

The WHO diagnostic criteria for systemic mastocytosis are listed in Table 15-9.

MAST CELL LEUKEMIA

Mast cell leukemia is the rarest form of aggressive systemic mastocytosis. Abnormal mast cells make up more than 20% of cells in marrow and usually over 10% of white cells in the blood

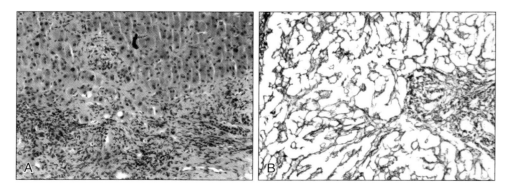

Fig. 15-77. Systemic mastocytosis: liver biopsy. **A,** There is a dense infiltrate of spindle-shaped mast cells in the periportal zone with extension of these neoplastic mast cells into the sinusoids. **B,** Reticulin staining shows periportal fibrosis and widespread thickening around the sinusoids. (Courtesy of Dr. Christopher McNamara.)

TABLE 15-9.   WORLD HEALTH ORGANIZATION CRITERIA FOR DIAGNOSIS OF SYSTEMIC MASTOCYTOSIS

Major criteria

Multifocal, dense infiltrates of mast cells (15 or more mast cells in aggregates) detected in sections of bone marrow and/or other extracutaneous organ(s), and confirmed by tryptase immunochemistry or other special stains

Minor criteria

In biopsy sections of bone marrow or other extracutaneous organs, more than 25% of the mast cells in the infiltrate are spindle shaped or have atypical morphology, or of all mast cells in bone marrow aspirate smears, more than 25% are immature or atypical mast cells

Detection of *KIT* point mutation at codon 816 in bone marrow, blood, or other extracutaneous organ(s)

Mast cells in bone marrow, blood, or other extracutaneous organs that co-express CD117 with CD2 and/or CD25

Serum total tryptase persistently >20 ng/ml (unless there is an associated clonal myeloid disorder, in which case this parameter is not valid)

The diagnosis of systemic mastocytosis may be made if one major and one minor criterion are present or if three minor criteria are fulfilled

(Fig. 15-79, *A*). Trephine biopsies show extensive involvement similar to aggressive systemic mastocytosis (Fig. 15-79, *B* to *D*). The initial manifestation of the disease is similar to other forms of aggressive systemic mastocytosis with flushing, hypotension, and diarrhea. Later there is multiple organ involvement with weight loss, bone pain, hepatomegaly, and splenomegaly. Plasma tryptase levels are extremely high.

MAST CELL SARCOMA

Mast cell sarcoma is an exceedingly rare tumor with only a few well-documented cases. At presentation it may be a localized tumor with an invasive growth pattern and pleomorphic immature cytology. All reported cases have evolved into an aggressive form of systemic mastocytosis. Images from a primary skin mast cell sarcoma are shown in Fig. 15-80.

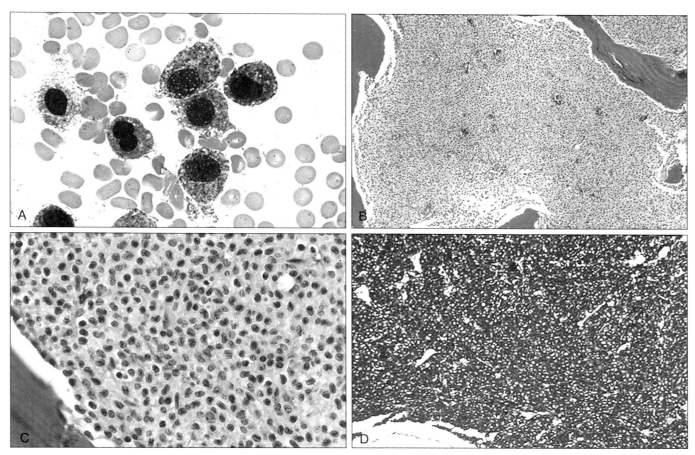

Fig. 15-79. Mast cell leukemia. **A,** Peripheral blood film shows numerous mast cells, some with defective granulation and one with a bilobed nucleus. **B,** Bone marrow trephine biopsy shows a diffuse sheet-like proliferation of neoplastic mast cells. **C,** At higher magnification, the cells have a clear cell appearance resulting from poor granulation of the immature leukemic mast cell population. **D,** Immunohistologic staining shows strong positivity for mast cell tryptase. (All images courtesy of Dr. James W. Vardiman.)

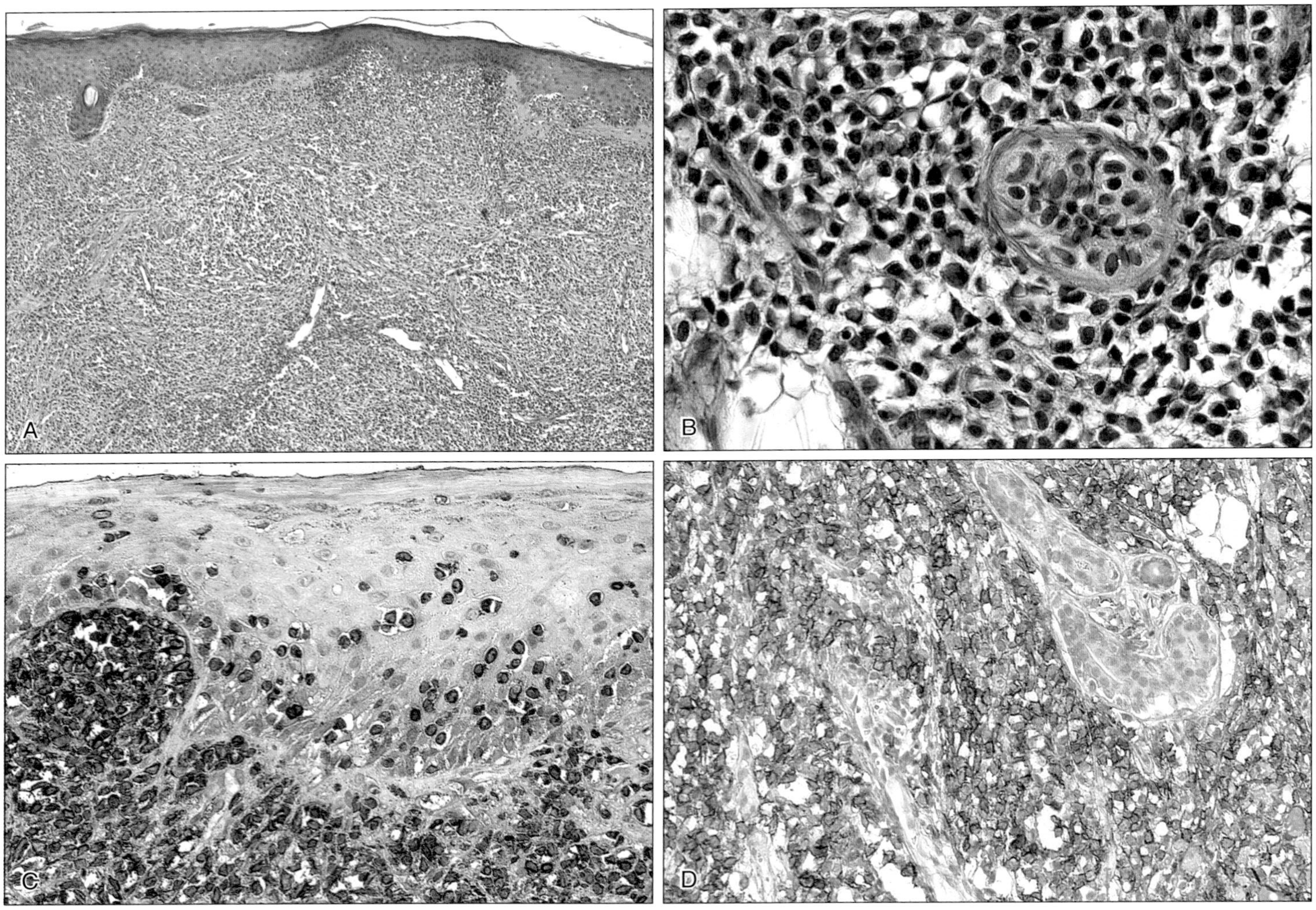

Fig. 15-80. Mast cell sarcoma. **A,** Sheets of malignant mast cells occupy the dermis with extension into the subcutaneous tissue. **B,** At higher magnification the tumor consists of pleomorphic, oval, and polygonal neoplastic cells that show no evidence of mast cell differentiation in the H & E–stained section. There is invasion of subcutaneous fat, and the malignant cells are seen within a lymphatic or venous vascular space. **C,** Immunohistologic staining for mast cell tryptase identifies the mast cell origin of the malignant cells. The tumor cells are seen migrating through the epidermis (epidermotrophism). **D,** Immunohistologic staining for CD117 is also positive in the malignant mast cells, which in this image are adjacent to sweat glands in the superficial subcutaneous fat. (All images courtesy of Professor H-P. Horny.)

EXTRACUTANEOUS MASTOCYTOMA

Extracutaneous mastocytoma, also rare and mostly reported in the lung, is a tumor of typical mature mast cells similar to those seen in cutaneous mastocytoma.

PROGNOSIS

The prognosis in mastocytosis is variable. Cutaneous mastocytosis in children usually resolves before or during puberty, but in adults regression is rare and skin involvement is often associated with systemic disease. There is no satisfactory cure for systemic mastocytosis. Although patients with indolent forms and skin involvement may have a normal life expectancy, those with aggressive disease have a life expectancy of weeks or, at best, less than a year.

HISTIOCYTIC DISORDERS

INTRODUCTION

This chapter includes discussion of both reactive proliferative conditions and the histiocytic and dendritic cell neoplasms.

HEMOPHAGOCYTIC SYNDROME

The hemophagocytic syndrome is the most frequently seen proliferative disorder of macrophages and is more common than malignant tumors of histiocytes. The syndrome occurs in a familial primary form with a recessive inheritance pattern that affects infants and young children and in an acquired secondary form. Sporadic cases are seen in association with the genetic immune deficiencies Chediak-Higashi syndrome, Griscelli syndrome and X-linked lymphoproliferative syndrome.

The hemophagocytic syndrome is not a clonal or neoplastic disease but is probably a reactive proliferative disorder related to an excessive production of monocyte-stimulating cytokines (e.g., interleukins 1, 2, and 10), tumor necrosis factor α and interferon γ, and chemokines (e.g., MIP-1a, Mig, and IP-10). Infection with Epstein–Barr virus or

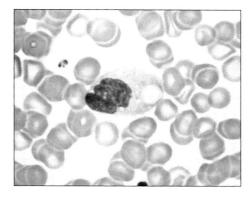

Fig. 16-1. Hemophagocytic syndrome: blood film showing a phagocytosed red cell inside a monocyte.

another virus is frequently the initiating event. There is uncontrolled macrophage activation and enhanced phagocytic activity.

Defects of performin and other proteins of the cytolytic pathway have been associated with defective T-cell function and the hemophagocytic syndrome. In the primary inherited form, mutations in the performin gene at locus 10q24 and defects in performin synthesis have been found in up to 40% of affected patients. Similar defects have also been found in patients treated later in life with presumed acquired disease. Less common mutations in primary inherited hemophagocytic syndrome include those of the *UNC13D* gene at locus 17q25 and the *STX11* gene at locus 6q24. An external cause (e.g., infection) is probably necessary to initiate or trigger the activation of the disease.

The acquired form may be precipitated by viral, bacterial, fungal, or protozoan infections, and is also seen in immunocompromised patients, in connective tissue or autoimmune disorders, and in patients with lymphoma or leukemia. Previously similar clinical conditions labeled as hemophagic lymphohistiocytosis and histiocytic medullary reticulosis are now considered part of this syndrome. Although most patients previously diagnosed with malignant histiocytosis would now be classified as having large cell malignant lymphoma, many had features identical to the hemophagocytic syndrome.

Patients with hemophagocytic syndrome have fever, pancytopenia, liver dysfunction, or neurologic symptoms. Phagocytosis of red cells by monocytes may be seen in the blood film (Fig. 16-1). Fibrinogen levels are usually low, and prolongation of the activated partial thromboplastin time (APTT) may indicate an associated coagulopathy. Serum ferritin and triglyceride levels are elevated. Special studies may show low or absent natural killer (NK) cell activity. Bone marrow aspirates show histiocytic hyperplasia and hemophagocytosis (Figs. 16-2 to 16-4). Trephine biopsies may show extensive replacement of other hematopoietic cells by sheets of hyperplastic histiocytes (Fig. 16-5). The bone marrow features in a patient with virus-associated hemophagocytic syndrome are illustrated in Fig. 16-6. Liver biopsy may show hemophagocytosis, histiocytic infiltration, and areas of necrosis (Fig. 16-7). Histiocytic proliferation also occurs in the spleen, lymph nodes, and other tissues. In the familial form there is often central nervous system involvement (Fig. 16-8).

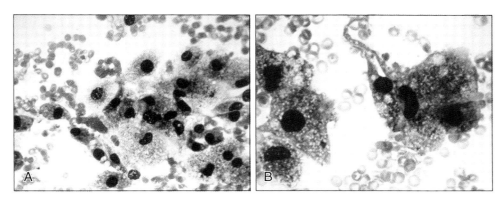

Fig. 16-2. Hemophagocytic syndrome. **A,** Bone marrow aspirate in a 64-year-old man with pancytopenia, hepatomegaly, and splenomegaly showing abnormal histiocytes in the cell trail. **B,** At high power the cells show considerable nuclear pleomorphism and abundant vacuolated cytoplasm.

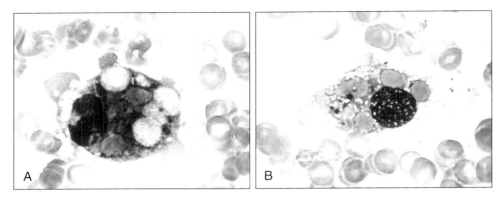

Fig. 16-3. Hemophagocytic syndrome. **A** and **B,** Bone marrow aspirate images showing prominent red cell phagocytosis in abnormal histiocytes.

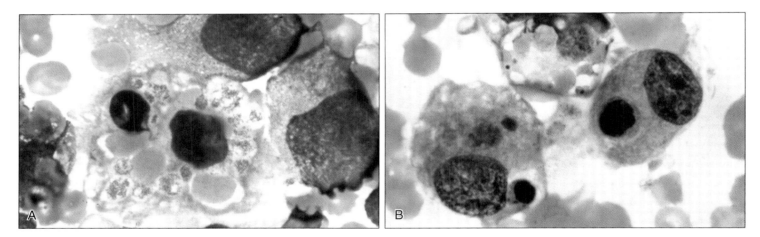

Fig. 16-4. Famialial hemophagocytic syndrome. **A** and **B,** Bone marrow aspirate images showing two abnormal histiocytes with phagocytosed red cells, platelets, and lymphocytes. (Courtesy of Dr. Imashuku.)

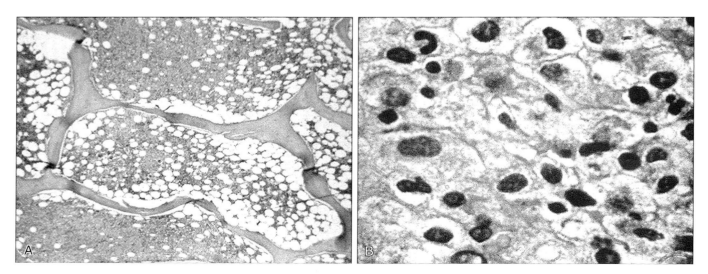

Fig. 16-5. Hemophagocytic syndrome: trephine biopsy in the same case shown in Fig. 16-2. **A,** There is extensive replacement of normal intertrabecular hematopoietic tissue by sheets of abnormal histiocytes. **B,** At higher magnification the cells are pleomorphic with hyperchromatic nuclei and abundant vacuolated cytoplasm.

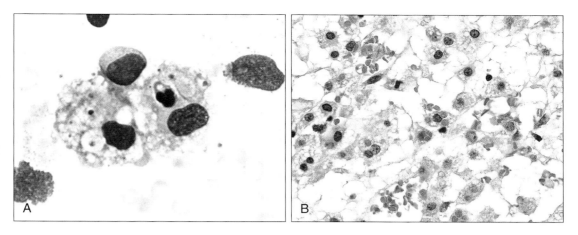

Fig. 16-6. Virus-associated hemophagocytic syndrome. **A,** Bone marrow aspirate showing two histiocytes that have engulfed red cells and erythroblasts. **B,** Bone marrow trephine biopsy showing replacement of normal architecture by erythrophagocytic histiocytes. (*A,* Courtesy of Dr. S. Knowles. *B,* Courtesy of Professor K. A. MacLennan.)

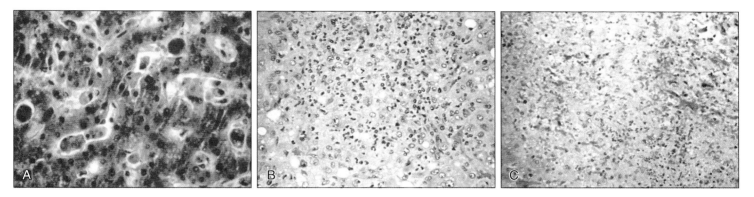

Fig. 16-7. Hemophagocytic syndrome: liver biopsies in different patients. **A,** This image shows sinusoidal Küpffer cell erythrophagocytosis. **B,** Infiltration of parenchymal cells by abnormal histiocytes. **C,** Associated areas of liver cell necrosis.

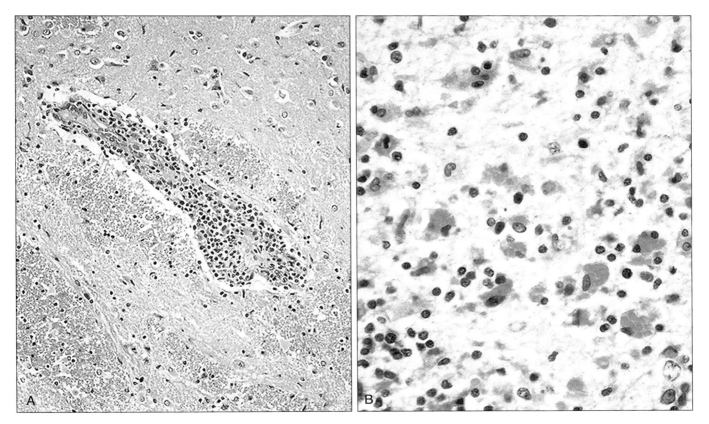

Fig. 16-8. Familial hemophagocytic syndrome. **A,** Section of brain at necropsy showing a collection of lymphocytes in the perivascular (Virchow–Robin) space. **B,** Higher magnification shows histiocytes that contain both red cells (erythrophagocytosis) and lymphocytes (lymphophagocytosis). (*A* and *B,* Courtesy of Dr. J. E. McLaughlin.)

XANTHOGRANULOMA

Xanthogranuloma is an uncommon histiocytic "tumor" arising in the first five years of life. Yellowish to reddish nodular "tumors" measuring up to several cm in diameter are usually solitary and are most frequent in the skin of the head and neck region, although other skin regions, mucus membranes, or almost any site in the body may be involved. Less commonly there are multiple tumors. Systemic spread from the primary site is rarely seen. Xanthogranuloma is most probably a reactive proliferation and there is usually a spontaneous involution. Histologically the skin "tumors" show intradermal collections of histiocytes with eosinophilic or vacuolated cytoplasm with variable numbers of Touton type giant cells (Figs. 16-9 and 16-10). Some lesions show small numbers of neutrophils, eosinophils, lymphocytes, or plasma cells. In establilshed lesions lipid accumulation (Fig. 16-11) and xanthoma cells are prominent. The histiocytes show positivity for CD45, CD68, CD4, and HLA-Dr and are negative for CD1a.

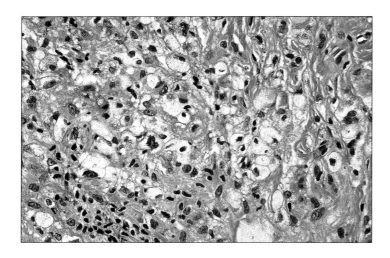

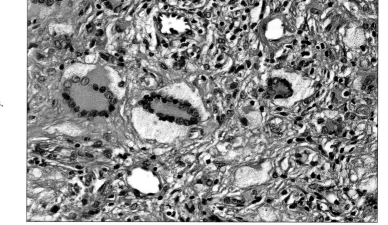

Fig. 16-9. Xanthogranuloma: skin biopsy showing an established lesion consisting of histiocytes, lymphocytes, and xanthoma cells. (Courtesy of Professor P. H. McKee.)

Fig. 16-10. Xanthogranuloma: skin biopsy showing multinucleated giant cells, which are a characteristic feature. (Courtesy of Professor P. H. McKee.)

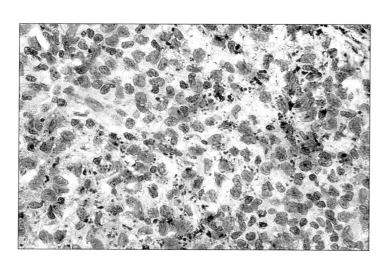

Fig. 16-11. Xanthogranuloma: skin biopsy. The presence of lipid can be identified in frozen sections stained with oil red O. (Courtesy of Professor P. H. McKee.)

ROSAI–DORFMAN DISEASE

Rosai–Dorfman disease, or sinus histiocytosis with massive lymphadenopathy, is a rare condition seen most frequently in young blacks. It is characterized by lymphadenopathy, fever, leucocytosis, and hypergammaglobulinemia. It is thought to be the result of an abnormal reaction to a viral infection. The cervical nodes are usually involved (Fig. 16-12). Histologically the nodes show marked sinusoidal dilation by macrophages with foamy cytoplasm (Fig. 16-13) and plasma cells. There is

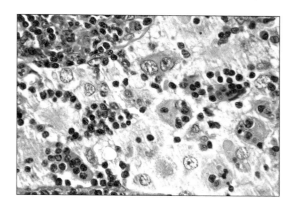

Fig. 16-14. Rosai–Dorfman disease: lymph node biopsy. High-power view showing characteristic histiocytes with engulfment of lymphocytes. (Courtesy of Professor K. A. MacLennan.)

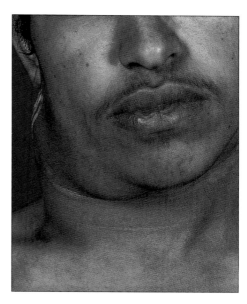

Fig. 16-12. Rosai–Dorfman disease: massive painless cervical lymphadenopathy in a teenager from the Middle East. This resolved spontaneously over a 2-year period.

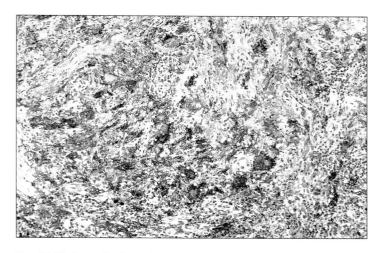

Fig. 16-15. Rosai–Dorfman disease: lymph node biopsy. The histiocytes are S-100 positive. (Courtesy of Professor P. H. McKee.)

often evidence of engulfment of lymphocytes by the hyperplastic histiocytes (Fig. 16-14). Immunohistologic staining demonstrates strong positivity for S-100 (Fig. 16-15). Although the disease may follow a protracted course, recovery is usually spontaneous and total.

HISTIOCYTIC AND DENDRITIC CELL NEOPLASMS

The 2008 World Health Organization (WHO) histologic classification of histiocytic and dendritic cell tumors is shown in Table 16-1. Table 16-2 lists the characteristic immunophenotypic marker patterns of histiocytes and accessory dendritic cells which help to identify the tumor type.

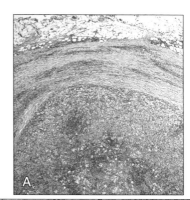

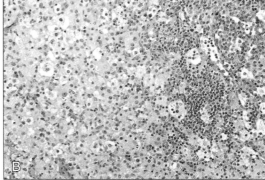

Fig. 16-13. Rosai–Dorfman disease. **A,** Lymph node biopsy showing marked capsular and pericapsular fibrosis. The sinuses are distended by a proliferation of histiocytes. This condition may occasionally be confused with a histiocytic lymphoma. **B,** Higher-power view shows a confluent mass of histiocytes with abundant vacuolated cytoplasm. There is a focal collection of lymphocytes and residual medullary cords.

TABLE 16-1.	WORLD HEALTH ORGANIZATION CLASSIFICATION OF TUMORS OF THE HISTIOCYTIC SYSTEM
Histiocytic sarcoma	
Langerhans cell histiocytosis	
Langerhans cell sarcoma	
Interdigitating dendritic cell sarcoma	
Follicular dendritic cell sarcoma	
Fibroblastic reticular cell tumor	
Indeterminate dendritic cell tumor	
Disseminated juvenile xanthogranuloma	

TABLE 16-2.   IMMUNOPHENOTYPES OF THE HISTIOCYTIC TUMORS

	CD68	LYS	CD1a	S100	FDC (CD21, 35)
Histiocytic sarcoma	+	+	−	−/+	−
Langerhans cell tumor/sarcoma	+	+/−	+	+	−
Interdigitating cell tumor/sarcoma	+/−	−	−	+	−
Follicular dendritic cell tumor/sarcoma	+/−	−	−	−/+	+

After Pileri SA: *Histopathology* 41:1–29, 2002.
LYS, Lysozyme.

HISTIOCYTIC SARCOMA

Histiocytic sarcoma is a rare tumor associated with an aggressive clinical course. Most cases occur in adults. The most common presenting feature is lymphadenopathy, closely followed by gastrointestinal or skin involvement. Fever, weight loss, blood pancytopenia, hepatomegaly, and splenomegaly may be present in those with systemic involvement through metastatic spread.

Characteristic histologic features of the malignant cells are depicted in Fig. 16-16. The cells are large and polymorphic with round or oval nuclei and abundant eosinophilic or foamy cytoplasm. The neoplastic cells are associated with a dense reticulin fiber network (Fig. 16-17). They must be differentiated from large cell lymphomas by the demonstration of histiocytic markers, such as lysozyme (Fig. 16-18), CD68, CD110, or CD14. Images from a further case of histiocytic sarcoma are shown in Fig. 16-19.

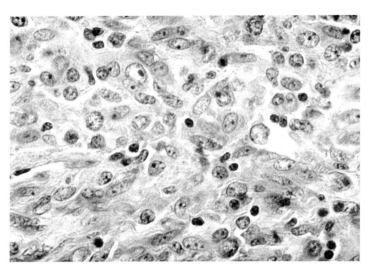

Fig. 16-16. Histiocytic sarcoma: histologic section of lymph node showing replacement of normal architecture by abnormal histiocytic cells with abundant cytoplasm.

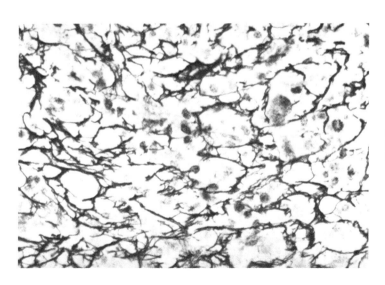

Fig. 16-17. Histiocytic sarcoma. Silver impregnation staining of the case in Fig. 16-16 shows a prominent dense reticulin fiber network surrounding individual tumor cells.

Fig. 16-18. Histiocytic sarcoma. Immunoperoxidase staining for lysozyme of the case in Fig. 16-16 shows a proportion of positive cells indicating a monocytic-histiocytic origin. The cells were also positive for α_1-antitrypsin.

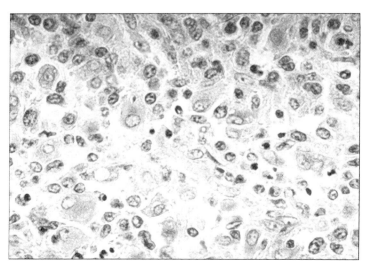

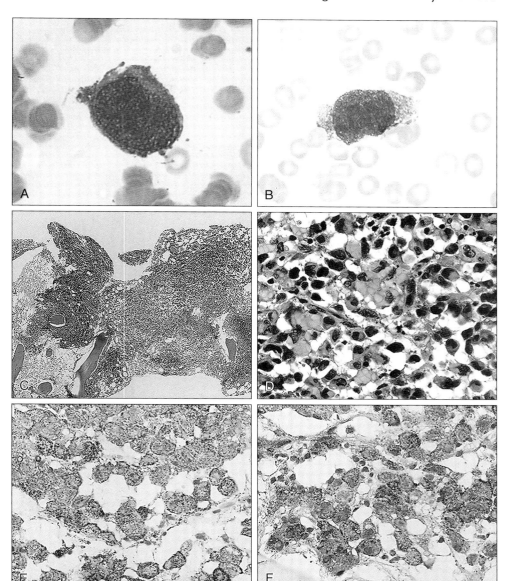

Fig. 16-19. Histiocytic sarcoma. **A** and **B,** Two examples of the large atypical monocytoid cells in peripheral blood. **C,** Trephine biopsy showing extensive replacement of hematopoietic tissue and fat by tumor. **D,** At higher magnification the atypical monocytoid cells are pleomorphic with hyperchromic nuclei and abundant cytoplasm, which in some cells show vacuolation. **E,** Immunoperoxidase staining shows cytoplasmic positivity for CD68 and lysozyme **(F);** the cells are also positive for CD45. (Courtesy of Professor P. G. Isaacson.)

LANGERHANS CELL HISTIOCYTOSIS

Langerhans cell histiocytosis comprises the diseases previously known as histiocytosis X: Letterer–Siwe disease, Hand–Schuller–Christian disease, and eosinophilic granuloma of bone. Langerhans cells are distinguished on electron microscopy by the presence of Birbeck granules (Fig. 16-20) and by immunohistologic positivity for CD1a and S100. Normal Langerhans cells are antigen-presenting cells, but the neoplastic cells of Langerhans cell histiocytosis are primitive dendritic cells and have lost this function. Small numbers of families have had more than one relative affected, and the disease has occurred in several sets of monozygotic and dizygotic twins. Although these family clusters support a role for genetic factors, no chromosomal abnormalities have been established. A number of studies have suggested that, like other pediatric clonal neoplastic proliferations, Langerhans cell histiocytosis may require a two-step mutational process.

In Langerhans cell histiocytosis the neoplastic cells, sometimes associated with eosinophils, lymphocytes, neutrophils, and macrophages, infiltrate a wide variety of organs, especially the skin, bone, lymph nodes, liver, spleen, and bone marrow. The disease may involve a single system or involve multiple systems. The central nervous

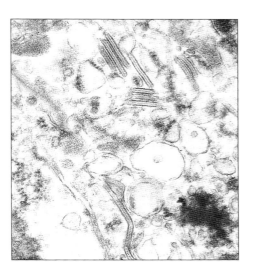

Fig. 16-20. Langerhans cell histiocytosis: Birbeck granules in the cytoplasm. These are rod-shaped structures with a central striated line that terminates in some cases in a vesicular dilation, which gives a tennis racquet appearance. They may arise secondary to receptor-mediated endocytosis and are not present in normal monocytes and non-Langerhans macrophages. (Courtesy of Professor P. Lanzkowsky.)

system, lungs, and gastrointestinal tract may also become involved. Multisystem disease usually affects children initially in the first 3 years of life, with hepatomegaly, splenomegaly, lymphadenopathy, and eczematoid skin eruptions (Fig. 16-21). Localized lesions occur frequently in the skull (Figs. 16-22 to 16-24), ribs, and long bones. Involvement of the central nervous system may result in degenerative changes in the cerebellum (Fig. 16-25). In familial forms of Langerhans cell histiocytosis, the disease may involve white matter of the cerebral hemispheres (Fig. 16-26). Diabetes insipidus may follow disease in the hypothalamus and pituitary stalk (Fig. 16-27). Lung involvement causes extensive fibrocystic changes resulting in a characteristic radiographic "honeycomb lung" (Fig. 16-28).

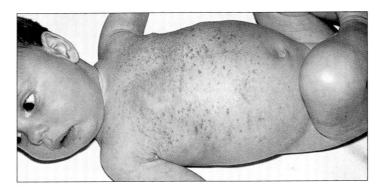

Fig. 16-21. Multisystem Langerhans cell histiocytosis: typical hemorrhagic eczematoid rash in a 10-month-old child. (Courtesy of Dr. M. D. Holdaway.)

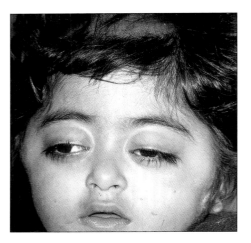

Fig. 16-22. Multisystem Langerhans cell histiocytosis: prominent bossing of the frontal bone and proptosis in a child with multiple skull deposits. (Courtesy of Dr. U. O'Callaghan.)

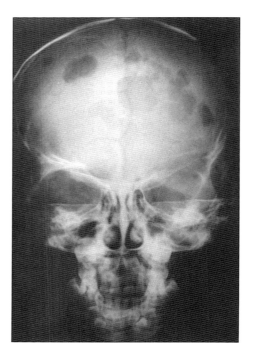

Fig. 16-23. Multisystem Langerhans cell histiocytosis: skull x-ray showing the presence of numerous osteolytic lesions. (Courtesy of Dr. S. Imashuku.)

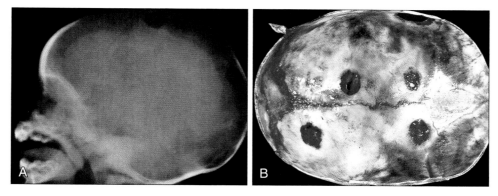

Fig. 16-24. Multisystem Langerhans cell histiocytosis: skull of an infant seen radiographically **(A)** and at necropsy **(B)** shows the typical osteolytic deposits in the vault.

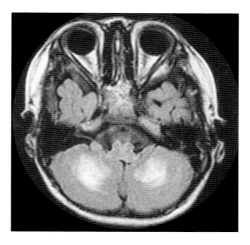

Fig. 16-25. Multisystem Langerhans cell histiocytosis: magnetic resonance imaging (MRI) scan showing increased signal in the cerebellum indicating cerebellar degeneration. (Courtesy of Dr. S. Imashuku.)

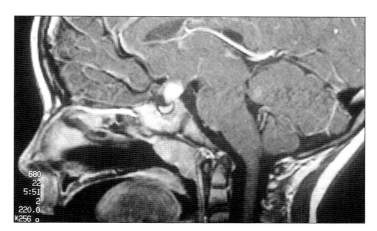

Fig. 16-27. Multisystem Langerhans cell histiocytosis: magnetic resonance imaging (MRI) showing thickened pituitary stalk with absent posterior pituitary signal on T1-weighted images. (Courtesy of Dr. D. K. H. Webb.)

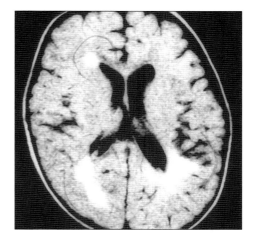

Fig. 16-26. Multisystem Langerhans cell histiocytosis: magnetic resonance imaging (MRI) scan showing increased signal in the white matter of the occipital and frontal lobes in a patient with the familial form of the disease. (Courtesy of Dr. S. Imashuku.)

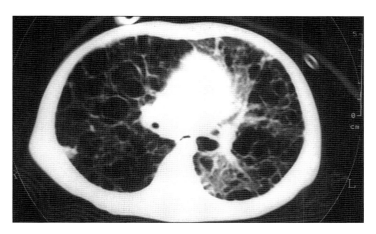

Fig. 16-28. Multisystem Langerhans cell histiocytosis: magnetic resonance imaging (MRI) scan showing extensive fibrocystic changes in the lungs ("honeycomb lung"). (Courtesy of Dr. S. Imashuku.)

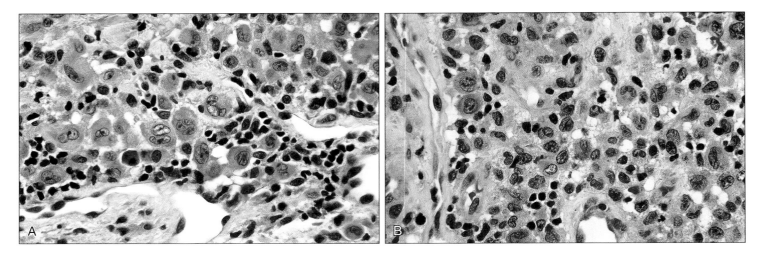

Fig. 16-29. Multisystem Langerhans cell histiocytosis: skin biopsy. **A,** This field shows typical coffee bean vesicular nuclei. **B,** A nucleus with a nuclear groove is present in the center of the field. (Courtesy of Professor P. H. McKee.)

Typical histologic features in skin biopsies are shown in Figs. 16-29 to 16-31. Langerhans cells are recognized by their characteristically grooved, folded, or lobulated nuclei with fine chromatin and inconspicuous nucleoli and moderately abundant cytoplasm. Bone marrow aspirates may occasionally show cells with typical Langerhans cell features (Fig. 16-32), but evidence of involvement is more easily seen in trephine biopsies. In localized disease in bone, the Langerhans cells are associated with eosinophils (Fig. 16-33). Biopsy of later localized osteolytic bone lesions shows sheets of lipid-laden foam cells (Fig. 16-34).

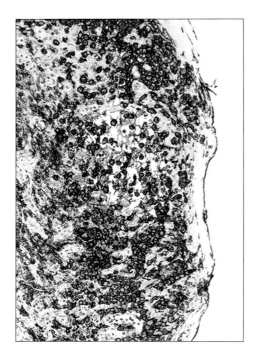

Fig. 16-31. Multisystem Langerhans cell histiocytosis: skin biopsy. CD1a is also strongly positive. (Courtesy of Professor P. H. McKee.)

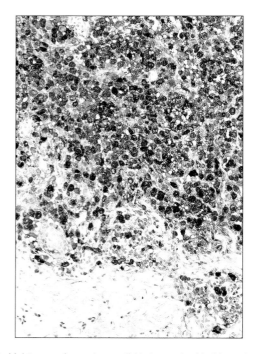

Fig. 16-30. Multisystem Langerhans cell histiocytosis: skin biopsy. Immunohistologic staining shows a uniform expression of S-100 in tumor cells. (Courtesy of Professor P. H. McKee.)

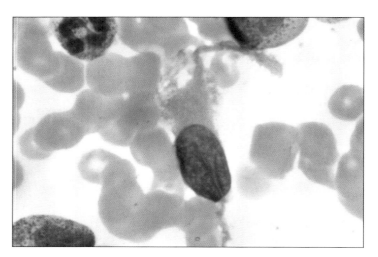

Fig. 16-32. Multisystem Langerhans cell histiocytosis: bone marrow aspirate showing a Langerhans cell with a central nuclear groove. (Courtesy of Dr. S. Imashuku.)

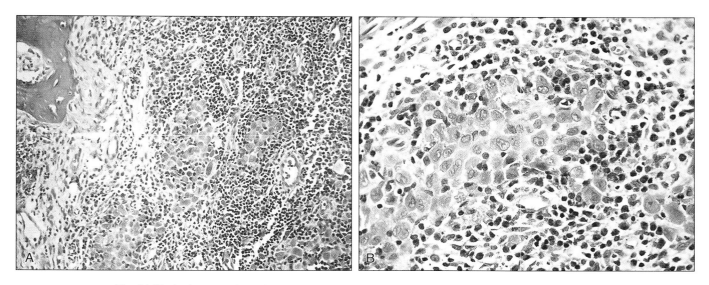

Fig. 16-33. Single-system Langerhans cell histiocytosis: trephine biopsy of a 28-year-old man with skeletal lesions shows replacement of normal hematopoietic tissue by sheets of histiocytes and eosinophils **(A)**; higher-power view of the abnormal histiocytes and eosinophils **(B).**

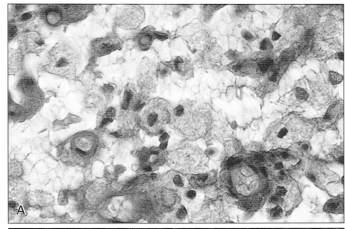

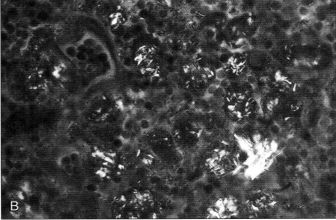

Fig. 16-34. Multisystem Langerhans cell histiocytosis: frozen sections of a skeletal lesion stained using the Sudan IV technique and viewed under normal **(A)** and polarized **(B)** light. The staining reaction indicated accumulation in the cytoplasm of neutral fat and cholesterol.

LANGERHANS CELL SARCOMA

Langerhans cell sarcoma is exceedingly rare. It has been reported in both adults and children. Multisystem involvement includes lymph nodes, liver, spleen, lung, and bone. Histology (Fig. 16-35) shows large cells with malignant features including hyperchromatic nuclei and prominent nucleoli. There may be nuclear grooves similar to those found in Langerhans cell histiocytosis, and there is a high mitotic rate. Birbeck granules are present on electron microscopy. Immunohistologic staining shows S-100 and focal CD1a positivity and, in some cases, positivity for CD68, CD45, and lysozyme.

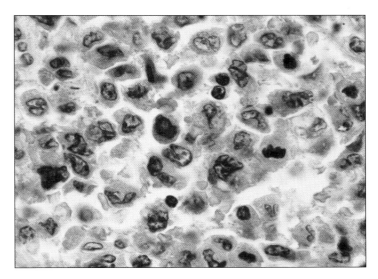

Fig. 16-35. Langerhans cell sarcoma: high-power histologic section showing pleomorphic cells resembling Langerhans cells with nuclear folding and eosinophilic cytoplasm, but also showing malignant features such as nuclear hyperchromatism, prominent nucleoli, and multinuclearity. There are numerous mitoses. (Courtesy of Dr. L. M. Weiss.)

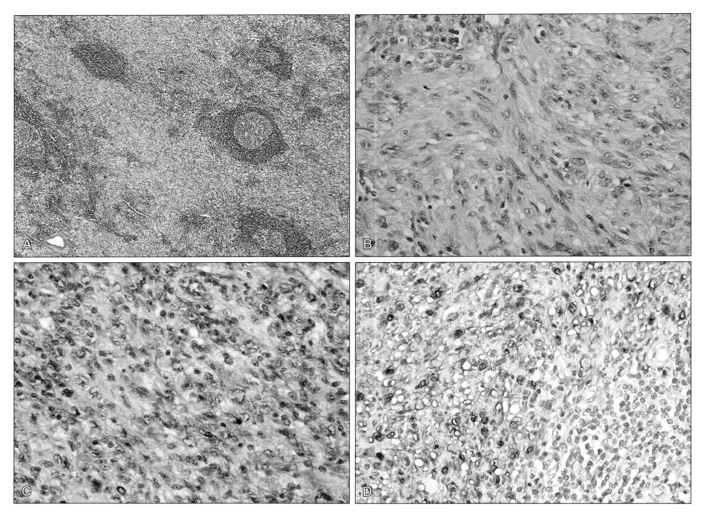

Fig. 16-36. Interdigitating dendritic cell sarcoma: lymph node biopsy. **A,** A low-power image shows extensive paracortical tumor with residual lymphoid follicles. **B,** At higher power many of the tumor cells are spindle shaped with indistinct borders and bland nuclei with a vesicular chromatin pattern. **C,** In other areas the tumor cells are rounded and more pleomorphic, and some have single nucleoli. **D,** Immunohistologic staining with S-100 shows positivity for the tumor cells, but there is no labeling of cells in the residual lymphoid follicle on the lower right. (Courtesy of Dr. David Ellis.)

INTERDIGITATING DENDRITIC CELL SARCOMA

Interdigitating dendritic cell sarcoma is another exceedingly rare tumor. Asymptomatic lymph node involvement is most common, but some cases have involved skin tumors. In some patients there is an aggressive clinical course with fever, weight loss, hepatomegaly, splenomegaly, and gastrointestinal involvement. Histologic examination of excised lymph nodes shows a paracortical distribution of tumor cells with residual lymphoid follicles (Fig.16-36, *A*). The neoplastic dendritic cells form fascicles and whorls of oval and spindled cells with areas of more rounded larger cells (Fig. 16-36, *B* and *C*). The tumor cells consistently show S-100 positivity (Fig. 16-36, *D*) and are negative for the markers used to identify follicular dendritic cells, CD21 and CD35.

FOLLICULAR DENDRITIC CELL SARCOMA

Follicular dendritic cell tumors are also rare. In 10% to 20% of cases there has been an association with Castleman's disease. Over half the cases described present with asymptomatic lymphadenopathy. Cervical sites are most common, with fewer patients having

axillary, mesenteric, mediastinal, or retroperitoneal nodal involvement. Other documented sites include the tonsil, spleen, oral cavity, gastrointestinal tract, liver, soft tissues, skin, and breast. Compared with interdigitating dendritic cell sarcomas, follicular dendritic tumors are typically indolent and tend to be localized with a potential for local spread or recurrence with less frequent spread to distant sites.

Histologic examination of excised nodes (Fig. 16-37, *A* and *B*) shows neoplastic ovoid and spindle-shaped cells often in fascicles, storiform, or whorling patterns. Residual lymphocytes are scattered throughout the tumor cells or in perivascular locations. Immunohistologic stains show positivity for one or more of the follicular dendritic cell markers CD21, CD35, and CD23 (Fig. 16-37, *C*).

INDETERMINATE DENDRITIC CELL TUMOR

This very rare tumor is thought to derive from the precursor cells of Langerhans cells. There is a diffuse dermal and subcutaneous infiltrate of neoplastic ovoid and spindle-shaped cells that express S100 protein and CD1a but lack Birbeck granules on electron microscopy.

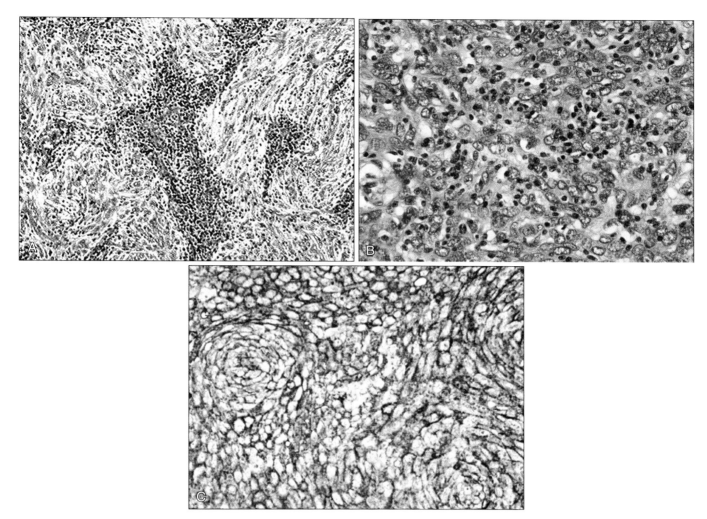

Fig. 16-37. Follicular dendritic cell tumor: lymph node biopsy. **A,** At low power there are sheets, fascicles, and whorls of spindle and oval tumor cells with perivascular collections of residual lymphocytes. **B,** In a higher-power view the cells show mild atypia with vesicular nuclei and indistinct cytoplasmic outlines. Occasional cells have multiple nuclei. Small numbers of small lymphocytes are scattered within the tumor. **C,** Immunostaining with CD21 shows strong positivity and outlines a prominent whorl of tumor cells on the left. (Courtesy of Dr. L. M. Weiss.)

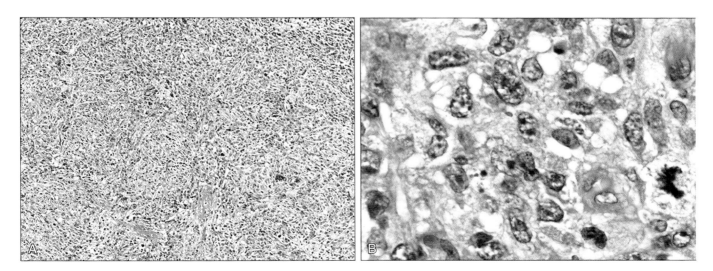

Fig. 16-38. Dendritic cell sarcoma. **A,** Lymph node biopsy showing complete replacement of normal architecture by pleomorphic oval- and spindle-shaped cells with some areas showing a storiform ("cartwheel") appearance. **B,** At higher magnification, the cells show irregular vesicular nuclei and pale cytoplasm within distinct borders. A prominent mitotic figure is seen here. Immunostaining was not carried out.

FIBROBLASTIC RETICULAR CELL TUMOR

Tumors arising from the fibroblastic reticular (dendritic) stromal support cells of lymph nodes, spleen and tonsil are very rare. These tumors show a whorled pattern of oval and spindle cells in a collagenous background. Immunostaining shows variable positivity for CD21, CD35, vimentin, desmin, smooth muscle actin, CD68, and cytokeratin.

BLASTIC PLASMACYTOID DENDRITIC CELL NEOPLASM

This tumor, previously known as blastic NK/T-cell lymphoma and hematodermic dendritic cell tumor (Fig. 16-39), is rare and has an aggressive course. The tumor usually occurs in the skin. In most patients there is involvement of bone marrow (Fig. 16-40), lymph nodes, and peripheral blood. The skin shows a dermal infiltrate of medium-sized lymphoid cell resembling lymphoblasts.

Tumor cells express CD4 and CD56, and the primitive hematopoietic marker TdT is usually positive (see Fig. 16-39). T-cell receptor genes are germline and the tumor cells are negative for Epstein–Barr virus. Chemotherapy similar to that used in acute leukemia usually induces remission, but relapse and resistance to further chemotherapy is common. The median survival is about 14 months.

In the current (2008) WHO classification this tumor is listed with acute leukemias.

DISSEMINATED JUVENILE XANTHOGRANULOMA

Disseminated and visceral forms of juvenile xanthogranuloma are rare and most occur in infants and children. There is evidence of clonality in some cases. Erdheim-Chester disease is a rare adult form with bone and lung involvement.

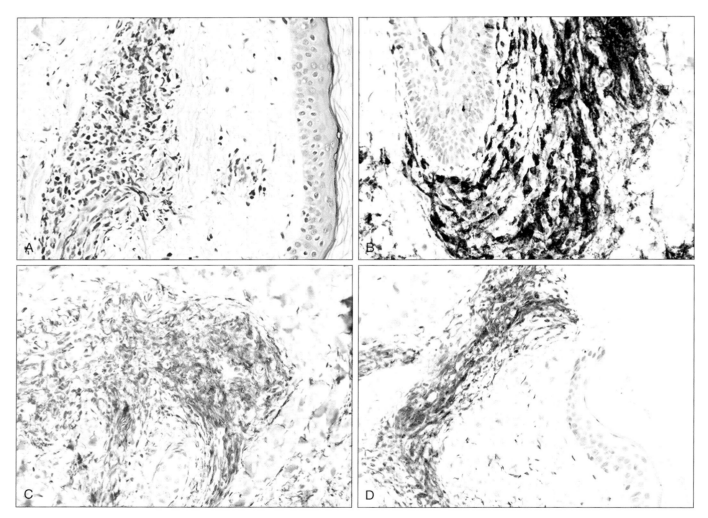

Fig. 16-39. Blastic plasmacytoid dendritic cell neoplasm. There is a dermal infiltrate of medium-sized atypical cells (A). The cells show positivity for CD4 (B), CD56 (C), and the primitive hematopoietic cell marker TdT (D). (Courtesy of Professor P.G. Isaacson.)

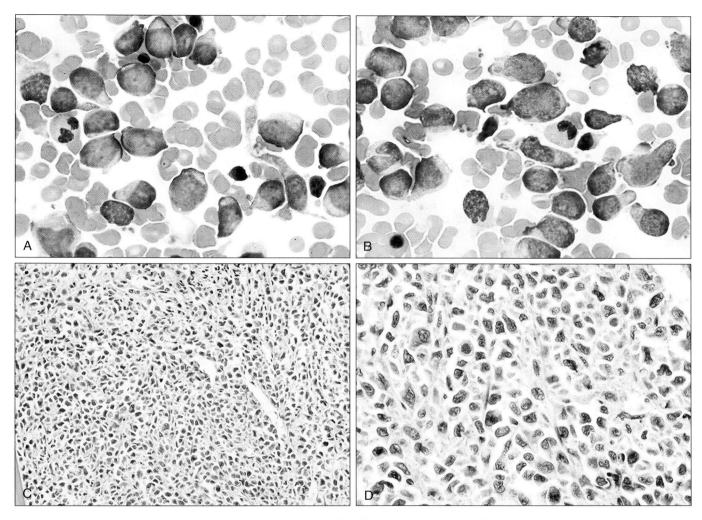

Fig. 16-40. Blastic plasmacytoid dendritic cell neoplasm. The bone marrow aspirate (**A** and **B**) shows numerous blast forms, some of which have plasmacytoid features. The trephine biopsy (**C** and **D**) shows almost complete replacement of normal hematopoietic cells by the neoplastic primitive cells. (Courtesy of Dr. Wendy Erber.)

APLASTIC AND DYSERYTHROPOIETIC ANEMIAS

APLASTIC ANEMIA

Aplastic (hypoplastic) anemia comprises pancytopenia caused by hypoplasia of the marrow. It may be transient, as following cytotoxic therapy, but the term is usually used to denote the chronic forms of the condition. The condition may be inherited (Table 17-1) or acquired (Table 17-2).

In about half of the acquired cases, no cause can be found. The response to antilymphocyte globulin (ALG) or cyclosporin in a substantial proportion of these idiopathic cases, however, suggests that an immune mechanism may be involved. The success of bone marrow transplantation implies that the hematopoietic microenvironment of the marrow is intact, at least in the majority of cases.

The cause of the anemia in about a third of patients appears to be damage by a drug or toxin to the hematopoietic stem cells, which are then reduced in number as they lose their ability to self-renew and proliferate. The drugs most frequently associated with aplastic anemia are the sulfonamides, chloramphenicol, and gold; however, a wide range of drugs has been implicated. In some patients these drugs give rise to only a selective neutropenia or thrombocytopenia. Aplastic anemia may also be caused by radiation or infection, particularly viral hepatitis (non-A, non-B, non-C).

The anemia is mildly macrocytic or normocytic. The clinical features are those of anemia, hemorrhage caused by thrombocytopenia, or infections because of neutropenia. Bleeding is usually into the skin, as petechiae or ecchymoses, or into or from interior surfaces (Fig. 17-1) but may also occur into internal organs (Fig. 17-2), with cerebral hemorrhage being the major risk. Infections are usually bacterial (Fig. 17-3), but viral (Fig. 17-4), fungal (Fig. 17-5), and protozoal infections may also occur, particularly later in the disease.

TABLE 17-1.   INHERITED APLASTIC ANEMIA: CAUSES

Pancytopenia

Fanconi anemia (FA)
Dyskeratosis congenita (DC)
Shwachman–Diamond syndrome (SDS)
Reticular dysgenesis
Pearson syndrome
Familial aplastic anemia (autosomal and X-linked)
Myelodysplasia

Single cytopenia

Anemia: Diamond–Blackfan anemia (DBA)
Neutropenia: severe congenital neutropenia including Kostmann syndrome
Thrombocytopenia: congenital amegakaryocytic thrombocytopenia (CAMT); with absent radii (TAR)

TABLE 17-2.   ACQUIRED APLASTIC ANEMIA: CAUSES

Idiopathic
Secondary:

Drugs – hypersensitivity (e.g., chloramphenicol, gold, sulfonamides)

Drugs – cytotoxics (e.g., busulfan, cyclophosphamide)

Irradiation

Infection: postviral hepatitis

Toxins: e.g., insecticides, benzene

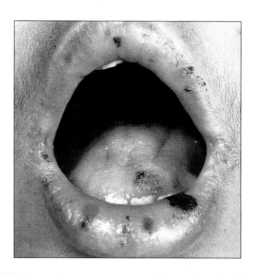

Fig. 17-1. Aplastic anemia: spontaneous mucosal hemorrhages in a 10-year-old boy with severe congenital (Fanconi) anemia. (Hb, 7.3 g/dl; white blood cell count [WBC], 1.1 × 10⁹/L [neutrophils, 21%; lymphocytes, 77%]; platelets <5.0 × 10⁹/L.)

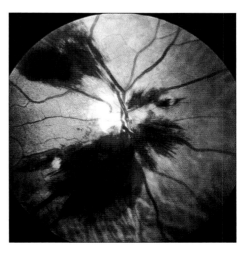

Fig. 17-2. Aplastic anemia: retinal hemorrhages in a patient with acquired disease and profound thrombocytopenia.

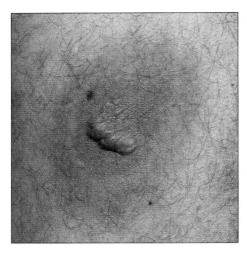

Fig. 17-3. Aplastic anemia: purple discoloration and blistering of the skin caused by infection with *Pseudomonas aeruginosa.*

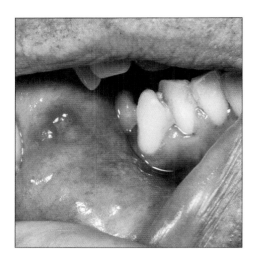

Fig. 17-4. Aplastic anemia: ulceration of the buccal mucosa associated with severe neutropenia. Herpes simplex virus was grown from the ulcers. (Total leukocyte count, 0.8 $\times$ 10^9/L; neutrophils, 20%.)

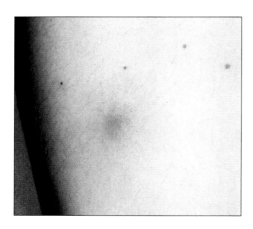

Fig. 17-5. Aplastic anemia: raised, erythematous skin nodule from infection with *Candida albicans,* which was also present in the bloodstream. The patient, a 27-year-old woman, had previously been treated with antibacterial agents for prolonged periods of fever caused by bacterial infections.

INHERITED APLASTIC ANEMIA

Fanconi Anemia

The inherited forms of aplastic anemia may be associated with other somatic congenital defects, as in the Fanconi syndrome, an autosomal recessive inherited disease that is genetically and phenotypically heterogeneous. It is defined by cellular hypersensitivity to deoxyribonucleic acid (DNA) cross-linking agents (e.g., diepoxybutane and mitomycin C). There are random chromosomal breaks with endoreduplication, and chromatid exchange can be demonstrated in peripheral lymphocytes. Patients may be mildly or severely affected with many congenital anomalies; the disease often progresses to myelodysplasia and acute myeloid leukemia. Skeletal, renal, and other defects may be present, as well as hyperpigmentation, small stature from birth, and hypogonadism (Figs. 17-6 to 17-11).

The Fanconi anemia (FA) proteins exist in various complexes in the cytoplasm and nucleus. They fall into 13 complementation groups (Table 17-3). The complex in the nucleus acts to facilitate the monoubiquitination of *FANCD2,* which then protects cells from genetic damage and death following exposure to cross-linking agents

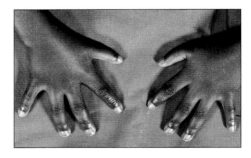

Fig. 17-6. Fanconi anemia. The hands of the child shown in Fig. 17-10 show symmetric abnormalities of the thumbs, resulting in their resemblance to fingers. (Courtesy of Dr. B. Wonke.)

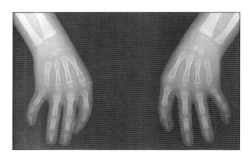

Fig. 17-7. Fanconi anemia: radiograph showing absent thumbs.

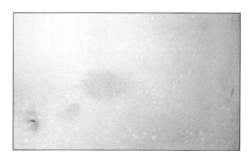

Fig. 17-8. Fanconi anemia: café-au-lait spot, pigmentation, and punctate areas of depigmentation over the abdominal wall. (Courtesy of Professor E. C. Gordon-Smith.)

(Fig. 17-12). Cytoplasmic complexes also exist and these act to suppress apoptosis. The ataxia-telangiectasia mutated *(ATM)* protein phosphorylates *FANCD2* at serine 222 in response to double-stranded DNA breaks caused by ionizing radiation. *FANCD1* is the breast cancer susceptibility gene *BRAC2; FANCN* is *PALB2* (partner of *BRAC2*) and *FANCJ* is *BRIP1* (partner of *BRAC1*). Cells lacking functioning *BRAC1* or *BRAC2* inaccurately repair damaged DNA and are hypersensitive to DNA cross-linking agents.

In addition to *ATM,* the FA proteins interact with other proteins, mutations of which are responsible for the rare genetic chromosome instability syndromes, including the ataxia telangiectasia (AT)–like disorder, Bloom syndrome, Nijmegen breakage syndrome, and Seckel syndrome. Defects of the FA genes have also been found in a variety of human cancers in people without FA.

At least 20% of patients with FA develop malignant disease, most frequently acute myeloid leukemia or myelodysplasia but also head and neck or gynecologic squamous cell tumors and also esophageal, liver, brain, skin, and renal tumors.

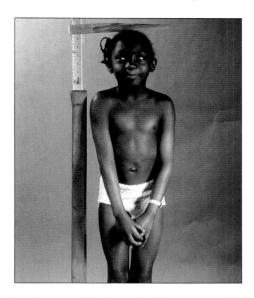

Fig. 17-10. Fanconi anemia. This 9-year-old child shows typical short stature of 1.06 m (42 inches). (Courtesy of Dr. B. Wonke.)

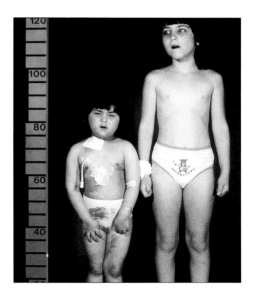

Fig. 17-9. Fanconi anemia. The 6-year-old patient shows short stature and a minor degree of microcephaly compared with her normal older sister, who was human leukocyte antigen (HLA) identical and the donor for bone marrow transplantation.

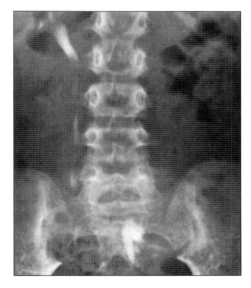

Fig. 17-11. Fanconi anemia. Intravenous pyelogram of the child shown in Fig. 17-10 shows a normal right kidney but a left kidney that is abnormally placed in the pelvis.

TABLE 17-3.	FANCONI ANEMIA: COMPLEMENTATION GROUP AND CHROMOSOME LOCATION OF 13 PROTEINS, MUTATION OF WHICH MAY RESULT IN FANCONI ANEMIA			
Complementation group (gene)	**Approximate % of FA patients**	**Chromosome location**	**Protein (amino acids)**	**Exons**
A *(FANCA)*	65	16q24.3	1455	43
B *(FANCAB)*	2	Xp22.2	859	10
C *(FANCC)*	10	9q22.3	558	14
D1 *(FANCD1)*	2	13q12.3	3418	27
D2 *(FANCD2)*	2	3p25.3	1451	44
E *(FANCE)*	4	6p21.3	536	10
F *(FANCF)*	4	11p15	374	1
G *(FANCG)*	10	9p13	622	14
I *(FANCI)*	2	15q25-26	1328	?
J *(FANCJ/BRIPI)*	2	17q23.1	1249	20
L *(FANCL)*	2	2p16.1	375	14
M *(FANCM)*	<1	14q21.3	2048	23
N *(FANCN/PALB2)*	2	16	1186	13

Courtesy of Professor I. S. Dokal.
FA, Fanconi anemia.

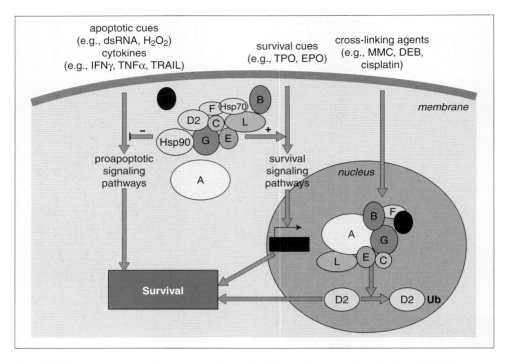

Fig. 17-12. Fanconi anemia: nuclear core complex, which facilitates the monoubiquitination of *FANCD2* protecting cells from genetic damage and death following exposure to cross-linking agents. The Fanconi proteins are shown in lettered ovals. (Adapted from Bagby GC: *Blood* 107:4196, 2006.)

Dyskeratosis Congenita

A less common association of the congenital form of aplastic anemia is dyskeratosis congenita (DC), in which there is skin pigmentation, nail dystrophy (Figs. 17-13 and 17-14), and mucosal leukoplakia (see Figs. 17-13 and 17-15). There may also be epiphora, telangiectasia, and alopecia, as well as mental retardation, growth failure, pulmonary disease, hypogonadism, dental caries and/or loss, and skeletal abnormalities; in contrast to FA, the chromosomal pattern is normal.

The mutations in three different genes *(DKC1, TERC,* and *TERT)* are now known to underlie DC. *DKC1* codes for dyskerin; *TERC* for the ribonucleic acid (RNA) component of telomerase; and *TERT* for the catalytic component of telomerase (Fig. 17-16). Dyskerin is involved in the ribonucleoprotein complexes involved in RNA modification (Fig. 17-17). All patients with DC have very short telomeres,

below the first percentile for a healthy control group of the same age range measured in total lymphocytes or T or B cells. The severity of the disease, age of onset, and spectrum of clinical manifestations vary with which of the genes is mutated and with the exact mutation. *DKC1* is located on the X chromosome (Xq28) and males, who have the genetic abnormality in affected families, all show the disease, whereas the female carriers are normal or have only mild disease. Hoyeraal–Hreidarrsson syndrome (HH) is a rare severe variant of DC, manifesting in early childhood and characterized by fetal growth retardation, mental retardation, combined immunodeficiency, and aplastic anemia. Mutations in the *DKC1* gene have been identified in some but not all cases.

DC usually is inherited in a dominant fashion in families with DC resulting from *TERC* or *TERT* gene mutations. The disease is often

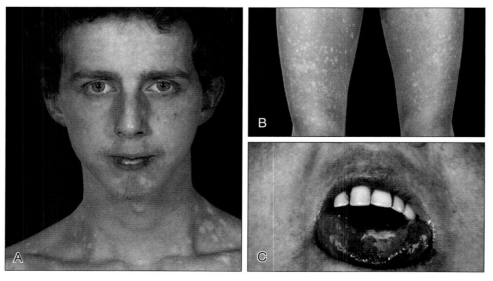

Fig. 17-13. Dyskeratosis congenita (DC): face **(A)**, skin pigmentation **(B)**, mouth **(C)**.

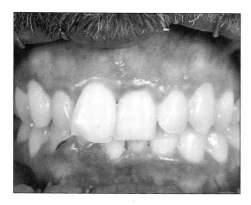

Fig. 17-14. Dyskeratosis congenita. This 24-year-old man with long-standing aplastic anemia has irregularities of tooth size and shape and of the gum margins.

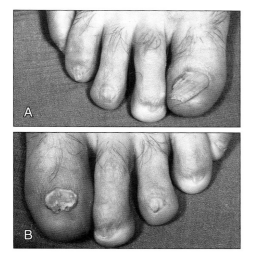

Fig. 17-15. Dyskeratosis congenita. **A** and **B,** The feet of the patient shown in Fig. 17-14 show grossly abnormal nails and excessive hair in an abnormal distribution.

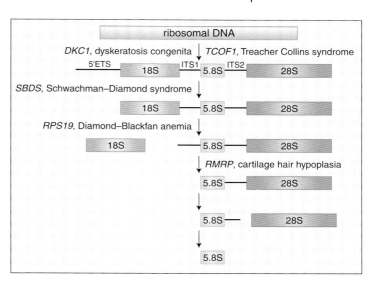

Fig. 17-17. The sites in ribosomal RNA processing at which the enzymes *DKC1, TCOF1, SBOS, RPS19,* and *RMRP* act and the diseases associated with their inherited deficiencies. The different RNA species have roles in cell stress response, proliferation, and apoptosis. (Adapted from Liu JM, Ellis SR: *Blood* 107:4585, 2006, Fig. 2.) See also Ganapathi KA, Shimamura A: *Brit J Haemat* 141:376, 2008.

Schwachman–Diamond Syndrome (SDS)

This autosomal recessive disease results from a mutation in the *SBDS* gene on 7q11 and is characterized by pancreatic insufficiency with fat malabsorption and neutropenia. Some cases also show thrombocytopenia, and 30% to 50% of patients have pancytopenia with a hypocellular marrow. It may be accompanied by short stature, metaphysical chondrodysplasia, and mental retardation. It progresses to myelodysplasia (Fig. 17-18) or acute myeloid leukemia in a significant proportion of patients.

Reticular Dysgenesis

This X-linked recessive disease is characterized by thrombocytopenia, granulocytopenia, and often anemia. The gene involved is unknown.

Other rare syndromes include Seckel syndrome, resulting from mutation of the *ATR* gene (and the *RAD3*-related gene). The syndrome manifests with growth failure, microcephaly, abnormal facies, and occasional pancytopenia. The cartilage-hair hypoplasia syndrome with anemia and neutropenia is also recessive (gene RMRP is at 9p-21-p12).

milder than *DKC1* mutations and with later onset. Some carriers do not express the disease, and the inheritance pattern may seem autosomal, recessive, or sporadic. Aplastic anemia, liver lesions, and pulmonary fibrosis are the prominent manifestations. The disease with *TERC* or *TERT* mutations often shows genetic anticipation, the disease manifesting at an earlier age in a more severe form in successive generations.

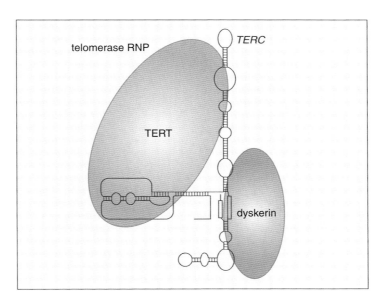

Fig. 17-16. Components of the catalytically active telomerase ribonucleoprotein complex including *TERT,* the telomerase RNA *TERC,* and dyskerin. Mutation of one of the three components of telomerase results in dyskeratosis congenita. (Adapted from Bessler M et al: *Haematologica* 92:1010, 2007, Fig. 1.)

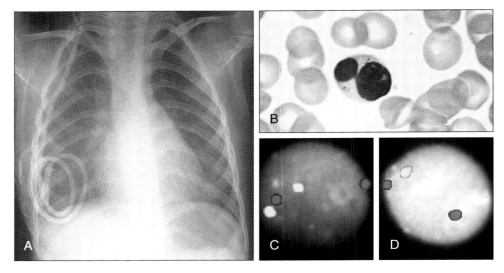

Fig. 17-18. Scwachman–Diamond syndrome transformed to myelodysplasia. **A,** Chest radiograph showing characteristic "cupping" deformity in the ribs. **B,** Peripheral blood showing Pelger neutrophil. **C, D,** Fluorescence in situ hybridization technique showing control **(C)** and patient with monosomy 7 **(D)** (*red,* internal control; *yellow,* chromosome 7 centromeric probe). (Courtesy of Professor O. P. Smith.)

Bone Marrow Appearances

Bone marrow fragments show reduced cellularity (Fig. 17-19), with fat spaces occupying >75% of the marrow. The trails are also reduced in cellularity, with particularly low numbers of megakaryocytes and often a predominance of lymphocytes and plasma cells. The hypoplasia is best shown by trephine biopsy (Fig. 17-20). There may be areas of normal cellularity despite the overall hypocellularity (Fig. 17-21), and lymphoid follicles may be prominent (Fig. 17-22). Marrow hypoplasia can also be detected by magnetic resonance imaging (MRI) scanning (Fig. 17-23).

As therapy differs according to the degree of aplasia, a standard classification of severity has been adopted. Criteria for severe disease are as follows:

- $<50 \times 10^5$/L reticulocytes
- $<10 \times 10^9$/ L platelets
- $<0.5 \times 10^9$/L granulocytes in peripheral blood
- >80% of the remaining cells in the marrow are nonmyeloid

When any three of these four conditions persists for more than 2 weeks, the patient is categorized as having severe aplastic anemia.

During the recovery phase, cellularity increases to normal (Fig. 17-24); the platelet count is usually the last of the blood cell counts

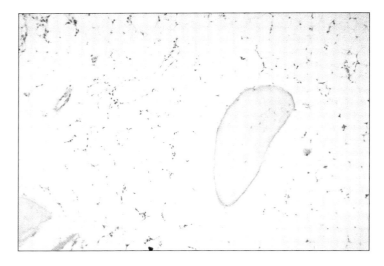

Fig. 17-20. Aplastic anemia: trephine biopsy of posterior iliac crest showing gross hypocellularity with replacement by fat.

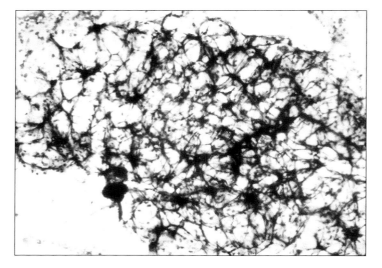

Fig. 17-19. Aplastic anemia: low-power view of bone marrow fragment showing severe reduction of hemopoietic cells and an increase in fat spaces.

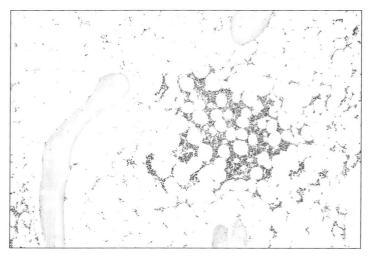

Fig. 17-21. Aplastic anemia: trephine biopsy showing some hematopoietic cellular foci in an otherwise grossly hypocellular marrow.

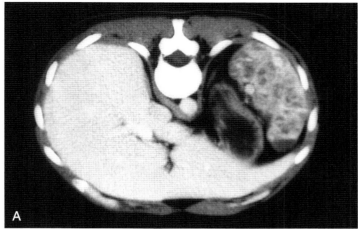

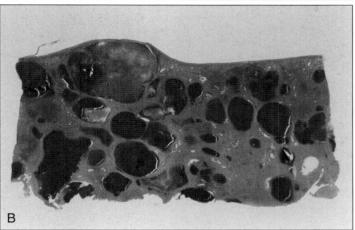

Fig. 17-25. Splenic peliosis in acquired aplastic anemia treated with oxymetholone and prednisolone. These are large blood-filled cavities that may or may not be lined by sinusoidal cells. They are randomly distributed and range from 1 mm to several centimeters in diameter. **A,** Computed tomography (CT) scan showing multiple filling defects in spleen. **B,** Low-power view of section of spleen showing multiple vascular lobes. (Courtesy of Dr. S. Imashuku.)

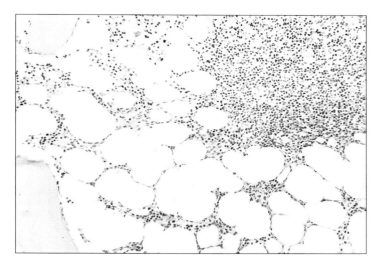

Fig. 17-22. Aplastic anemia: higher-power view of the biopsy shown in Fig. 17-20, showing grossly hypocellular marrow with a remaining lymphoid follicle in the upper right field.

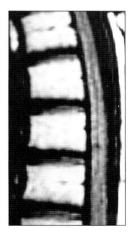

Fig. 17-23. Magnetic resonance imaging: dorsal vertebrae in T1 sequence. In aplastic anemia a marked increase in signal intensity can be observed in comparison with that of the spinal cord.

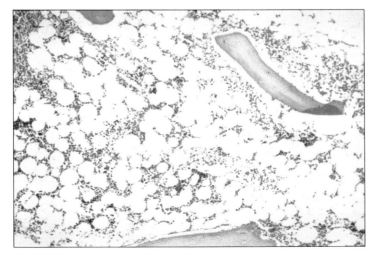

Fig. 17-24. Aplastic anemia: trephine biopsy (same case as shown in Fig. 17-20), showing partial recovery of cellularity 4 weeks after treatment with antilymphocyte globulin. Peripheral blood cell counts also rose moderately.

to recover completely. Overt paroxysmal nocturnal hemoglobinuria (PNH) or a subclinical PNH defect may develop transiently or chronically, and some of these patients may have aplasia of the marrow.

Treatment

Once diagnosed, the cause of severe aplastic anemia must be eliminated if possible. The patient is managed with support care (e.g., platelets, antibiotics, blood transfusions). If a human leukocyte antigen (HLA)–matching sibling is available, allogeneic stem cell transplantation is considered. A hematologic recovery is promoted by antilymphocyte globulin (ALG) in 40% to 50% of cases; cyclosporin may also be of benefit, and the combination of ALG and cyclosporin with corticosteroids is moderately more effective than these drugs used alone. Androgens are used in some cases but may be associated with liver and splenic damage (Fig. 17-25).

RED CELL APLASIA

The causes of pure red cell aplasia are listed in Table 17-4. Like aplastic anemia it may be congenital (familial) or acquired. In the congenital Diamond-Blackfan anemia (DBA) (Figs. 17-26 and 17-27) skeletal defects occur without renal or chromosomal abnormalities. Alterations of ribosomal subunit proteins underlie the disease. One gene responsible for 25% of cases is located on chromosome 19q13 and codes for the ribosomal protein S19. The heterozygous mutation

TABLE 17-4.   RED CELL APLASIA:
CAUSES

Congenital
Diamond–Blackfan syndrome
Acquired
Primary

Autoimmune:
  immunoglobulin inhibitors of erythroid
  precursors or of erythropoietin
T-cell inhibition of erythroid precursors
transient erythroblastopenia of childhood

Secondary
Tumors: thymoma

Lymphoma:
  Hodgkin
  non-Hodgkin
chronic lymphocytic leukemia
large granular lymphocytic leukemia
acute lymphoblastic leukemia
other tumors

Infections: parvovirus (transient) human immunodeficiency virus viral hepatitis infectious mononucleosis others
Immune disorders: systemic lupus erythematosus rheumatoid arthritis
Drugs and chemicals (e.g., benzene,   diphenylhydantoin, isoniazid)
Nutritional deficiencies: riboflavin vitamin B_{12} or folate deficiency

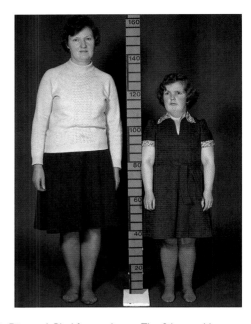

Fig. 17-27. Diamond–Blackfan syndrome. The 24-year-old woman on the *right* had received corticosteroid therapy as an infant and child to reduce the need for blood transfusions. This led to stunted growth (compare her normal mother). The patient had received over 100 units of blood and developed transfusional hemosiderosis with enlargement of the liver and spleen.

may also be present in clinically unaffected family members. There is a functional defect in ribosomal assembly, faulty cleavage of ribosomal RNA, with arrested maturationi of the 18s RNA species resulting in a decreased number of mature ribosomes (Fig. 17-17). Mutations of other ribosomal genes occur in other families with DBA. These include RPS24 at 10q-22-23, RPS17 at 15q and RPL 35a at 3q which codes for a protein necessary for 28s and 5.8s RNAs, 60s subunit biogenesis. Other families appear to have a defect of a gene on chromosome 8p23. The acquired form may be idiopathic or may appear in conjunction with another disease, such as a thymoma (Figs. 17-28 and 17-29). A transient form of red cell aplasia occurs in the course of chronic and other hemolytic anemias but is best recognized in sickle cell anemia. This form is the result of parvovirus B19 infection, with selective damage by the virus to bone marrow red cell progenitors. It is likely that a similar red cell aplasia occurs in normal subjects

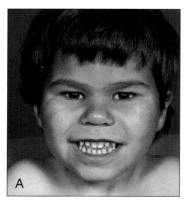
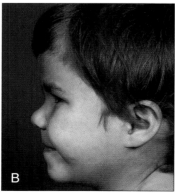

Fig. 17-26. Diamond–Blackfan syndrome. **A** and **B,** Three-year-old boy with congenital red cell aplasia shows the typical facies, with a sunken bridge of the nose. He was treated with blood transfusions and subsequently corticosteroids to which he made a partial response and became transfusion independent. His mental development is normal, but his growth has been partly retarded because of the corticosteroid therapy. (Hb, 6.1 g/dl; WBC, 7.2 × 10⁹/L [neutrophils, 55%; lymphocytes, 41%]; monocytes, 4%; platelets, 289 × 10⁹/L.)

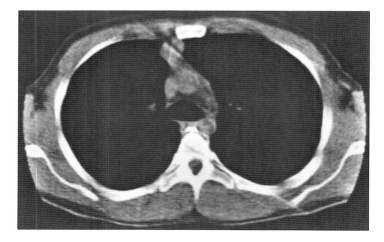

Fig. 17-28. Acquired red cell aplasia: upper mediastinal computed tomography scan showing a thymoma as a retrosternal mass of irregular outline. The patient, a 62-year-old man, had developed myasthenia gravis and pure red cell aplasia, which required regular blood transfusions. (Courtesy of Dr. R. Dick.)

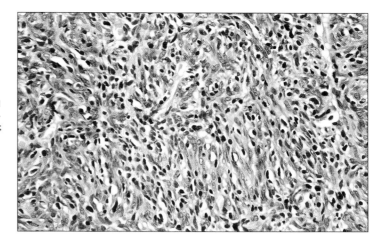

Fig. 17-29. Red cell aplasia: section of thymoma showing spindle cells and epithelial cells. The thymoma was removed surgically from a patient with severe red cell aplasia (Hb, 6.1 g/dl) and neutropenia (WBC, 3.2 × 10⁹/L; neutrophils, 0.4 × 10⁹/L; platelets, 168 × 10⁹/L). (H & E.) (Courtesy of Dr. J. E. McLaughlin.)

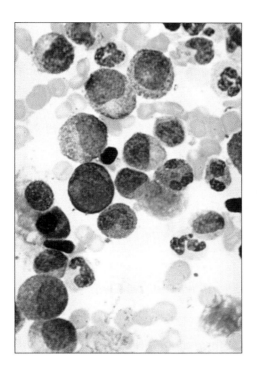

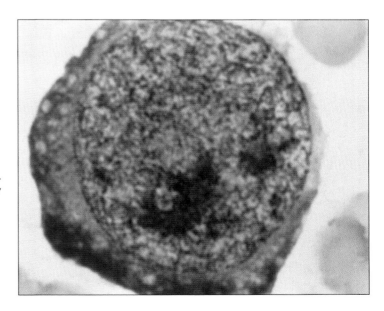

Fig. 17-30. Acquired red cell aplasia: bone marrow aspirate cell trail shows normal numbers of granulocytes and their precursors, but an absence of erythroblasts.

Fig. 17-31. Acquired red cell aplasia: bone marrow aspirate in parvovirus B19 infection showing a giant proerythroblast with cytoplasmic vacuolation and poorly defined intranuclear viral inclusions. (Courtesy of Professor E. C. Larkin.)

with this infection but is not clinically apparent because of the longer red cell life span. In all forms the bone marrow is of normal cellularity, but there is a relative absence of erythroid precursors (Fig. 17-30). In parvovirus B19 infection, giant proerythroblasts may be a feature (Fig. 17-31).

Pure red cell aplasia occasionally responds to thymectomy or other immunosuppressive therapy, corticosteroids, Rituximab, or cyclosporin. If severe, it usually needs regular blood transfusions and iron chelation therapy.

CONGENITAL DYSERYTHROPOIETIC ANEMIAS

The congenital dyserythropoietic anemias (CDAs) are rare autosomal recessive diseases characterized clinically by anemia, often with jaundice as a result of ineffective erythropoiesis and shortened red cell survival, and morphologically by abnormal red cell precursors in the bone marrow. The anemia is usually macrocytic, and the reticulocyte count may be raised, but is low relative to the degree of anemia.

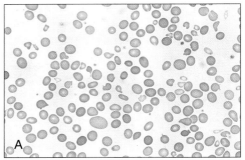
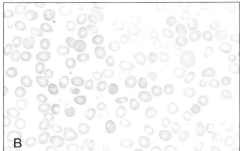

Fig. 17-32. Congenital dyserythropoietic anemia (type 1): peripheral blood film showing oval macrocytes, poikilocytes, and small fragmented cells. The platelets and granulocytes are normal.

Fig. 17-33. Congenital dyserythropoietic anemia (type 1): bone marrow aspirate showing erythroid hyperplasia, megaloblastic erythropoiesis, and binucleate erythroblasts (**A**); examples of cells with internuclear bridges (**B** and **C**).

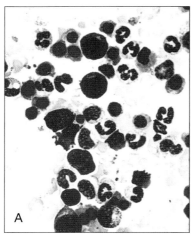
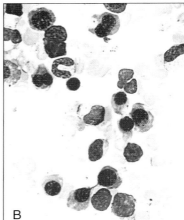
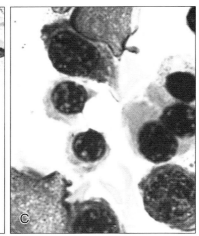

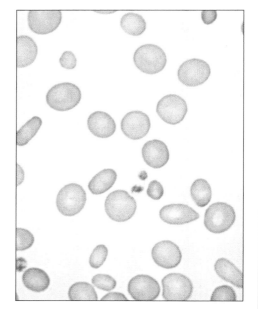

Fig. 17-34. Congenital dyserythropoietic anemia (type II): peripheral blood film showing marked red cell anisocytosis and poikilocytosis.

Fig. 17-35. Congenital dyserythropoietic anemia (type II). **A–E,** Selected high-power views of bone marrow aspirate showing multinucleate erythroblasts.

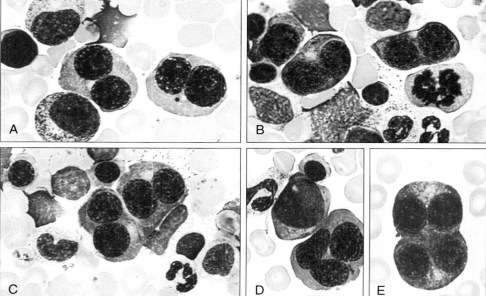

The diseases are divided into three main groups according to the appearance of the bone marrow. In CDA I (Figs. 17-32 and 17-33), megaloblastic changes and internuclear chromatin bridges are prominent. In the most frequent type, CDA II—also known as hereditary erythroblast multinuclearity with positive acidified serum test (HEMPAS)—there are binucleate and multinucleate erythroblasts (Figs. 17-34 and 17-35). The cells lyse in acidified serum from about 30% of normal subjects, but not in the patient's serum (Fig. 17-36). This is because a naturally occurring immunoglobulin M (IgM) complement-binding antibody is present, but the antigen on HEMPAS red cells recognized by this antibody is not known. The pathogenesis is an enzyme defect in glycosylation of membrane glycoproteins. Defects in alpha-mannosidase II and N-acetylglucosaminyl transferase II have been detected. CDA III (Figs. 17-37 and 17-38) is characterized by multinuclearity and gigantoblasts. The existence of a type IV CDA, similar to a type II CDA but with a negative acid lysis test, has been postulated.

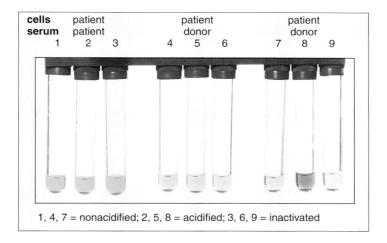

1, 4, 7 = nonacidified; 2, 5, 8 = acidified; 3, 6, 9 = inactivated

Fig. 17-36. Congenital dyserythropoietic anemia (HEMPAS, type II). In the samples from some normal donors, the affected red cells show complement-dependent lysis in fresh acidified serum at 37 °C, but not in the patient's own serum.

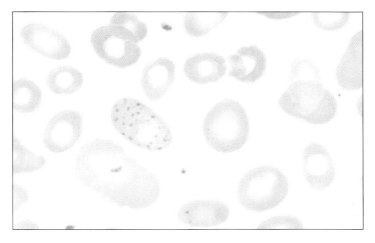

Fig. 17-37. Congenital dyserythropoietic anemia (type III). Peripheral blood film shows gross macrocytosis, anisocytosis, poikilocytosis, and punctate basophilia. (Courtesy of Dr. I. M. Hann.)

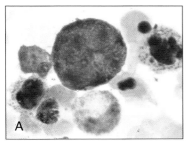
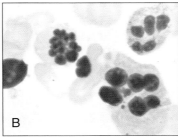
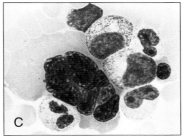
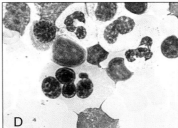

Fig. 17-38. Congenital dyserythropoietic anemia (type III). **A–D,** Selected high-power views of bone marrow aspirate showing multinucleate erythroblasts and karyorrhexis. (Courtesy of Dr. I. M. Hann.)

CHRONIC LYMPHOID LEUKEMIAS

The chronic lymphoid leukemias are included with the mature B- or T-cell neoplasms in the World Health Organization (WHO) (2008) classification (Table 18-1). In this chapter, those diseases classified primarily as leukemias are described; Chapters 19 to 22 deal with the lymphomas and myeloma.

TABLE 18-1.	CHRONIC LYMPHOID LEUKEMIAS: WHO (2008) CLASSIFICATION
Mature B cell neoplasms	
Chronic lymphocytic leukemia/ small lymphocytic lymphoma	
B-cell prolymphocytic leukemia	
Hairy cell leukemia	
Hairy cell leukemia variant	
Mature T cell neoplasms	
T-cell prolymphocytic leukemia	
T-cell large granular lymphocytic leukemia	
Adult T-cell leukemia/lymphoma	

CHRONIC B-CELL LEUKEMIAS

CHRONIC LYMPHOCYTIC LEUKEMIA

Chronic lymphocytic (lymphatic) leukemia (CLL) is predominantly a disease of the elderly and is characterized by greater than $5.0 \times 10^9/L$ monoclonal lymphocytes in the peripheral blood. The cells accumulate

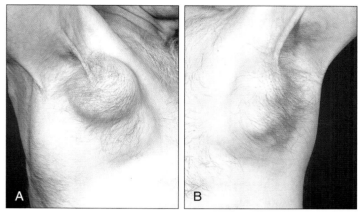

Fig. 18-2. Chronic lymphocytic leukemia. **A, B,** Bilateral axillary lymphadenopathy (same patient as shown in Fig. 18-1).

in the blood, spleen, liver, and lymph nodes. The cells are a monoclonal population of immature B lymphocytes with low-density surface immunoglobulin (Ig). Prolymphocytes (see Fig. 18-29) are also seen in variable proportions in the peripheral blood, the proportion increasing with more advanced disease in some cases.

Symmetric enlargement of the superficial lymph nodes is found except in early-stage patients (Figs. 18-1 and 18-2) and, rarely, there is also tonsillar involvement (Fig. 18-3). In advanced disease, there is both splenomegaly and hepatomegaly, and patients with thrombocytopenia may show bruising and extensive skin purpura (Fig. 18-4). Infections frequently result from immunoglobulin deficiency, neutropenia, lymphoid dysfunction, and immunosuppressive therapy. In many patients herpes zoster (Figs. 18-5 and 18-6) or herpes simplex (Fig. 18-7) infections may be associated, and oral candidiasis and other infections are also a frequent occurrence (Fig. 18-8).

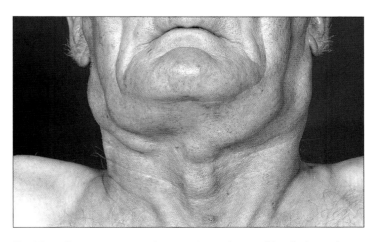

Fig. 18-1. Chronic lymphocytic leukemia: bilateral cervical lymphadenopathy in a 65-year-old man. (Hb, 12.5 g/dl; WBC, 150 × 10⁹/L [lymphocytes, 140 × 10⁹/L]; platelets, 120 × 10⁹/L.)

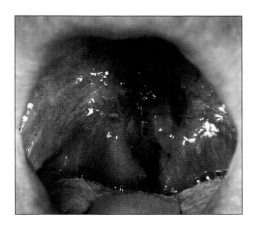

Fig. 18-3. Chronic lymphocytic leukemia: massive enlargement of the pharyngeal tonsils (same patient as shown in Fig. 18-1).

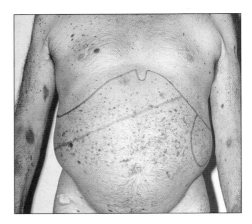

Fig. 18-4. Chronic lymphocytic leukemia: purpuric hemorrhage and abdominal swelling in a 54-year-old man. The extent of liver and splenic enlargement is indicated. (Hb, 10.9 g/dl; WBC, 250 × 10⁹/L [lymphocytes, 245 × 10⁹/L]; platelets, 35 × 10⁹/L.)

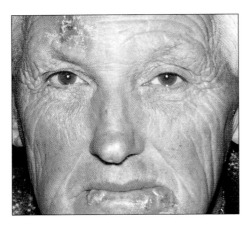

Fig. 18-7. Chronic lymphocytic leukemia: herpes simplex eruptions of the lower lip and of the skin of the forehead.

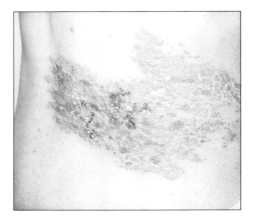

Fig. 18-5. Chronic lymphocytic leukemia: herpes zoster infection in a 68-year-old woman.

The blood count in CLL reveals an absolute lymphocytosis (between 5.0×10^9 and 200×10^9/L is usual), and the peripheral blood has a characteristic lymphoid morphology (Figs. 18-9 and 18-10). If the monoclonal lymphocyte population is less than 5.0×10^9/L the term *monoclonal B-cell lymphocytosis* is used providing there are no other clinical or laboratory abnormalities. In advanced disease a normochromic anemia and thrombocytopenia often occurs. About 10% of patients develop a secondary warm-type autoimmune hemolytic anemia (Fig. 18-11), and in a smaller number of cases an autoimmune thrombocytopenia occurs. An increasing proportion of patients diagnosed with CLL are asymptomatic, and the diagnosis is made only when a routine blood test is performed. Rarely, the lymphocytes show crystalline deposits of immunoglobulin (Fig. 18-12).

Bone marrow examination shows extensive replacement of normal marrow elements by lymphocytes, reaching 30% to 95% of the marrow cell total. Trephine biopsies (Fig. 18-13) show nodular, interstitial, or diffuse collections of abnormal cells. Patients with nodular or interstitial histology have a better prognosis. Immunohistology typically shows the cells to be B cells, C19+, CD20+, CD23+, and CD79+, also expressing CD5 (Fig. 18-14). In patients with autoimmune hemolytic anemia or thrombocytopenia, the spleen is sometimes removed and shows a characteristic histology (Fig. 18-15).

Apoptosis
In vivo, CLL cells have a long life span, expressing BCL-2. The cells rapidly die in culture unless apoptosis is prevented by incubation with stroma or certain cytokines (e.g., interleukin 4 [IL-4]) (Fig. 18-16).

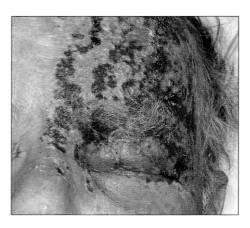

Fig. 18-6. Chronic lymphocytic leukemia: herpes zoster infection in the territory of the ophthalmic division of the fifth cranial nerve.

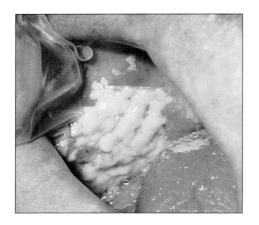

Fig. 18-8. Chronic lymphocytic leukemia: extensive *Candida albicans* infection of the buccal mucosa of a 73-year-old woman.

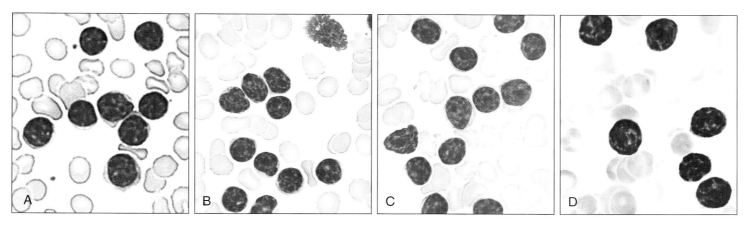

Fig. 18-9. Chronic lymphocytic leukemia. **A–D,** Lymphocytes from the peripheral blood of four different patients show thin rims of cytoplasm, condensed coarse chromatin, and only rare nucleoli.

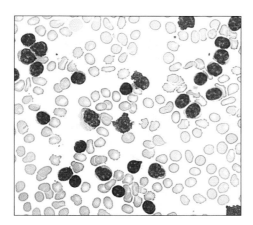

Fig. 18-10. Chronic lymphocytic leukemia: peripheral blood film showing the increased numbers of lymphocytes and occasional characteristic "smudge" cells. (Hb, 9.0 g/dl; WBC, 190 × 10⁹/L; platelets, 70 × 10⁹/L.)

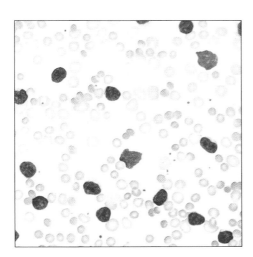

Fig. 18-11. Chronic lymphocytic leukemia with autoimmune hemolytic anemia: peripheral blood film shows increased numbers of lymphocytes, red cell spherocytosis, and polychromasia. The direct antiglobulin test was strongly positive with IgG on the surface of the cells. (Hb, 8.3g/dl; reticulocytes, 150 × 10⁹/L; WBC, 110 × 10⁹/L [lymphocytes, 107 × 10⁹/L]; platelets, 90 × 10⁹/L.)

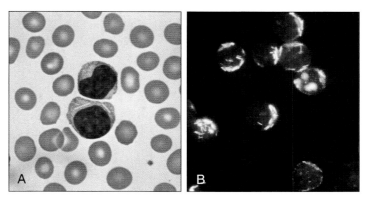

Fig. 18-12. Chronic lymphocytic leukemia: the clonal B cells show crystalline deposits of immunoglobulin. **A,** Jenner-Giemsa stain. **B,** Immunofluorescence. (A, B, Courtesy of Professor T. J. Hamblin.)

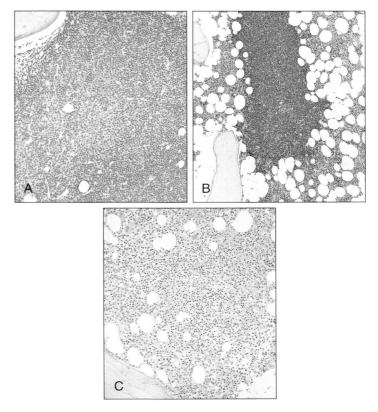

Fig. 18-13. Chronic lymphocytic leukemia: trephine biopsies showing **(A)** a marked diffuse increase in marrow lymphocytes (closely packed cells with small dense nuclei); **(B)** a nodular pattern of lymphocyte accumulation (in a different patient); and **(C)** interstitial infiltration.

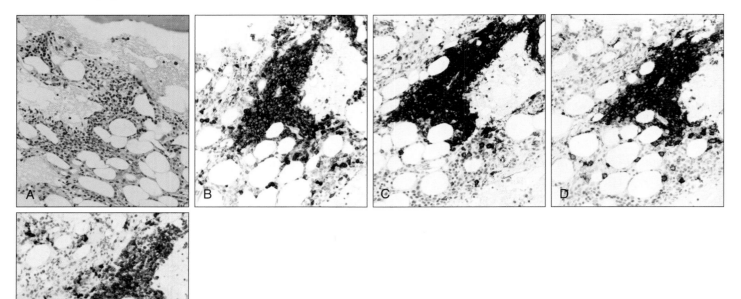

Fig. 18-14. Chronic lymphocytic leukemia: **(A)** residual disease after alemtuzimab therapy, trephine biopsy. Immunohistology shows that the disease is **(B)** CD5+, **(C)** CD20+, **(D)** CD23+, and **(E)** CD79+.

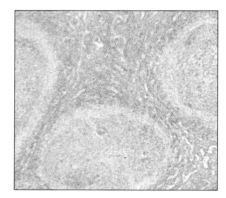

Fig. 18-15. Chronic lymphocytic leukemia: histologic section of spleen in a patient with secondary autoimmune hemolytic anemia. There is expansion of lymphoid tissue in the periarterial sheaths of the white pulp and obvious red cell entrapment in the reticuloendothelial cords and splenic sinuses.

Cytogenetics

Frequent chromosomal changes detected by fluorescent in situ hybridization (FISH) on interphase cells in CLL are as follows: deletions or translocations of the long arm of chromosome 13 at band q14 (55%) (Fig. 18-17), trisomy 12 (+12) (15%), mutations or deletions of the ataxia-telangiectasia (ATM) gene located at 11q22-23 (18%), structural abnormalities of 17p13 (which involve the p53 gene) (5% to 10%), and deletions or translocations of 6q21 (10%), especially in patients in blastic transformation. Deletion 13q14 is associated with deletion of two micro–ribonucleic acids (micro-RNAs), mir-15a, mir-16-1, which may be relevant to the disease process. ATM is involved in control of P53 expression, but 17p deletions imply a worse prognosis compared with 11q deletions.

Membrane Markers

The results of different membrane markers in chronic B-cell leukemias are shown in Table 18-2. Figure 18-18 shows a flow chart illustrating the different phenotypes of the main diseases, and typical

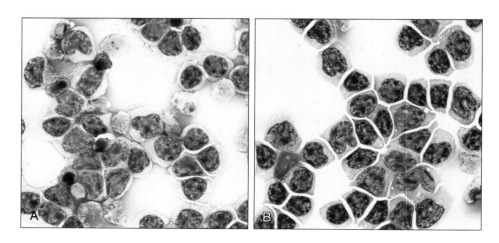

Fig. 18-16. Chronic lymphocytic leukemia. **A,** Death of some cells (small, darkly stained chromatin) by apoptosis after 30 hours' culture in medium and plasma. **B,** Prevention of apoptotic cell death by IL-4 addition to culture (10 days). (Courtesy of Dr. P. Panayiotides.)

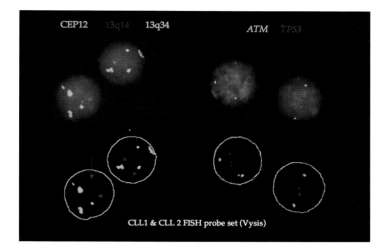

Fig. 18-17. Chronic lymphocytic leukemia: FISH panel (Vysis) screening for the most frequent genetic changes. CLL panel 1 consists of probe CEP 12 (green) for the centromere of chromosome 12 and two probes for chromosome 13 (red and blue). CLL panel 2 consists of probes for the ATM gene (green) and P53 gene (red). In this case the patient showed heterozygous deletion of 13q14 (arrowed) but no other abnormality. The second set of images circled in yellow are the nuclei stained with DAPI to enhance visualization of the FISH signals. (Courtesy of Dr. E. Necheva.)

TABLE 18-2.   CHRONIC B-CELL LEUKEMIAS: MEMBRANE IMMUNOPHENOTYPIC PATTERNS

	CLL	PLL	HCL	HCL-V	SMLZ	FL	MCL	PCL
SIg	+/–	++	++	++	++	+	+	– (cyt Ig+)
CD5	+	–	–	–	–	–	+	–
CD19/CD20/37	+	+	+	+	+	+	+	–
FMC7/CD22	–/+	+	+	+	+	+	++	–
CD23	+	–/+	–	–	–/+	–/+	–	–
CD25	–	–	++	–	–/+	–	–	–
CD38	–/+	–	–/+	–/+	–	–/+	–	++
CD103/CD123	–	–	+	–	–	–	–	–
HLA-DR	+	+	+	+	+	+	+	–
CD79b	–/+	++	–/+	?	++	++	++	?

SIg, surface immunoglobulin
CLL, B-cell chronic lymphocytic leukemia
PLL, prolymphocytic leukemia
HCL-V, hairy cell leukemia variant
SMLZ, splenic lymphoma marginal zone (± villous lymphocytes)
FL, follicular lymphoma
MCL, mantle cell lymphoma
PCL, plasma cell leukemia

Adapted from Dighiero G, Hamblin TJ: *Lancet* 371:1017, 2008.

findings on fluorescent activated cell sorting (FACS) analysis in CLL are shown in Fig. 18-19. A scoring system using a selection of five of these markers has been used to distinguish CLL from other chronic B-lymphoid diseases. Characteristically, in CLL a score of 4 or 5 is obtained: weak expression of SmIg (score 1), negative staining for FMC7 (score 1) and CD79b (score 1), and positive staining for CD5 (score 1) and CD23 (score 1). B-cell disorders other than CLL usually score 0 to 2.

Clinical Staging
According to the extent of involvement of different lymphoid organs and the presence or absence of anemia and thrombocytopenia from bone marrow failure, CLL may be divided into a number of clinical

stages (Table 18-3). The stage, sex of patient, presence or absence of autoimmune hemolytic anemia or positive direct antiglobulin test, and peripheral blood lymphocytic doubling time all have prognostic significance (Table 18-4).

Prognostic Markers
Abnormalities detected by molecular or biochemical tests also give prognostic information. The V heavy (VH) and V light (VL) chain genes undergo somatic hypermutation in the germinal centers. In

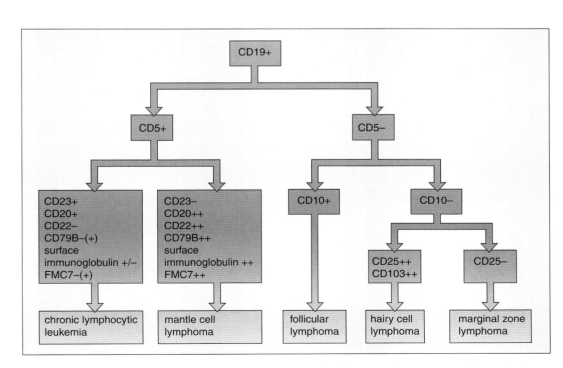

Fig. 18-18. Chronic B-cell leukemias: differential diagnosis of CLL from other frequent causes of monoclonal B-cell lymphoma. (Adapted from Dighiero G, Hamblin TJ: *Lancet* 371:1017, 2008.)

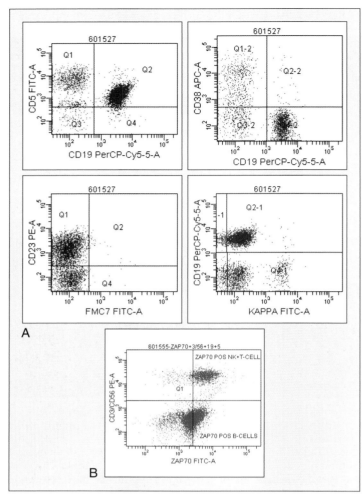

Fig. 18-19. Chronic lymphocytic leukemia: immunophenotype analysis by fluorescent activated cell sorting (FACS). **A,** In this case the cells are CD19+, CD5+, CD23+, CD38−, FMC7−, kappa light chain +. **B,** In this case the cells are ZAP 70+, CD3+, CD56+. (Courtesy of Immunophenotyping Laboratory, Royal Free Hospital.)

TABLE 18-4. CHRONIC LYMPHOCYTIC LEUKEMIA: CLINICAL AND LABORATORY PROGNOSTIC MARKERS

Prognostic factor	Good	Bad
Stage	Binet A (Rai 0-1)	Binet B,C (Rai 2-4)
Sex	Female	Male
Histology	Nodular or interstitial	Diffuse
Direct antiglobulin test	Negative	Positive
Chromosomes	Deletion 13q14	Trisomy 12*, del 17p13, p53 mutations, del 11q22-23 (ATM)
Lymphocyte doubling time	>1 year	<6 months
VH immunoglobulin genes	Hypermutated	Unmutated
VH family	Not VH 1-6, VH 3-21	VH 1-69, VH 3-21
ZAP expression	Low	High
CD38 expression	Low	High
Telomeres	Long (negative)	Short (positive)
CLLU.I expression	Low	High
CD49d expression	Low	High
Lipoprotein lipase	High	Low
Serum thymidine kinase	Low	High
Serum β_2 microglobulin	Low	High
Serum CD23	Low	High

*Trisomy 12 is not a prognostic indicator in some recent trials using fludarabine-containing regimens

CLL, the VH genes are mutated in at least 50% of cases. These cases usually show a favorable clinical course. The VH family used in the clonal population may also be of prognostic significance (see Table 18-4). Other prognostic markers include CD38 and ZAP-70 (a tyrosine kinase) expression, as well as serum levels of biologic markers of disease burden (see Table 18-4). Cytogenetic analysis (see Fig. 18-17) gives important prognostic data. Gene array studies may also give prognostic information, genes coding for inhibitors of cell adhesion and motility being downregulated in disease progression.

Chronic Lymphocytic Leukemia: Mixed Cell Types
Mixed cell cases include those showing a dimorphic population of small lymphocytes and prolymphocytes (greater than 10% and less than 55%) (CLL/PLL) (Figs. 18-20 and 18-21) and those showing a spectrum of small to large lymphocytes with less than 10% prolymphocytes. Some of the cases resemble typical CLL in clinical and laboratory features and in clinical course. Others show greater splenomegaly and markers more typical of PLL, are more refractory to therapy, and follow a more aggressive course than typical CLL. Some cases manifest with a mixed pattern that remains stable, but in others prolymphocytic transformation gradually progresses.

Richter's Syndrome (Diffuse Large Cell Transformation)
Some cases of CLL transform into a more aggressive stage, with the local formation (often retroperitoneal) of a mass of high-grade, diffuse large cell lymphoma. This may be clonally related or unrelated (usually Epstein-Barr virus [EBV] related) to the original disease. There may be circulating "immunoblastic" cells if "immunoblastic" transformation is present in the marrow (Figs. 18-22 to 18-25). There is usually loss of CD5 and CD23 expression and the cells often express ZAP-70, CD38 and show unmutated IgVH genes. Structural changes and mutations of p53, unusual in chronic-phase CLL, are frequent at this stage. Positron emission tomography (PET) scanning may reveal the site of disease transformation (Fig. 18-26). The serum lactate dehydrogenase level is increased. Richter's transformation is also described in Hodgkin's disease, diffuse large B-cell lymphoma, and B-cell EBV-related lymphoma.

TABLE 18-3. CHRONIC LYMPHOCYTIC LEUKEMIA: CLASSIFICATION OF CLINICAL STAGES

Rai classification of chronic lymphocytic leukemia	
Stage 0	Lymphocytes >5 x 10⁹/L and >40% of bone marrow cells
Stage I	As Stage 0, with enlarged lymph nodes
Stage II	As Stages 0 or I, with enlarged liver and/or spleen
Stage III	As Stages 0, I, or II, with Hb <10 g/dl
Stage IV	As Stages 0, I, II, or III, with platelets <100 x 10⁹/L

Revised international (Binet) classification of chronic lymphocytic leukemia	
Group A (good prognosis)	Hb >10 g/dl
	Platelets >100 x 10⁹/L
	< three sites of palpable organ enlargement
Group B (intermediate prognosis)	Hb >10 g/dl
	platelets >100 x 10⁹/L
	≥ three sites of palpable organ enlargement (one site = spleen or liver, or lymph nodes in the neck, axillae, or groin)
Group C (bad prognosis)	Hb <10 g/dl
	platelets <100 x 10⁹/L

Rai classification, modified from Kai KR, Saritsky A, Cronkite EP, et al: Clinical staging of chronic lymphocytic leukemia, *Blood* 46:219-234, 1975.

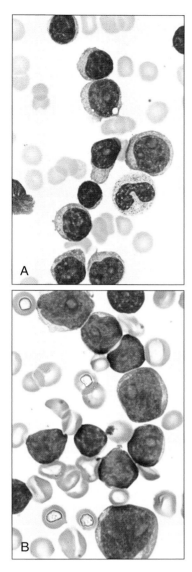

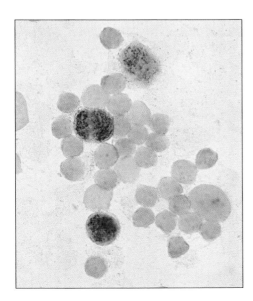

Fig. 18-20. Chronic lymphocytic leukemia. **A, B,** Mixed cell type. The circulating lymphoid cells include greater than 10% but less than 55% prolymphocytes.

Fig. 18-21. Chronic lymphocytic leukemia: mixed cell (CLL/PLL) type. Immuno-peroxidase reaction using anti-Ki-1 (CD30) monoclonal antibody to detect proliferating cells. A positive reaction is seen in these cells. (Courtesy of Professor D. Catovsky.)

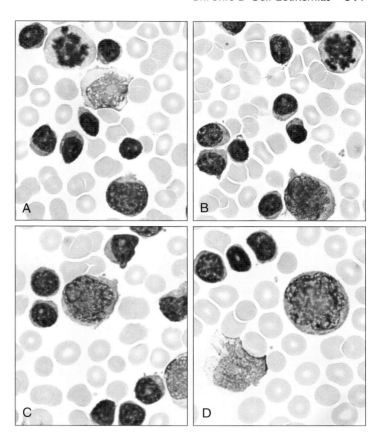

Fig. 18-22. Chronic lymphocytic leukemia. **A–D,** Richter's syndrome (large cell transformation). Peripheral blood films showing typical small lymphocytes, large blast cells, and mitotic cells.

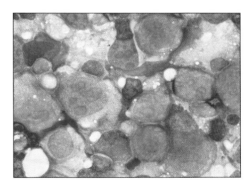

Fig. 18-23. Chronic lymphocyte leukemia: Richter's syndrome. Imprint from enlarged lymph node showing large "immunoblastic" cells with multiple prominent nucleoli and a few residual small lymphocytes. (Courtesy of Professor D. Catovsky.)

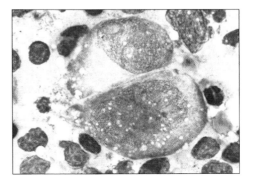

Fig. 18-24. Chronic lymphocytic leukemia: Richter's syndrome. Imprint from lymph node showing two large immunoblasts surrounded by small lymphocytes.

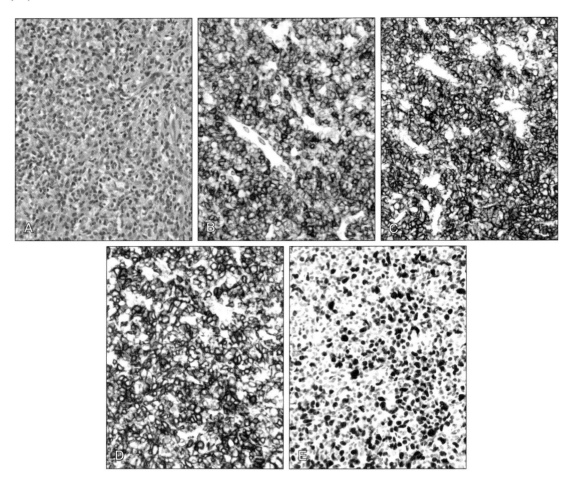

Fig. 18-25. Richter's syndrome: diffuse large B-cell lymphoma arising in chronic lymphocytic leukemia. Axillary node core biopsy. **A,** Mixture of small lymphocytes and large cells with irregular nuclear contours and prominent nucleoli. **B,** Immunostain for CD5; the small and large cells are CD5+. This is unusual as typically the transformed cells in CLL lose CD5 expression. **C,** The cells are CD20+. **D,** The cells are CD23+. **E,** MIBI staining shows a high proliferation rate among the tumor cells. (Courtesy Dr. A. Ramsay.)

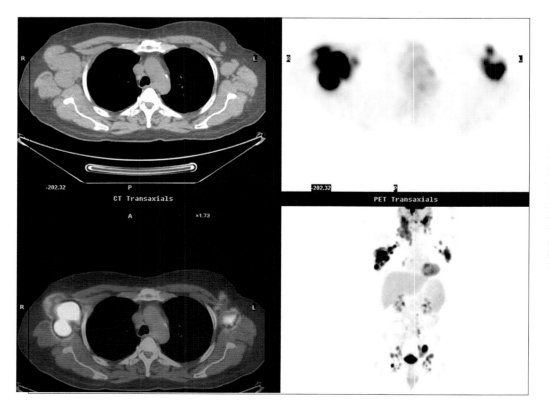

Fig. 18-26. Chronic lymphocytic leukemia: Richter's syndrome. Axial CT, FDG PET, fused PET/CT, and maximum intensity projection (MIP) images showing massive, active axillary lymphadenopathy, right greater than left. Biopsy of the right axillary mass showed diffuse large B-cell lymphoma, CD5+, in a patient with long-standing multitreated CLL. There is also active disease in the cervical, pharyngeal, and pelvic lymph nodes, implying Richter's transformation at multiple sites.

PROLYMPHOCYTIC LEUKEMIA

Prolymphocytic leukemia, a variant of CLL, usually occurs in the elderly and is associated with marked splenomegaly, absolute lymphocytosis (usually over 100×10^9/L), and minimal lymph node enlargement. Electron microscopy shows characteristic differences (Figs. 18-27 and 18-28), and the blood film shows larger lymphocytes than are found in classic CLL (Fig. 18-29). In the majority of patients, surface marker studies indicate a B-cell origin of prolymphocytes, although the nature of the normal equivalent cell is unknown. Marker studies help to distinguish PLL from CLL by the stronger expression of surface Ig, FMC7 and cytoplasmic CD22, and weaker expression of CD5. In the mixed cell type more of the cells in the peripheral blood are proliferating (see Fig. 18-21). The prognosis is worse than in CLL.

HAIRY CELL LEUKEMIA

Patients with hairy cell leukemia (HCL) usually have pancytopenia and splenomegaly without lymphadenopathy. The characteristic cells, of B-lymphocyte origin, are seen in the peripheral blood (Figs. 18-30 and 18-31) and may also be found in large numbers in marrow aspirates or from splenic imprints in patients who have undergone splenectomy (Fig. 18-32). Hairy cells also show characteristic cytochemical reactions (Fig. 18-33).

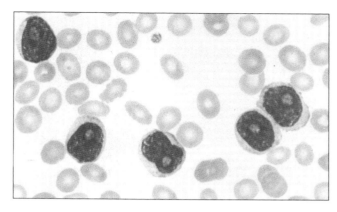

Fig. 18-29. B-cell prolymphocytic leukemia: blood film showing prolymphocytes that have prominent central nucleoli and an abundance of pale cytoplasm. A high density of surface immunoglobulin confirmed their B-cell nature.

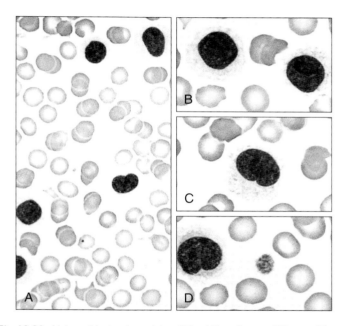

Fig. 18-30. Hairy cell leukemia: peripheral blood films showing **(A)** typical "hairy" cells, which have round or oval nuclei and a moderate amount of finely mottled, pale gray cytoplasm with irregular serrated ("hairy") edges; the chromatin is less dense than in typical small lymphocytes; **(B–D)** at higher magnification the nucleoli are clearly visible. (Hb, 9.4 g/dl; WBC, 25×10^9/L [hairy cells, 23.5×10^9/L]; platelets, 90×10^9/L.)

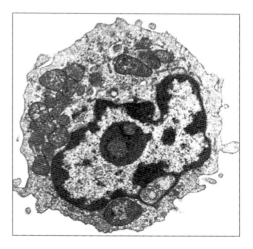

Fig. 18-27. B-cell prolymphocytic leukemia: the B prolymphocyte is characterized by its relatively large size, moderately abundant cytoplasm, chromatin condensed in the periphery of the nucleus, and a prominent nucleolus. (Courtesy of D. Robinson and Profesor D. Catovsky.)

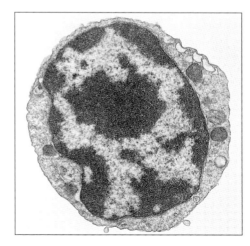

Fig. 18-28. B-cell chronic lymphocytic leukemia: compared to Fig. 18-27, this cell is smaller and has less cytoplasm (high nuclear/cytoplasmic [N/C] ratio) and more marked nuclear chromatin with no visible nucleolus. (Courtesy of D. Robinson and Professor D. Catovsky.)

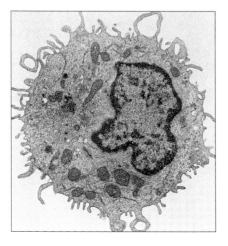

Fig. 18-31. Hairy cell leukemia: hairy cell from the peripheral blood. Typical features are the abundant cytoplasm, low N/C ratio, and cytoplasmic projections or villi that give the cell a "hairy" appearance ($\times$ 9200). (Courtesy of D. Robinson and Professor D. Catovsky.)

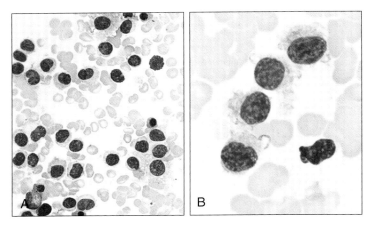

Fig. 18-32. Hairy cell leukemia: **(A)** bone marrow aspirate showing a predominance of hairy cells in the cell trail; **(B)** splenic imprints showing typical nuclear and cytoplasmic features of the abnormal hairy cells.

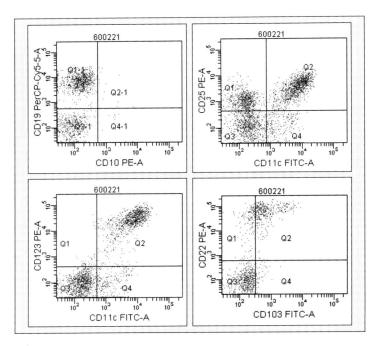

Fig. 18-35. Hairy cell leukemia. FACS scan of peripheral blood cells. The hairy cells are typically CD11c+, CD19+, CD20+, CD22+, CD25+, CD103+, CD123+, CD10−, CD23−, and FMC7−. (Courtesy of Immunophenotyping Laboratory, Royal Free Hospital, London.)

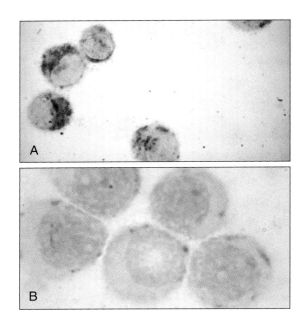

Fig. 18-33. Hairy cell leukemia: typical cytochemical findings of hairy cells include **(A)** a strongly positive reaction to tartaric acid–resistant acid phosphatase (TRAP) and **(B)** a fine granular positivity with crescentic accumulation at one side of the nucleus following alpha-naphthyl butyrate esterase staining.

In many patients the marrow is difficult to aspirate and trephine biopsy is necessary for diagnosis. In these cases, interstitial or diffuse infiltration by hairy cells and a dense reticulin fiber pattern are usually seen (Fig. 18-34). The nuclei of the cells are widely spaced giving a "frog spawn"–like appearance. The cells show a characteristic phenotype in the peripheral blood (Fig. 18-35) and by immunohistology (Fig. 18-36). The cells are typically CD11c, CD19, CD20, CD22, CD25, and CD103 positive and CD10, CD23, and FMC7 negative. DBA44 is an antibody useful for detecting hairy cells in small numbers in tissue sections.

Histologic sections of the spleen (Figs. 18-37 and 18.38) and liver (Figs. 18-39 and 18-40) may demonstrate unusual vascular "lakes" caused by hairy cell infiltration of these organs.

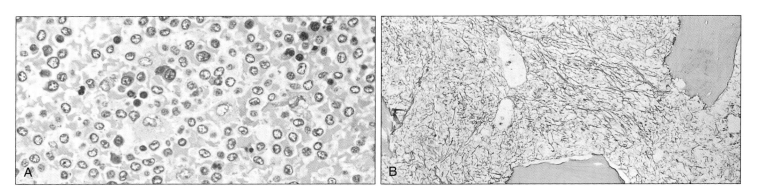

Fig. 18-34. Hairy cell leukemia. **A,** Bone marrow trephine biopsy showing extensive replacement of normal hematopoietic tissue by discrete mononuclear hairy cells. The nuclei are typically surrounded by a clear zone of cytoplasm, which is accentuated by a contraction artifact in vitro. (Methacrylate section.) **B,** Showing increased fiber density and thickness in the reticulin fiber pattern. (Silver impregnation technique.)

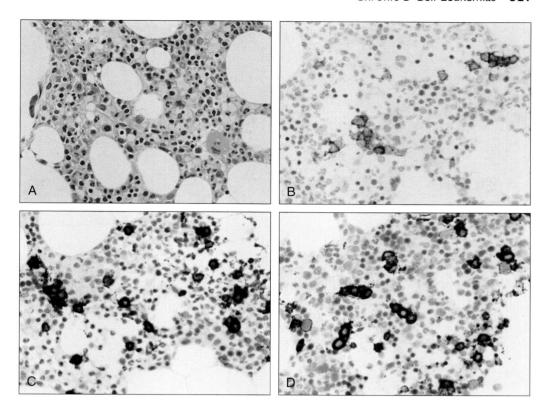

Fig. 18-36. Hairy cell leukemia: bone marrow trephine biopsy. **A,** Many discrete cells with clear cytoplasm present. Immunohistology shows the cells are **(B)** CDHc+, **(C)** CD20+, and **(D)** CD103+. The cells are also DBA44+ (not shown).

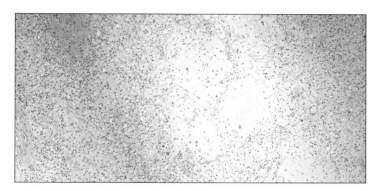

Fig. 18-37. Hairy cell leukemia: histologic section of spleen showing hairy cell infiltration of reticuloendothelial cords and sinuses. Numerous blood "lakes" are seen in the center of the field.

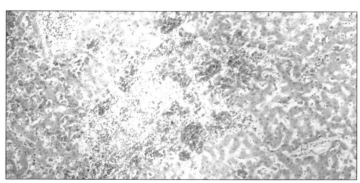

Fig. 18-39. Hairy cell leukemia: histologic section of liver shows hairy cell infiltration of sinusoids and portal tracts. There is sinusoidal ectasia and pseudoangiomatous transformation of hepatic blood vessels.

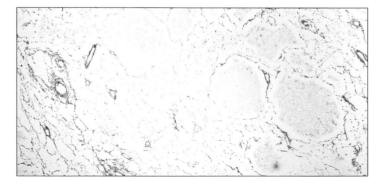

Fig. 18-38. Hairy cell leukemia: histologic section of spleen (same case as shown in Fig. 18-37) showing more clearly the reticulin fiber pattern outlining the abnormal venous "lakes." The presence of these structures may explain the extensive splenic red cell pooling that occurs in this disease. (Silver impregnation technique.)

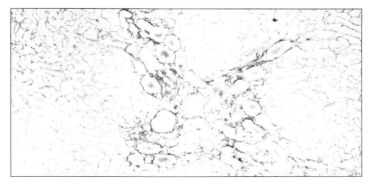

Fig. 18-40. Hairy cell leukemia: histologic section of liver (same case as shown in Fig. 18-39) showing the reticulin fiber pattern clearly, confirming the gross distortion of hepatic vascular architecture. It is thought that attachment of large numbers of hairy cells to the sinusoidal lining cells causes cell damage that results in these characteristic vascular abnormalities in the liver and spleen. (Silver impregnation technique.)

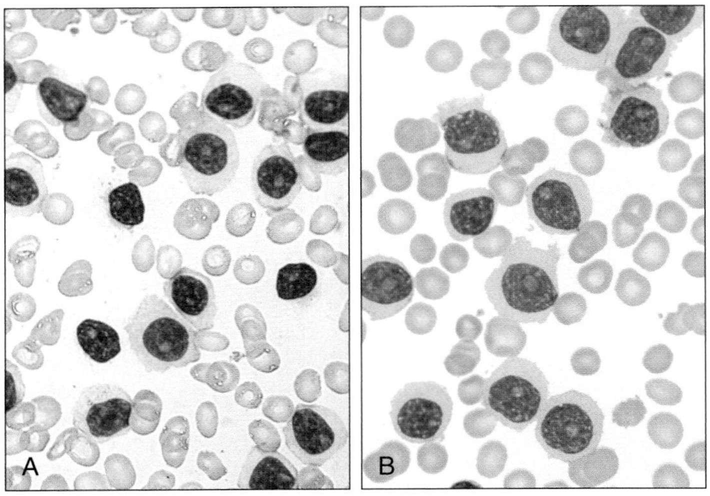

Fig. 18-41. Hairy cell leukemia variant. **A, B,** Peripheral blood films showing cells with a prominent nucleolus, abundant pale cytoplasm, and an irregular cytoplasmic border. (Courtesy of Professor D. Catovsky.)

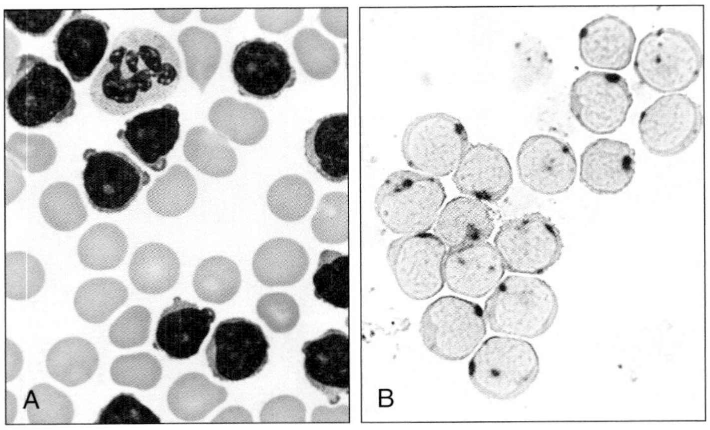

Fig. 18-42. Prolymphocytic leukemia (T-cell type): blood films showing **(A)** prolymphocytes, each with a prominent central nucleolus and a single neutrophil. Cell marker studies showed positive reactions with anti–T-cell antisera (CD2+, CD3+, CD4+, CD5+, CD7+, CD8−, CD25+) and an absence of surface immunoglobulin; **(B)** "clump" positivity of these cells using acid phosphatase staining. (Hb, 10.5 g/dl; WBC, 240 × 10⁹/L; platelets, 60 × 10⁹/L.) (Courtesy of Professor D. Catovsky.)

Hairy Cell Leukemia Variant

The rare cases of HCL variant usually manifest with a white cell count greater than 40 × 10⁹/L and splenomegaly. The cells show a prominent nucleolus (Fig. 18-41) and are usually CD25 and TRAP negative (see Fig. 18-33).

LEUKEMIA/LYMPHOMA SYNDROMES

In many cases classified as B-cell lymphomas or myeloma, there is "spillover" of the malignant clonal cells into the peripheral blood. This is seen particularly in follicular lymphoma, lymphoplasmacytic lymphoma, mantle cell lymphoma, diffuse large cell lymphoma, plasma cell leukemia (closely related to myeloma), and splenic marginal zone lymphoma when, if more than 20% of the circulating cells are villus lymphocytes, the condition has been termed by hematologists as "splenic lymphoma with villus lymphocytes" (see Fig. 19-19). The B-cell leukemia/lymphoma conditions are discussed and illustrated in Chapter 19, T-cell syndromes in Chapter 20, and plasma cell leukemia in Chapter 22.

CHRONIC T-CELL LEUKEMIAS

The T-cell diseases that manifest primarily as leukemia described here are listed in Table 18-1, and their membrane immunophenotypes are shown in Table 18-5. The T-cell lymphomas, including Sézary syndrome, are discussed in Chapter 20.

T-CELL PROLYMPHOCYTIC LEUKEMIA

T-cell prolymphocytic leukemia usually manifests similar to B-cell PLL (B-PLL) with a high white cell count (greater than 100 × 10⁹/L), but is often associated with widespread lymphadenopathy, splenomegaly, serous effusions, and skin lesions, and runs an aggressive course. The cells resemble those of B-PLL but may have a more irregular outline, a higher N/C ratio, and an inconspicuous nucleolus (Figs. 18-42 and 18-43). Two thirds of the cases show inv(14) (see Fig. 20-49), with similar breakpoints in 14q11 and 14q32. ATM mutations are frequent. Most are CD4+, CD8− (see Table 18-5).

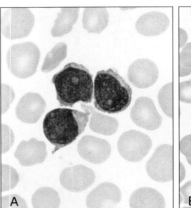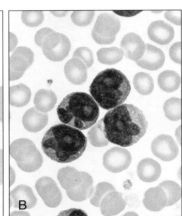

Fig. 18-43. T-cell prolymphocytic leukemia. **A, B,** Small cell type with scant cytoplasm and irregular nuclear outline.

TABLE 18-5.   CHRONIC T-CELL LEUKEMIAS: MEMBRANE IMMUNOPHENOTYPIC PATTERNS

	LGLL*	T-PLL	ATLL	Sézary syndrome
CD2	+	+	+	+
CD3	+	+/−	+	+
CD5	−	+	+	+
CD7	−/+	++	−	−
CD4		+	+	+
CD8	+	+/−	−	−
CD25	−	−/+	++	−
CD56/57	+	−	−	−

LGLL, large granular lymphocyte leukemia
T-PLL, T-cell prolymphocytic leukemia
ATLL, adult T-cell leukemia–lymphoma
*Approximately 15% of LGLL have an NK phenotype (CD3−, CD56+)

Note: These marker patterns are usual, but variant patterns also occur.

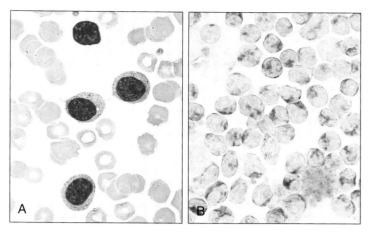

Fig. 18-44. Large granular lymphocytic leukemia: peripheral blood films showing **(A)** abnormal lymphocytes and **(B)** characteristic "clump" positivity in the Golgi zone using acid phosphatase staining.

LARGE GRANULAR LYMPHOCYTIC LEUKEMIA

In large granular lymphocytic leukemia patients usually have chronic neutropenia, anemia, and T-cell lymphocytosis, which persists for more than 3 months. Some patients show seropositive rheumatoid arthritis and splenomegaly. T-cell receptor gene rearrangement analysis shows that the cells are usually clonal, but the disease often runs a benign course. The cells may be large and have abundant cytoplasm and show multiple fine or coarse azurophil granules (Figs. 18-44 and 18-45). Some of the cells are positive for tartrate-resistant acid phosphatase. In the majority of cases the cells are positive for T-cell markers CD3+ and CD8+ and show T-cell receptor α/β rearrangement but are usually CD4− (see Fig. 18-45). Figure 18-46 shows the immunophenotype of a rare CD4+ case. Other rare cases show rearrangement of the T-cell γ/δ receptor rather than the α/β receptor. Approximately 15% of cases have an immunophenotype of natural killer cells (CD3−, CD56+, CD57+).

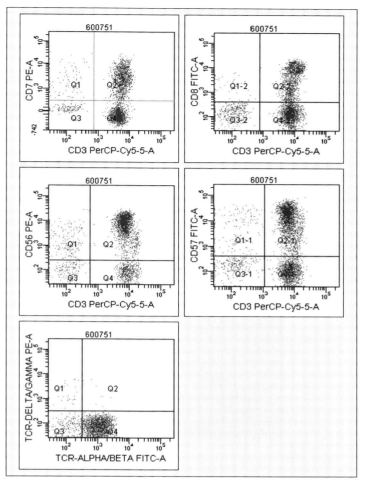

Fig. 18-46. Large granular lymphocytic leukemia. FACS analysis. In this rare type, the cells are CD3+, CD4+, CD8+, CD56+, CD57+, and TCR α/β receptor positive. More usually (as in Fig. 18-45), the cells are CD8+, CD4−. (Courtesy of the Immunophenotyping Laboratory, Royal Free Hospital.)

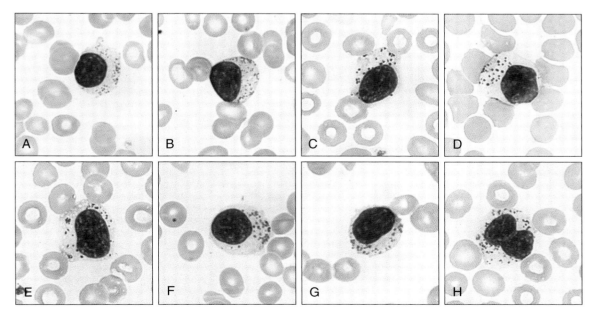

Fig. 18-45. Large granular lymphocytic leukemia. **A–H,** Peripheral blood films showing representative large lymphocytes with multiple coarse, azurophilic, cytoplasmic granules. Immunologic marker studies showed the cells to be CD8+, CD4−, CD3+, CD16+, and CD57+. The patient had splenomegaly, chronic neutropenia, and lymphocytosis. (Absolute lymphocyte count, 9.4×10^9/L.)

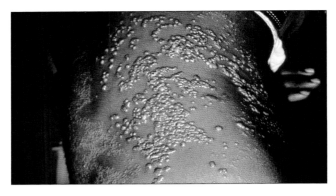

Fig. 18-47. Adult T-cell leukemia/lymphoma syndrome: extensive involvement of the skin. (Courtesy of Dr. J.W. Clark.)

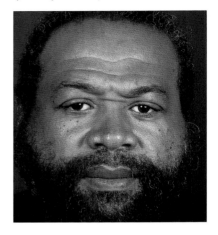

Fig. 18-48. Adult T-cell leukemia/lymphoma in a 42-year-old male patient. He was diagnosed in Jamaica 5 years earlier to have paraplegia because of spinal disease. He had firm swelling of the salivary glands, but no superficial lymphadenopathy. (Hb, 12.3 g/dl; WBC, 28 × 10⁹/L; platelets, 134 × 10⁹/L; serum positive for anti–HTLV-I; serum calcium normal; no skin rash.)

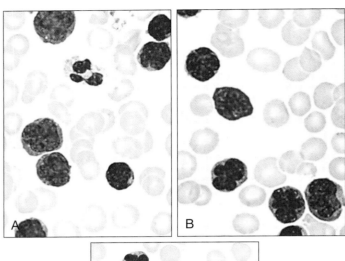

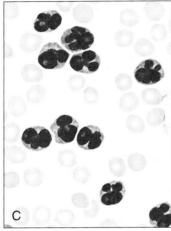

Fig. 18-49. Adult T-cell leukemia/lymphoma syndrome. **A–C,** Peripheral blood films showing the characteristic abnormal lymphocytes with convoluted nuclei.

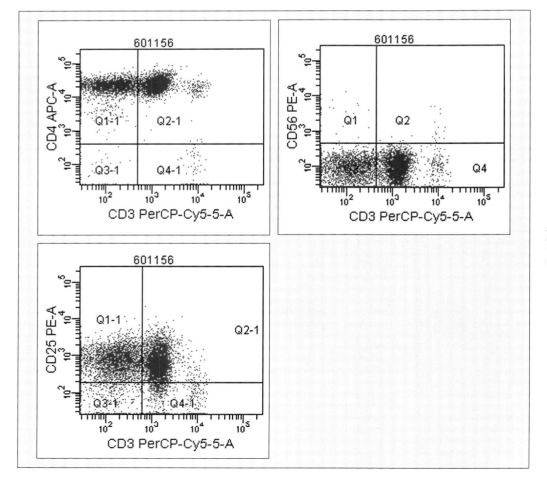

Fig. 18-50. Adult T-cell leukemia/lymphoma syndrome FACS analysis. The cells are CD3+, CD4+, CD25+, and CD56−. (Courtesy of the Immunophenotyping Laboratory, Royal Free Hospital.)

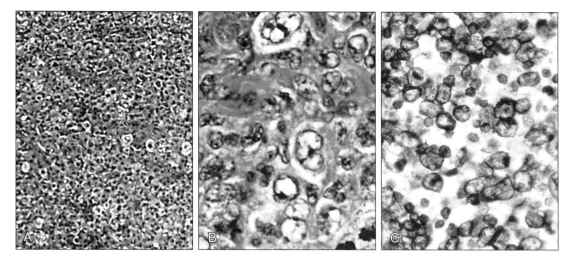

Fig. 18-51. Adult T-cell lymphoma/leukemia syndrome: histologic sections of lymph node showing **(A)** replacement of normal architecture by pleomorphic lymphoid cells; **(B)** occasional bizarre polylobulated giant cells and prominent mitotic figures at high magnification; and **(C)** paraffin-stained (immunophosphatase) section for CD3. (Courtesy of Professor D.Y. Mason.)

ADULT T-CELL LEUKEMIA/LYMPHOMA

Adult T-cell leukemia/lymphoma is an unusual lymphoproliferative malignancy that occurs predominantly in Japan and in blacks of the West Indies and other Caribbean countries and of the United States (Figs. 18-47 and 18-48). Typically, the lymphoma evolves rapidly with early involvement of the lymph nodes, skin (see Fig. 18-47), blood (Fig. 18-49), and bone marrow. The cells are CD4+, CD3+, CD25+ (Fig. 18-50).

The white cell count varies widely with between 10% and 80% of tumor cells. The neoplastic lymphoid cells vary in size and have an irregular nucleus, often with marked convolutions (Figs. 18-49 and 18-51). Associated hypercalcemia may lead to death in coma. The disease is caused by a C-type RNA retrovirus, human T-cell lymphoma/leukemia virus I (HTLV-I). The life cycle of a typical retrovirus is illustrated in Fig. 18-52. Invasion of the host cell causes cell proliferation, but there is no consistent integration site and no identified oncogene activation.

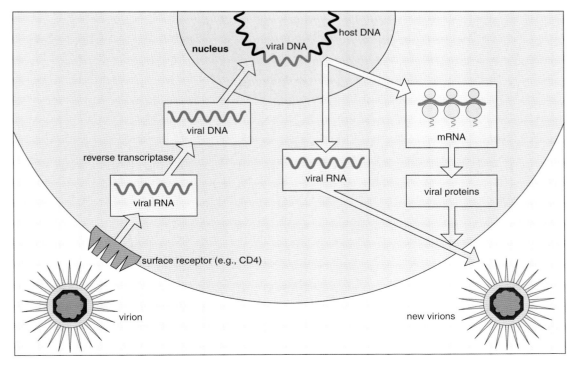

Fig. 18-52. Replication of a retrovirus within a host cell.

NON-HODGKIN LYMPHOMAS: MATURE B-CELL NEOPLASMS

WRITTEN WITH PROFESSOR ELIAS CAMPO

INTRODUCTION

The term *malignant lymphoma* embraces all neoplastic diseases that originate in the lymph nodes or extranodal lymphatic tissue. They comprise Hodgkin lymphoma (discussed in Chapter 21), which is relatively uniform in histology, and the large heterogeneous category known as the non-Hodgkin lymphomas, which vary from highly proliferating and rapidly fatal disorders to indolent (although often incurable) malignancies that may be well tolerated for 10 to 20 years or more. It has been known for many years that non-Hodgkin lymphomas represent monoclonal expansions of B or T cells or natural killer (NK) cells. Evidence of this comes from both expression of a single type of immunoglobulin (Ig) on the cell surface and/or within the cytoplasm and also from studies of Ig or T-cell receptor gene rearrangement. It is possible to find a normal counterpart for many types of non-Hodgkin lymphoma. The large number of these diseases reflects the rich diversity of much of the maturation stages and subpopulations of reactive human lymphoid cells. The Reed-Sternberg cells characteristic of a Hodgkin lymphoma are also clonal in origin, deriving from B cells.

Sometimes the difference between lymphomas, in which lymph node, spleen, or other solid tumor is present, and lymphoid leukemias (acute and chronic), with dominant bone marrow disease, is imprecise because lymphomas can be leukemic and leukemias can be lymphomatous (e.g., they can manifest as solid tumor deposits). A single lymphoproliferative disease can be categorized as two clinical manifestations, for example, chronic lymphocytic leukemia and small lymphocytic lymphoma merge into each other, their cell phenotypes and genotypes being identical. Also lymphoblastic lymphomas of precursor B or T cells are now classified with B-cell lineage acute lymphoblastic leukemia (ALL) or T-cell ALL, respectively, and treated as such (Chapter 12).

TABLE 19-1.   THE WORLD HEALTH ORGANIZATION CLASSIFICATION (2008) OF THE MATURE B-CELL NEOPLASMS

Chronic lymphocytic leukemia/small lymphocytic lymphoma

B-cell prolymphocytic leukemia	Nodal marginal zone lymphoma
Splenic marginal zone lymphoma	*Pediatric nodal MZL*
Hairy cell leukemia	Follicular lymphoma
Splenic lymphoma/leukemia, unclassifiable	*Pediatric follicular lymphoma*
Splenic diffuse red pulp small B-cell lymphoma	Primary cutaneous follicle center lymphoma
Hairy cell leukemia-variant	Mantle cell lymphoma
Lymphoplasmacytic lymphoma	Diffuse large B-cell lymphoma, not otherwise
Waldenström macroglobulinemia	specified
Heavy chain diseases	T cell/histiocyte-rich large B-cell lymphoma
Alpha heavy chain disease	Primary DLBCL of the CNS
Gamma heavy chain disease	Primary cutaneous DLBCL, leg type
Mu heavy chain disease	*EBV + DLBCL of the elderly*
Plasma cell myeloma	Lymphomatoid granulomatosis
Solitary plasmacytoma of bone	Primary mediastinal (thymic) large B-cell
Extraosseous plasmacytoma	lymphoma
Extranodal marginal zone lymphoma of mucosa-	Intravascular large B-cell lymphoma
associated lymphoid tissue (MALT lymphoma)	ALK positive large cell lymphoma

Plasmablastic lymphoma

Primary effusion lymphoma

Large B-cell lymphoma arising in HHV8-associated multicentric Castleman disease

Burkitt lymphoma
B-cell lymphoma, unclassifiable, with features intermediate between diffuse large B-cell lymphoma and Burkitt lymphoma
B-cell lymphoma, unclassifiable, with features intermediate between diffuse large B-cell lymphoma and classical Hodgkin lymphoma

GEOGRAPHIC VARIATION

The frequencies of some types of non-Hodgkin lymphoma vary markedly between the different parts of the world. For example, two lymphoma categories that are common in Western countries, Hodgkin lymphoma and follicular lymphoma, are much rarer in Eastern and less developed countries, whereas large B-cell lymphomas and T-cell neoplasms are more frequent in the latter areas. Some subtypes of non-Hodgkin lymphoma that are only rarely seen in Western countries are found at much higher frequency elsewhere, and this may be partly accounted for by local patterns of exposure to

viruses and other pathogens (Table 19-2). In each of these instances the infectious agent presumably provides a stimulating effect on lymphoid cell growth, but how this interacts with other cellular mechanisms to induce neoplastic transformation is unclear.

CHROMOSOME ABNORMALITIES

The molecular etiology of lymphomas has been shown by the study of chromosome alterations (Table 19-3), and in many instances the consequences of these alterations have been identified

TABLE 19-2.   LYMPHOMA AND INFECTIOUS AGENTS: GEOGRAPHIC DISTRIBUTION

Lymphoma type	Infectious agent	Geographic distribution
Viruses		
Burkitt	Epstein–Barr virus and malaria	Endemic form—areas with malaria in Africa and New Guinea
Nasal type NK/T cell (angiocentric)	Epstein–Barr virus	Asia, Mexico, Central and South America
Lymphoplasmacytic; cryoglobulinemia; rarely lymphomas of liver, salivary glands	Hepatitis C	Mediterranean
Primary effusion lymphoma; solid tumors arising in Castleman's disease or *de novo* in nodular or extranodal tissues (large cell immunoblastic or anaplastic)	Human herpes virus 8 (HHV-8) usually in conjunction with HIV	Non-HIV associated in Mediterranean area (high prevalence of HHV-8 infection)
Adult T-cell leukemia/lymphoma	Human T-cell leukemia virus – type 1 (HTLV-1)	Japan, Caribbean, Central Africa
Bacteria		
Extranodal marginal zone B-cell lymphoma of mucosa associated lymphoid tissue (MALT)	*Helicobacter pylori*	High incidence in North-East Italy
Immunoproliferative small intestinal disease (IPSID)	*Helicobacter pylori*	Middle East, South Africa
Cutaneous B-cell	*Borrelia burgdorferi*	

TABLE 19-3.   NON-HODGKIN LYMPHOMA: CHROMOSOME TRANSLOCATIONS AND THEIR GENETIC CONSEQUENCES

Neoplasm	Translocation	Genes involved	Consequences
B-cell neoplasms			
Burkitt's	t(8;14)(q24;q32)	MYC and IgH	Activation of c-MYC (DNA-binding protein)
	t(2;8)(q11;q24)	MYC IgK	Activation of c-MYC (DNA-binding protein)
	t(8;14)(q24;q32)	MYC Igγ	Activation of c-MYC (DNA-binding protein)
MALT	t(11;18)(q21;q21)	AP12 and MALT1	Reduced apoptosis
	t(1;14)(p24;q32)	BCL-10	More aggressive disease
	t(14;18)(q32;q21)	IgH-MALT1	
	t(3;14)(p14;q32)	IgH-FOXP1	
Follicular	t(14;18)(q32;q21)	IgH and BCL-2	Activation of BCL-2 (apoptosis inhibitor)
Mantle cell	t(11;14)(q13;q32)	CCND1 and IgH	Activation of cyclin D1
Diffuse large B-cell	t(3;14)(q27;q32)	BCL-6	Extranodal disease; better prognosis
	t(14;18)(q32;q21)	IgH and BCL-2	Activation of BCL-2 (apoptosis inhibitor)
T-cell neoplasms (See Chapter 20)			
Peripheral T-cell lymphoma	Complex rearrangements	TCR*	
Anaplastic large cell	t(2;5)(p23;q35)	ALK and NPM	Creation of hybrid NPM–ALK tyrosine kinase

*T cell receptor genes are also usually clonally rearranged in enteropathy-type T-cell lymphoma, subcutaneous panniculitis-like T-cell lymphoma, mycosis fungoides, and Sézary syndrome cells and other T-cell neoplasms

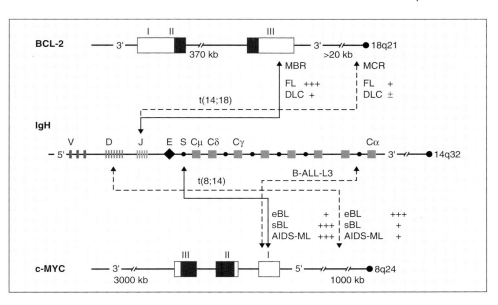

Fig. 19-1. Non-Hodgkin lymphoma: molecular analysis of common breakpoints found in reciprocal translocations involving IgH and BCL-2 (follicular lymphoma) or IgH and c-MYC (in Burkitt's lymphoma). Exons of BCL-2 and c-MYC are represented by rectangles with roman numeral designation above. Coding regions of BCL-2 and c-MYC are solid red rectangles. (MBR, major breakpoint cluster region; MCR, minor breakpoint cluster region; V, variable region; D, diversity region; J, joining region; E, enhancer; S, switch region; C, constant regions of IgH genes; FL, follicular lymphoma; DLC, diffuse large B-cell lymphoma type; ALL, acute lymphoblastic leukemia; eBL, endemic Burkitt's lymphoma; sBL, sporadic Burkitt's lymphoma; AIDS-ML, AIDS-related malignant lymphoma; +++, majority of cases; +, minority of cases; ±, some cases.)

at the deoxyribonucleic acid (DNA) level (Fig. 19-1). Other diseases (e.g., mantle cell lymphoma, ALK positive, and anaplastic large cell lymphoma) are defined on the basis of a genetic abnormality.

In the past, following the terminology of Rappaport from the 1960s, many large cell non-Hodgkin lymphomas were referred to as "histiocytic," but it is now evident that the vast majority of neoplasms arising from the monocyte-phagocyte system manifest as leukemias. The latter are summarized in Chapter 16 and T-cell lymphomas in Chapter 20. This chapter discusses the largest group, the mature B-cell lymphomas.

MATURE B-CELL NEOPLASMS

These tumors make up 85% on the non-Hodgkin lymphomas. Follicular lymphoma and diffuse large B-cell lymphoma are the most frequent subtypes in Western counties. The diseases are clonal and resemble phenotypically different B-cell subpopulations at various stages of maturation (Fig. 19-2, Table 19-4).

The major risk factors for mature B-cell neoplasms are abnormalities of the immune system, particularly immune deficiency or autoimmune diseases. Immune deficiency may be caused by human immunodeficiency virus (HIV) infection (see Chapter 11);

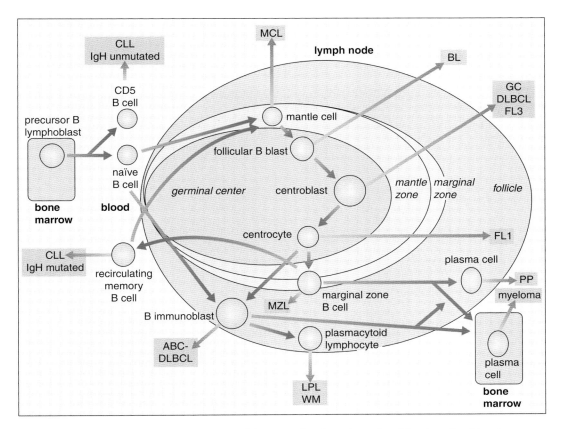

Fig. 19-2. Suggested lymphoid cell of origin of the mature B-cell neoplasms. For diffuse large B-cell lymphoma (DLBCL) two types, one arising from the germinal center (GC), the other from an activated peripheral blood B cell (ABC), have been identified by gene array and immunohistologic markers. Chronic lymphocytic leukemia (CLL) may originate from a cell with mutated IgH genes or from an antigen experienced cell with unmutated IgH genes. FL1, FL3, follicular lymphoma grades 1 and 3; LPL, lymphoplasmacytic lymphoma; MCL, mantle cell lymphoma; MZL, marginal zone lymphoma; PP, peripheral plasmacytoma; WM, Waldenstrom's macroglobulinemia. (See also Fig. 4-69.)

TABLE 19-4A. IMMUNOPHENOTYPE OF MATURE B-CELL NEOPLASMS

Disease	CD19, CD20, CD22, CD79a	SIg	CD10	CD23	BCL-2	BCL-6	MUM1	CD5	Additional antibodies
Chronic lymphocytic leukemia/ small cell lymphocytic lymphoma	+	Weak	–	+	+	–	–	+	FMC7–, CD79b–, CD43–
B-prolymphocytic leukemia	+	+	–	–	+	+/–	+/–	+/–	
Hairy cell leukemia	+	+	–	–	+/–	–	+/–	–	DBA44+, CD25+, CD11c+, CD103+, CD123+, Annexin I+
Lymphoplasmacytic lymphoma	+	+ cyt Ig +/– –	–	–	+	–	+	–	
Myeloma (plasmacytoma)	– CD79a +/–	– Cyt Ig +	–	–	–	–	+	–	CD138+
Splenic, nodal, and extranodal marginal zone lymphoma	+	+	–	–	+	–	+/–	–	CD21+, CD35+, CD43+/–
Follicular lymphoma	+	+	+/–	+/–	+	–	–	–	HGAL+
Mantle cell lymphoma	+	+	–	–	+	–	–	+	Cyclin D1+, FMC7+
Diffuse large B-cell lymphoma (GC type)	+ (variable)	+/–	+	+/–	+/–	+/–	–	–	MIBI +/–, HGAL+
Diffuse large B-cell lymphoma (ABC type)	+ (variable)	+/–	–	+/–	+/–	+	+	–	MIBI +/–, HGAL+
Mediastinal B-cell lymphoma	+/–	+	–	+/–	+/–	+/–	+/–	–	CD30+, CD45+
Burkitt lymphoma	+	+	+	–	–	+	–	–	MIBI nearly 100%, HGLA+

Key : S = surface, Cyt = cytoplasmic, HGAL = human germinal center–associated lymphoma protein.
MUM1 is expressed on plasma cells and later stages of B-cell development. MIBI detects the Ki-67 antigen, a proliferation marker.

TABLE 19-4B. IMMUNOLOGIC MARKERS OF VALUE IN CLASSIFYING THE MATURE B-CELL NEOPLASMS

Reagent	Normal distribution of staining	Clinical utility in mature B-cell lymphoid malignancy	Comments
CD5	T cells and minor B-cell subset	Expression on B cells: CLL, MCL	–
CD10	Immature T cells and B cells, subset of mature T cells and B cells, and neutrophils	Germinal center-like phenotype: FL, DLBCL, BL; frequently present in ALL	–
CD19	All B cells, including lymphoblasts, mature B-lymphoid cells, and most plasma cells	Indicates B-cell lineage; may demonstrate abnormal intensity in B-cell neoplasms; usually absent in plasma cell neoplasms	Aberrant expression on myeloid cells in AML or MDS
CD20	Acquired during maturation of precursor B cells (hematogones); mature B-lymphoid cells positive; absent on most BM plasma cells; minor T-cell subset	Supports B-cell lineage; intensity often differs between subtypes: CLL/SLL dim, FL brighter; aberrant expression on ALL or PCN	Present on occasional T-cell lymphoid neoplasms
CD45	All B cells (weaker intensity on precursors and plasma cells), all T cells (weaker intensity on precursors)	Useful in distinguishing mature lymphoid neoplasms (bright intensity) from ALL and PCN (weak intensity to negative)	–
Kappa and lambda, surface	Mature B cells	Immunoglobulin light chain reaction	–
CD9*	Precursor B cells, activated T cells, platelets	Precursor B-cell ALL	–
CD11c*	Some B cells, some T cells	Hairy cell leukemia CD11c (+ br) Hodgkin lymphoma	Frequent weaker expression on CLL, MCL and others
CD15*	Myeloid and monocytic cells	May be aberrantly expressed in B-cell neoplasia	More frequently seen in ALL than in mature neoplasm

TABLE 19-4B.   IMMUNOLOGIC MARKERS OF VALUE IN CLASSIFYING THE MATURE B-CELL NEOPLASMS—cont'd

Reagent	Normal distribution of staining	Clinical utility in mature B-cell lymphoid malignancy	Comments
CD22*	Cytoplasmic expression in early B cells; surface expression acquired during maturation of precursor B cells	Indicates B-cell lineage in ALL and mature lymphoid neoplasms; intensity often differs between subtypes of mature B-cell neoplasm: CLL/SLL dim	Cross reactivity of some clones with monocytes and basophils
CD23*	Weak intensity expression on resting B cells and increased with activation	Distinguish CD5+ B-cell lymphoid neoplasms; CLL/SLL+	–
CD25*	Activated B cells and T cells	Hairy cell leukemia in combination with CD11c and CD103	–
CD13*	Myeloid and monocytic cells	May be aberrantly expressed in B-cell neoplasia	More frequently seen in ALL than in mature neoplasms
CD33*	Myeloid and monocytic cells	May be aberrantly expressed in B-cell neoplasia	More frequently seen in ALL than in mature neoplasms
CD34*	B-cell and T-cell precursors and myeloblasts	ALL	Also AML
CD38*	Precursor B cells (hematogones), normal follicle center B cells, immature and activated T cells, plasma cells (bright intensity), myeloid and monocytic cells, and erythroid precursors	Bright intensity staining may indicate plasmacytic differentiation; prognostic marker in CLL/SLL	–
CD43*	T cells, myeloid, monocytes, small B-cell subset	Aberrant expression in CLL, MCL, some MZL	–
CD58*	Leukocytes including bright intensity staining of precursors and decreased intensity with maturation	Distinction of ALL from normal precursor B-cell (hematogones) including detection of minimal residual disease	–
CD79a and b*	Cytoplasmic staining in precursor B cells, plasma cells positive, variable expression mature B cells	Indicates B-cell lineage in ALL and mature lymphoid neoplasms; intensity often differs between subtypes of mature B-cell neoplasm; CLL/SLL dim CD79b	CD79a staining has been reported in some T-ALL and rare mature T-cell lymphoid neoplasms
CD103*	B-cell subset, intramucosal T cells	Hairy cell leukemia and some MZL	Also EATCL
FMC-7*	B cells	Distinguish CD5+ lymphoid neoplasms: CLL−, MCL often positive. Also HCL+	
BCL-2*	T cells, some B cells; negative normal germinal center cells	Distinguish CD10+ lymphoid neoplasms; FL+, DL−, BL−	Variable staining in DLBCL
Kappa and lambda, cytoplasmic	Plasma cells	Light chain restriction in cells with plasmacytic differentiation	Most flow cytometric assays detect surface and cytoplasmic Ig
Zap-70*	T cells, NK cells, precursor B cells	Prognostic marker in CLL/SLL	–
TdT*	B-cell and T-cell precursors	ALL	Also some AML
cIgM*	First Ig component in precursor B cells; expressed by subset of plasma cells and mature B cells	IgM-producing neoplasms that might be associated with Waldenstrom macro-globulinemia	–

Reagents included in this table are recommended in the consensus guidelines.
+ indicates usually positive; − usually negative; b, bright or strong intensity; Ig, immunoglobulin; TdT, terminal deoxynucleotidyl transferase; cIg, cytoplasmic immunoglobulin; −, not applicable; EATCL, enteropathy associated T cell lymphoma.
*These reagents may be considered for secondary evaluation, after other reagents listed have been used in the initial evaluation.

may occur after allogeneic transplantation, particularly when immunosuppressive drugs are used (see Chapter 23); or the immune deficiency may be primary. MALT lymphomas of the salivary glands or thyroid are examples of lymphomas associated with autoimmune disease (see p. 341).

Epstein-Barr virus (EBV) underlies 100% of endemic, 10% to 25% of sporadic, and 40% of HIV-associated Burkitt's lymphoma (and probably many cases of Hodgkin lymphoma). Human herpes virus 8 (HHV-8) (previously called Kaposi sarcoma herpes virus) is

associated in HIV-infected patients with primary effusion lymphoma and lymphomas arising in multicentric Castleman's disease (see p. 357). Hepatitis C virus underlies some cases of lymphoplasmacytic lymphoma associated with cryoglobulinemia and some lymphomas of the liver and salivary glands.

Helicobacter pylori, by stimulating an immune response to its bacterial antigens, is thought to be responsible for gastric mucosa associated lymphoid tissue (MALT) lymphomas, and *Borrelia burgdorferi* has been implicated in cutaneous MALT lymphoma.

TABLE 19-5. COTSWOLD REVISION
OF THE ANN ARBOR
STAGING CLASSIFICATION

Stage	Definition
I	Involvement of a single lymph node region or lymphoid structure (e.g. spleen, thymus, Waldeyer ring).
II	Involvement of two or more lymph node regions on the same side of the diaphragm (the mediastinum is a single site; hilar lymph nodes are lateralized); the number of anatomic sites should be indicated by suffix (e.g. II$_3$)
III	Involvement of lymph node regions or structures on both sides of the diaphragm.
III$_1$	With or without splenic, hilar, celiac or portal nodes.
III$_2$	With paraaortic, iliac or mesenteric nodes.
IV	Involvement of extranodal site(s) beyond those designated E.

E$_1$ involvement of a single extranodal site, or contiguous or proximal to known nodal site of disease.

CLINICAL FEATURES AND DIAGNOSIS

The clinical presentation of non-Hodgkin lymphoma is more variable than that of Hodgkin lymphoma and the pattern of tumor spread is not as regular. Staging is with the Ann Arbor system (Table 19-5) but is less useful than in Hodgkin lymphoma. Furthermore, a greater proportion of patients have disease in organs other than lymph nodes or have leukemic manifestations. The median age of presentation of low grade and large cell B lymphomas is 55 to 60 years. Patients with indolent histology do not usually have B symptoms (fever 38° C or more, night sweats, or loss of more than 10% of body weight in 6 months), but these features are common in those with aggressive histology.

Patients may have asymmetric, painless enlargement of lymph nodes in one or more peripheral node regions (Fig. 19-3). This presentation is often associated with widespread involvement of lymph nodes (e.g., mesenteric or retroperitoneal) that is not detectable on routine clinical examination (Fig. 19-4). The liver and spleen may also be enlarged (Figs. 19-5 and 19-6).

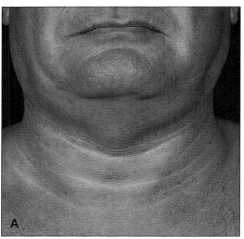 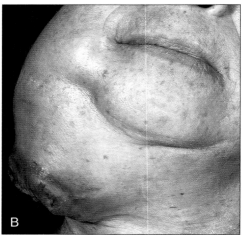 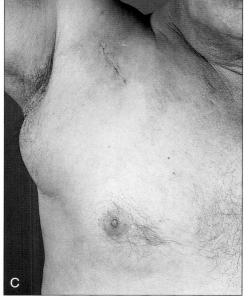

Fig. 19-3. Non-Hodgkin lymphoma. **A,** Bilateral cervical lymphadenopathy in a patient with CLL/small lymphocytic lymphoma. **B,** Massive enlargement of lymph nodes in the left submandibular area, with extensive ulceration of the overlying skin in a patient with diffuse large B-cell lymphoma. **C,** Massive enlargement of axillary nodes with mass extending subcutaneously and also intramuscularly in the right infraclavicular and supraclavicular regions in a patient with diffuse large B-cell lymphoma.

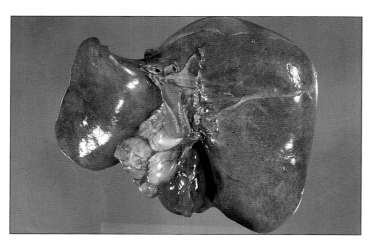

Fig. 19-4. Diffuse large B-cell lymphoma: enlarged porta hepatis lymph nodes seen at autopsy.

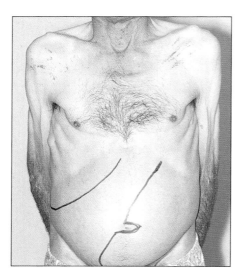

Fig. 19-5. Non-Hodgkin lymphoma: massive enlargement of the spleen and hepatomegaly in CLL/small lymphocytic lymphoma. (Hb, 9.5 g/dl; WBC, 6.0 × 10^9/L; lymphocytes, 2.7 × 10^9/L; platelets, 80 × 10^9/L.)

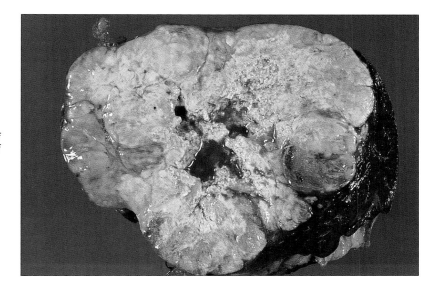

Fig. 19-6. Diffuse large B-cell lymphoma: macroscopic appearance of spleen removed at laparotomy, showing widespread replacement of splenic tissue by pale tumor and extensive areas of necrosis.

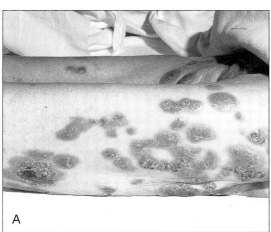

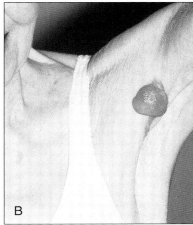

Fig. 19-7. Non-Hodgkin lymphoma: cutaneous deposits in **(A)** advance diffuse large B-cell lymphoma and **(B)** follicular lymphoma.

At least 10% of patients with B-cell non-Hodgkin lymphoma have extranodal disease that includes skin (Fig. 19-7) and soft tissues (Fig. 19-8). When the gastrointestinal tract is involved, patients may have acute abdominal symptoms. However, in some instances extranodal involvement represents a tumor that derives from lymphocytes such as those in the gastrointestinal tract, such as MALT lymphoma (see Fig. 19-30); jaw (e.g., Burkitt's lymphoma, see Fig. 19-82); and are locally spread from these sites (Fig. 19-9). Some B-cell (and T-cell) lymphomas show a predilection for certain tissues, which sometimes reflect the distribution of the normal counterpart from which they derive (Table 19-6).

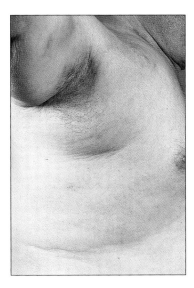

Fig. 19-8. Non-Hodgkin lymphoma: diffuse large B-cell lymphoma invading the anterior and lateral chest wall by direct spread into muscle from the axillary lymph nodes.

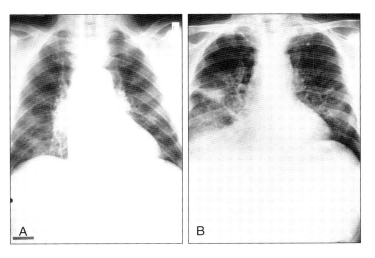

Fig. 19-9. Non-Hodgkin lymphoma: chest radiographs showing **(A)** bilateral hilar lymph node enlargement and **(B)** interstitial and confluent shadowing particularly in the lower and middle zones caused by lymphomatous infiltration (as shown by biopsy) in a patient with MALT lymphoma.

TABLE 19-6. DISTRIBUTION OF SOME LYMPHOID NEOPLASMS AND THEIR CELLS OF ORIGIN

Neoplasm	Cell of origin and its localization
Mycosis fungoides and/or Sézary syndrome	Epidermal associated T cell
MALT lymphoma	Mucosa and/or epithelium associated B cell
Splenic marginal zone lymphoma	Splenic B cells
Follicular lymphoma	Germinal center
Myeloma	Bone marrow plasma cell
Nasal (angiocentric) lymphoma	Nasopharyngeal T/NK EBV + cell
Enteropathy-associated T cell lymphoma	Small intestinal intraepithelial T cell
Hepatosplenic lymphoma	γ/δ T cell in splenic red pulp and liver

Lymphoblastic neoplasms of B-cell type usually manifest as a leukemia (see B-ALL, p. 210) and are not included by the World Health Organization (WHO) as mature B-cell neoplasms. They typically express markers, such as terminal deoxynucleotidyl transferase (TDT) and CD10, found on early B cells. The CD79a antigen is of value, since it is often the only B-cell marker expressed by these cells that is detectable in paraffin-embedded tissue. Although bone marrow and blood involvement is common, a minority of cases manifest as localized solid tumors, usually in lymph nodes. The disease, though aggressive, can be cured, particularly when it occurs in children.

IMAGING

Imaging plays an important part in diagnosing and assessing the distribution (staging) of non-Hodgkin lymphoma. For example, involvement of intrathoracic and intraabdominal sites can be evaluated by computed tomography (CT) scanning (Figs. 19-10 and 19-11).

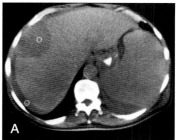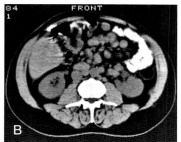

Fig. 19-10. Non-Hodgkin lymphoma: CT scans through the abdomen show **(A)** hepatic and splenic enlargement and a prominent radiolucent focus in the right lobe of the liver (ascitic fluid is present and contrast medium is present in the gut) and **(B)** mesenteric and some para-aortic lymph node enlargement.

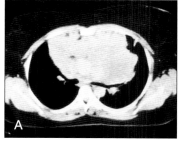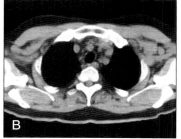

Fig. 19-11. Non-Hodgkin lymphoma: CT scans through the midthorax show **(A)** gross enlargement of anterior mediastinal, paratracheal, and hilar nodes in T-lymphoblastic lymphoma now classified with acute T-cell ALL; **(B)** anterior mediastinal and paratracheal lymph node enlargement in follicular lymphoma.

Magnetic resonance imaging (MRI) is particularly useful for detecting central nervous system (CNS) disease (see Fig. 11-52).

Positrons are positively charged electrons produced by decay of certain radionuclides. They travel a few millimeters before colliding with an electron where the two particles annihilate each other. Two equal protons are produced, which can be detected by a positron emission tomography (PET) camera. 18-Fluorodeoxyglucose (FDG) is used as radionuclide in oncology and detects increased glucose

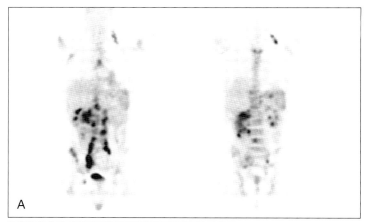

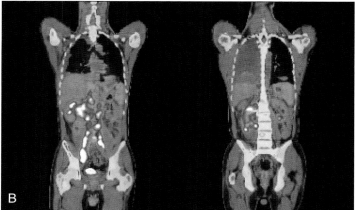

Fig. 19-12. Non-Hodgkin lymphoma. **A,** Coronal FDG PET. Diffuse large B-cell lymphoma showing abnormal FDG uptake in lymph nodes above and below the diaphragm, as well as a focus within the spleen and the bone marrow involvement (lumbar spine and right pelvis). **B,** Fused FDG PET/CT images. A right pleural effusion is also noted on the CT component. (Courtesy of Professor G. Cook.)

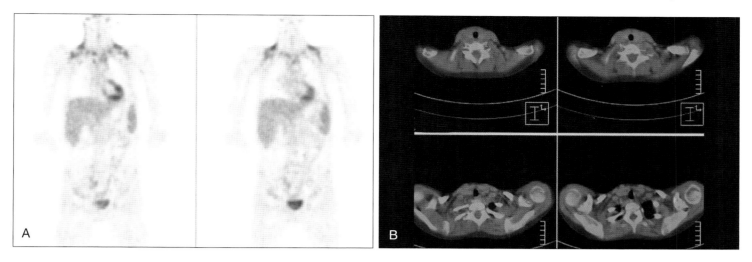

Fig. 19-13. Non-Hodgkin lymphoma. **A,** Coronal FDG PET slices of a patient with diffuse large B-cell lymphoma following chemotherapy showing symmetric activity in the supraclavicular fossae. **B,** Fused FDG PET/CT transaxial slices showing that the FDG activity is confined to fat and therefore represents physiologic brown fat activity rather than active lymphoma. (Courtesy of Professor G. Cook.)

metabolism by the tumor compared with normal tissues. Compared with CT or MRI, PET scanning has the advantage of differentiating active tumor from residual scar tissue.

PET scanning combined with CT is valuable for initial staging (Fig. 19-12) and in detecting residual disease, or confirming remission or restaging after chemotherapy or radiotherapy (Fig. 19-13) or for detecting relapse or transformation to low- or high-grade disease (Fig. 19-14).

DIAGNOSIS

Diagnosis depends on clinical features, the histologic pattern and cytology, the immunologic phenotype (see Tables 19-4, *A* and *B*), and the genetic abnormality detected by conventional cytogenetics, fluorescent in situ hybridization (FISH) analysis, or molecular genetic techniques (see Table 19-3).

Histologic diagnosis of lymph node, bone marrow, or extranodal mass tissue is essential. Fine-needle aspirates were used to exclude or

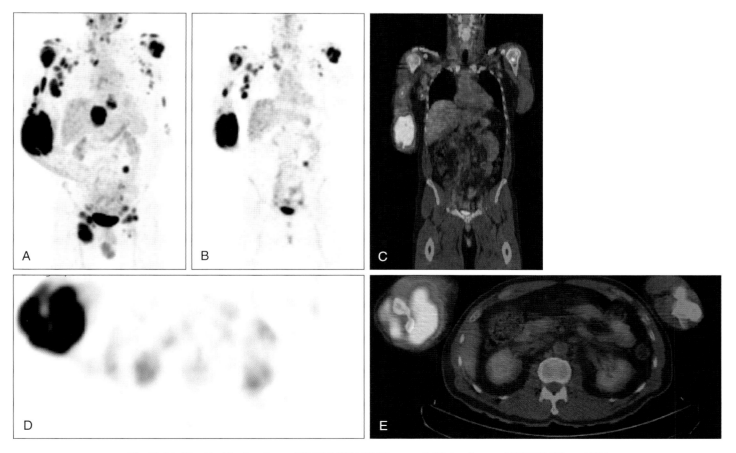

Fig. 19-14. Non-Hodgkin lymphoma: **(A)** FDG PET MIP, **(B)** coronal, **(C)** fused coronal PET/CT, **(D)** axial PET, and **(E)** axial fused PET/CT through elbow. The patient had a previous diagnosis of follicular lymphoma with lymph nodes above and below the diaphragm and bone marrow involvement **(A)** with a sudden increase in size of nodal tissue at the right elbow, which on biopsy proved to be due to transformed high-grade diffuse B-cell lymphoma. (Courtesy of Professor G. Cook.)

TABLE 19-7. IMMUNOPHENOTYPIC FEATURES OF SPLENIC MARGINAL ZONE LYMPHOMA COMPARED WITH OTHER LOW-GRADE B-CELL LEUKEMIAS AND LYMPHOMAS

	SMZL	CLL	MCL	FL	HCL	HCL-v	MALT
Flow cytometry							
Strong SigM	+++	+/−	+++	+++	+++	+++	+++
CD5	+	+++	+++	Neg	Neg	Neg	Neg
CD23	+	+++	Neg	+	Neg	Neg	Neg
FMC7	+++	Neg	+++	+++	+++	+++	+++
CD11c	++	Neg	Neg	Neg	+++	+++	Neg
CD103	Neg	Neg	Neg	Neg	+++	++	Neg
CD123	Neg	Neg	Neg	Neg	+++	Neg	Neg
CD25	+	Neg	Neg	Neg	+++	Neg	Neg
CD27	++	Neg	+++	+++	Neg	++	+
Immunohistochemistry							
DBA44	++	+	Neg	Neg	+++	+++	Neg
IgM, IgD	+++	+++	+	+	+++	+	+
CD10	Neg	Neg	Neg	+++	Neg	Neg	Neg
BCL6	Neg	Neg	Neg	+++	Neg	Neg	Neg
CCND1	Neg	Neg	+++	Neg	+	Neg	Neg
CD5	+/−	+++	+++	Neg	Neg	Neg	Neg
CD43	+/−	+++	+++	Neg	Neg	Neg	+
CD23	Neg	+++	Neg	+	Neg	Neg	Neg
CD27	++	+++	+++	+++	Neg	++	+
Annexin A1	Neg	Neg	Neg	Neg	+++	Neg	Neg

Abbreviations: CLL, chronic lymphocytic leukemia; FL, follicular lymphoma; HCL, hairy cell leukemia; HCL-v, hairy cell leukemia variant; MALT, mucosa-associated lymphoid tissue; MCL, mantle-cell lymphoma; Neg, less than 10% of cases positive; +, 11–35% positive cases;++, 36–75% positive cases; +++, > 75% positive cases; SMZL, splenic marginal zone lymphoma.

(Adapted from Matutes E et al: Leukemia, 22:487-495, 2008)

suggest lymphoma or demonstrate infection in those with unexplained lymphadenopathy. It is essential, however, to perform ultrasound or CT-guided core biopsy or an excision biopsy of a large node or extranodal mass or in some cases splenectomy or bone marrow trephine to obtain adequate material for histology, including immunophenotyping.

Other laboratory findings may include cytopenias due to marrow involvement, hypersplenism or the anemia of chronic disorders but anemia may also be autoimmune, especially in those with low-grade disease. There may be circulating lymphoma cells. This is more common in late-stage disease. Serum lactate dehydrogenase (LDH) is raised in aggressive disease where it is of prognostic significance (Table 19-9). Paraproteins are found in serum in the indolent B-cell lymphomas, for example, small lymphocytic, lymphoplasmacytic, and splenic marginal zone lymphomas, and more rarely in large cell lymphomas.

SMALL LYMPHOCYTIC LYMPHOMA

This disease in the tissue is equivalent to chronic lymphocytic leukemia (CLL). Histologically there is a replacement of lymph node architecture by a monotonous infiltration of small cells with round nuclei with densely clumped heterochromatin (Figs. 19-15, *A*, and 19-16). In some cases these are clusters of larger cells that form pseudofollicles or proliferation centers with regularly distributed pale areas in a background of small darker cells (Fig. 19-15, *B*). Occasionally the neoplastic cells differentiate to a plasma cell stage, but this should not prompt a diagnosis of lymphoplasmacytic lymphoma. Also there may be some larger cells (prolymphocytes) and paraimmunoblasts/large cells with round or oval nuclei, dispersed chromatin, and a central nucleus. There may be diffuse or focal involvement of the bone marrow (Figs. 19-17 and 19-18). If there are more than 5.0×10^9/L circulating lymphocytes, the disease is classified as CLL. Like CLL, the cells are B cells expressing CD5 and CD23 and weak surface immunoglobulin (see Table 19-7).

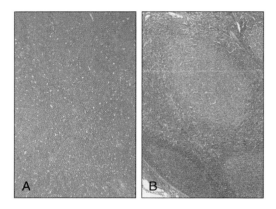

Fig. 19-15. Small lymphocytic lymphoma: **(A)** lymph node shows a diffuse pattern of involvement, with total replacement of the normal architecture by a uniform population of neoplastic lymphocytes; **(B)** lymph node showing a nodular or parafollicular pattern.

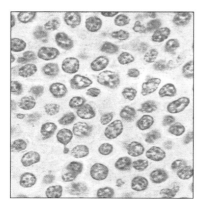

Fig. 19-16. Small lymphocytic lymphoma: a predominance of small lymphocytes with round nuclei that contain densely clumped heterochromatin.

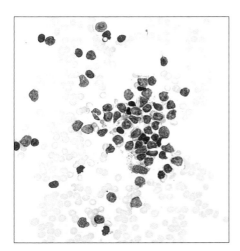

Fig. 19-17. Small lymphocytic lymphoma: bone marrow aspirate showing dominance of neoplastic lymphocytes in the cell trail.

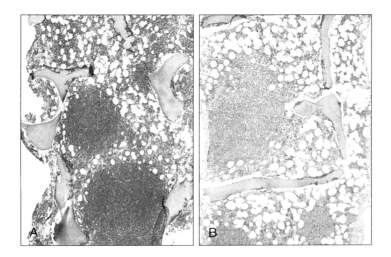

Fig. 19-18. Small lymphocytic lymphoma. **A, B,** Bone marrow trephine biopsies from two patients, showing extensive focal deposits of lymphoma cells.

SPLENIC MARGINAL ZONE LYMPHOMA

This is a primary splenic disease of the elderly. The spleen may be massively enlarged and bone marrow involvement is usual, but lymphadenopathy is rare. A small monoclonal serum paraprotein occurs in about a third of cases, and warm-type autoimmune hemolytic anemia or immune thrombocytopenia is frequent. The peripheral blood shows a moderate lymphocytosis (up to 25 × 10⁹/L), and if the cells have an irregular plasma membrane with villi, often confined to one pole of the cell, the disease has been termed by hematologists as splenic lymphoma with villus lymphocytes (Fig. 19-19). Cytogenetic abnormalities include trisomy 3 and structural abnormalities including allelic loss of chromosome 7q31-32.

Histologically the neoplastic lymphocytes surround and infiltrate the germinal centers in the white pulp (Figs. 19-20 and 19-21). There may be a population of larger tumor cells at the periphery of the germinal center. The red pulp is also infiltrated with nodules of larger cells surrounded by small lymphocytes,

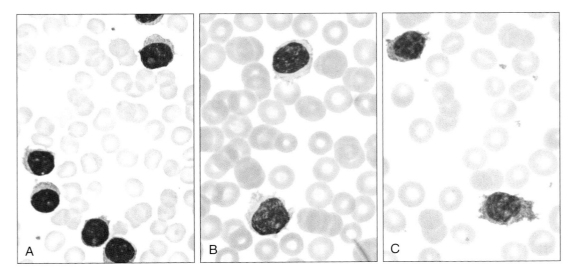

Fig. 19-19. Splenic marginal zone lymphoma. **A–C,** Peripheral blood films on a case with villus lymphocytes showing characteristic cells with irregular plasma membranes with short and thin villi often concentrated at one or two poles of the cells; the cells are larger than in typical CLL, the nucleus is round or ovoid, and sometimes eccentric with a clumped chromatin pattern. (*A,* Courtesy of Professor D. Catovsky; *B, C,* courtesy of Professor M. Peetermans.)

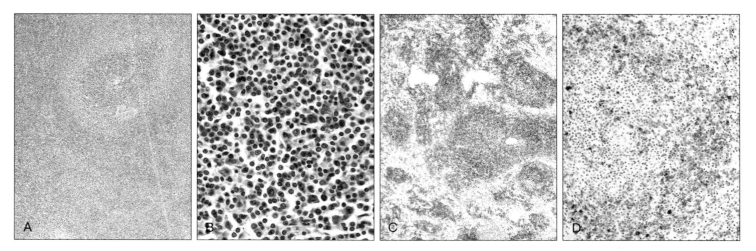

Fig. 19-20. Splenic marginal zone lymphoma. **A,** H&E. The white pulp is expanded with an increase of the marginal zone by neoplastic cells with paler cytoplasm surrounding a residual germinal center. **B,** H&E. Detail of the characteristic biphasic pattern of small lymphocytes and scattered larger cells. **C,** Immunostain: the neoplastic cells are CD20 positive and infiltrate the white and red pulp. **D,** Immunostain: the neoplastic cells are IgD positive.

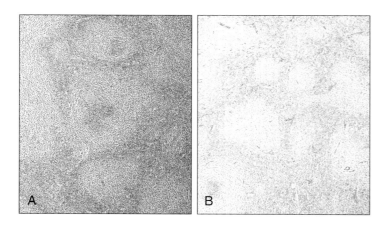

Fig. 19-21. Splenic marginal zone lymphoma. **A,** Splenic pulp showing predominant involvement of the white pulp areas by a uniform population of lymphoplasmacytic cells with clumped nuclear chromatin and a population of nucleolated cells, arranged in nodules with "margination" (larger tumor cells at the periphery and smaller, germinal center cells at the center). **B,** Reticulin stain reveals the nodular distribution of the infiltrate. (Courtesy of Dr. S. Hamilton-Dutoit.)

Fig. 19-22. Splenic marginal zone lymphoma: bone marrow trephine biopsies showing **(A)** nodular infiltrate; **(B)** diffuse interstitial infiltration by lymphocytes with lymphoplasmacytic forms. (Courtesy of Professor K. A. MacLellan.)

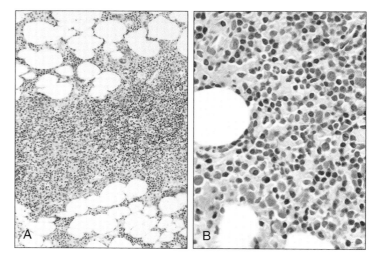

which usually invade sinuses. The cells may also show some lymphoplasmacytic forms. The lymphocytes have the immunophenotype SIgM+, IgD+/−, cytoplasmic Ig−/+, CD19, CD20, CD22, CD79a+, CD5−, CD10−, CD23−, and CD43+/−. The bone marrow shows nodular or interstitial infiltration (Fig. 19-22). The disease is quite different from the other two marginal zone lymphomas, MALT lymphoma and nodal marginal zone lymphoma (see below).

LYMPHOPLASMACYTIC LYMPHOMA/ WALDENSTROM'S MACROGLOBULINEMIA

In this disease, also called immunocytoma in the Kiel classification, the B lymphocytes differentiate toward plasma cells (Fig. 19-23). In the cells with plasmacytic figures, IgM is detectable in the cytoplasm or in the intranuclear inclusions, "Dutcher bodies," which also stain positive for PAS (Fig. 19-24). A paraprotein is usually present in the serum, and when this is IgM and there is bone marrow involvement

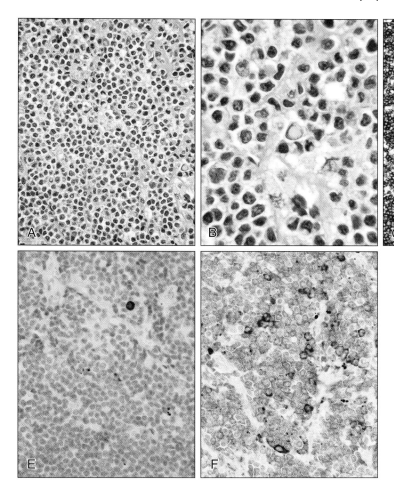

Fig. 19-23. Lymphoplasmacytic lymphoma. **A,** H&E: the tumor is composed of small lymphocytes, plasmacytoid cells, and mature plasma cells. **B,** Detail of neoplastic cytology with Dutcher bodies in the tumor plamacytoid cells. **C,** Immunostain: the neoplastic cells are strongly positive for CD79a. **D, E,** Immunostain kappa **(D)** and lambda **(E)** light chains: the neoplastic cells show kappa light chain restriction. **F,** Immunostain: the neoplastic cells express IgM.

the disease may be termed Waldenstrom's macroglobulinemia. This is often associated with hyperviscosity (Fig. 19-29) or cryoglobulinemia (Fig. 22-61).

The lymphocyte infiltration may replace the normal architecture or be interfollicular with sparing of the sinuses. Pseudofollicles, neoplastic follicles, and marginal zone or monocytoid B cells are absent. The cells, small lymphocytes, plasmacytoid lymphocytes, and plasma cells (Fig. 19-25) may circulate in the peripheral blood (Fig. 19-26) and can be detected as a diffuse or nodular infiltration in the bone marrow (Figs. 19-27 and 19-28) or lymph nodes.

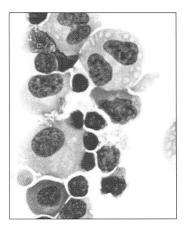

Fig. 19-25. Fine-needle aspirate showing lymphoplasmacytic lymphoma. (May-Grünwald-Giemsa stain.) Some of the cells show plasma cell differentiation with blue cytoplasm with pale staining perinuclear zone ("hof") and eccentric nucleus.

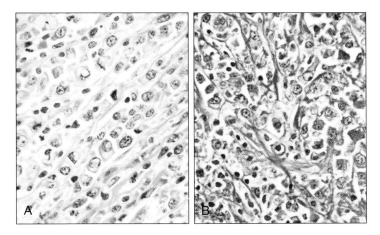

Fig. 19-24. Lymphoplasmacytic lymphoma. **A,** Diffuse sheet of small lymphoid cells, some with plasmacytoid differentiation. **B,** A periodic acid–Schiff (PAS) stain shows more marked plasma cell differentiation (center) with an intranuclear inclusion (Dutcher body; these pink intranuclear inclusions are commonly encountered in lymphoplasmacytic lymphoma). Small scattered lymphocytes and lymphoplasmacytoid cells are also present.

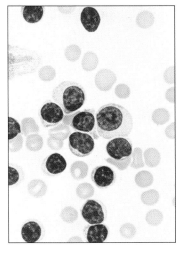

Fig. 19-26. Lymphoplasmacytic lymphoma in leukemic phase: peripheral blood film.

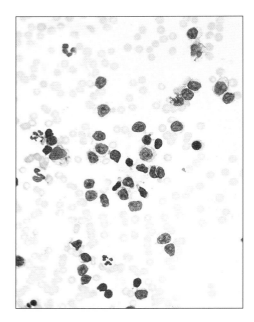

Fig. 19-27. Lymphoplasmatic lymphoma/Waldenström's macroglobulinemia: bone marrow cell trail shows a predominance of lymphocytes and lymphoplasmacytoid cells.

The cells are CD5, CD10, CD23, and BCL6 negative but express BCL-2 and MUM1. The disease may transform into a large cell lymphoma.

HYPERVISCOSITY SYNDROME

The hyperviscosity syndrome may complicate lymphoplasmacytic lymphoma. It is characterized by loss of vision, CNS symptoms, a hemorrhagic diathesis, and heart failure; the most severely affected patients may be in coma. The retina may show a variety of changes, including engorged veins, hemorrhages, exudates, and blurred optic discs (Fig. 19-29). The causes of hyperviscosity are listed in Table 22-5.

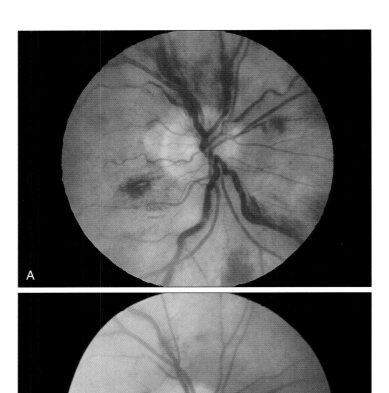

Fig. 19-29. Lymphoplasmacytic lymphoma/Waldenström's macroglobulinemia: hyperviscosity syndrome. The patient complained of blurred vision, headache, and dizziness. **A,** The retina before plasmapheresis shows gross distention of vessels, particularly the veins, which show bulging and constriction (the "linked sausage effect") and areas of hemorrhage. **B,** Following plasmapheresis, the vascular diameters are normal and the hemorrhagic areas have cleared.

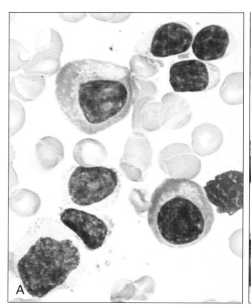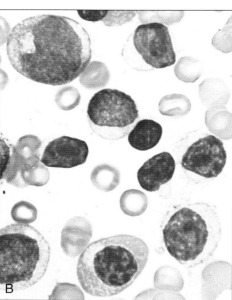

Fig. 19-28. Lymphoplasmacytic lymphoma/Waldenström's macroglobulinemia bone marrow aspirate. **A, B,** The cells have features varying between those of lymphocytes and plasma cells. The chromatin patterns in the larger nuclei are more open and primitive.

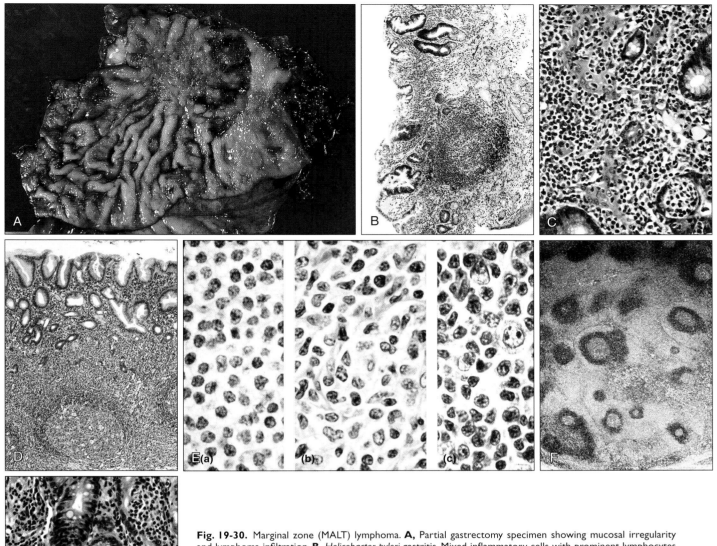

Fig. 19-30. Marginal zone (MALT) lymphoma. **A,** Partial gastrectomy specimen showing mucosal irregularity and lymphoma infiltration. **B,** *Helicobacter pylori* gastritis. Mixed inflammatory cells with prominent lymphocytes infiltrate around a reactive B-cell follicle. **C,** Gastric MALT lymphoma: lymphoepithelial lesions with lymphocytes surrounding and infiltrating epithelial structures. **D,** Gastric MALT lymphoma: the tumor cells surround reactive follicles and infiltrate the mucosa. The follicle has a "starry sky" appearance. **E,** Gastric MALT lymphoma. Cytology: (a) tumor cells resembling centrocytes with abundant cytoplasm; (b) characteristic small to medium-sized cells with irregular nuclei, inconspicuous nucleoli, and abundant pale cytoplasm; (c) cells resembling small lymphocytes with scattered larger cells. **F,** Gastric MALT lymphoma: gastric lymph node: the tumor cells are largely in the marginal zone of the follicles and interfollicular areas. **G,** Gastric MALT lymphoma: transformation to diffuse large B-cell lymphoma in the lower field with residual MALT lymphoma in the superficial aareas. (*B–G*, Courtesy of Professor P. Isaacson.)

EXTRANODAL MARGINAL ZONE B-CELL LYMPHOMA OF MUCOSA ASSOCIATED LYMPHOID TISSUE (MALT) LYMPHOMA

This small cell lymphoma arises in extranodal tissues of the gastro-intestinal tract in at least 50% of cases (Fig. 19-30) or in other extranodal sites, for example, skin (Fig. 19-31) or glandular epithe-lial tissues such as lung, thyroid, breast, and salivary glands (Figs. 19-32 and 19-33). The neoplasm is derived from B cells associated with epithelial tissues. It usually arises against a background of reactive lymphoid tissue in which non-neoplastic germinal centers are prominent.

Gastric MALT lymphoma recapitulates the histology of Peyer's patches. Infection with *Helicobacter pylori* is thought to induce a T-cell reaction against bacterial antigens, which stimulates a B-lymphoid proliferation in the stomach. Elimination of the infection may cause regression of the lymphoma or of the preced-ing polyclonal lymphoid proliferation. The autoimmune disease Sjogren's syndrome may underlie salivary gland MALT and Hashimoto's disease MALT lymphoma of the thyroid.

The cells are heterogeneous including marginal centrocyte-like cells with irregular nuclei, monocytoid cells, small lymphocytes, and scattered large cells. The tumor cells are CD19+, CD20+, CD22+, and CD79a+ B cells that are CD10−, CD23−, and CD43+/−.

The cells infiltrate the marginal zone of reactive B follicles and interfollicular areas. Plasma cell differentiation may be present. Epithelial tissues may be invaded to form lymphoepithelial lesions (see Fig. 19-33). The bone marrow is less frequently involved in MALT lymphomas than in splenic marginal zone lymphoma. Transformation to a diffuse large B-cell lymphoma may occur. An immunoproliferative small intestinal disease (IPSID) is now termed a subtype of MALT lymphoma. It was previously called alpha chain disease.

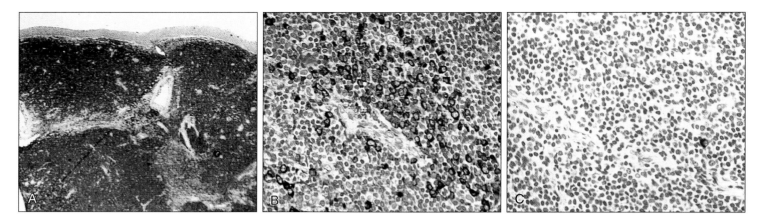

Fig. 19-31. Marginal zone (MALT) lymphoma of the skin. **A,** Low-power view of immunoperoxidase (CD20) stain showing extensive B-cell infiltrate. **B, C,** Clonality of tumor cells (showing plasma cell differentiation) shown by **(B)** kappa positivity and **(C)** rare lambda positivity.

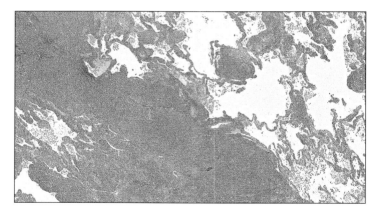

Fig. 19-32. Marginal zone (MALT) lymphoma in the lung: low-power view of a histologic section shows sheets of neoplastic lymphocytes at the edge of the tumor infiltrating the surrounding lung along bronchovascular bundles and alveolar septae.

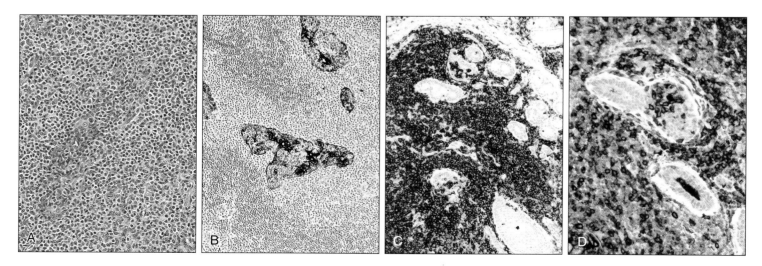

Fig. 19-33. Marginal zone (MALT) lymphoma of salivary gland. **A,** Sheets of marginal zone B cells and formation of lymphoepithelial lesions. **B,** Immunoperoxidase stain for low-molecular-weight cytokeratin (MNF116) shows positive staining of normal epithelial cells infiltrated by lymphoma. **C,** Immunostain showing CD20+ tumor cells surrounding and invading epithelial structures. **D,** The tumor cells express IgM. (*C, D,* Courtesy of Dr. A. Ramsay.)

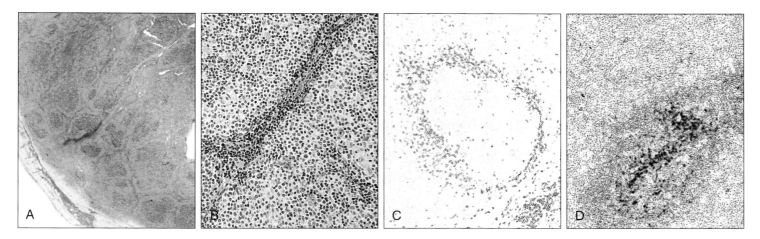

Fig. 19-34. Nodal marginal zone B-cell lymphoma. **A,** H&E: the neoplastic cells infiltrate the interfollicular area. **B,** H&E: perivascular infiltrate of monocytoid cells with pale cytoplasm. **C,** Immunostain: the neoplastic cells are IgD negative whereas the residual mantle cuff is positive. The tumor cells grow in the perifollicular areas. **D,** Immunostain: CD10 staining highlights the residual germinal center of the follicle colonized by CD10-negative tumor cells.

NODAL MARGINAL ZONE B-CELL LYMPHOMA

This is a rare disease involving peripheral lymph nodes and only occasionally bone marrow or blood. The marginal zones and interfollicular areas are infiltrated by neoplastic marginal zone B cells (Fig. 19-34). These include centrocyte-like cells, monocytoid B cells, and small lymphocytes with scatted large blast cells. The cells may surround small blood vessels. The cells may colonize germinal centers of the follicles. The immunophenotype is similar to that of MALT lymphomas. In some cases the cells are uniformly monocytoid and this has been termed monocytoid B-cell lymphoma (Fig. 19-35).

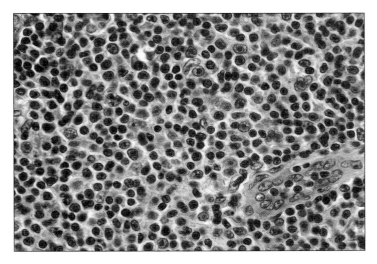

Fig. 19-35. Nodal marginal zone lymphoma (monocytoid B-cell lymphoma): lymph node shows an admixture of small to medium-sized B cells with abundant clear cytoplasm and scanty, admixed, large, transformed lymphoid cells. A venule with high endothelial cells is present, as typically encountered in this form of lymphoma.

FOLLICULAR LYMPHOMA

These tumors account for 35% of all adult non-Hodgkin lymphomas in Western countries and about 20% worldwide. They are the neoplastic equivalent of the normal germinal center. The translocation t(14;18)(q32;q21) involving BCL-2 and IgH genes is present in greater than 80% of cases (Fig. 19-36). Two different breakpoint sites occur on chromosome 18. The major breakpoint region is in 80% to 90% of translocations and a minor cluster region in the remainder (see Table 19-3 and Fig. 19-1).

The tumor is composed of centrocytes and centroblasts. They are graded histologically on the proportion of centroblasts present: grade 1, 0 to 5 centroblasts per high-power field; grade 2, 6 to 15 centroblasts per high-power field; and grade 3, greater than 15 centroblasts per high-power field (Fig. 19-37). Grade 3 is further subdivided into a and b, which is entirely composed of centroblasts. This subdivision is now included in the WHO classification. Grade 3b cases are often treated as high-grade large cell lymphomas.

Centrocytes are small to medium-sized cells with angular or elongated nuclei, indistinct nucleoli, and scant pale cytoplasm (see Fig. 19-37). Centroblasts are larger with a rounded or oval nucleus and prominent nucleoli, many of which are adjacent to the nuclear membrane. The scant cytoplasm in basophilic (see Fig. 19-37).

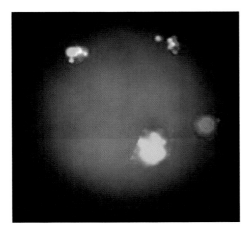

Fig. 19-36. Follicular lymphoma. FISH analysis using probes to chromosomes 14 (green) and 18 (red) demonstrating the translocation t(14;18)(q32;q21) by the two fusion product. (Courtesy of Dr. W. Erber.)

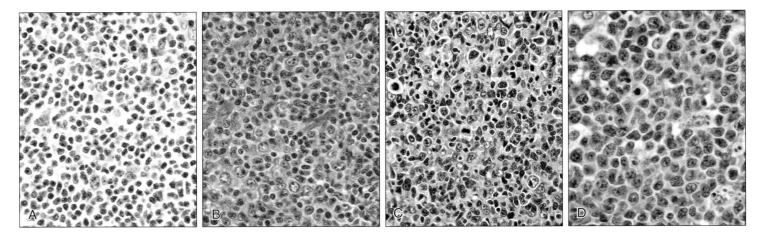

Fig. 19-37. Follicular lymphoma. **A,** Grade 1: the neoplastic population is monotonous, with scattered (less than 5%) centroblasts. **B,** Grade 2: there are more than 5 but less than 15 centroblasts per high-power field (HPF) with admixed centrocytes. **C,** Grade 3A; there are more than 15 centroblasts/HPF with admixed centrocytes. **D,** Grade 3B; monotonous population of large cells ("centroblasts").

The neoplastic follicles may be poorly defined and lack a mantle zone. There may be diffuse areas with sclerosis and involvement of interfollicular areas. Immunohistology shows that cells are usually SIg+ (usually IgM), CD10+, BCL-2+, BCL6+, CD5−, and CD43− (Fig. 19-38). This is in contrast to the normal germinal follicles in which the BCL-2 is negative (Fig. 19-39). The follicular nature of the disease is well seen at low power and can be demonstrated by staining follicles positive for one or other immunoglobulin light chain (Fig. 19-40) or for CD20 (Fig. 19-41, *A*) or by negative staining of the tumor cells for CD3, which is positive in surrounding reactive T cells (Fig. 19-41, *B*). Marrow involvement may be diffuse or paratrabecular (Figs. 19-43 and 19-44).

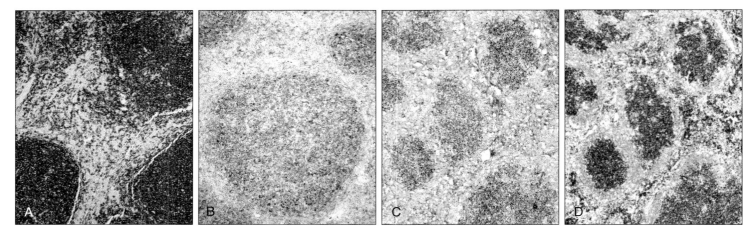

Fig. 19-38. Follicular lymphoma: CD20 immunostain. **A,** The neoplastic cells are diffusely positive for B-cell markers. **B,** Immunostain: the neoplastic cells are diffusely positive for CD10, a germinal center marker, and are located in the follicular and interfollicular areas. **C,** The neoplastic cells are positive for BCL-6, a germinal center marker. **D,** Immunostain: the neoplastic cells are positive for BCL-2.

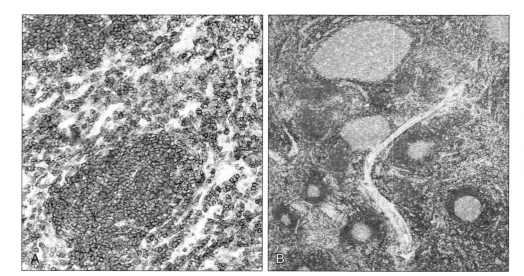

Fig. 19-39. Immunohistologic detection of BCL-2 protein in reactive and neoplastic lymphoid cells. **A,** A follicular lymphoma is positive, reflecting activation of the BCL-2 gene by the (14;18) translocation. **B,** In reactive lymphoid tissue unstained germinal centers are surrounded by numerous positive mantle zone B and T cells.

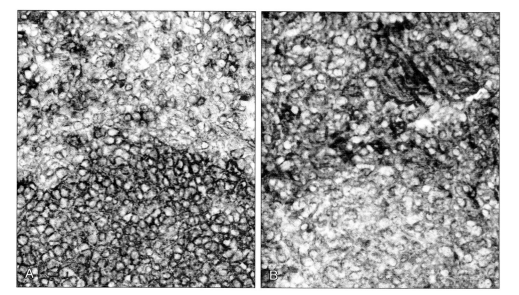

Fig. 19-40. Follicular lymphoma: demonstration of monoclonality by immunostaining: a lymph node biopsy shows **(A)** cytoplasmic positivity for k light chains in the malignant lymphoid nodule; **(B)** no labeling for λ light chains in the nodule (lower field).

About 20% of patients initially have non-bulky localized disease, but in the majority, the disease is at a more advanced stage at presentation, often with circulating lymphoma cells (Fig. 19-42) and with liver, spleen, and bone marrow involvement (Figs. 19-43 and 19-44). There may also be involvement of soft tissues, for example, skin (Fig. 19-45) or gastrointestinal tract.

A rare cytologic variant contains numerous signet ring cells (Fig. 19-45, *B*). Other types show marginal zone differentiation at the periphery of the follicle or foci of monocytoid B cells or rarely plasmacytic differentiation. The disease may transform to a diffuse large cell lymphoma, often with B-cell symptoms, a raised serum LDH, and a localized, rapidly expanding mass that may be detected by CT or PET scanning (see Fig. 19-14) and shows the histology of a diffuse large cell lymphoma.

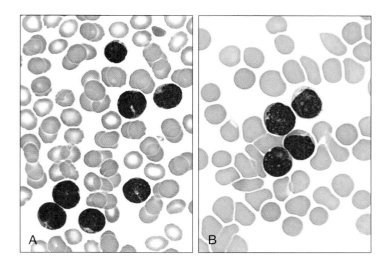

Fig. 19-42. Follicular lymphoma: peripheral blood shows presence of small lymphoid cells with nuclear clefts, diffuse nuclear chromatin, and scant, darkly staining cytoplasm.

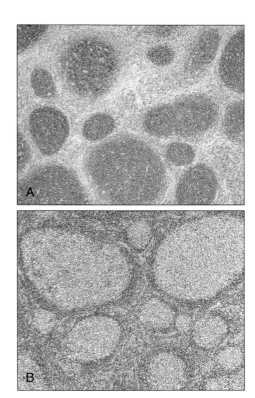

Fig. 19-41. Follicular lymphoma: immunostain. **A,** CD20 expressed in tumor cells. **B,** CD3 is confined to reactive T cells.

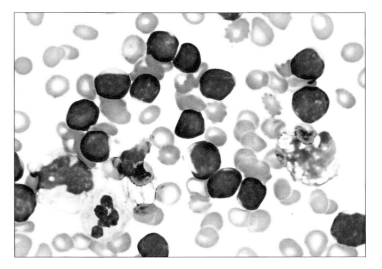

Fig. 19-43. Follicular lymphoma: bone marrow aspirate shows infiltration by small lymphocytes with diffuse nuclear chromatin. (Courtesy of Dr. W. Erber.)

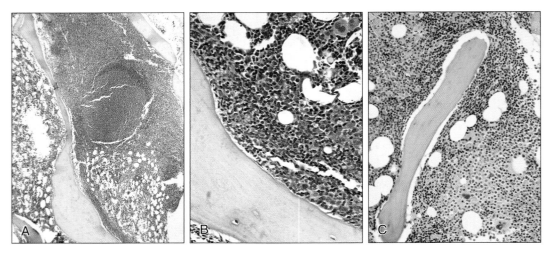

Fig. 19-44. Follicular lymphoma. **A,** Bone marrow trephine biopsy shows almost complete replacement of normal hematopoietic tissue in the upper field and a paratrabecular collection of neoplastic lymphoid cells below. **B,** Higher power shows the demarcation between the paratrabecular centrocytes and centroblasts and the normal hematopoietic cells and fat. **C,** Diffuse marrow infiltration with cells concentrated in paratrabecular zones. (*C,* Courtesy of Dr. W. Erber.)

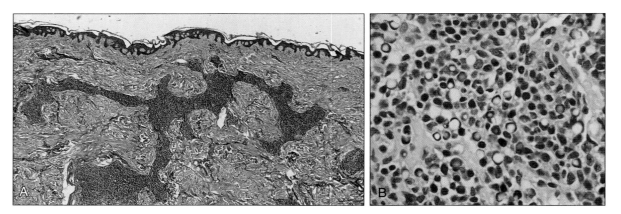

Fig. 19-45. Follicular lymphoma: **(A)** skin involvement with sheets of tumor cells in the dermis; **(B)** rare "signet ring" variety.

TABLE 19-8.   CUTANEOUS B-CELL LYMPHOMAS

Primary cutaneous marginal B-cell lymphoma
Primary cutaneous follicle center lymphoma
Primary cutaneous diffuse large B-cell lymphoma, leg type
Primary cutaneous diffuse large B-cell lymphoma, other
Intravascular large B-cell lymphoma
Blastic plasmacytoid dendritic cell neoplasm

(Adapted from Kim YH et al: *Blood*, 110:479-484, 2007.)

PRIMARY CUTANEOUS FOLLICLE CENTER LYMPHOMA

Table 19-8 gives classification of the primary cutaneous B-cell lymphomas.

Cutaneous follicular lymphoma tends to occur in the upper half of the body, has a follicular pattern, and is composed of centrocytes and centroblasts. The cells are CD20 and CD10 positive but often BCL-2 negative (Fig. 19-46). In diffuse follicle center lymphoma there is also a mixture of centrocytes and centroblasts but the histology resembles that of diffuse large B-cell lymphoma. The clinical course is indolent. In this disease the cells are SIg+, CD10+, BCL-2+, and BCL-6+.

MANTLE CELL LYMPHOMA

This is a small B-cell lymphoma of low-grade histology with, however, an aggressive clinical course. It occurs predominantly in males and is associated with a characteristic cytogenetic abnormality, the t(11;14) reciprocal translocation (Fig. 19-47). This causes overexpression of cyclin D1 (see Fig. 19-49) as the oncogene on chromosome 11 (BCL-1 or PRAD-1) encodes a D cyclin involved in cell cycle control.

The disease usually manifests with lymphadenopathy and splenomegaly; spleen and bone marrow involvement are usual. The disease may be found at extranodal sites, especially in the gastrointestinal tract (it is one cause of lymphomatous polyposis; Fig. 19-48). The neoplastic cells are usually monomorphic of small to medium size with an irregular or cleaved nucleus without nucleoli (Figs. 19-49 and 19-50) or have a more blastic appearance. The growth pattern often shows a nodular (Fig. 19-51) and the neoplastic cells tend to home to mantle zones of lymphoid follicles. Scattered histiocytes may give a "starry sky" appearance.

The disease is frequently present in blood or bone marrow. The cells are of medium size with nuclear indentations or clefts (Figs. 19-52 to 19-55). It must be distinguished from the other CD5+ B-cell disorder chronic lymphocytic leukemia by the expression of cyclin D1, the characteristic cytogenetic abnormality, the absence of CD23 expression, and the presence usually of FMC7. A simple prognostic index has been proposed to include the white cell count, the

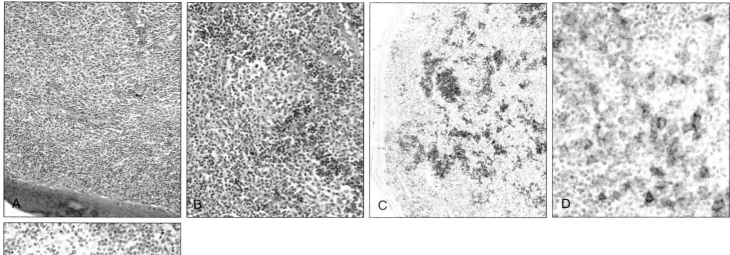

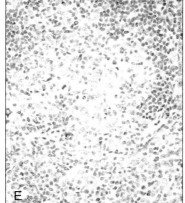

Fig. 19-46. Cutaneous follicle center lymphoma. **A,** H&E: low power showing a follicular growth pattern and extensive infiltration of the dermis. **B,** More detail of the follicular growth pattern. **C,** Immunostain: the neoplastic cells are CD20 positive. **D,** Immunostain: the neoplastic cells are CD10 positive. **E,** Immunostain: the neoplastic cells are BCL-2 negative.

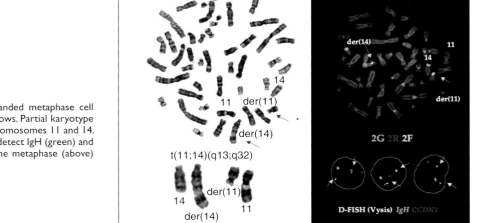

Fig. 19-47. Mantle cell lymphoma cytogenetics. *Left,* G-banded metaphase cell with abnormal products of the t(11;14) indicated by red arrows. Partial karyotype below shows the normal and rearranged homologues of chromosomes 11 and 14. *Right,* FISH analysis using D (double) FISH (Vysis) probes to detect IgH (green) and CCDN1 (red) loci shows the fusion signals (arrowed) in the metaphase (above) and interphase (below). (Courtesy of Dr. E. Nacheva.)

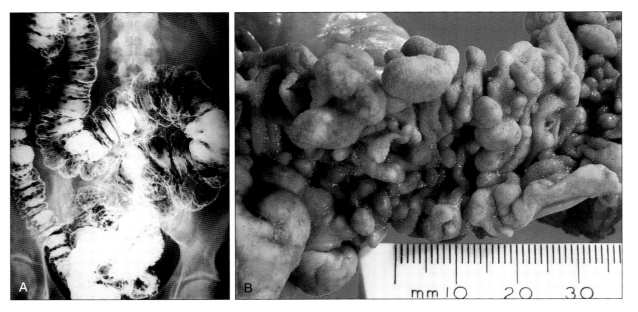

Fig. 19-48. Mantle cell lymphoma; lymphomatous polyposis affecting the ileocecal region. **A,** Barium study shows mucosal and mural involvement. **B,** Macroscopic appearances showing the presence of multiple mucosal polyps that range in size from a few millimeters to a few centimeters.

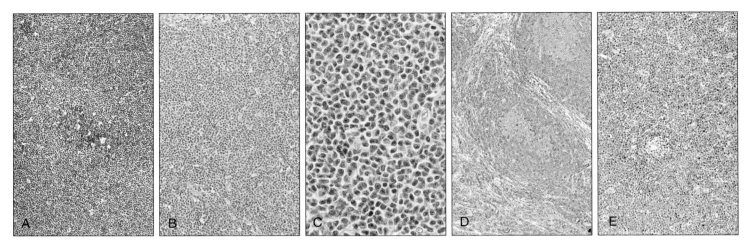

Fig. 19-49. Mantle cell lymphoma. **A,** At low power the neoplasm is seen surrounding a naked reactive germinal center, which gives a characteristic mantle zone distribution. **B,** Medium power view shows diffuse growth pattern with some hyaline fibrosis around small vessels. **C,** At high power irregular small lymphoid cells (small cleaved cells, centrocytes) typical of mantle cell lymphoma are seen. No large lymphoid cells are present (see also Fig. 19-52). **D,** Immunostain for CD5 shows strong positivity. **E,** Immunostain for cyclin D1 shows characteristic nuclear positivity.

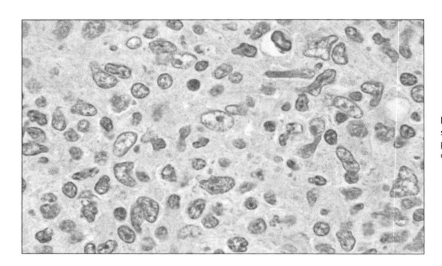

Fig. 19-50. Mantle cell lymphoma: lymph node biopsy. Large cells are seen with considerable nuclear pleomorphism and pale indistinct cytoplasm; the deformed nuclei have a light chromatin pattern and may contain nucleoli.

Fig. 19-51. Mantle cell lymphoma: immunostaining for CD20 reveals a nodular growth pattern.

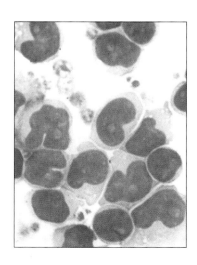

Fig. 19-52. Mantle cell lymphoma: fine-needle aspirate showing small and medium-sized cells with convoluted and angular nuclei, indistinct nucleoli, and pale cytoplasm.

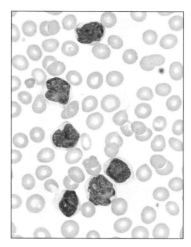

Fig. 19-53. Mantle cell lymphoma: peripheral blood film showing medium-sized lymphocytes with irregular nuclear contours and scant pale cytoplasm. (Courtesy of Dr. W. Erber.)

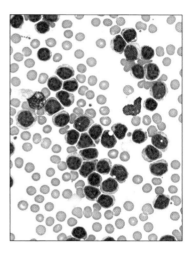

Fig. 19-54. Mantle cell lymphoma: bone marrow aspirate showing diffuse infiltration with medium-sized lymphoid cells with scanty pale cytoplasm, nuclei, some clefted, with indistinct nucleoli. (Courtesy of Dr. W. Erber.)

ECOG performance status, age, and serum LDH (Hoster E et al: *Blood* 111:558-565, 2008). Mantle cell lymphoma does not transform to large cell lymphoma but increased mitoses, nuclear size, and polymorphism may occur in late-stage disease.

DIFFUSE LARGE B-CELL LYMPHOMA

Diffuse large B-cell lymphoma (DLBCL), which accounts for 30% of all non-Hodgkin lymphomas, has received various subclassifications. The Kiel scheme postulated two main categories: "centroblastic" and "immunoblastic" (Figs. 19-56 and 19-57, *A* and *B*) but no survival differences were found between the two groups, which were in some cases difficult to separate histologically (Fig. 19-57, *C*) or by cell appearance in fine-needle aspirates (Fig. 19-58). The WHO has combined these types, which both show diffuse proliferation of large cells, at least twice the size of a normal lymphocyte, with vesicular nuclei, prominent nucleoli, and usually basophilic cytoplasm (Figs. 19-56 to 19-58).

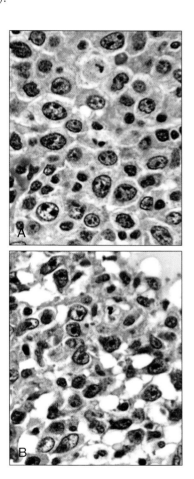

Fig. 19-56. Diffuse large B-cell lymphoma, H&E. **A,** Centroblastic variant, membrane-bound nucleoli can be observed in the tumor cells of this variant. **B,** Immunoblastic variant; nearly all of the neoplastic cells show a prominent central nucleolus.

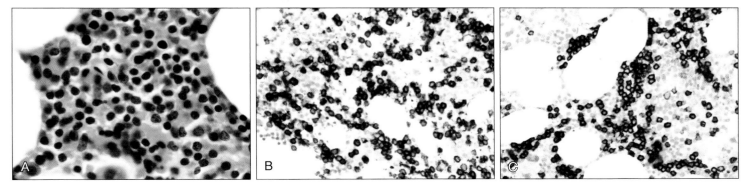

Fig. 19-55. Mantle cell lymphoma. Bone marrow trephine biopsy: **(A)** infiltration with lymphoid cells showing angulated nuclei that stain positively for **(B)** CD5 and **(C)** CD20. (Courtesy of Dr. W. Erber.)

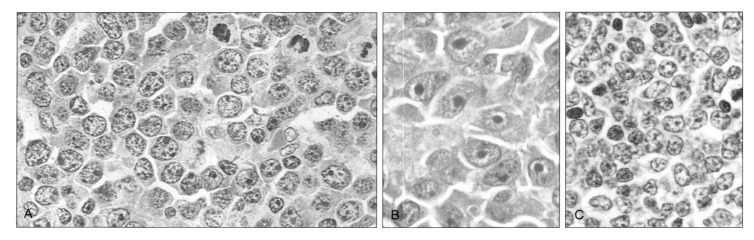

Fig. 19-57. Diffuse large B-cell lymphoma at higher magnification. **A,** The neoplastic cells are much larger than normal lymphocytes and have a round nucleus with prominent nucleoli, many of which are adjacent to the nuclear membrane ("centroblasts"). A number of mitotic figures are seen. **B,** The large cells show prominent central nucleoli ("immunoblasts"). **C,** The round or oval nuclei have delicate, evenly distributed chromatin with one to three nucleoli, either central or near the nuclear membrane, and scant cytoplasm.

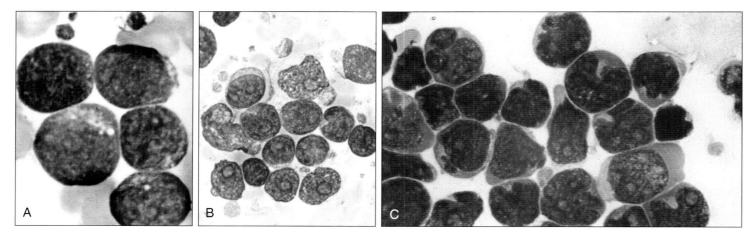

Fig. 19-58. Diffuse large B-cell lymphoma: fine-needle lymph node aspirate showing **(A)** "centroblasts," **(B)** "immunoblasts," and **(C)** pleomorphic large cells with irregular nuclear outline, nuclear clefts, and prominent nucleoli.

The disease may be nodal or extranodal in up to 40% of cases including the gastrointestinal tract, skin, central nervous system, bone, testes, ovary, lung, liver, and spleen. The incidence of the disease is increasing both in association with HIV infection and independently of this.

Gene array studies (Fig. 19-59) and immunophenotyping (see Table 19-4) can distinguish two main subgroups: one appearing to arise from germinal center B cells (GC type), which is CD10+, MUM1−, and HGAL+, and the other appears to arise from an activated cell (ABC type), which is CD10−, MUM1+, and HGAL−. Both types express pan B-cell markers CD19, CD20, CD27, and CD79a to a varying degree (Fig. 19-60). Prognosis appears to be more favorable in the GC type of tumor. In some cases CD5 is expressed, and BCL-2 is positive in 30% to 50% of cases. The proliferation fraction measured by Ki-67 (MIB1) staining is usually greater than 40%.

As well as the frequent centroblastic and immunoblastic histologic appearance, two other histologic subtypes, anaplastic or T-cell rich (discussed later), occur less frequently. The cells may be anaplastic without the t(2;5) translocation, which results in expression of the anaplastic lymphoma kinase (ALK) protein (see later).

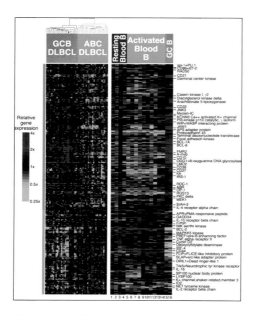

Fig. 19-59. Diffuse large B-cell lymphoma: gene array studies. The left-hand panel shows gene expression data in the two subgroups (germinal center and activated B cell); the right-hand panel shows expression data in normal B-cell samples (for full details see Alizadeh AA et al: *Nature* 403:503-511, 2000). (Courtesy of Professor L. M. Staudt.)

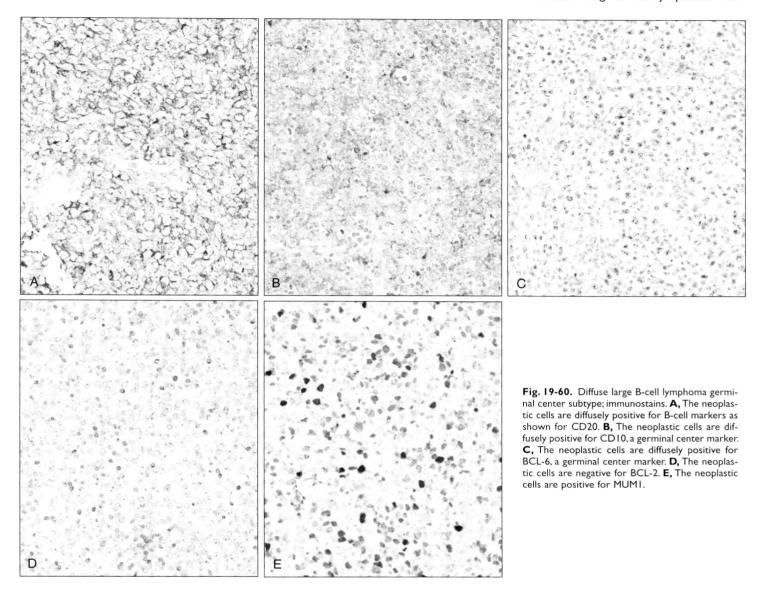

Fig. 19-60. Diffuse large B-cell lymphoma germinal center subtype; immunostains. **A,** The neoplastic cells are diffusely positive for B-cell markers as shown for CD20. **B,** The neoplastic cells are diffusely positive for CD10, a germinal center marker. **C,** The neoplastic cells are diffusely positive for BCL-6, a germinal center marker. **D,** The neoplastic cells are negative for BCL-2. **E,** The neoplastic cells are positive for MUM1.

Molecular studies show rearrangement of the BCL-6 gene at 3q27 in one third of cases and mutations within the gene in additional cases. BCL-6 is a transcription factor of the zinc finger family that is involved in maintaining B cells in a germinal center–like state, inhibiting B-cell differentiation. Cytogenetically, t(3;4) (q27;q22) may be found. The t(14;18) (q32;q21) translocation, the genetic hallmark of follicular lymphoma, is also found in 20% to 30% of de novo DLBCL. The 8q24/MYC rearrangement found in Burkitt's lymphoma may also occur in DLBCL in 10% to 15% of cases and may be a secondary event in this tumor.

The disease may be localized or widespread with involvement of the bone marrow (Figs. 19-61 to 19-63) and peripheral blood (Fig. 19-64). Other tissues may be infiltrated, for example, thyroid (Fig. 19-65) and brain (Fig. 19-66). Involvement of extranodal sites is included as a poor prognostic factor in the international prognostic index (IPI) (Table 19-9).

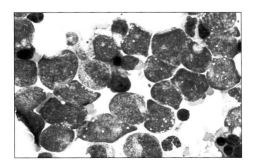

Fig. 19-61. Diffuse large B-cell lymphoma: bone marrow aspirate showing large cells with abundant dark blue, cytoplasmic, and nuclear vacuoles and nuclei with open chromatin and prominent nucleoli. (Courtesy of Dr. W. Erber.)

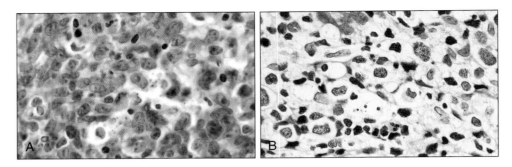

Fig. 19-62. Diffuse large B-cell lymphoma: bone marrow trephine biopsy. **A,** Low power: pleomorphic large cells with vesicular nuclei, prominent nucleoli, and apoptotic forms replacing hematopoietic marrow. **B,** High power: mixture of "centroblasts" and "immunoblasts" infiltrating bone marrow. (Courtesy of Dr. W. Erber.)

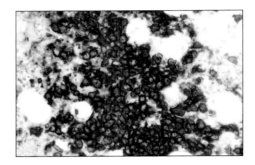

Fig. 19-63. Diffuse large B-cell lymphoma, bone marrow trephine biopsy: immunostain showing infiltrate of large cells, CD20 positive. (Courtesy of Dr. W. Erber.)

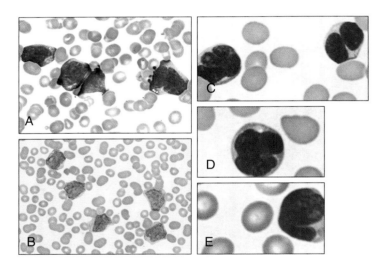

Fig. 19-64. Diffuse large B-cell lymphoma: peripheral blood films showing large lymphoid cells that are **(A)** dark and **(B)** paler blue with vacuolated cytoplasm and irregularly shaped nuclei occupying most of the cell, and prominent nucleoli. **C, D, E,** Bizarre cells in terminal, widely disseminated "centroblastic" lymphoma. (*A, B,* Courtesy of Dr. W. Erber.)

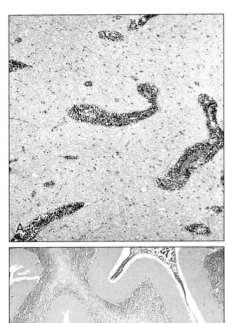

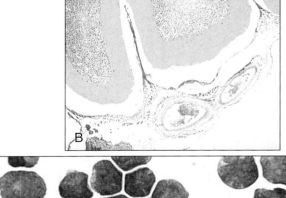

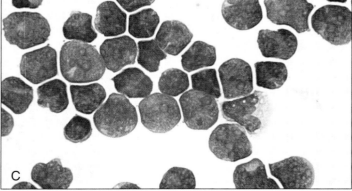

Fig. 19-66. Diffuse large B-cell lymphoma in the brain: sections of brain in CNS relapse showing **(A)** nodular invasion along perivascular spaces and **(B)** extensive involvement of the meninges. A similar pattern of involvement occurs in primary lymphoma of the brain. **C,** Cerebrospinal fluid: cytospin preparation shows typical large lymphoid cells with prominent nucleoli. (*A, B,* Courtesy of Dr. B. B. Berkeley.)

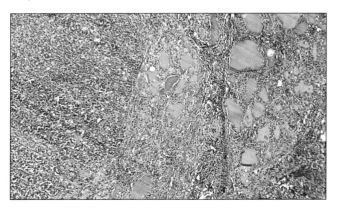

Fig. 19-65. Diffuse large B-cell lymphoma of the thyroid: a histologic section shows sheets of neoplastic cells (left) and remaining colloid-filled acini (right). Immunoperoxidase staining for light chains confirmed the monoclonality of the tumor cells.

TABLE 19-9.   INTERNATIONAL
PROGNOSTIC INDEX FOR
AGGRESSIVE LYMPHOMAS

Unfavourable
Age > 60 years
Poor performance status (ECOG ≥ 2)
Advanced Ann Arbor stage (III-IV)
Extranodal involvement ≥ 2 sites
High serum LDH (> normal)

T-CELL–RICH DIFFUSE LARGE B-CELL LYMPHOMA

In T-cell–rich diffuse large B-cell lymphoma, the histology is dominated by CD3+ T cells, and the large neoplastic B cells (less than 10% of the total) are best detected by immunohistology (Figs. 19-67 and 19-68). The pattern is diffuse.

LYMPHOMATOID GRANULOMATOSIS

This is an angiocentric lymphoproliferative disease of extranodal sites composed of EBV+ B cells mixed with reactive and inflammatory cells and T cells (Fig. 19-69). It may progress to a diffuse large B-cell lymphoma. The most common site involved is lung, but other soft tissues may be affected. It occurs especially in immunosuppressed individuals. Blood vessel infiltration occurs often with vascular damage and necrosis.

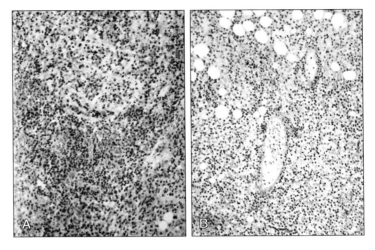

Fig. 19-69. Lymphomatoid granulomatosus: lung sections **(A)** showing prominent blood vessels with **(B)** thickened walls and areas of necrosis. (Elastic van Giesen stain.) (Courtesy of Dr. J. E. McLaughlin.)

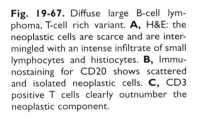

Fig. 19-67. Diffuse large B-cell lymphoma, T-cell rich variant. **A,** H&E: the neoplastic cells are scarce and are intermingled with an intense infiltrate of small lymphocytes and histiocytes. **B,** Immunostaining for CD20 shows scattered and isolated neoplastic cells. **C,** CD3 positive T cells clearly outnumber the neoplastic component.

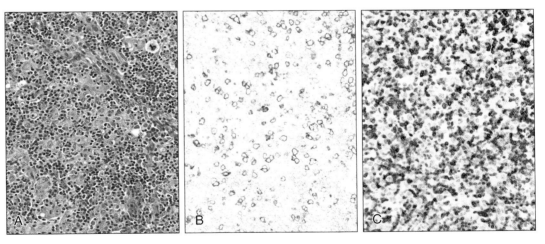

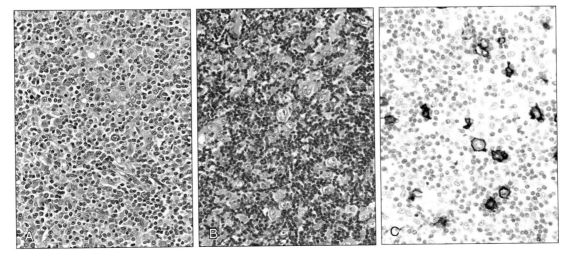

Fig. 19-68. Diffuse large B-cell lymphoma, T-cell rich: **(A)** low-power view showing diffuse architecture with scattered large cells admixed with numerous small lymphocytes; **(B)** high-power view showing large blast cells with immunoblastic cytology; **(C)** immunostain for CD20 showing neoplastic large B cells.

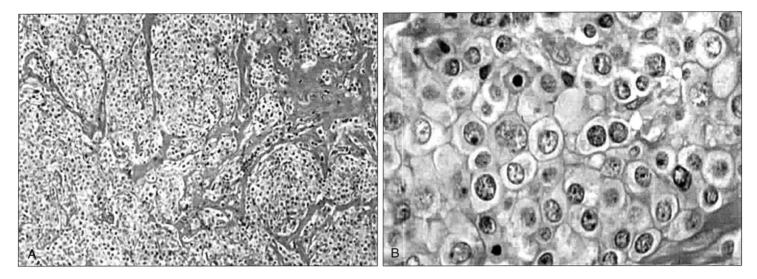

Fig. 19-70. Primary mediastinal (thymic) large B-cell lymphoma. **A,** Typical fibrosis between the sheets of tumor cells. **B,** The cells, abundant pale cytoplasm, and centroblast-type nuclei.

PRIMARY MEDIASTINAL (THYMIC) LARGE B-CELL LYMPHOMA

This is a large cell disease, manifesting as a large anterior mediastinal mass, sometimes with superior vena cava obstruction. There is usually dense fibrosis, which may compartmentalize the tumor (Fig. 19-70, *A*). Thymic remnants and scattered benign lymphocytes and eosinophils may be present. The tumor cells usually have abundant pale cytoplasm and centroblast-type nuclei (Fig. 19-70, *B*). The immunophenotype is of a B-cell tumor, CD10 negative, with weak or absent expression of surface immunoglobulin. The tumor may spread locally to neighboring viscera or more distally, especially to extranodal sites (e.g., kidney, lung, skin, and brain).

INTRAVASCULAR LARGE B-CELL LYMPHOMA

This is a rare type of extranodal B-cell lymphoma characterized by the presence of tumor cells only in the lumina of the small vessels (Fig. 19-71). It occurs particularly in the skin, CNS, lung, kidneys, or bone marrow (Figs. 19-72 and 19-73). Cells are large with vesicular nuclei, prominent nucleoli, and frequent mitosis. They express pan B-cell antigens and rarely CD5.

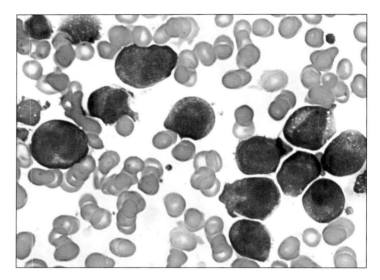

Fig. 19-72. Intravascular large B-cell lymphoma: bone marrow aspirate showing infiltration of large cells with irregular nuclei, open chromatin, and vacuoles (mainly cytoplasmic). (Courtesy of Dr. W. Erber.)

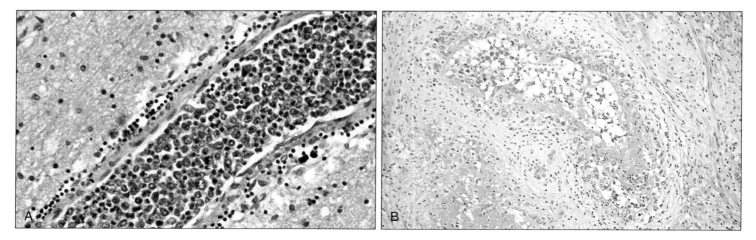

Fig. 19-71. A, Intravascular large B-cell lymphoma. The neoplastic cells fill the intraparenchymatous vessels of the brain. **B,** Section of cervix showing vascular distention by large lymphoid cells.

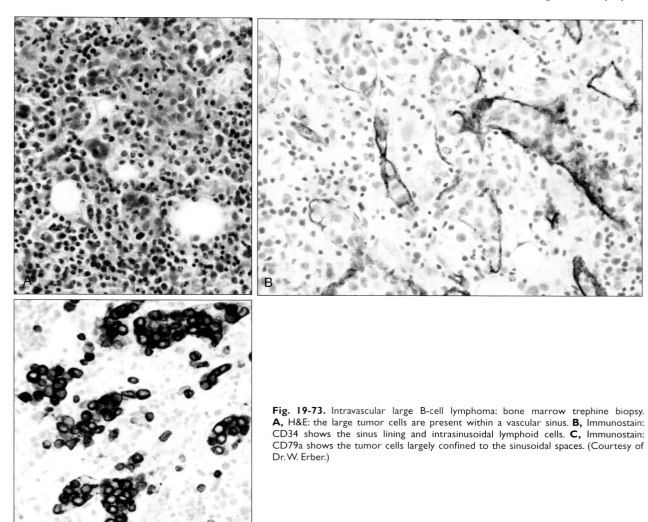

Fig. 19-73. Intravascular large B-cell lymphoma: bone marrow trephine biopsy. **A,** H&E: the large tumor cells are present within a vascular sinus. **B,** Immunostain: CD34 shows the sinus lining and intrasinusoidal lymphoid cells. **C,** Immunostain: CD79a shows the tumor cells largely confined to the sinusoidal spaces. (Courtesy of Dr. W. Erber.)

PRIMARY CUTANEOUS DIFFUSE LARGE B-CELL LYMPHOMA, LEG TYPE

This tumor is composed of large monomorphic B cells that infiltrate the dermis (Fig. 19-74). The cells are BCL-2+, CD10+. Prognosis is worse than for primary cutaneous follicle center lymphoma.

ALK-POSITIVE DIFFUSE LARGE B-CELL LYMPHOMA

This tumor is different from the T/Null ALK-positive anaplastic large cell lymphoma. It is composed of large B cells that lack CD20 but express CD138 and ALK due to t(2;17) or t(2;5)

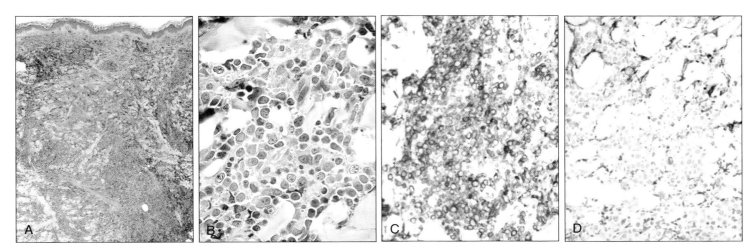

Fig. 19-74. Primary cutaneous diffuse large B-cell lymphoma: leg type. **A,** H&E: the neoplastic cells are infiltrating the dermis and extending to the subcutis. The epidermis is spared. **B,** H&E: the neoplastic cells are large and monomorphic. **C,** Immunostain: the neoplastic cells are strongly positive for BCL2. **D,** Immunostain: the neoplastic cells are negative for CD10.

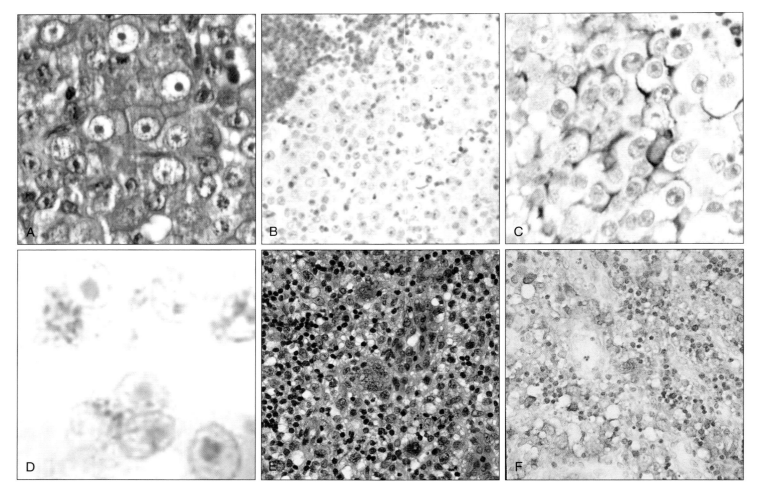

Fig. 19-75. Diffuse large B-cell lymphoma: ALK+. **A,** H&E: the neoplastic cells are very large and grow in a cohesive pattern with an immunoblastic morphology. **B,** Immunostain with CD79a; the neoplastic cells are negative for B-cell markers. **C,** Immunostain: the neoplastic cells are positive for CD138, a plasma cell marker. **D,** Immunostain: ALK is positive with a cytoplasmic granular pattern, suggestive of the Clathrin translocation. **E,** H&E DLBCL, anaplastic variant. This should not be confused with ALK+ DLBCL. **F,** The cells are CD30+ but ALK−.

translocation, which induces formation of a chimeric protein nucleophosmin-anaplastic lymphoma kinase (NPM-ALK) that has enhanced ALK tyrosine kinase activity. Chromosome aberrations involving ALK result in ALK expression in both cytoplasm and nuclei (Fig. 19-75).

PLASMABLASTIC LYMPHOMA

In this high-grade lymphoma, the tumor cells show plasma cell differentiation but retain the morphology of a large lymphoid cell histologically (Fig. 19-76) or by cytology (Fig. 19-77). Like myeloma, the cells express CD138 but lack CD20.

Fig. 19-76. Plasmablastic lymphoma. **A,** H&E: The neoplastic cells are large with prominent centrally located nucleoli. The cytoplasm is amphophilic with a paranuclear hof. **B,** Immunostain: the neoplastic cells are strongly positive for CD138.

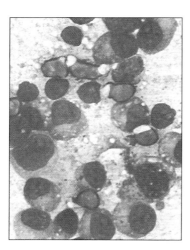

Fig. 19-77. Plasmablastic lymphoma. Fine-needle aspirate; the large lymphoid cells show plasmablastic and plasmacytic forms.

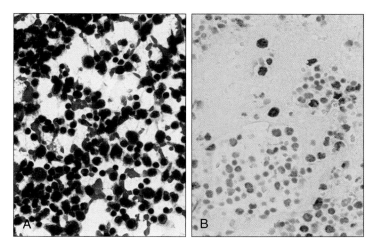

Fig. 19-78. Primary effusion lymphoma. **A,** Papanicolaou stain: large neoplastic cells in a pleural effusion. **B,** The LANA-1 HHV-8–associated antigen is strongly positive in the nuclei of the neoplastic cells.

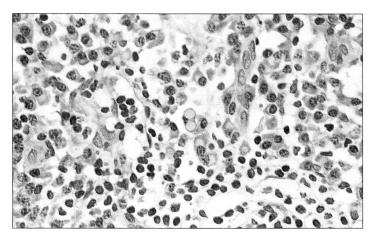

Fig. 19-80. Castleman's disease (angiofollicular hyperplasia), plasma cell variant: high-power view showing plasma cells, many of which contain Russell bodies; other fields showed typical follicular hyalinization.

PRIMARY EFFUSION LYMPHOMA

Primary effusion lymphoma (PEL) causes serous effusions, especially pleural, pericardial, or peritoneal, usually without tumor masses. It is associated with infection with the human herpes virus 8 (HHV-8), previously called Kaposi sarcoma herpes virus (KHSV). Co-infection with Epstein-Barr virus is common. Rarely cases with similar morphology and clinical presentation that are HHV-8 negative have been reported. The majority of cases of PEL are HIV positive, but negative cases occur especially in elderly males in the Mediterranean area or other areas where HHV-8 is frequent. HHV-8 infection may also underlie large B-cell lymphomas with a similar morphology to PEL cells arising in extranodal tissues arising in Castleman's disease (see below).

The PEL cells have a characteristic morphology with immunoblastic, anaplastic, and plasmablastic cells and regardless of the morphologic type express a plasma cell–related phenotype and usually stain positive for HHV-8 (Fig. 19-78). Vacuoles are common. Pan-B markers are negative but CD30, CD38, and CD138 are usually positive. In some cases, solid tumors, also HHV-8 positive, precede the development of PEL or occur after its resolution.

LARGE B-CELL LYMPHOMA ARISING IN HHV8 ASSOCIATED MULTICENTRIC CASTLEMAN'S DISEASE

Multicentric Castleman's disease may underlie HHV-8 positive diffuse large B-cell lymphoma. The disease typically affects mediastinal and axillary lymph nodes. In the hyaline and vascular variant these are increased reactive follicles and prominent hyalinized central arterial and whorls of mantle lymphocytes (Fig. 19-79). Patients with this variant are typically HIV negative, asymptomatic with localized disease that does not recur after surgical resection. In the rarer plasma cell type (usually HIV associated) in which a marked increase in interfollicular plasma cells occurs (Fig. 19-80), the disease is usually multicentric and progressive with fever, weight loss, anemia, neutropenia, and thrombocytopenia. There may be marrow plasmacytosis and polyclonal gammaglobulinemia and evolution to DLBCL and associated Kaposi sarcoma. HHV-8 infection is associated with transformation to Kaposi sarcoma or diffuse large B-cell lymphoma (Fig. 19-81).

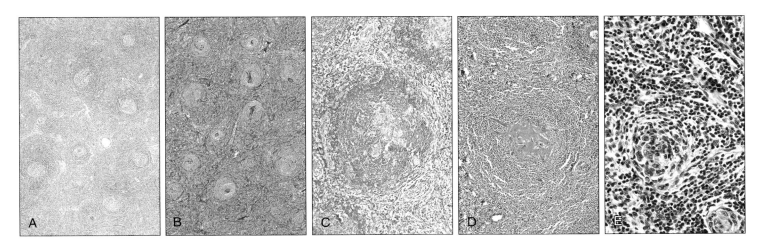

Fig. 19-79. Castleman's disease (angiofollicular hyperplasia): low-power views of a lymph node biopsy show increased follicular centers with prominent central arterioles and whorls of mantle lymphocytes in sections stained using **(A)** H&E and **(B)** silver impregnation for reticulin. At higher power, **(C)** prominent vascular proliferation in the center of a follicle, **(D)** extensive hyalinization of central vessels, and **(E)** whorling of mantle lymphocytes are seen. (*E,* Courtesy of Dr. J. E. McLaughlin.)

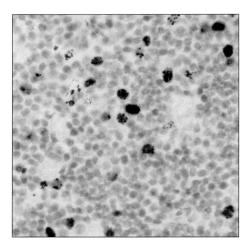

Fig. 19-81. Castleman's disease immunostain: scattered HHV-8–positive cells in an HIV-positive patient. (Courtesy of Dr. M. Heller.)

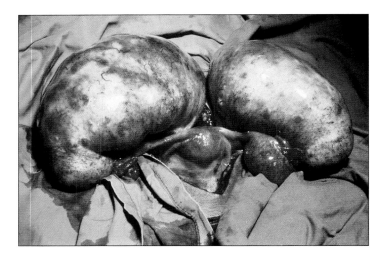

Fig. 19-83. Burkitt's lymphoma: gross bilateral involvement of the ovaries.

BURKITT'S LYMPHOMA.

Burkitt's lymphoma was first found in young African children and has an unusual predilection in them for massive jaw lesions (Fig. 19-82); extranodal abdominal involvement and ovarian, intestinal, kidney, or breast tumors also occur (Fig. 19-83). The disease is now known to be endemic in equatorial Africa, sporadic throughout the world, and associated with immunodeficiency. All three types are associated with a high incidence of CNS disease and to a variable degree with EBV infection.

The most frequent underlying cytogenetic change is t(8;14) (q24;q32) (Fig. 19-84). This involves the MYC oncogene and IgH gene, and MYC is involved in the less frequent t(2;8) and t(8;22) translocations that also involve, respectively, the immunoglobulin λ and kappa light chains. BCL-2 and BCL-6 translocations are not present.

The cells are medium sized with basophilic cytoplasm and lipid-filled vacuoles. The nuclei are round with nucleoli. The tumor has a high proliferation rate with frequent mitoses and apoptotic cells. Macrophages dispersed throughout the tumor cells give a "starry sky" appearance (Fig. 19-85). Rare cases manifest purely with acute leukemia with bone marrow involvement and circulating blasts (see Chapter 12).

The immunophenotype is of a mature B-cell neoplasm that is SIgM+, CD10+, BCL6−, BCL2, CD5−, CD23−, and TDT−. MIB1 staining approaches 100% (Fig. 19-86). The serum LDH is high, reflecting the high cell turnover rate. In most endemic African cases EBV DNA is found in the malignant cells. Sporadic cases in Western countries that occur mainly in children and young adults are histologically and phenotypically identical. They may arise in the absence of immune impairment, and EBV is only identifiable in 10% to 25% of cases.

The distinction between Burkitt's lymphoma and diffuse large B-cell lymphoma may be difficult in some cases. For those with DLBCL with Burkitt-like morphology, MYC rearrangement, and a proliferation fraction of 100%, atypical Burkitt's lymphoma is diagnosed and they are treated as for Burkitt's lymphoma although the outcome is poorer. Some cases of Burkitt's lymphoma show plasmacytoid differentiation, especially in immunodeficiency states.

PARANEOPLASTIC PEMPHIGUS

This is a rare autoimmune skin and mucosal disease, most commonly associated with non-Hodgkin lymphoma (80%), Castleman's disease, and rarely solid tumors. There is blistering of the skin and ulceration and scarring of mucosal membranes, for example, of the mouth

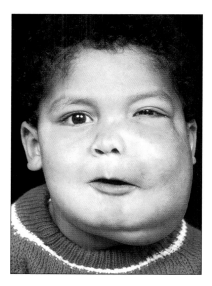

Fig. 19-82. Burkitt's lymphoma: characteristic facial swelling caused by extensive tumor involvement of the mandible and surrounding soft tissues. (Courtesy of Professor J. M. Chessells.)

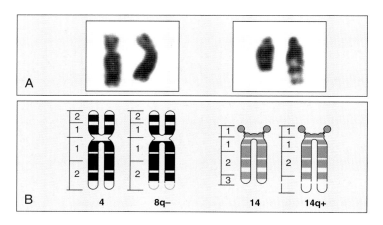

Fig. 19-84. Burkitt's lymphoma. **A,** Partial karyotypes of G-banded chromosomes 8 and 14 from a child. The translocated chromosomes are on the right in each pair. The cellular oncogene c-MYC moves with the translocated portion of chromosome 8 and is juxtaposed to the Ig heavy-chain locus. **B,** A systematized description of the structural aberration. More rarely, cases of Burkitt's lymphoma show (8;22) or (2;8) translocations, involving, respectively, the k and γ light chain genes. (Courtesy of Professor L. M. Secker-Walker.)

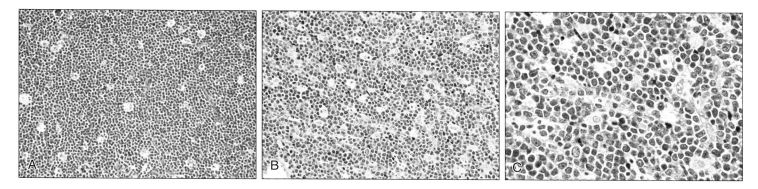

Fig. 19-85. Burkitt's lymphoma. **A,** H&E: diffuse infiltration of a lymph node with a "starry sky" appearance. **B,** diffuse infiltration with a prominent "starry sky" appearance and many mitotic figures and apoptotic cells. **C,** At high power the cells are uniform in size and contain multiple basophilic nucleoli.

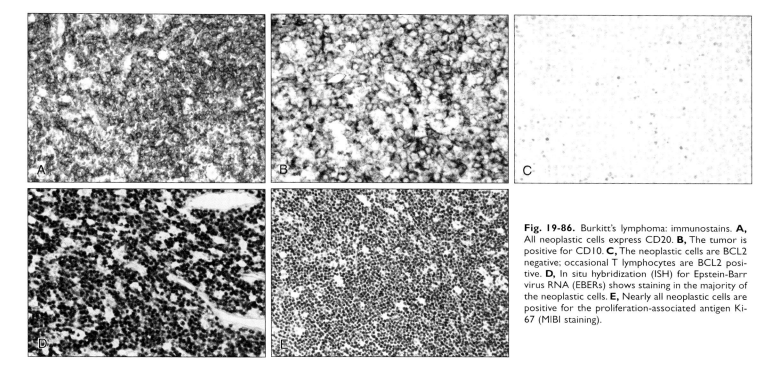

Fig. 19-86. Burkitt's lymphoma: immunostains. **A,** All neoplastic cells express CD20. **B,** The tumor is positive for CD10. **C,** The neoplastic cells are BCL2 negative; occasional T lymphocytes are BCL2 positive. **D,** In situ hybridization (ISH) for Epstein-Barr virus RNA (EBERs) shows staining in the majority of the neoplastic cells. **E,** Nearly all neoplastic cells are positive for the proliferation-associated antigen Ki-67 (MIBI staining).

(Fig. 19-87). The conjunctivae may ulcerate and scar. The prognosis is poor. Antibodies to proteins expressed at epithelial cell junctions, desmoglein I and III, and members of the plakin family are found in serum. Antibodies to bullus pemphigoid antigen 2 and to an unknown 170-kd antigen are unique to the condition. The patient illustrated in Fig. 19-87 had all of the clinical and laboratory features of paraneoplastic pemphigus, in his case with underlying systemic mastocytosis.

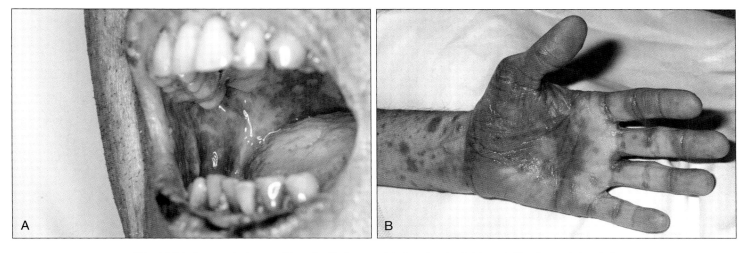

Fig. 19-87. Paraneoplastic pemphigus. **A,** Oral mucosal lesion showing bright red, bleeding, and denuded mucosa. **B,** Skin showing thin-walled blisters and widespread violaceous plaques.

PERIPHERAL T-CELL DISORDERS

MATURE T-CELL AND NATURAL KILLER–CELL NEOPLASMS

T-cell and natural killer (NK)–cell neoplasms differ, as do B-cell tumors, in terms of the maturation stage from which they arise. However, there is also a greater degree of subdivision into different local populations (e.g., cutaneous T cells associated with the skin lymphomas, T cells associated with the gastrointestinal tract with enteric lymphomas, etc.). The World Health Organization Classification of these neoplasms is shown in Table 20-1. For some unknown reason there is a greater frequency of these tumors in Eastern Asia than in Europe and the United States, where they account for less than 20% of non-Hodgkin lymphoma. As in the case of B-cell neoplasms, those diseases diagnosed by hematologists rather than histopathologists (aggressive NK-cell leukemia, T-cell prolymphocytic leukemia, T-cell

large granular cell leukemia, adult T-cell leukemia/lymphoma) are discussed in Chapters 12 and 18. In this chapter, discussion of the primary skin T-cell lymphomas is followed by discussion of the remaining T-cell lymphomas listed in the WHO classification.

PRIMARY CUTANEOUS T-CELL LYMPHOMAS

The T-cell lymphomas that occur in the skin (Table 20-2) are a heterogeneous group with clinical and biologic features different from systemic T-cell lymphomas. Mycosis fungoides and Sézary syndrome are well known and make up over 60% of all cutaneous T-cell lymphomas. Some of the more recently recognized conditions are classified as provisional entities as they are rare tumors and their clinical and biologic behavior is not yet well established. Correct diagnosis of cutaneous T-cell lymphomas requires close correlation between clinical, histologic, and phenotypic features.

MYCOSIS FUNGOIDES

The classic form of mycosis fungoides is the most common primary cutaneous T-cell lymphoma. Most patients are elderly, and there is a male predominance. The disease usually has a long natural history and evolves through three stages:

1. The first stage is a premycotic stage with lesions similar to eczema or psoriasis (Fig. 20-1).
2. The second stage is an infiltrative or plaque stage (Fig. 20-2).
3. The third stage is a nodular or tumor stage associated with deeper invasion by the tumor (Fig. 20-3) and infiltration of lymph nodes and other organs (e.g., liver, spleen, and lungs). Bone marrow involvement is rare.

TABLE 20-1. WHO CLASSIFICATION OF MATURE T-CELL LYMPHOMAS (2008)

T-cell prolymphocytic leukaemia

T-cell large granular lymphocytic leukaemia

Chronic lymphoproliferative disorder of NK-cells

Aggressive NK ceil leukaemia

Systemic EBV positive T-cell lymphoproliferative disease of childhood

Hydroa vacciniforme-like lymphoma

Adult T-cell leukaemia/lymphoma

Extranodal NK/T cell lymphoma, nasal type

Enteropathy-associated T-cell lymphoma

Hepatosplenic T-cell lymphoma

Subcutaneous panniculitis-like T-cell lymphoma

Mycosis fungoides

Sézary syndrome

Primary cutaneous CD30 positive T-cell lymphoproliferative disorders

Lymphomatoid papulosis

Primary cutaneous anaplastic large cell lymphoma

Primary cutaneous gamma-delta T-cell lymphoma

Primary cutaneous CD8 positive aggressive epidermotropic cytotoxic T-cell lymphoma

Primary cutaneous CD4 positive small/medium T-cell lymphoma

Peripheral T-cell lymphoma, NOS

Angioimmunoblastic T-cell Lymphoma

Anaplastic large cell lymphoma, ALK positive

Anaplastic large cell lymphoma, ALK negative

TABLE 20-2. WHO CLASSIFICATION OF PRIMARY CUTANEOUS LYMPHOMAS

Mycosis fungoides and variants

Sézary syndrome

Lymphomatoid papulosis

Primary cutaneous anaplastic large cell lymphoma

Subcutaneous panniculitis-like T-cell lymphoma

Primary cutaneous gamma-delta T-cell lymphoma

Primary cutaneous CD8 positive aggressive epidermotropic cytotoxic T-cell lymphoma

Primary cutaneous CD4 positive small/medium T-cell lymphoma

Primary cutaneous peripheral T-cell lymphoma, not otherwise specified

Extranodal NK/T cell lymphoma, nasal type

Hydroa vacciniforme-like lymphoma

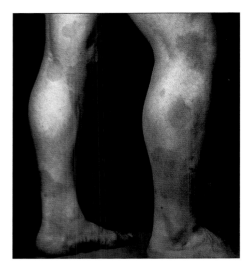

Fig. 20-1. Mycosis fungoides: typical eczematoid lesions at presentation.

The skin lesions show dermal and epidermotrophic infiltrates of small to medium-sized cells with convoluted or cerebriform nuclei (Fig. 20-4). Localized pockets of these cells in the epidermis ("Pautrier microabscesses," Fig. 20-5) are characteristic but are not seen in all cases. The cells express pan T-cell antigens (Fig. 20-6) and are usually positive for CD2, CD3, CD5, and TCRβ. The T-cell receptor genes are rearranged in most patients. There are no specific cytogenetic abnormalities, but patients with advanced disease may have complex karyotypes.

Folliculotrophic Mycosis Fungoides (Mycosis Fungoides–Associated Follicular Mucinosis).

This variant of mycosis fungoides is characterized by a follicular infiltrate, often with sparing of the epidermis. Most cases show mucinous degeneration of the hair follicles (Fig. 20-7). There is preferential involvement of the head and neck. The immunophenotype is similar to classic mycosis fungoides. Isolated CD30-positive blast cells may be seen.

Pagetoid Reticulosis

In this localized and nonfatal variant of mycosis fungoides, patients have a slowly progressive solitary psoriaform or hyperkeratotic plaque usually on the arms or legs. There is epidermal hyperplasia with a Pagetoid infiltration of atypical cells with convoluted nuclei (Fig. 20-8).

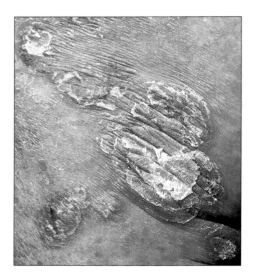

Fig. 20-2. Mycosis fungoides: these psoriasiform plaques appeared 6 months later (same patient as shown in Fig. 20-1).

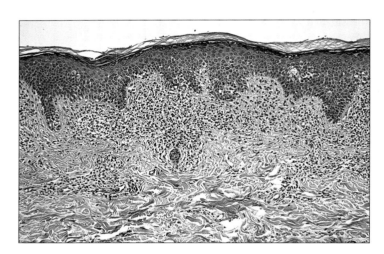

Fig. 20-4. Mycosis fungoides: there is a bandlike dermal infiltrate with atypical lymphocytes in the basal epidermis. (Courtesy of Dr. David Weedon and Dr. Geoffrey Strutton.)

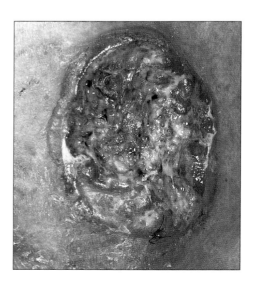

Fig. 20-3. Mycosis fungoides: extensive ulceration of the abdominal skin indicative of the invasive tumor stage.

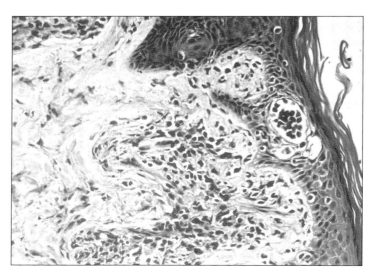

Fig. 20-5. Mycosis fungoides: typical histologic pattern, showing a focal intraepidermal collection of abnormal lymphoid cells (Pautrier's abscess) and similar groups of tumor cells in the papillary dermis.

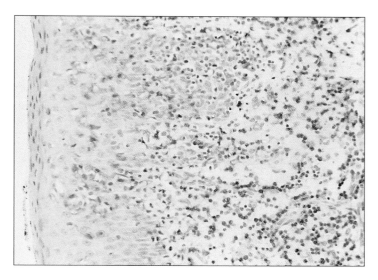

Fig. 20-6. Mycosis fungoides: malignant lymphoid cells in a skin biopsy show cytoplasmic positivity for the T-cell marker CD45RO (antibody UCHL1). (Courtesy of Dr. J. E. McLaughlin.)

The neoplastic cells may be positive for either CD3 and CD4 or CD3 and CD8 with variable expression of CD30.

Granulomatous Slack Skin Disease

Granulomatous slack skin disease is an extremely rare cutaneous T-cell lymphoma characterized by the development of laxity in the major skin folds and granulomatous infiltrates of neoplastic T cells (Fig. 20-9).

SÉZARY SYNDROME

In Sézary syndrome there is erythroderma, generalized lymphadenopathy, and characteristic neoplastic T cells (Sézary cells) in blood, skin, and lymph nodes. Traditionally this rare disease of adults has been considered a leukemic and aggressive variant of mycosis fungoides. The erythroderma (Fig. 20-10) is often associated with exfoliation and intense pruritis. The atypical cells in the blood usually exceed $1.0 \times 10^9/L$ and have markedly convoluted nuclei and may be small (Lutzner cells) or large (classical Sézary cells) (Figs. 20-11 and 20-12). The cytoplasm may show PAS-positive granules (Fig. 20-13), and electron microscopy defines the deeply clefted cerebriform nuclei (Fig. 20-14). Lymphoid marker studies show positivity for CD2,

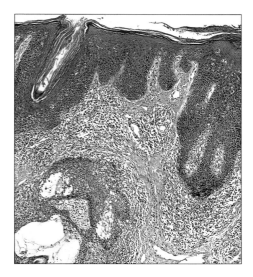

Fig. 20-7. Folliculotrophic mycosis fungoides (follicular mucinosis): there is a folliculotrophic infiltrate of neoplastic lymphocytes and mucinous degeneration of the hair follicle. (Courtesy of Dr. David Weedon and Dr. Geoffrey Strutton.)

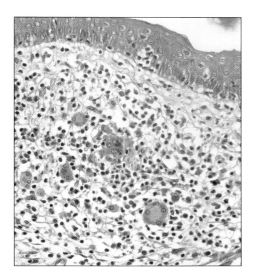

Fig. 20-9. Granulomatous slack skin disease: there is an intraepidermal and dermal lymphoid infiltrate and characteristic multinucleated histiocytic giant cells. Elastophagocytosis was present in other fields of the biopsy. (Courtesy of Professor Elias Campo.)

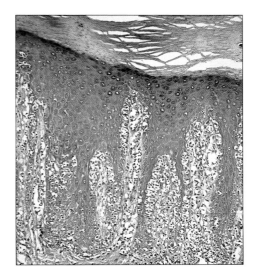

Fig. 20-8. Pagetoid reticulosis: there is a marked epidermotrophism of atypical lymphocytes. (Courtesy of Dr. David Weedon and Dr. Geoffrey Strutton.)

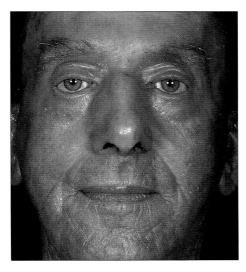

Fig. 20-10. Sézary syndrome: erythroderma in advanced disease.

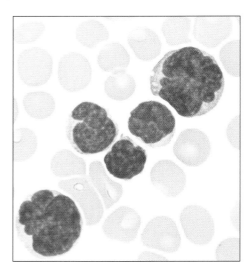

Fig. 20-11. Sézary syndrome: abnormal cells in the peripheral blood have characteristic, cerebriform, large, and clefted nuclei with fine chromatin pattern and scanty cytoplasm. (Courtesy of Professor D. Catovsky.)

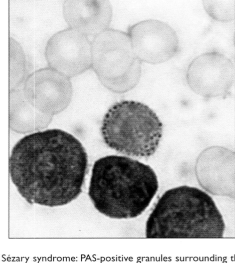

Fig. 20-13. Sézary syndrome: PAS-positive granules surrounding the nucleus in a lymphocyte with convoluted nucleus. (Courtesy of Dr. P. M. Canfield.)

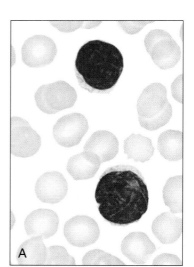

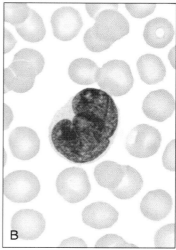

Fig. 20-12. Sézary syndrome. **A,** Small cell type (Lutzner cell)—the cells show grooved nuclear chromatin with a high nuclear-to-cytoplasm (N/C) ratio. **B,** Large cell type with grooved nuclear pattern, densely clumped chromatin, and lower N/C ratio. (Courtesy of Professor D. Catovsky.)

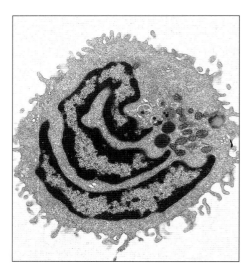

Fig. 20-14. Mycosis fungoides–Sézary syndrome: electron micrograph of an abnormal T lymphocyte from the peripheral blood shows a deeply clefted nucleus (× 8,000). (Courtesy of Dr. E. Matutes and Professor D. Catovsky.)

CD3, TCRβ, and CD5 and in most cases CD4. The 2008 World Health Organization (WHO) Classification suggests that one or more of the following criteria are required for a diagnosis of Sézary syndrome: an absolute blood count of Sézary cells of $1.0 \times 10^9/L$, an expanded CD4+ T-cell population resulting in a CD4/CD8 ratio of more than 10, and a loss of one or more T-cell antigens. The skin lesions are similar to those of mycosis fungoides with epidermal and dermal infiltrates of convoluted lymphocytes.

PRIMARY CUTANEOUS ANAPLASTIC T-CELL LYMPHOMA

The usual presenting features are solitary skin nodules or tumors. Multifocal cutaneous lesions are seen in only 20% of cases. The lesions have a tendency for partial or complete spontaneous regression with frequent relapses. Late involvement of regional nodes occurs only in a minority of patients. Skin biopsies show an exstensive dermal infiltrate of atypical lymphoid cells (Fig. 20-15, *A*). The cytologic features (Fig. 20-15, *B*) are similar to nodal or systemic anaplastic large cell lymphoma, but multinucleated giant cells are often more conspicuous. Strong positivity for CD30 is seen in most of the neoplastic cells (Fig. 20-15, *C*). CD4 and cytotoxic granule–associated

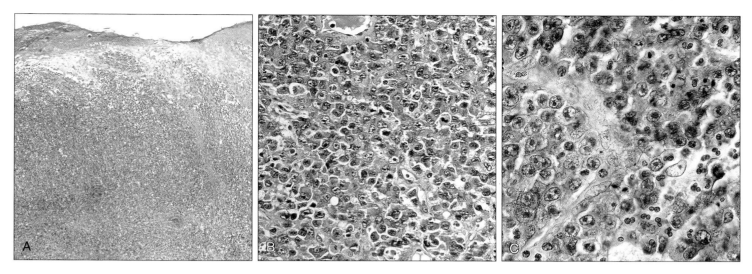

Fig. 20-15. Primary cutaneous anaplastic large cell lymphoma: skin biopsy showing **(A)** an extensive dermal infiltrate of atypical lymphoid cells. The infiltrating large neoplastic cells are pleomorphic with prominent nucleoli **(B)**, and immunostaining for CD30 shows positive cytoplasmic and Golgi zone staining **(C)**. (*A,* Courtesy of Dr. Shona McDowell. *B,* and *C,* Courtesy of Dr. David Weedon and Dr. Geoffrey Strutton.)

proteins (granzyme B, perforin, TIA-1) are usually positive. In contrast to nodal and systemic anaplastic T-cell tumors, the primary cutaneous tumors are negative for epithelial membrane antigen (EMA) and ALK protein. TCR genes are clonally rearranged.

LYMPHOMATOID PAPULOSIS

This chronic recurrent atypical lymphoproliferative disorder is characterized by the appearance and spontaneous regression of multiple skin papules, some of which may show ulceration. Although not classified as a lymphoma in the 2008 WHO classification, there are close similarities to cutaneous anaplastic large cell lymphoma. In most patients the condition has a benign course over many years, but a late evolution to systemic lymphoma occurs in 5%. Biopsy shows dermal infiltrates of atypical neoplastic lymphocytes (Fig. 20-16, *A*) sometimes resembling Reed-Sternberg cells (Fig. 20-16, *B*). CD30, CD4, and cytotoxic granule proteins are positive in the majority of cases. There is usually a variable associated population of inflammatory cells. In less than 10% of cases (Type B), the infiltrate is epidermotrophic with predominantly cerebriform cells similar to mycosis fungoides. The cells in this subgroup are CD3 and CD4 positive but

negative for CD30. Clonal rearrangement of T-cell receptor genes is demonstrated in approximately 70% of cases.

SUBCUTANEOUS PANNICULITIS-LIKE NK-/T-CELL LYMPHOMA

Subcutaneous nodules up to several centimeters in diameter are the usual presenting features of this rare lymphoma.

Sections show a subcutaneous neoplastic infiltrate of polymorphic lymphocytes, many with hyperchromatic nuclei. The cells surround or "rim" individual fat cells, and there are often foci of apoptotic and necrotic cells (Fig. 20-17). The neoplastic cell population has an $\alpha\beta$ cytotoxic T-cell phenotype with positivity for CD8 and cytotoxic granule molecules granzyme B, perforin, and TIA-1 (Fig. 20-18). T-cell receptor genes are rearranged, and there is no evidence of involvement by Epstein-Barr virus (EBV). The disease has an aggressive course. Dissemination to regional lymph nodes and other organs is unusual but may occur late in the disease. Release of cytokines and chemokines may produce a hemophagocytic syndrome (see p. 283) with fever, pancytopenia, and hepatosplenomegaly.

Fig. 20-16. Lymphomatoid papulosis: the dermal infiltrates **(A)** at higher magnification **(B)** are a mixture of small lymphocytes and atypical large cells similar to those seen in anaplastic large cell lymphoma. Some cells are multinucleated and others resemble Reed-Sternberg cells. (Courtesy of Dr. David Weedon and Dr. Geoffrey Strutton.)

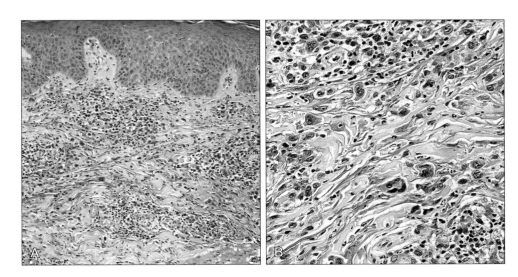

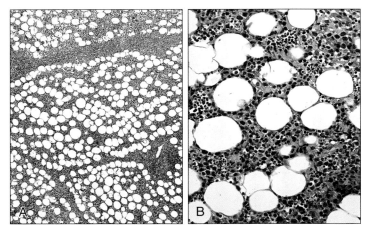

Fig. 20-17. Subcutaneous panniculitis-like T-cell lymphoma: **(A)** low-power view showing lymphomatous infiltration between fat cells; **(B)** lymphomatous infiltration between fat cells with areas of apoptosis by lymphoma cells.

CUTANEOUS γδ T-CELL LYMPHOMA

In this rare tumor there is a clonal proliferation of mature activated γδ T cells with a cytotoxic phenotype. Patients usually have disseminated plaques or ulcerated nodules or tumors. There may be involvement of mucosal and other extranodal sites, and occasionally there is a hemophagocytic syndrome. Pleomorphic small to large cells infiltrate the subcutaneous tissue and dermis (Fig. 20-19). In frozen sections the cells are TCR δ positive (if only paraffin sections are available, absence of βF1 may indicate a γδ phenotype). Most patients have aggressive disease resistant to therapy, and the median survival is about 15 months.

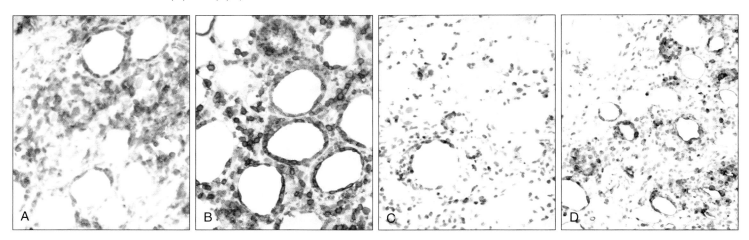

Fig. 20-18. Subcutaneous panniculitis-like T-cell lymphoma: immunoperoxidase staining. **A,** CD3. **B,** CD8. **C,** Granzyme B. **D,** Perforin. (Courtesy of Dr. Graeme Taylor.)

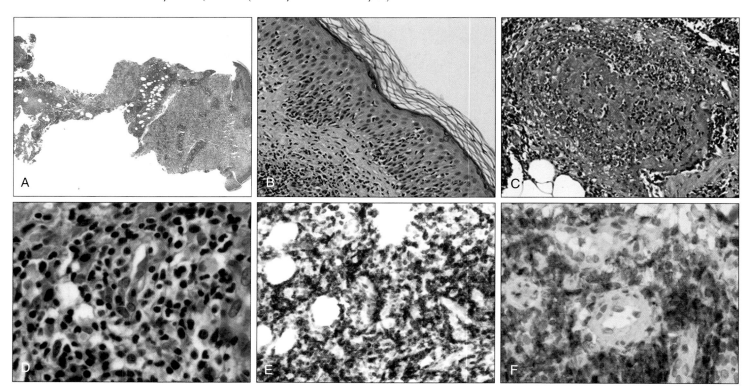

Fig. 20-19. Cutaneous γδ T-cell lymphoma: **(A),** infiltrates of neoplastic lymphoid cells involve both the dermis and subcutaneous fat. Focal collections of atypical lymphocytes also involve the epidermis **(B),** and there is angiocentricity and angiodestruction **(C).** At higher magnification the cells are predominantly small and medium-sized lymphocytes **(D).** The neoplastic cells show immunoreactivity for CD3 **(E)** and TCRδ1 **(F).** (All images courtesy of Professor Elias Campo.)

Fig. 20-20. Primary cutaneous aggressive epidermotrophic CD8+ T-cell lymphoma: skin biopsy. **A,** The infiltrate of atypical cells is almost wholly intraepidermal. **B,** The lymphoma cells express CD8. (Courtesy of Dr. Phillip McKee.)

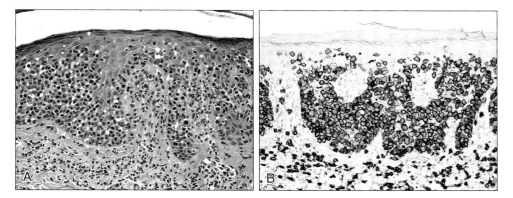

PRIMARY CUTANEOUS AGGRESSIVE EPIDERMOTROPHIC CD8+ T-CELL LYMPHOMA (PROVISIONAL CATEGORY)

These lymphomas usually manifest as disseminated eruptive papules, nodules, and tumors showing central ulceration or as hyperkeratotic plaques. Occasionally there is involvement of the oral mucosa. Histologically the tumor cells are epidermotrophic (Fig. 20-20); invasion and destruction of adnexal structures, angiocentricity, and angioinvasion may be present. The tumor cells vary in size with pleomorphic or blastic nuclei. Immunohistology shows positivity for βF1, CD3, CD8, granzyme B, perforin, TIA1, and CD45RA. EBV is usually negative. Systemic dissemination occurs and the prognosis is poor with a medium survival of less than 3 years.

PRIMARY CUTANEOUS SMALL/MEDIUM CD4+ T-CELL LYMPHOMA (PROVISIONAL CATEGORY)

In this lymphoma the presenting plaque or tumor, commonly found on the face, neck, or upper trunk, is usually solitary with an indolent growth pattern. Occasionally there are multiple lesions, but systemic dissemination is rare. The small to medium-sized lymphocytes infiltrate the dermis and sometimes the upper subcutaneous tissues (Fig. 20-21). Occasionally there is focal epidermotrophism. The immunophenotype is CD3+ and CD4+. CD8, CD30, and the cytotoxic proteins are not expressed. The prognosis is favorable with a 60% to 80% 5-year survival rate. Demonstration of TCR gene rearrangement and an abnormal T-cell phenotype are useful in excluding pseudo–T-cell lymphomas.

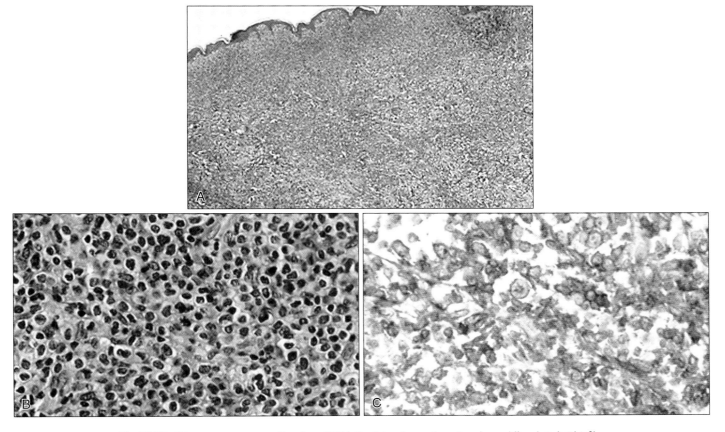

Fig. 20-21. Primary cutaneous small/medium CD4+ T-cell lymphoma: there is a dense diffuse lymphoid infiltrate throughout the entire dermis **(A)**, and at higher magnification the cells are predominantly small and medium-sized lymphocytes **(B)** with positivity for CD4 **(C)**. (All images courtesy of Professor Elias Campo.)

PRIMARY CUTANEOUS PERIPHERAL T-CELL LYMPHOMA UNSPECIFIED

The designation primary cutaneous lymphoma unspecified is reserved for cutaneous T-cell tumors that fail to conform to criteria consistent with either the well-defined cutaneous T-cell neoplasms or the two provisional entities. The neoplastic cells are usually large and pleomorphic. In all cases mycosis fungoides, lymphomatoid papulosis, and anaplastic large cell lymphoma must be excluded by differences in both clinical and histologic features.

EXTRANODAL NK-/T-CELL LYMPHOMA, NASAL TYPE

This angiocentric lymphoma is rare in the United States and Europe, but is much more common in Asia and often involves the nose, palate, and skin, but other soft tissues, including the gut, may also be involved. There is a tendency to invade the walls of blood vessels, accompanied in many cases by blockage of vessels by lymphoma cells, often associated with ischemic necrosis of normal and neoplastic tissue (Fig. 20-22). Cutaneous infiltration is usually dermal and may also involve subcutaneous tissue. The neoplastic cells are variable in size with irregular or oval nuclei, and there is typically necrosis (Fig. 20-23). The cell morphology is highly variable, and admixed inflammatory cells may cause difficulty in diagnosing early cases. The neoplastic cells are probably of NK-cell rather than T-cell origin: surface CD3 is absent in many cases (although cytoplasmic CD3 epsilon chain is present) and CD56 is often expressed (Fig. 20-24). The cytotoxic proteins granzyme B, perforin, and TIA-1 are also positive. EBV is almost always present in the neoplastic cells (Fig. 20-25). The most frequently found cytogenetic abnormalities are del(6) (q21;q25) and inv(6)(p10).

The cutaneous form is an aggressive tumor with a poor prognosis and a median survival less than 1 year. In some cases there is an associated hemophagocytic syndrome. This lymphoma is closely related to aggressive NK-cell leukemia that may also have extensive cutaneous involvement. Nasal disease may have a more protracted course.

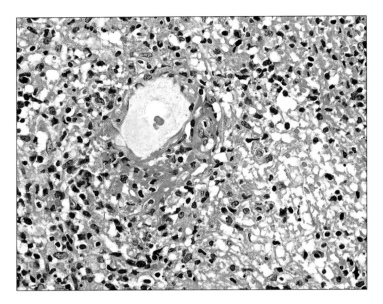

Fig. 20-23. T/NK nasal type (angiocentric) lymphoma: typical lesion with angiocentricity and marked necrosis. (Courtesy of Professor R. Liang.)

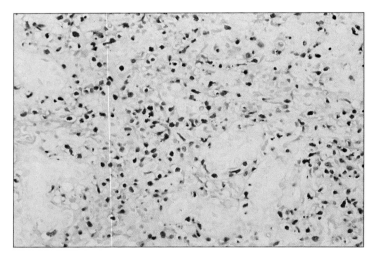

Fig. 20-24. T/NK nasal type (angiocentric) lymphoma: positive immunoperoxidase stain for CD56. (Courtesy of Professor R. Liang.)

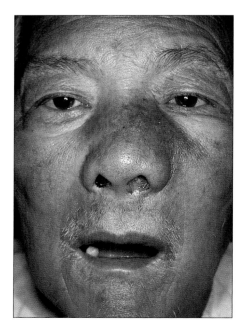

Fig. 20-22. T/NK nasal type (angiocentric) lymphoma: midline nasal swelling. (Courtesy of Professor R. Liang.)

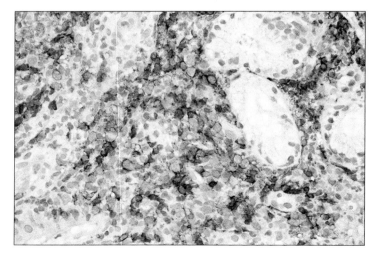

Fig. 20-25. T/NK nasal type (angiocentric) lymphoma: positive immunoperoxidase stain for EBER. (Courtesy of Professor R. Liang.)

HYDROA VACCINIFORME–LIKE T-CELL LYMPHOMA

This exceptionally rare pediatric lymphoma has been reported mainly from South America, Japan, and Korea. The lymphoma occurs on sun-exposed skin of the face and extremities and also on covered skin with edema, blistering, and ulceration simular to the benign form of hydroa vacciniforme (Fig. 20-26, *A*). There is associated fever, wasting, lymphadenopathy, anemia, and leucopenia. Skin biopsies (Fig. 20-26, *B–F*) show superficial and deep perivascular and periappendageal lymphoid infiltrates that often extend into subcutaneous fat. There is ballooning degeneration of the overlying epidermis. The neoplastic cells are predominantly cytotoxic T cells positive for CD3, CD4, CD8, cytotoxic granules, and EBV. There is a monoclonal rearrangement of the T-cell receptor gene.

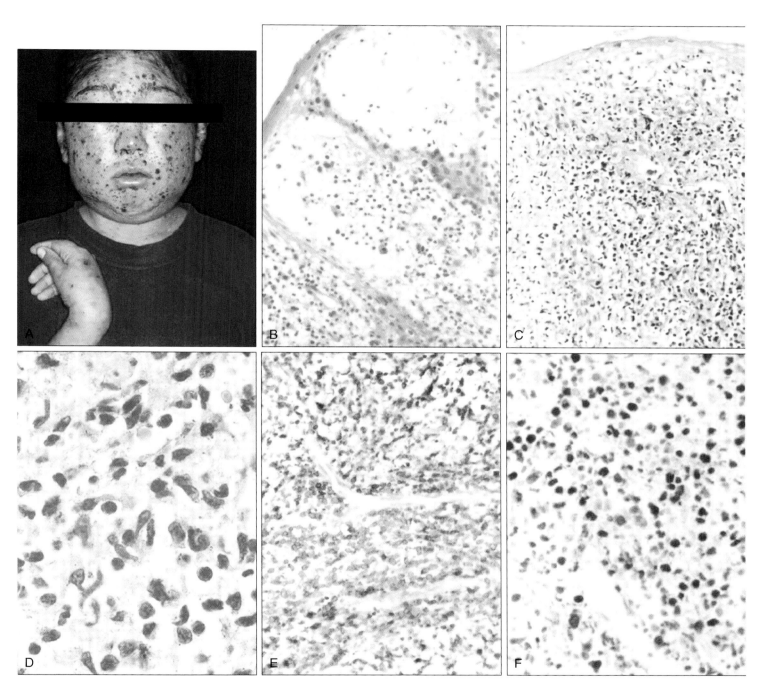

Fig. 20-26. Hydroa vacciniforme-like T-cell lymphoma: **(A),** Typical vacciniform skin eruptions in an 8-year-old Peruvian boy. Skin biopsy showing blisters **(B),** an atypical dermal infiltrate with epidermotrophism and spongiosis **(C),** cytologic detail of pleomorphic neoplastic cells **(D),** and immunopositivity for CD3 **(E)** and EBER **(F).** (All images courtesy of Dr. Carlos Barrionuevo.)

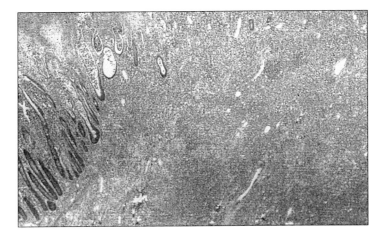

Fig. 20-27. Enteropathy-associated T-cell lymphoma: ulceration of small intestinal mucosa and infiltration into the smooth muscle below.

INTESTINAL AND/OR ENTEROPATHY-ASSOCIATED T-CELL LYMPHOMA

Small intestinal lymphomas have long been recognized as a complication of gluten-induced enteropathy (celiac disease). They were first thought to be a heterogeneous group of tumors, but later studies suggested a histiocytic origin. In the early 1980s it became clear that they were T-cell lymphomas of widely varying morphology.

This neoplasm is often associated with small bowel ulceration. The typical histologic features of celiac disease, though often present, may be absent because of the phenomenon of "latency" recently recognized in celiac patients. In keeping with this, some patients have a history of documented celiac disease, whereas others have the lymphoma. Typical histologic appearances are shown in Figs. 20-27 to 20-29. The neoplastic cells express CD3, CD7, CD8 (occasionally), and, in most cases, the CD103 integrin molecule found on normal intestinal T lymphocytes. Most patients have HLA DQA1*0501, DQB1*0201 characteristic of celiac disease. An association with EBV has been found in some cases, especially in South and Central America. TCR β and γ genes are clonally rearranged. The clinical outlook is poor since the neoplasm is frequently multifocal.

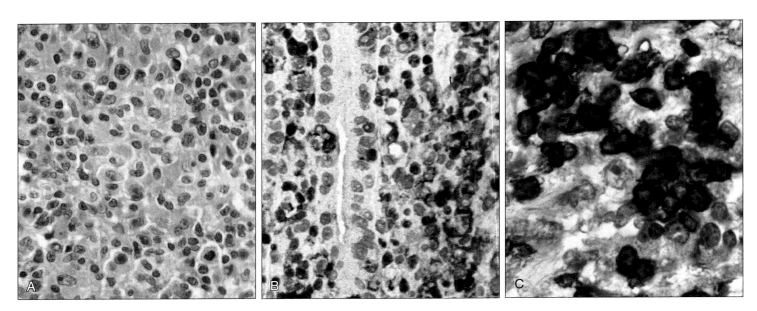

Fig. 20-28. Enteropathy-associated T-cell lymphoma. **A,** High-power view showing pleomorphic and polymorphic infiltration of lymphoid cells. **B, C,** APAAP immunoalkaline phosphatase stain shows that some but not all of the neoplastic cells express CD3.

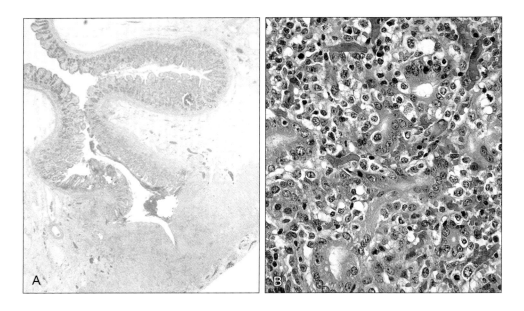

Fig. 20-29. Enteropathy-associated T-cell lymphoma. **A,** Deep fissure formation and a flat, small intestinal mucosa. **B,** Infiltration of small intestinal crypts by neoplastic cells.

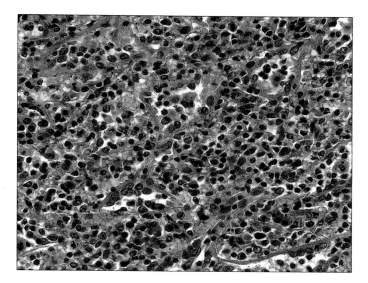

Fig. 20-30. Hepatosplenic γδ T-cell lymphoma: infiltration of splenic pulp cords by medium-sized lymphoma cells. The cells showed clonal T-cell receptor γ and δ rearrangements.

HEPATOSPLENIC T-CELL LYMPHOMA

This rare form of lymphoma representing less than 5% of all T-cell neoplasms is predominantly a disease of young adults and has a male predominance. There is an increased incidence in immunosuppressed patients following organ transplantation. The tumor is derived from cytotoxic T cells usually of the δT-cell receptor subtype. Marked sinusoidal infiltration of the spleen (Fig. 20-30), liver, and bone marrow are characteristic features. The neoplastic cells are medium-sized lymphocytes with a high nuclear-to-cytoplasm ratio. Patients have hepatosplenomegaly with no peripheral lymphadenopathy. There is usually anemia, thrombocytopenia, and leukocytosis. The atypical T cells are seen in the blood (Fig. 20-31), especially in the later stages of the disease. Infiltration of bone marrow may be seen in aspirates (Fig. 20-32) and trephine biopsies. The immunophenotype is usually CD3 and TCRδ1 positive and CD4, CD5, and CD8 negative. The cells express the cytotoxic protein TIA1, but perforin is usually negative. There is rearrangement of the TCRδ gene. Isochromosome 7q is almost always present. There is no evidence of EBV involvement. Less commonly, variant cases express the αβ T-cell receptor (Fig. 20-33). These lymphomas are aggressive, with a median survival of less than 2 years.

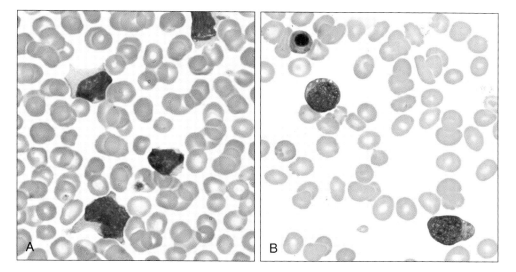

Fig. 20-31. Hepatosplenic T-cell lymphoma: peripheral blood film. In **(A)** the atypical lymphocytes show large nuclei and abundant cytoplasm while in another patient **(B)** the cells are more blastic in appearance with basophilic cytoplasm. (Courtesy of Dr. Wendy Erber.)

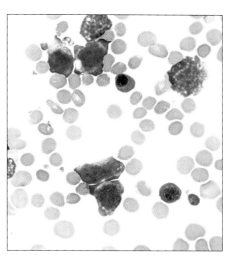

Fig. 20-32. Hepatosplenic T-cell lymphoma: bone marrow aspirate in same patient as Fig. 20-33, B. The four large lymphoma cells show a vesicular chromatin pattern, nucleoli, and basophilic cytoplasm. (Courtesy of Dr. Wendy Erber.)

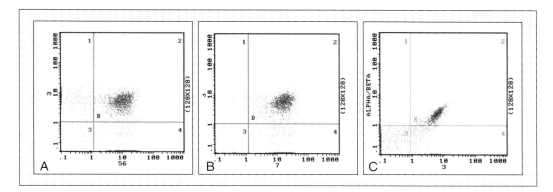

Fig. 20-33. Hepatosplenic T-cell lymphoma: flow cytometry [**(A)** CD3/CD56, **(B)** CD3/CD7, and **(C)** αβ/CD3] shows the neoplastic T-cells are positive for CD3, CD7, and CD56 and express the αβ T-cell receptor. (Courtesy of Dr. Wendy Erber.)

ANGIOIMMUNOBLASTIC LYMPHADENOPATHY

Angioimmunoblastic T-cell lymphoma was initially thought of as an abnormal immune reaction, but is now considered as a category of peripheral T-cell lymphoma in which the neoplastic cells are mixed with and obscured by a complex histologic picture that includes proliferating vessels, epithelioid histiocytes, plasma cells, eosinophils, and hyperplastic clusters of follicular dendritic cells (Fig. 20-34). The neoplastic cells are of variable morphology and include atypical "clear" cells with indented nuclei and abundant pale cytoplasm. Immunohistology shows positivity for the T-cell markers CD3 and CD4 (Fig. 20-35, A and B) and CD8. CD10 may also be positive. Hyperplastic clusters of follicular dendritic cells (CD21+) may be prominent (Fig. 20-35, C). EBER positivity may identify EBV-positive B cells (Fig. 20-35, D). T-cell receptor genes are rearranged in 75% of cases. The most frequent cytogenetic abnormalities are trisomy 3, trisomy 5, and an additional X chromosome. There is frequently involvement of bone marrow (Fig. 20-36), and occasionally the neoplastic T cells are seen in blood films (Fig. 20-37).

The disease is most frequent among the elderly and may manifest at multiple extranodal sites. Patients often have systemic symptoms such as weight loss, fever, skin rash (Fig. 20-38), and a polyclonal hypergammaglobulinemia. The disease is moderately aggressive, patients may die from infective complications, and a high-grade lymphoma (usually of T-cell but occasionally of B-cell type) may emerge. The median survival is less than 3 years.

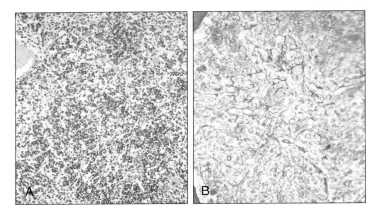

Fig. 20-36. Angioimmunoblastic T-cell lymphoma: bone marrow trephine biopsy shows **(A)** extensive replacement of hemopoietic cells by abnormal lymphoid tissue, and **(B)** silver impregnation staining outlines the characteristic arborizing vascular pattern of the condition.

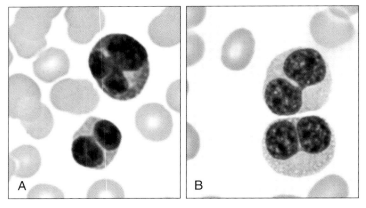

Fig. 20-37. Angioimmunoblastic T-cell lymphoma: peripheral blood film. **A** and **B,** The atypical lymphoid cells show nuclear lobation and segmentation. (Courtesy of Dr. Wendy Erber.)

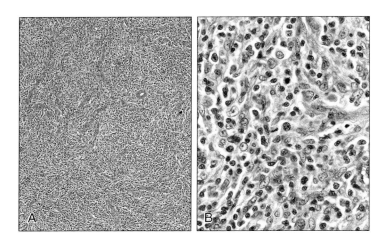

Fig. 20-34. Angioimmunoblastic T-cell lymphoma: **A,** Low-power view showing prominent arborizing vascular pattern. **B,** High-power view showing clear cell cytology of the neoplastic T cells.

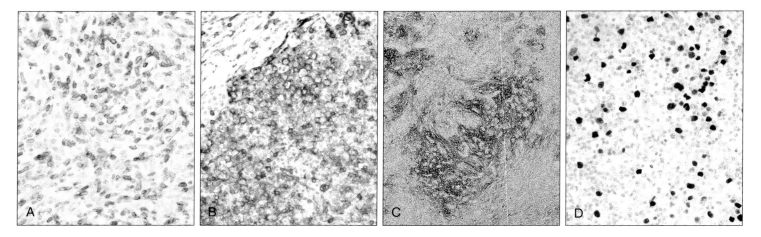

Fig. 20-35. Angioimmunoblastic T-cell lymphoma: immunoperoxidase staining. The neoplastic T-cells show positive staining for CD3 **(A)** and CD4 **(B)**. CD21 positivity identifies perivascular proliferation of follicular dendritic cells **(C)**. Numerous cells are positive for EBER **(D)**. By double staining most of these EBER positive cells are CD20 positive B cells. (**B,** and **D,** Courtesy of Dr. Graeme Taylor.)

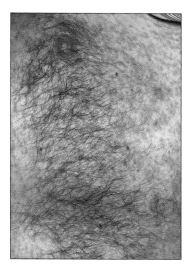

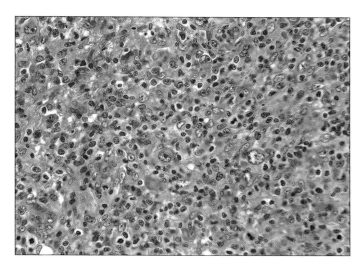

Fig. 20-38. Angioimmunoblastic T-cell lymphoma: skin appearances of a 65-year-old man with fever, an erythematous rash, and lymphadenopathy. He subsequently died of a high-grade lymphoma.

Fig. 20-39. Anaplastic large cell T-cell lymphoma: high-power view showing typical cytologic features with large cells with prominent nucleoli, abundant cytoplasm, and prominent Golgi zones.

ANAPLASTIC LARGE CELL LYMPHOMA: ALK POSITIVE

In the 1980s, a monoclonal antibody ("Ki-1") raised against a Hodgkin cell line was found to react with the tumor cells in a group of non-Hodgkin large cell lymphomas. These neoplasms tended to share unusual morphologic features (cohesive "pseudo-carcinomatous" growth pattern, sinusoidal invasion, large bizarre cells with abundant cytoplasm, and pleomorphic, often horseshoe-shaped nuclei), and the term *anaplastic large cell lymphoma* was designated for these tumors. The (2;5)(q23;q35) chromosomal translocation was subsequently found to be associated with these lymphomas.

This translocation creates the NPM-ALK fusion gene, encoding a hybrid tyrosine kinase. Variant translocations include t(1;2), t(2,3), and t(2;22), all of which are ALK positive. Typical biopsy appearances are shown in Fig. 20-39. The tumor cells are positive for CD30 on the cell membrane and in the Golgi region (Fig. 20-40, *A*) and their distribution is often perivascular (Fig. 20-40, *B*). ALK

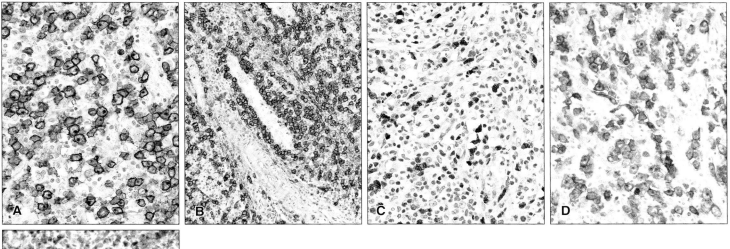

Fig. 20-40. Anaplastic large cell T-cell lymphoma: immunoperoxidase staining. **A,** Positive cell membrane and Golgi zone staining for CD30. **B,** CD30 positivity showing perivascular accumulation of tumor cells. **C,** The neoplastic cells show nuclear positivity for ALK 1. **D,** The cells are also positive for EMA. **E,** Positivity for granzyme B. (*D* and *E,* Courtesy of Dr. Graeme Taylor.)

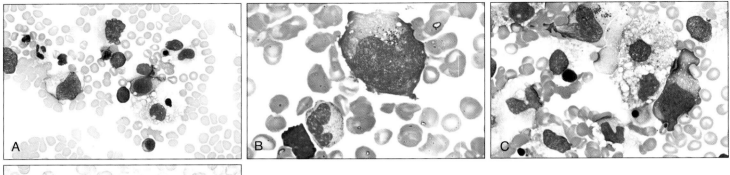

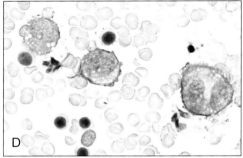

Fig. 20-41. Anaplastic large cell T-cell lymphoma: bone marrow aspirate. **A–C,** MGG stain. The tumor cells are large and pleomorphic with prominent nucleoli and pale cytoplasm. The two large vacuolated cells are histiocytes. **D,** Immunoperoxidase staining shows membrane positivity for CD30 in the large neoplastic cells. (Courtesy of Dr. Wendy Erber.)

staining is usually both cytoplasmic and nuclear (Fig. 20-40, *C*). One or more T-cell antigens, EMA, and the cytotoxic-associated antigens granzyme B, perforin, and TIA-1 are positive in the great majority of cases (Fig. 20-40, *D* and *E*). CD3 is negative in most cases. Approximately 90% of these tumors show clonal rearrangement of the T-cell receptor. EBV sequences are absent.

Anaplastic large cell lymphoma is most frequent in the first three decades of life. It accounts for approximately 3% of adult non-Hodgkin lymphomas and up to 30% of childhood lymphomas. The disease involves both lymph nodes and extranodal sites. Bone marrow involvement (Figs. 20-41 to 20-43) is present in up to 30% of cases if immunostaining for CD30, EMA, and ALK is employed. In occasional patients large neoplastic T cells are seen in blood films (Fig. 20-44). Chemotherapy is often curative. The overall 5-year survival rate in ALK-positive anaplastic large cell lymphoma is close to 80%.

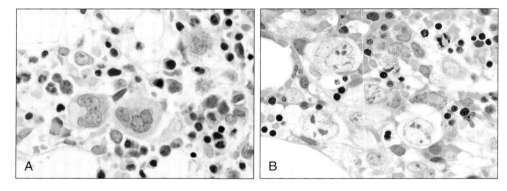

Fig. 20-42. Anaplastic large cell T-cell lymphoma: bone marrow trephine biopsy. **A,** The lymphoma cells are large with prominent nucleoli and abundant agranular cytoplasm. **B,** In this patient there was an associated hemophagocytic syndrome. The large lymphoma cells show cytoplasm with prominent large vacuoles. (Courtesy of Dr. Wendy Erber.)

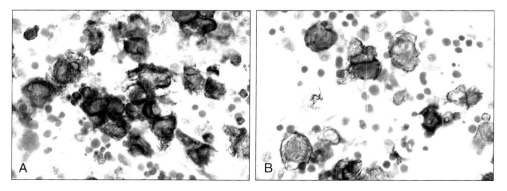

Fig. 20-43. Anaplastic large cell T-cell lymphoma: immunoperoxidase staining, same case as Fig. 20-42, *B*. **A,** Positive staining for CD3. **B,** Positive staining for CD30. (Courtesy of Dr. Wendy Erber.)

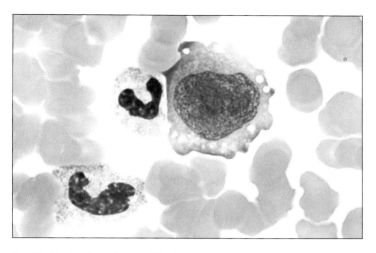

Fig. 20-44. Anaplastic large cell T-cell lymphoma: peripheral blood film showing two band form neutrophils and a very large atypical lymphoma cell with multiple nucleoli, a vesicular nuclear chromatin pattern, and abundant pale vacuolated cytoplasm. (Courtesy of Dr. Wendy Erber.)

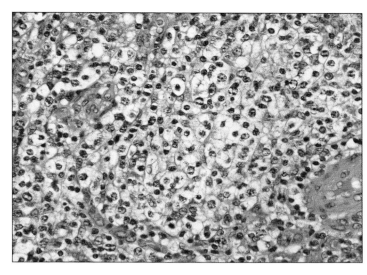

Fig. 20-45. Peripheral T-cell lymphoma unspecified: high-power view of a peripheral T-cell lymphoma of clear type showing a focus of neoplastic T cells with water-clear cytoplasm, which are commonly encountered in malignant lymphomas of peripheral T-cell lineage.

ANAPLASTIC LARGE CELL LYMPHOMA: ALK NEGATIVE

ALK-negative cases of anaplastic large cell lymphoma are less well characterized and are classified as provisional in the WHO 2008 Classification. Patients are generally older, and the disease has a more aggressive course and less favorable prognosis. The histologic appearances are similar to ALK-positive disease, and the neoplastic cells are generally larger and more pleomorphic. There are no differences in phenotypic or molecular markers.

PERIPHERAL T-CELL LYMPHOMA, UNSPECIFIED

Although a number of well-defined categories of T-cell neoplasia have come to be recognized over the years (e.g., mycosis fungoides and those described previously), many T-cell lymphomas have features that do not match these entities. They were often referred to as "pleomorphic" or "polymorphic" T-cell neoplasms, reflecting their wide variation in cell morphology. The REAL scheme created a single category of "peripheral T-cell lymphoma." The word "unspecified" was added to indicate that this category might comprise several entities. These unspecified tumors make up half of all T-cell lymphomas

seen in Western countries. The majority of patients are adults with lymphadenopathy, but often there is generalized disease with involvement of bone marrow, liver, spleen, and skin.

These neoplasms typically show diffuse infiltrates with replacement of normal lymph node architecture. The neoplastic cells are a mixture of small and large pleomorphic cells, often with irregular nuclei. Clear cells (Fig. 20-45) and Reed-Sternberg–like cells are often present. There may be a marked infiltration of nonneoplastic cells, including macrophages and eosinophils. Rare variant morphologic patterns are recognized. In the first, clusters of epithelioid histiocytes, characteristic of so-called Lennert's or lymphoepithelioid T-cell lymphoma, are seen (Fig. 20-46). In the T-zone variant the infiltrate is interfollicular with preservation or even hyperplasia of follicles (Fig. 20-47). These variants do not appear to have any specific clinical features. A variety of patterns of T-cell antigen expression are found (Fig. 20-48), CD4 being more frequent than CD8. In large cell tumors CD30 may be expressed. Positivity for cytotoxic granules is rare in nodal disease, and EBV is usually not present in tumor cells. TCR genes are clonally rearranged in most cases. Complex karyotypes are often found. An example of inv(14) is shown in Fig. 20-49. The peripheral blood is often involved (Fig. 20-50), and occasionally there is a hemophagocytic syndrome (see p. 283). Involvement of skeletal muscle is shown in Fig. 20-51.

Fig. 20-46. Peripheral T-cell lymphoma unspecified showing nodular accumulations of macrophages. **A, B,** This appearance is given the title "lymphoepithelioid lymphoma" in the Kiel scheme (and is also sometimes known as "Lennert's lymphoma"), although no evidence indicates that this entity can be differentiated from other T-cell lymphomas. Clumps of epithelioid cells are interspersed with a mixed population of small and large lymphocytes with occasional mitoses and large atypical cells that resemble Reed-Sternberg cells. The small cells show irregular angular nuclei. The tumor T cells are thought to produce lymphokines that cause epithelioid cell formation from histiocytes. (Courtesy of Dr. J. E. McLaughlin.)

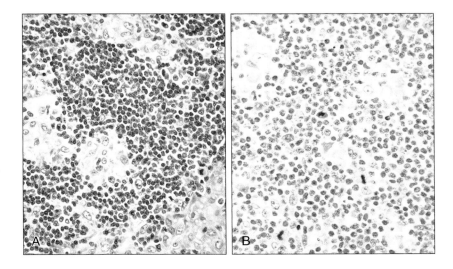

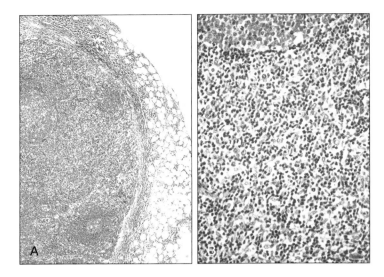

Fig. 20-47. Peripheral T-cell lymphoma unspecified. **A,** Expansion of paracortical region with wide separation of germinal follicles. **B,** High power shows many T lymphocytes with clear cytoplasm, eosinophils, and prominent venules. This pattern is referred to as "T-zone lymphoma" in the Kiel scheme, but there is no evidence that it is an entity that can be differentiated from other peripheral T-cell lymphomas. (Courtesy of Dr. J. E. McLaughlin.)

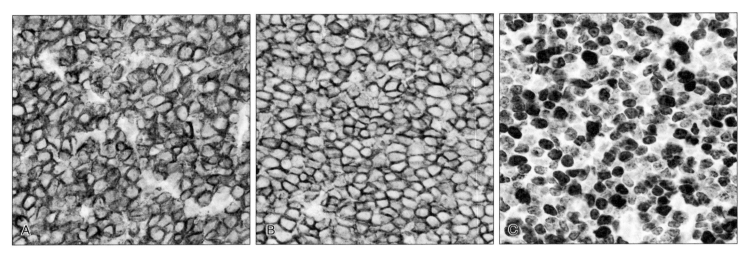

Fig. 20-48. Peripheral T-cell lymphoma unspecified: immunoperoxidase stains showing positivity for CD3 **(A)** and CD5 **(B).** A high proliferation rate is indicated with Ki-67 **(C).**

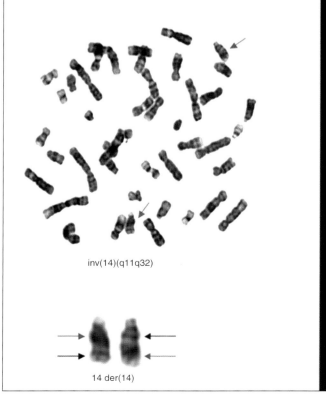

inv(14)(q11q32)

14 der(14)

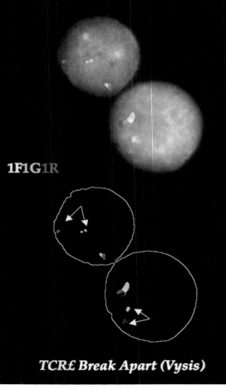

1F1G1R

TCR£ Break Apart (Vysis)

Fig. 20-49. Peripheral T-cell lymphoma unspecified: cytogenetics; inv (14). The left-hand panel shows a G-banded metaphase with arrows pointing to a normal chromosome 14 (at 6 o'clock) and an inverted chromosome 14 (1 o'clock), both shown enlarged below with arrows indicating the breakpoint positions. The right-hand panel shows interphase nuclei with FISH signals from TCRα dual color breakpoint (Vysis) probes. The signal pattern 1 fusion, 1 green, 1 red shows that one of the TCRα genes at 14q11 loci is rearranged (split signal indicated by arrows). Unprocessed images above, processed images below. (Courtesy of Dr. E. Nacheva.)

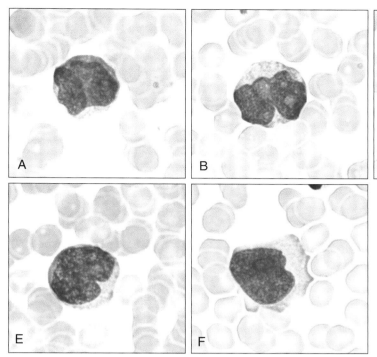

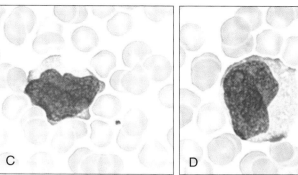

Fig. 20-50. Peripheral T-cell lymphoma unspecified: peripheral blood film in same case as Fig. 20-48 showing selected atypical lymphoma cells.

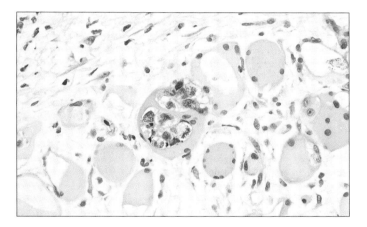

Fig. 20-51. Peripheral T-cell lymphoma unspecified: neoplastic cells are invading striated muscle.

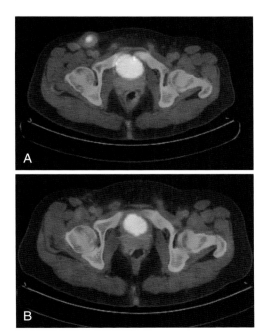

Fig. 20-52. Peripheral T-cell lymphoma unspecified. **A,** Right groin disease is indicated by axial fused FDG PET/CT. **B,** Following chemotherapy the corresponding image shows a complete metabolic response. (Courtesy of Dr. Garry Cook.)

Positron emission tomography is useful in detecting sites of involvement and the effectiveness of therapy (Fig. 20-52). The prognosis of these unspecified T-cell lymphomas is highly variable.

The phenotypes of the principal T-cell and NK-cell lymphomas discussed in this chapter are summarized in Table 20-3.

SYSTEMIC EBV+ T-CELL LYMPHOPROLIFERATIVE DISEASE OF CHILDHOOD

This extremely rare, fulminant, and fatal lymphoproliferative disease associated with active EBV infection is characterized by hepatosplenomegaly, often without significant lymphadenopathy, fever, liver failure, pancytopenia, and a hemophagocytic syndrome.

TABLE 20-3.   T-CELL LYMPHOMAS (TCLs): TYPICAL PHENOTYPIC PATTERNS

Neoplasm	Immunophenotype (positive)
Mycosis fungoides	CD2, CD3, CD4, CD5, TCRβ
Sézary syndrome	CD2, CD3, CD4, CD5, TCRβ
Primary cutaneous anaplastic large TCL	CD30, CD4, CyAg
Lymphomatoid papulosis	CD30, CD4, CyAg
Subcutaneous panniculitis-like TCL	CD8, CyAg
Extranodal NK/T cell lymphoma, nasal type	CD56, CD3ε (CD3neg)
Primary cutaneous γδTCL	TCRδ1, CD3, variable CD56
Cutaneous aggressive epidermotrophic CD8+ cytotoxic TCL	βF1, CD3, CD8, CyAg
Cutaneous small–medium CD4+TCL	βF1, CD3, CD4
Enteropathy-type TCL	CD3, CD7, CD103, CyAg
Hepatosplenic TCL	CD3, CD56, TCRδ1, TIA1
Angioimmunoblastic TCL	CD3, CD4, CD10
Anaplastic large cell lymphoma	CD30, ALK, EMA, CyAg
Peripheral TCL unspecified	CD3, variable CD4, CD5, CD7

CyAg, antigens of cytotoxic proteins (TIA1, granzyme B, perforin); βF1, T-cell receptor β chain; CD3ε, CD3ε chain subunit.

HODGKIN LYMPHOMA

Hodgkin lymphoma is one of the most common categories of lymphoid neoplasia and is closely related to the other malignant lymphomas.

PRESENTATION AND EVOLUTION

In many patients the disease at presentation is localized to a single peripheral lymph node region, and studies of its natural history indicate that its subsequent progression is initially by direct contiguity within the lymphatic system.

With advanced disease, dissemination involves nonlymphatic tissue. The disease affects all age groups, but is particularly common in young and middle-aged adults. Most patients have a painless, asymmetric, firm, and discrete enlargement of the superficial lymph nodes (Figs. 21-1 and 21-2). Mediastinal disease, occasionally accompanied by an obstructed superior vena cava (Fig. 21-3), and involvement of retroperitoneal lymph nodes may be detected during staging procedures. Clinical splenomegaly occurs during the course of the disease in 50% of patients. Rarely, patients may have lymphatic obstruction (Fig. 21-4).

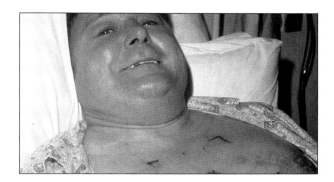

Fig. 21-3. Hodgkin lymphoma: cyanosis and edema of the face, neck, and upper trunk result from superior vena cava obstruction caused by mediastinal node involvement. The skin markings over the anterior chest indicate the field of radiotherapy.

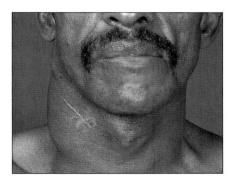

Fig. 21-1. Hodgkin lymphoma: right-sided cervical lymphadenopathy. The scar of previous biopsy incision is well healed.

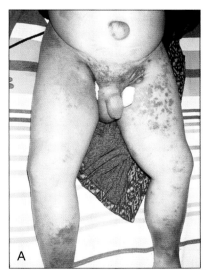

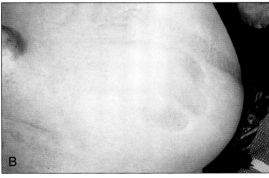

Fig. 21-4. Hodgkin lymphoma. **A,** Gross edema of the legs, genitals, and lower abdominal wall with umbilical herniation caused by lymphatic obstruction that resulted from extensive involvement of the inguinal and pelvic lymph nodes. A staphylococcal infection in the skin folds of the groin is present. **B,** A close-up view of "pitting" edema of the abdominal wall is shown.

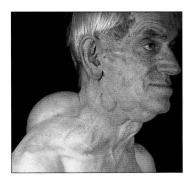

Fig. 21-2. Hodgkin lymphoma: massive cervical lymphadenopathy in a 73-year-old man with extensive disease.

The disease may involve the liver, skin (Fig. 21-5), and other organs, for example, the gastrointestinal tract or brain and, in rare patients, the retina (Fig. 21-6). Depressed cell-mediated immunity is also present and is associated with an increased incidence of infections, particularly herpes zoster (Fig. 21-7), fungal diseases, and tuberculosis.

Occasionally the first indication of Hodgkin lymphoma follows fine-needle aspiration of enlarged nodes (Figs. 21-8 and 21-9). The diagnosis is usually made from histologic examination of excised lymph nodes. The affected nodes are enlarged and show pale translucent cut surfaces (Fig. 21-10). Initially the nodes remain discrete, but later in the disease, they become matted together and there may be invasion of surrounding tissues. Hodgkin tissue in other organs has a similar pale, flesh-like appearance (Fig. 21-11).

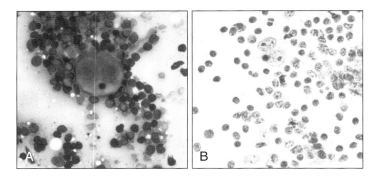

Fig. 21-8. Hodgkin lymphoma: fine-needle aspirates of involved lymph nodes showing Reed-Sternberg cells stained by **(A)** May-Grünwald-Giemsa and **(B)** Papanicolaou techniques.

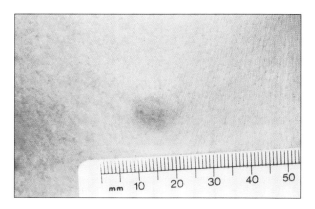

Fig. 21-5. Hodgkin lymphoma: a skin deposit approximately 1 cm in diameter is shown.

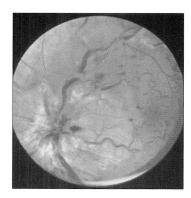

Fig. 21-6. Hodgkin lymphoma: extensive infiltration of the optic disc and surrounding retina.

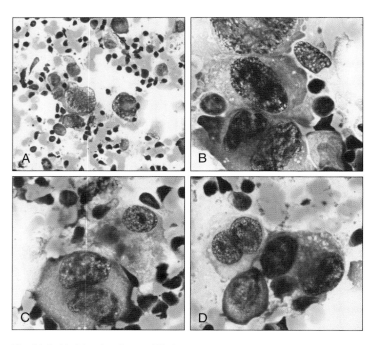

Fig. 21-9. Hodgkin lymphoma: **(A)** fine-needle aspirate of lymph node showing Reed-Sternberg cells, a mitotic figure, histiocytes, and lymphoid cells; **(B–D)** at higher magnification, further Reed-Sternberg cells from the same fine-needle aspirate.

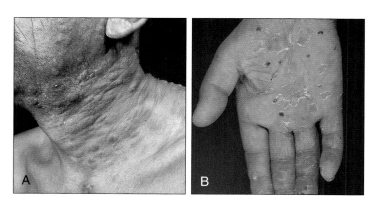

Fig. 21-7. Hodgkin lymphoma: **(A)** vesicular cutaneous eruption of the neck caused by herpes zoster; **(B)** atypical herpetic eruption of the palmar surface of the hand.

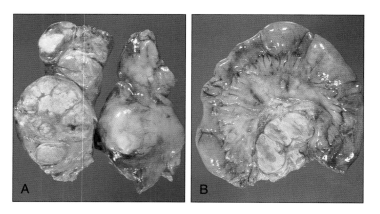

Fig. 21-10. Hodgkin lymphoma: **(A)** matted block of resected involved cervical nodes showing a cross section of the pale, translucent, fleshy tumor tissue with areas of fibrosis and necrosis; **(B)** para-aortic lymph nodes removed at necropsy showing in cross section the typical moist "fish-flesh" appearance of this tumor.

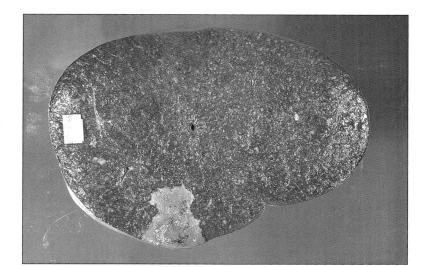

Fig. 21-11. Hodgkin lymphoma: cross section of a spleen removed at laparotomy shows a single large Hodgkin deposit adjacent to the capsule. Numerous scattered focal grayish-yellow areas up to 4 mm in diameter are also present.

HISTOLOGY

Hodgkin lymphoma is characterized by the presence of Reed-Sternberg cells, which are multinucleated cells, typically with prominent nucleoli and abundant violaceous cytoplasm (as seen in routine H & E stains; Figs. 21-12 to 21-14). The diagnosis of Hodgkin lymphoma is made when Reed-Sternberg cells are found against a background of lymphocytes, histiocytes, neutrophils, and eosinophils (Figs. 21-13 and

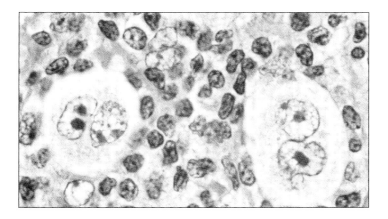

Fig. 21-12. Hodgkin lymphoma: high-power view of lymph node biopsy showing two typical multinucleate Reed-Sternberg cells surrounded by lymphocytes.

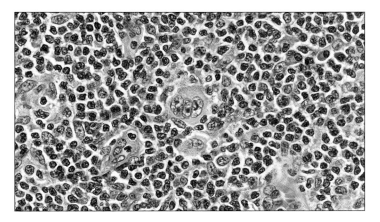

Fig. 21-13. Hodgkin lymphoma: lymph node biopsy showing multinucleate Reed-Sternberg cells surrounded by lymphocytes, histiocytes, neutrophils, and eosinophils.

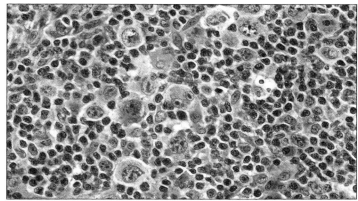

Fig. 21-14. Hodgkin lymphoma: lymph node biopsy showing multiple Reed-Sternberg cells surrounded by lymphocytes and other mononuclear cells in mixed cellularity disease.

21-14), which distinguishes the disease from other conditions (occasional viral infections, drug reactions, non-Hodgkin lymphomas) in which cells with cytologic features resembling Reed-Sternberg cells may be found.

THE HODGKIN REED-STERNBERG CELL

The Reed-Sternberg cells of classic Hodgkin lymphoma have a unique phenotype, usually being positive for both CD15 and CD30 (Fig. 21-15). They do not show phenotypes found in normal lymphocytes. Molecular studies relying on single-cell micromanipulation and amplification of ribonucleic acid (RNA) and genomic deoxyribonucleic acid (DNA) by polymerase chain reaction (PCR) have established a B-cell origin for Reed-Sternberg cells in most cases. Recurrent mutations involving genes of the I kappa B family are usually present. Most patients with the nodular sclerosis subtype of Reed-Sternberg cells have clonal rearrangement of the V, D, and J segments of the immunoglobulin heavy chain locus similar to mature B cells of germinal center or postgerminal center origin. However, in most cases the neoplastic Reed-Sternberg cells lose the phenotypic features of normal germinal center cells such as BCL-6 and only a minority show CD20. Somatic hypermutation usually results in a crippled cell with nonfunctioning immunoglobulin (Ig) variable regions and failure to transcribe RNA for immunoglobulin. The absence of immunoglobulin gene expression may result from impaired activation of the immunoglobulin promotors and enhancers due to lack of expression of B-cell transcription factors (e.g., Oct2, BOB.1).

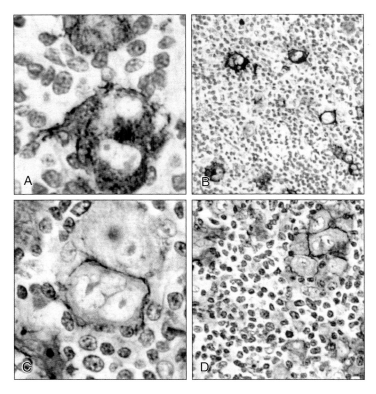

Fig. 21-15. Hodgkin lymphoma: abnormal mononuclear Hodgkin cells and binucleate Reed-Sternberg cells are positively labeled for **(A, B)** CD 15 and **(C, D)** CD30. (*A–D,* Immunoperoxidase stain.)

TABLE 21-1. HODGKIN LYMPHOMA: WORLD HEALTH ORGANIZATION HISTOLOGIC CLASSIFICATION

Type	Features
Nodular lymphocyte predominance Hodgkin lymphoma	Lymphocyte proliferation of irregular nodules that contain abnormal polymorphic B cells (LP or popcorn cells) Reed–Sternberg cells are absent
Classical Hodgkin lymphoma Nodular sclerosis	Tumor nodules surrounded by collagen bands extending from nodal capsule
Grades I and II (see text)	Characteristic 'lacunar cell' variant of Reed–Sternberg cell often seen
Mixed cellularity	Numerous Reed–Sternberg cells seen No sclerosis or fibrosis Intermediate numbers of lymphocytes
Lymphocyte rich	Scanty Reed–Sternberg cells; multiple small lymphocytes with few eosinophils and plasma cells; nodular and diffuse types
Lymphocyte depleted	'Reticular' pattern with predominant Reed–Sternberg cells and sparse lymphocytes or 'diffuse fibrosis' with disordered connective tissue, few lymphocytes, and infrequent Reed–Sternberg cells This subtype is very rarely diagnosed currently

It appears likely that activation of the nuclear factor kappa-B transcription factor signaling pathway may be a reason for the growth and survival of the Reed-Sternberg cells of classic Hodgkin lymphoma. Epstein-Barr virus (EBV) present in the majority of cases of mixed cellularity and lymphocyte depletion subtypes may contribute to nuclear factor kappa-B activation. The antiapoptotic action of nuclear factor kappa-B may help prevent these crippled cells from being negatively selected for apoptosis.

The presence of EBV in Sternberg-Reed cells varies from 75% in the mixed cellularity subtype to as low as 10% to 40% in nodular sclerosis Hodgkin lymphoma. In human immunodeficiency virus (HIV)–infected patients and those living in developing countries, positivity for EBV approaches 100%.

In Hodgkin lymphoma there are variable but nonspecific cytogenetic abnormalities. Aneuploidy and hypertetraploidy reflect the multinuclearity of the Reed-Sternberg cells. Many cases show 14q abnormalities, and fluorescent in situ hybridization (FISH) analysis has shown abnormalities in chromosome number in most cases. Intraclonal variability reflects chromosome instability.

CLASSIFICATION OF HODGKIN LYMPHOMA

The World Health Organization (WHO) histologic classification of Hodgkin lymphoma is shown in Table 21-1.

NODULAR SCLEROSING HODGKIN LYMPHOMA

In nodular sclerosing Hodgkin lymphoma, normal lymph nodal architecture is replaced by a nodular proliferation of tumor surrounded by birefringent collagen. This subtype accounts for about 70% of all cases of classic disease. The median age of presentation is 28 years, and the incidence is equal in males and females. Mediastinal involvement is present in 80% of cases and in over 50% there are large tumors. Most patients present with stage II disease, and B symptoms are present in approximately 40%.

Lymph node histology reveals classic Hodgkin lymphoma with a nodular growth pattern. Broad collagen bands surround the tumor (Fig. 21-16), and there is usually a fibrous thickening of the nodal capsule. The nodules contain variable numbers of Reed-Sternberg cells, small lymphocytes, and other nonneoplastic inflammatory cells, including eosinophils and neutrophils. A further diagnostic feature is the presence of the lacunar cells, which are Reed-Sternberg cell variants with friable cytoplasmic processes that open up into a "lake-like" appearance when subjected to routine processing (Fig. 21-17).

When Reed-Sternberg cells are particularly numerous, cohesive, or pleomorphic (the criteria are subjective but about 25% of the node or cells should be affected), the condition is believed to carry a worse prognosis and is graded by the British National Lymphoma Investigation group and WHO as Grade II. All other nodular sclerosis cases are Grade I. This grading is controversial, and many oncologists fail to find it of any prognostic value.

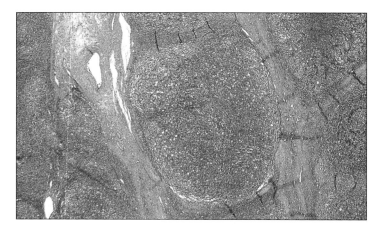

Fig. 21-16. Hodgkin lymphoma: lymph node biopsy showing abundant bands of collagenous connective tissue separating areas of abnormal Hodgkin tissue in the nodular sclerosis type.

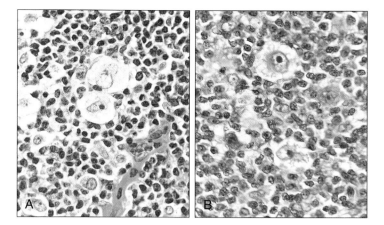

Fig. 21-17. Hodgkin lymphoma. **A, B,** High-power views of "lacunar" variants of Reed-Sternberg cells.

The Reed-Sternberg cells show the classic Hodgkin lymphoma phenotype with positivity for CD15 and CD30 (see Fig. 21-15). EBV encoded latent membrane protein (LMP 1) is less frequently positive (10% to 40%) than in other subtypes.

MIXED CELLULARITY HODGKIN LYMPHOMA

This subtype makes up 20% to 25% of classic Hodgkin lymphoma. There is a 70% male predominance, and an increased prevalence in HIV-infected patients and in developing countries. Mixed cellularity disease is often stage III or IV at presentation.

Histology of involved nodes show typical Reed-Sternberg cells in a diffuse or partly nodular mixed inflammatory background of lymphocytes, and variable numbers of eosinophils, neutrophils, histiocytes, and plasma cells (Fig. 21-18). Small granulomatous clusters of epithelioid histiocytes may be present.

The Reed-Sternberg cells show classic CD15 and CD30 phenotype. In 70% of patients the EBV encoded LMP 1 is positive (Fig. 21-19).

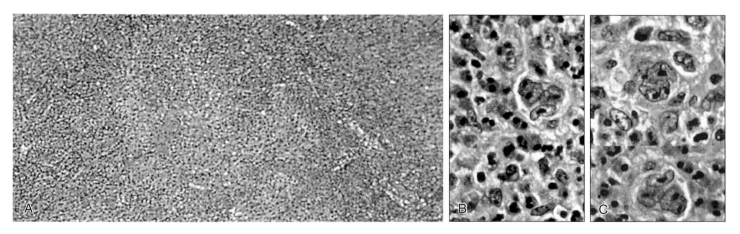

Fig. 21-18. Hodgkin lymphoma: mixed cellularity disease showing Reed-Sternberg cells surrounded by a mixed population of lymphocytes and eosinophils. **A,** Low power. **B, C,** Higher powers.

Fig. 21-19. Mixed cellularity Hodgkin lymphoma, **A,** In situ hybridization for EBV-encoded small nuclear RNAs (EBER1 and 2). Note the strong selective staining of the Hodgkin and Reed-Sternberg cells. **B,** Immunoalkaline phosphatase (APAAP) staining for the EBV-encoded latent membrane protein. Note the strong selective staining of the two Reed-Sternberg cells. (Courtesy of Professor H. Stein.)

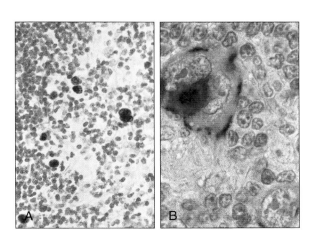

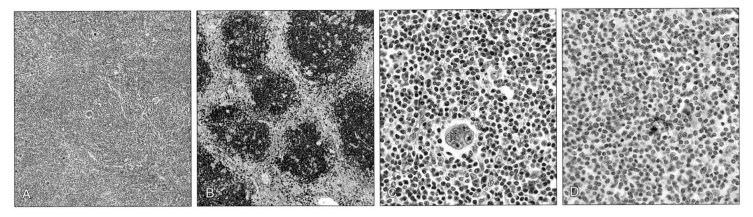

Fig. 21-20. Lymphocyte-rich classic Hodgkin lymphoma. **A,** Low-power view showing nodular growth pattern. **B,** Immunostain for CD20 shows that the nodules are composed of small B cells. **C, D,** Diffuse growth pattern—a high-power view **(C)** shows a single Reed-Sternberg cell in a sea of small lymphoid cells, and **(D)** immunostaining for CD30 highlights Hodgkin and Reed-Sternberg cells.

LYMPHOCYTE-RICH CLASSIC HODGKIN LYMPHOMA

The term *lymphocyte-rich classic Hodgkin lymphoma* is applied to morphologic variants characterized by an abundance of small lymphocytes with relatively scanty Reed-Sternberg cells and very few eosinophils and plasma cells. This variant makes up only 5% of all cases of Hodgkin lymphoma, peripheral lymph nodes are usually involved, and most patients have stage I or II disease without B symptoms. In the commoner nodular variant there is expansion of tumor in the mantle zones and attenuation of surrounding T-zones (Fig. 21-20, *A–C*). The sparsely distributed Reed-Sternberg cells show positivity for CD30 (Fig. 21-20, *D*) and CD 15 similar to that found in other subtypes of classic Hodgkin lymphoma. In the rarer diffuse variant there is no evidence of involvement of germinal centers, and isolated Reed-Sternberg cells may be surrounded by lymphocytes and histiocytes. The prognosis with modern therapy is better than that in other forms of classic Hodgkin lymphoma, and survival is similar to that of nodular lymphocyte-predominant Hodgkin lymphoma.

LYMPHOCYTE-DEPLETED HODGKIN LYMPHOMA

In lymphocyte-depleted Hodgkin lymphoma, Reed-Sternberg cells are present as sheets or clusters within a fibrous stroma containing small numbers of lymphocytes with no surrounding inflammatory cells (Fig. 21-21). In a fibrotic variant the fibrous stroma is dominant with only small numbers of Reed-Sternberg cells (see Fig. 21-29). These lymphocyte-depleted Hodgkin lymphomas are rarely diagnosed in current clinical practice and make up less than 5% of all Hodgkin lymphomas. Most lymphoma pathology groups that have reviewed their cases of this subtype and have applied immunostaining criteria have reclassified them as large B-cell lymphomas or anaplastic

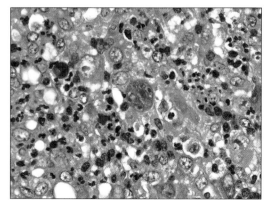

Fig. 21-21. Hodgkin lymphoma: lymphocyte depleted. Frequent Reed-Sternberg cells are present with a paucity of inflammatory cells.

large cell lymphoma. Lymphocyte-depleted Hodgkin lymphoma usually occurs in those over 50 years of age, with a high frequency of advanced disease, abdominal and bone marrow involvement, and B-category symptoms. It is often now associated with HIV infection, and there is a low complete remission rate and poor survival.

The Reed-Sternberg cells show a similar immunophenotype to other forms of classic Hodgkin lymphoma. The majority of HIV-positive patients are EBV infected, and immunostains for LMP1 are positive.

NODULAR LYMPHOCYTE-PREDOMINANT HODGKIN LYMPHOMA

Nodular lymphocyte-predominant Hodgkin lymphoma (NLPHL) is a distinct entity from classic Hodgkin lymphoma. It has always been recognized as quite separate from other types of Hodgkin lymphoma in view of its good prognosis with or without treatment and its unique histology (especially the lack of Reed-Sternberg cells). It usually manifests in older patients as stage I disease.

The lymph node histology shows replacement of normal architecture by a nodular or nodular and diffuse population of small lymphocytes, epithelioid histiocytes, and intermingling foci of atypical large neoplastic cells known as lymphocyte predominant cells (LP cells). These cells usually have a single nucleolus and scanty cytoplasm (Fig. 21-22, *A* and *C*). The nuclei of the largest cells are often polylobated to such an extent as to be called "popcorn" cells. The nucleoli of these giant cells are often multiple but smaller than those of classic Hodgkin lymphoma (Figs. 21-22, *C,* 21-31, and 21-32).

Unlike the Reed-Sternberg cell of classic Hodgkin lymphoma, the neoplastic cells of NLPHL show immunopositivity for the B-cell associated antigens CD19, CD20, CD22, CD79a (see Figs. 21-22, *B* and *D,* and 21-33, *A* and *B*); J chain and CD45 are demonstrated in most cases and EMA (Fig. 21-23, *A*) in over 50%. They also express the nuclear protein encoded by bcl-6 gene. Immunostaining shows expression of the transcription factor Oct2 (Fig. 21-23, *B*). The cells also express the Oct2 cofactor BOB.1 (Fig. 21-23, *C*) but are negative for both CD30 and CD15. Surrounding the neoplastic LP cells there is usually a corona of T cells, positive for CD3 (Fig. 21-22, *E*) and CD57.

Sensitive PCR techniques of isolated LP cells show rearranged and hypermutated immunoglobulin heavy chain genes (VH) and ongoing mutations. In most cases the rearrangements are functional and Ig mRNA transcripts are detectable. Nonspecific cytogenetic abnormalities in chromosome number similar to those found in classic Hodgkin lymphoma and other variable mutations are present in most cases studied.

The genetic, immunophenotypic, and cytologic features support a B-cell tumor arising from proliferating centroblasts of the germinal center.

Significant morphologic and phenotypic differences between Reed-Sternberg cells and the LP neoplastic cells of nodular lymphocyte predominant Hodgkin lymphoma are shown in Table 21-2.

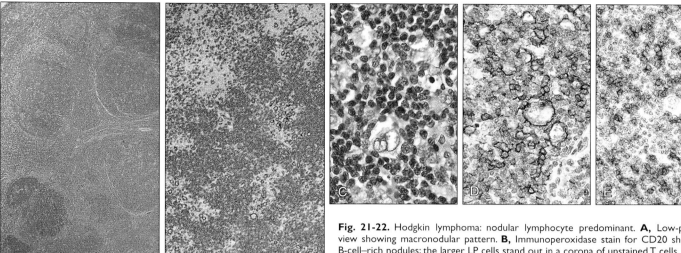

Fig. 21-22. Hodgkin lymphoma: nodular lymphocyte predominant. **A,** Low-power view showing macronodular pattern. **B,** Immunoperoxidase stain for CD20 showing B-cell–rich nodules; the larger LP cells stand out in a corona of unstained T cells. **C,** LP cells show large lobulated nuclei. **D,** LP cells showing strong CD20 membrane in immunostaining. **E,** Immunoperoxidase stain for CD3 showing corona of T cells surrounding LP cells.

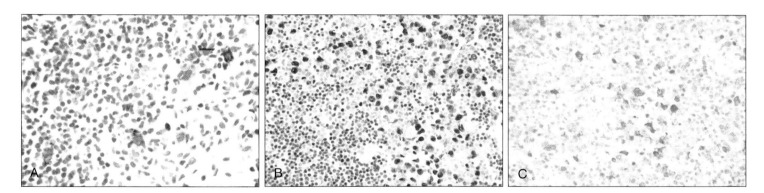

Fig. 21-23. Nodular lymphocyte-predominant Hodgkin lymphoma: immunostaining showing popcorn cell positivity for epithelial membrane antigen **(A).** There is also strong positive staining in popcorn cells for Oct2 **(B)** and BOB.1 **(C)** with weaker staining of the bystander B lymphocytes. (Courtesy of Dr. Graeme Taylor.)

TABLE 21-2.   HODGKIN LYMPHOMA: COMPARISON OF CLASSIC REED-STERNBERG CELLS WITH TYPICAL NEOPLASTIC CELLS OF THE NODULAR LYMPHOCYTE-PREDOMINANT SUBTYPE

	Classical HL	Nodular LPHL
Neoplastic cells	Reed–Sternberg (RS) cells, mononuclear and lacunar cells	LP cells with vesicular polylobated nuclei – popcorn cells
Associated cells	Lymphocytes, histiocytes, plasma cells, eosinophils	Lymphocytes and histiocytes
Sclerosis	Common	Rare
CD30, CD15	+	−
CD20	−/+	+
CD45, EMA, Oct2, BOB.1	−	+
J chain	−	+
Ig	Negative or positive polytypic (κ and λ) from passive absorption of tissue fluid Ig	Negative or monotypic
EBV	RS cells positive in over 50%	Infrequently positive
Associated lymphocytes	Predominantly T cells	Predominantly B cells
Ig genes (single-cell PCR)	Rearranged, clonal crippled	Rearranged, clonal, hypermutated, ongoing mutations

TABLE 21-3. HODGKIN LYMPHOMA: ANN ARBOR STAGING, AND LATER COTSWOLD AMENDMENTS

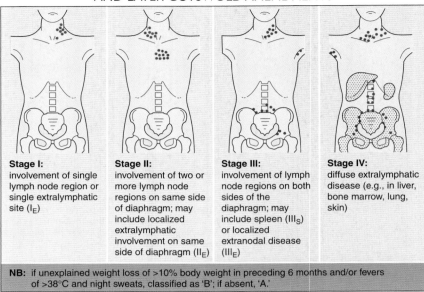

Stage I:	Stage II:	Stage III:	Stage IV:
involvement of single lymph node region or single extralymphatic site (I$_E$)	involvement of two or more lymph node regions on same side of diaphragm; may include localized extralymphatic involvement on same side of diaphragm (II$_E$)	involvement of lymph node regions on both sides of the diaphragm; may include spleen (III$_S$) or localized extranodal disease (III$_E$)	diffuse extralymphatic disease (e.g., in liver, bone marrow, lung, skin)

NB: if unexplained weight loss of >10% body weight in preceding 6 months and/or fevers of >38°C and night sweats, classified as 'B'; if absent, 'A.'

Modified from Hoffbrand AV, Pettit JE: *Essential haematology,* ed 3, Oxford, 1993, Blackwell Scientific.
Stage I: single lymph node region or lymphoid structure involvement (e.g., spleen, thymus, Waldeyer's ring). Stage II: two or more lymph node regions or lymphoid structures confined to one side of diaphragm. Stage III: lymph node regions or lymphoid structures above and below diaphragm (splenic involvement is included in this classification because it is often a prelude to widespread hematogenous spread). Stage IV: extranodal areas, including bone marrow and liver. The stage number is followed by either "A" (absence) or "B" (presence), referring to unexplained fever above 38°C (100.4°F), night sweats, and loss of more than 10% of body weight within 6 months. The subscript "E" indicates localized extranodal extension from a nodal mass; for example, IE describes mediastinal disease with contiguous spread to the lung or spinal theca. In the Cotswold classification Stage III is divided into Stage III1, "Involvement of splenic, celiac or portal nodes" and Stage III2, "Involvement of para-aortic, iliac or mesenteric nodes." The definition of bulk is nodal mass >10 cm diameter and mediastinal mass greater than one-third maximum diameter of chest.

STAGING TECHNIQUES

The prognosis and selection of the optimum treatment depends on accurate staging of the disease (Table 21-3). After thorough clinical examination, a number of laboratory and radiologic procedures are employed in the initial assessment (Table 21-4). Many patients have a normochromic normocytic anemia with a leukocytosis and/or eosinophilia, and bone marrow aspirates and trephine biopsies may provide diagnostic material (Figs. 21-24 to 21-33).

Mediastinal, hilar node, or lung involvement may be detected by chest radiography (Figs. 21-34 and 21-35), liver involvement by percutaneous biopsy, and para-aortic or pelvic lymph node involvement by abdominal radiography (Fig. 21-36). Computed tomography (CT) scanning (Fig. 21-37) and magnetic resonance imaging (MRI) are used in the search for thoracic, abdominal, and pelvic lymph node and organ involvement. Positron emission tomography (PET) scans also detect areas of involvement. They are particularly sensitive at detecting small areas of tumor and are able to distinguish active areas of disease from scar tissue following therapy (Figs. 21-38 to 21-41).

Previously used staging techniques such as lymphangiography (Figs. 21-42 and 21-43), other contrast x-ray methods (Figs. 21-44 and 21-45), gallium tomography (Fig. 21-46), and laparotomy with abdominal node and liver biopsy and splenectomy are very rarely employed today.

Text continues on page 393

TABLE 21-4. HODGKIN LYMPHOMA: LABORATORY AND RADIOLOGIC TECHNIQUES FOR STAGING PATIENTS

Laboratory	Full blood count Erythrocyte sedimentation rate Bone marrow aspirate and trephine biopsy Liver function LDH C-reactive protein
Radiology	Chest radiograph Computed tomography (thorax, abdomen, pelvis, neck)
Special tests	Magnetic resonance imaging Bone scan Positron-emission tomography

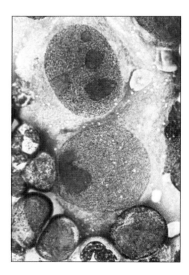

Fig. 21-24. Hodgkin lymphoma: high-power view of bone marrow aspirate, showing a Reed-Sternberg cell.

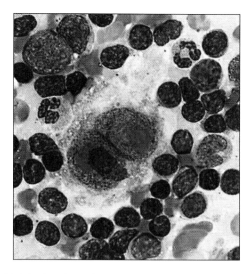

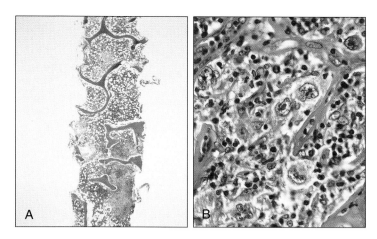

Fig. 21-25. Hodgkin lymphoma: bone marrow aspirate squash preparation showing a typical binucleate Reed-Sternberg cell surrounded by lymphoid cells, neutrophils, and monocytes. (Courtesy of Dr. Wendy Erber.)

Fig. 21-27. Hodgkin lymphoma: bone marrow trephine biopsy. **A,** Low-power view showing focal involvement. **B,** High-power view showing mononuclear Hodgkin cells.

Fig. 21-26. Hodgkin lymphoma: trephine biopsy **(A, B)** showing Hodgkin tissue replacing normal hematopoietic elements; **(C, D)** higher power showing fibrosis and Reed-Sternberg cells, which show immunopositivity for CD30 **(E).**

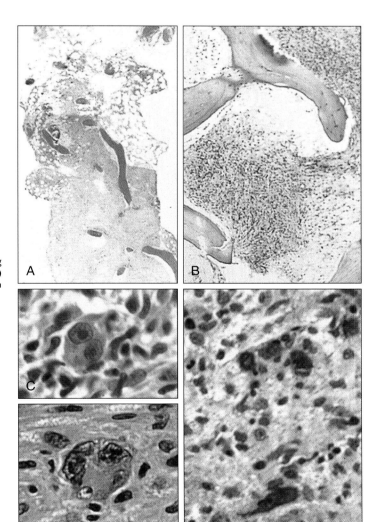

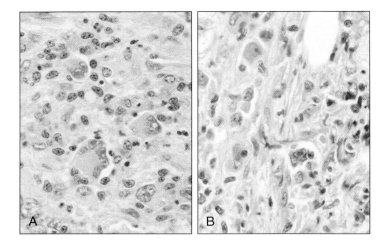

Fig. 21-28. Hodgkin lymphoma: bone marrow trephine biopsy in two patients **(A)** and **(B)** showing Reed-Sternberg and mononuclear Hodgkin cells with scattered lymphocytes and eosinophils and neutrophils in **(a).** (Courtesy of Dr. Wendy Erber.)

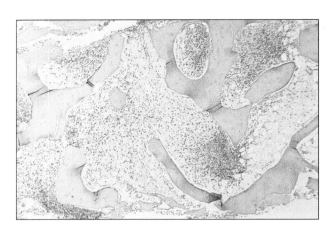

Fig. 21-29. Hodgkin lymphoma: trephine biopsy in the fibrotic variant of lymphocyte-depleted disease, showing almost complete replacement of hematopoietic tissue by Hodgkin deposits, along with abundant fibrous tissue in the intertrabecular space.

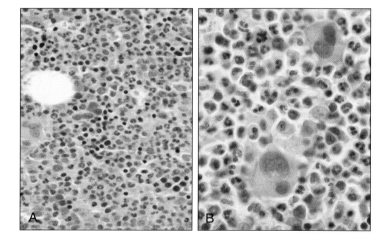

Fig. 21-30. Hodgkin lymphoma: Bone marrow trephine biopsy showing reactive hyperplasia of granulopoiesis with prominent neutrophils and eosinophils **(A).** No Reed-Sternberg cells were seen. At higher magnification **(B)** the large polylobated cells are megakaryocytes. (Courtesy of Dr. Wendy Erber.)

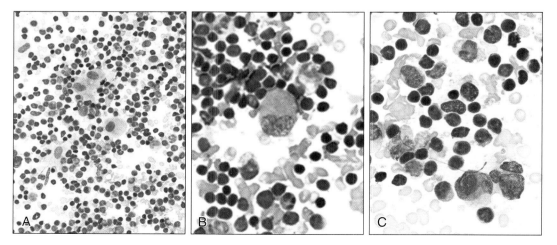

Fig. 21-31. Nodular lymphocyte predominant Hodgkin lymphoma: bone marrow aspirate showing LP cells surrounded by large numbers of lymphocytes **(A).** At higher magnification **(B** and **C)**, the characteristic vesicular polylobated nuclei of the larger LP or popcorn cells are evident. (Courtesy of Dr. Wendy Erber.)

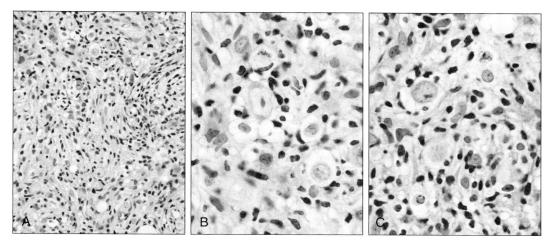

Fig. 21-32. Nodular lymphocyte-predominant Hodgkin lymphoma: bone marrow trephine biopsy showing LP cells and lymphocytes supported by a delicate fibrous stroma **(A).** At higher magnification (**B** and **C**), the large vesicular nuclei and relatively small nucleoli of the LP cells are evident. (Courtesy of Dr. Wendy Erber.)

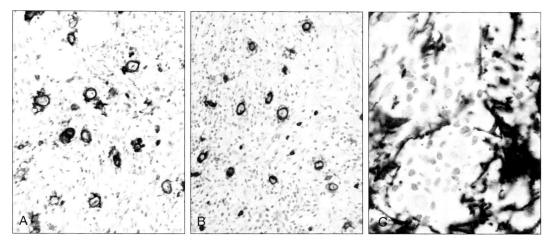

Fig. 21-33. Nodular lymphocyte-predominant Hodgkin lymphoma: bone marrow trephine biopsy. Immunostaining for CD20 **(A)** and CD 79a **(B)** shows strong positivity in the LP cells. With immunostaining for CD10 **(C)** the LP cells are negative but the supporting stroma is positive. (Courtesy of Dr. Wendy Erber.)

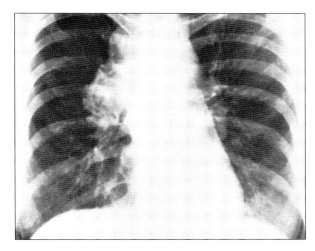

Fig. 21-34. Hodgkin lymphoma: chest radiograph showing prominent right paratracheal and hilar lymph node enlargement. The enlargement of the anterior mediastinal, subcarinal, and left hilar nodes is less marked and the proximal regions of both major bronchi are significantly narrowed. Contrast material in the apical lymph node on the left is from previous lymphangiography.

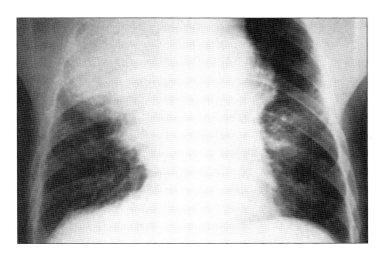

Fig. 21-35. Hodgkin lymphoma: chest radiograph showing widespread enlargement of hilar and mediastinal lymph nodes with associated collapse of the right upper lobe and infiltration or possibly pneumonic changes in the midzone of the left lung.

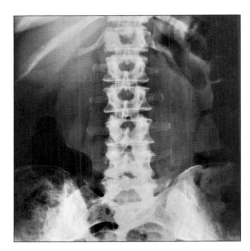

Fig. 21-36. Hodgkin lymphoma: plain abdominal radiograph showing bilateral massive para-aortic lymph node enlargement. (Courtesy of Dr. D. Nag.)

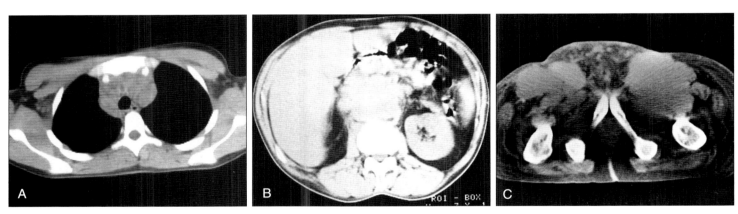

Fig. 21-37. Hodgkin lymphoma: CT scans of **(A)** chest showing paratracheal and anterior mediastinal lymph node enlargement; **(B)** abdomen showing massive para-aortic lymph node enlargement displacing the pancreas forward; **(C)** pelvis showing massive bilateral inguinal and pelvic lymphadenopathy with marked edema of the lower abdominal wall (same patient as Fig. 21-4).

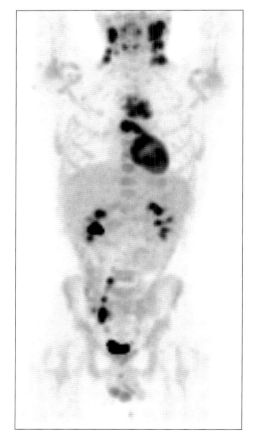

Fig. 21-38. Hodgkin lymphoma: fluorodeoxyglucose (FDG) PET maximum projection intensity (MIP) image of a 14-year-old boy with recurrent Hodgkin lymphoma indicating relapse of nodal disease in the neck, mediastinum, and right pelvis. (Courtesy of Dr. Garry Cook.)

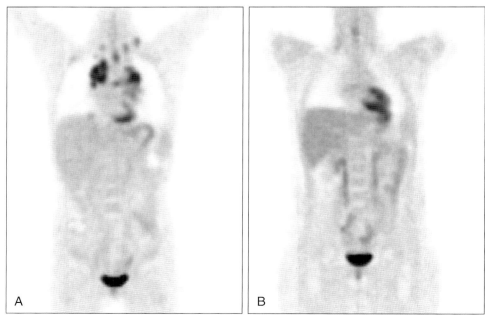

Fig. 21-39. Hodgkin lymphoma: FDG PET MIP image showing Hodgkin's disease before chemotherapy **(A)** and after 2 cycles of chemotherapy **(B)** showing a complete response and chemosensitivity. (Courtesy of Dr. Garry Cook.)

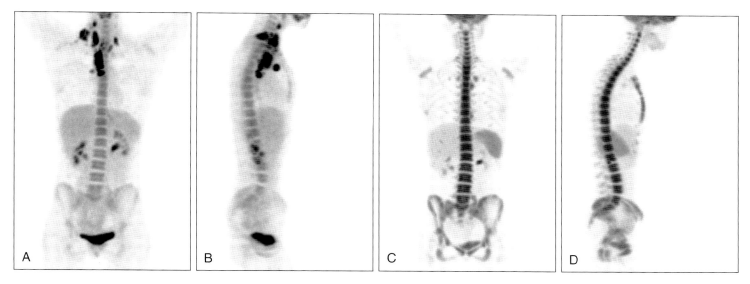

Fig. 21-40. Hodgkin lymphoma: FDG PET MIP coronal **(A)** and sagittal **(B)** images showing extensive cervical and mediastinal nodal involvement. Following chemotherapy, corresponding images **(C)** and **(D)** show no residual disease. Uptake in the skeleton reflects regeneration or rebound of bone marrow after chemotherapy. (Courtesy of Dr. Hamish Fraser.)

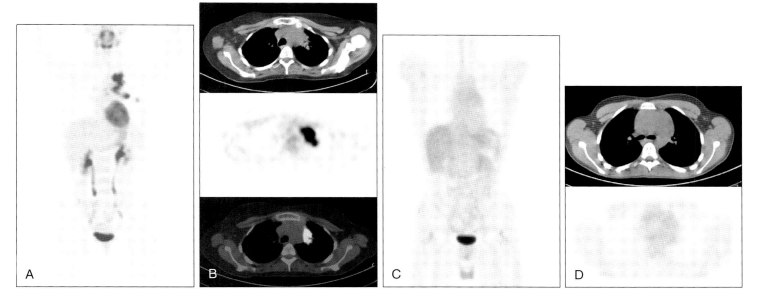

Fig. 21-41. Hodgkin lymphoma. **A,** FDG PET MIP image. **B,** CT, FDG PET, and fused axial slices through the mediastinum following chemotherapy showing persistent abnormal uptake in an anterior mediastinal mass indicating residual disease activity. Following more chemotherapy, FDG PET MIP image **(C)** and CT and FDG PET components of the PET/CT acquisition **(D)** show no abnormal uptake in an anterior mediastinal mass indicating scar tissue and no residual active Hodgkin lymphoma. (Courtesy of Dr. Garry Cook.)

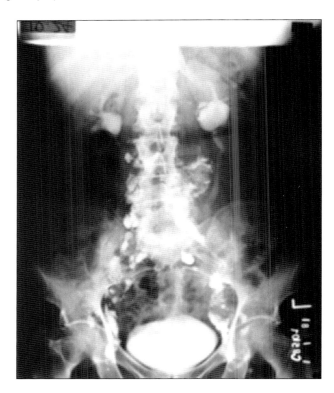

Fig. 21-42. Hodgkin lymphoma: lymphangiogram with intravenous pyelogram shows enlarged para-aortic lymph nodes (particularly on the left and lower left pelvis) with displacement of the ureter.

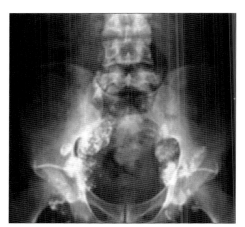

Fig. 21-43. Hodgkin lymphoma: lymphangiogram showing bilateral external iliac and lower para-aortic lymph node enlargement and filling defects.

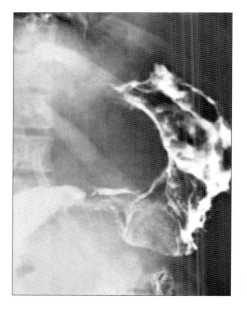

Fig. 21-44. Hodgkin lymphoma: barium meal demonstrating extensive mucosal and gastric wall involvement of the body and pylorus of the stomach. (Courtesy of Dr. D. Nag.)

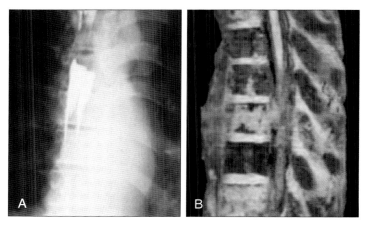

Fig. 21-45. Hodgkin lymphoma. **A,** Cisternogram showing partial block of contrast at the T4 level and a complete block at the lower part of T6. **B,** Sagittal section postmortem shows extradural extension of tumor from the body of T4 (uppermost) and more extensive cordal involvement at T7 and T9. There is patchy involvement of other vertebral bodies and spinous processes. Extensive paravertebral tumor is seen anteriorly below the T5 level.

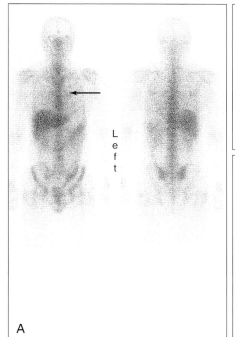

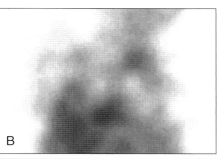

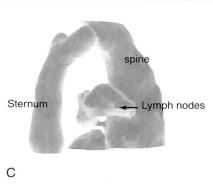

Fig. 21-46. Non-Hodgkin lymphoma: stage IIb. Postchemotherapy with residual mediastinal mass see on CT scan. **A,** Whole body scan 48 hours after injection of gallium-67 citrate, with subtle increased uptake in the mediastinum (arrow). **B,** Tomographic image shows uptake in mediastinum. **C,** Surface rendered tomographic image confirms presence of active disease in hilar lymph nodes. (Courtesy of Dr. A. J. W. Hilson.)

PROGNOSTIC FACTORS

Based on the analysis of large numbers of patients, a number of prognostic indices have been published for patients with Hodgkin lymphoma. For patients with localized disease, the European Organization for Research and Treatment of Cancer (EORTC) Index based on factors shown in Table 21-5 has been useful. For patients with advanced disease the International Prognostic Score or Hansclever index is widely used. In this latter index seven factors (Table 21-6) were identified, each of which was associated with an 8% reduction in the predicted 5-year disease-free progression rate.

TABLE 21-5.   HODGKIN LYMPHOMA: EUROPEAN ORGANIZATION FOR RESEARCH AND TREATMENT OF CANCER (EORTC) RISK FACTORS FOR LOCALIZED HODGKIN LYMPHOMA

Favorable
Patients must have all of the following features
Clinical stage I and II
Maximum of three nodal areas involved
Age <50 years
ESR <50 mm/h without B symptoms or ESR <30 mm/h with B symptoms
Mediastinal/thoracic ratio <0.35
Unfavorable
Patients have any of the following features
Clinical stage II with involvement of at least four nodal areas
Age >50 years
ESR >50 mm/h if asymptomatic or ESR >30 mm/h if B symptoms
Mediastinal/thoracic ratio >0.35

TABLE 21-6.   HODGKIN LYMPHOMA: INTERNATIONAL PROGNOSTIC INDEX (HANSCLEVER INDEX) FOR ADVANCED HODGKIN LYMPHOMA

Age >45 years
Male gender
Serum albumin <40 g/dl
Hemoglobin level <10.5 g/dl
Stage IV disease
Leucocytosis (white cell count $\geq$15 x 10^9/L)
Lymphopenia (<0.6 x 10^9/L or <8% of the white cell count)

The presence of each of the seven factors is associated with a reduction of five-year freedom from progression by about 8%. From Hasenclever D, Diehl V: *N Engl J Med* 339:1506-1514, 1998.

MYELOMA AND RELATED CONDITIONS

CHAPTER

22

PLASMA CELL MYELOMA

Table 22-1, *A*, classifies the plasma cell neoplasms. Plasma cell (multiple) myeloma is characterized by proliferation in the bone marrow of a clonal population of malignant plasma cells. There, cells produce cytokines that are responsible for bone loss and nearly always for monoclonal proteins that appear in plasma and often in urine. There are major interactions between the plasma cells and the marrow microenvironment (Fig. 22-1). Table 22-1, *B*, lists the criteria for

diagnosis of plasma cell myeloma, dominantly the triad of plasma cell infiltration of the bone marrow, presence of a paraprotein in serum and/or Bence-Jones protein in urine, and lytic bone lesions. The malignant neoplastic proliferation of plasma cells is in the bone marrow, usually making up over 30% of the marrow cell total in aspirates at presentation. In advanced disease the abnormal cell population may exceed half the total cell number (Fig. 22-2). The morphology of these cells is often abnormal, with more primitive features and a greater variation in size than found in classic plasma cells (Figs. 22-3 to 22-5).

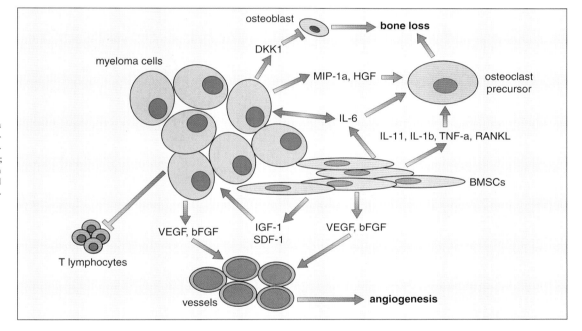

Fig. 22-1. Pathophysiology of plasma cell myeloma. DKKI, dickkop-1 protein; MIP.I, macrophage inhibitor factor; IGF-I, insulin-like growth factor; VEGF, vascular endothelial growth factor; BMSC, bone marrow stromal cell; RANK, receptor activator of nuclear factor-kappa B ligand.

TABLE 22-1.   PLASMA CELL NEOPLASMS
(WHO, 2008)

Monoclonal gammopathy of undetermined significance (MGUS)

Plasma cell myeloma
    Variants:
        Asymptomatic (smoldering) myeloma
        Nonsecretory myeloma
        Plasma cell leukemia

Plasmacytoma
    Solitary plasmacytoma of bone
    Extraosseous (extramedullary) plasmacytoma

Immunoglobulin deposition diseases
    Primary amyloidosis
    Systemic light and heavy chain deposition diseases

Osteosclerotic myeloma (POEMS syndrome)

Symptomatic plasma cell myeloma

M-protein in serum or urine[*]
Bone marrow clonal plasma cells or plasmacytoma[#]
Related organ or tissue impairment[^] (**CRAB**: hyper**c**alcemia, **r**enal insufficiency, **a**nemia, **b**one lesions)

Asymptomatic (smoldering) myeloma

M-protein in serum at myeloma levels (>30 g/L)
AND/OR
10% or more clonal plasma cells in bone marrow
No related organ or tissue impairment [end organ damage or bone lesions (CRAB: hypercalcemia, renal insufficiency, anemia, bone lesions)] or myeloma-related symptoms

[*]No level of serum or urine M-protein is included. M-protein in most cases is >30 g/L of IgG or >25 g/L of IgA or >1 g/24 hr of urine light chain but some patients with symptomatic myeloma have levels lower than these.

[#]Monoclonal plasma cells usually exceed 10% of nucleated cells in the marrow but no minimal level is designated because about 5% of patients with symptomatic myeloma have <10% marrow plasma cells.

[^]The most important criteria for symptomatic myeloma are manifestations of end organ damage including anemia, hypercalcemia, lytic bone lesions, renal insufficiency, hyperviscosity, amyloidosis or recurrent infections.

395

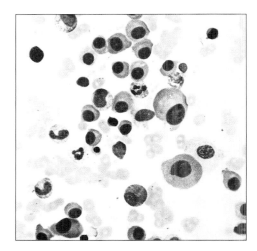

Fig. 22-2. Multiple myeloma: marrow cell trail. The majority of cells seen are atypical plasma cells.

Fig. 22-3. Multiple myeloma: abnormal plasma cells in marrow in two cases. **A,** Myeloma cells, one binucleate, with nucleoli, and one with a mitotic figure. **B,** The nuclei in a binucleate cell vary greatly in size. **C,** Abnormal cytoplasmic and nuclear vacuolation.

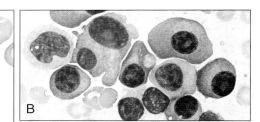

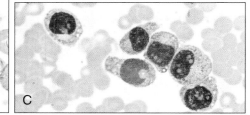

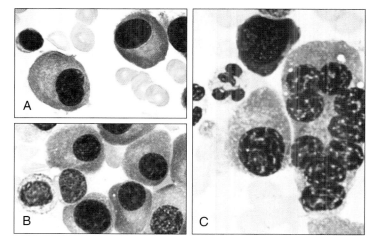

Fig. 22-4. Multiple myeloma: **(A–C)** abnormal plasma cells in bone marrow. Considerable variation occurs in nuclear size and cytoplasmic volume, and one of the myeloma cells is multinucleate **(C).**

Fig. 22-5. Multiple myeloma: "flaming" plasma cells in marrow with IgA M-protein in serum. There are numerous thesaurocytes, large plasma cells with small, sometimes pyknotic, nuclei, and expanded fibrillary cytoplasm, which also shows "flaming" of the cell rim (inset). Although "flaming" occurs most frequently with IgA production, it may also be seen with M-proteins of other classes.

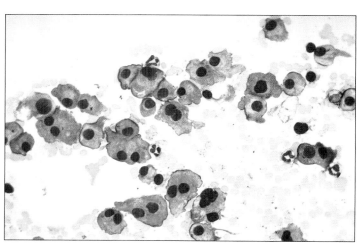

By flow cytometry the cells can be shown to express CD138 and light chain restriction, in this case kappa (Fig. 22-6). Multinucleate cells may be frequent. Flaming plasma cells are most frequent when the plasma cells secrete immunoglobulin A (IgA) (see Fig. 22-5). As a result of abnormal immunoglobulin deposits, inclusion bodies may occur in the cytoplasm (Figs. 22-7 and 22-8). Trephine biopsy shows a uniform infiltration by plasma cells and plasmablasts (Figs. 22-9 and 22-10), which stain positive for CD38 or CD138 (Fig. 22-11) but negative for CD19 or CD20. The cells express either kappa or lambda light chains (Fig. 22-12).

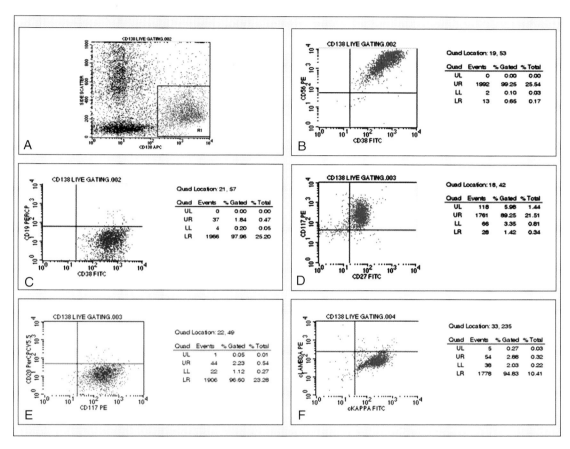

Fig. 22-6. Multiple myeloma. Flow cytometry shows a population of CD138, kappa light chain positive cells.

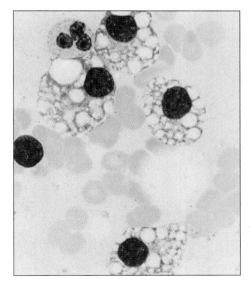

Fig. 22-7. Multiple myeloma: bone marrow aspirate showing abnormal plasma cells with many large cytoplasmic vacuoles ("Mott cells" or morular cells). Each vacuole is an accumulation of immunoglobulin. (Courtesy of Dr. M. Saary.)

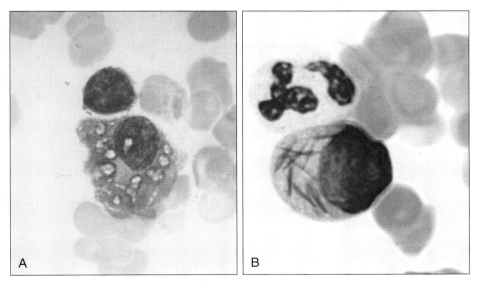

Fig. 22-8. Multiple myeloma: **A,** plasma cell showing crystalline pink inclusions of abnormal immunoglobulin. **B,** Plasma cell showing slender rod-like cytoplasmic inclusions. (A, Courtesy of Dr. R. Britt.)

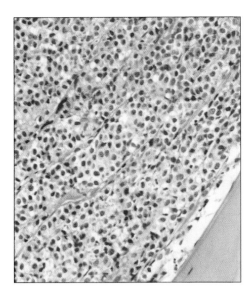

Fig. 22-9. Multiple myeloma: trephine biopsy shows almost complete replacement of hematopoietic tissue by sheets of abnormal plasma cells.

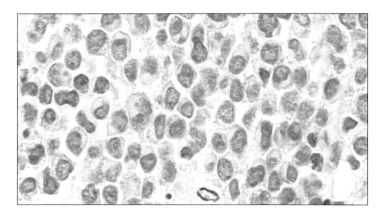

Fig. 22-10. Multiple myeloma/plasma cell leukemia: trephine biopsy showing almost complete replacement of hematopoietic cells by plasma cells and plasmablasts. (Courtesy of Dr. D. M. Swirsky.)

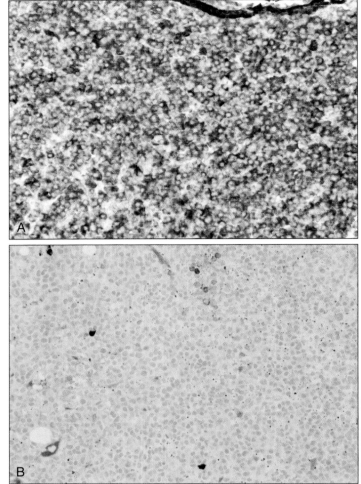

Fig. 22-12. Multiple myeloma: **(A)** immunostaining positive for kappa light chains, **(B)** immunostaining negative for lambda light chains.

The majority of patients produce a monoclonal protein (M-protein or paraprotein), which may be demonstrated in the serum and/or urine. Typically, the serum protein is increased and electrophoresis shows an abnormal paraprotein in the globulin region (Fig. 22-13).

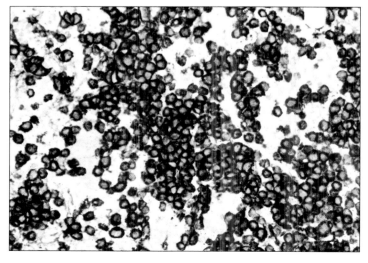

Fig. 22-11. Multiple myeloma: immunostaining that shows the malignant plasma cells are CD138 positive.

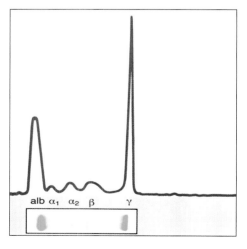

Fig. 22-13. Multiple myeloma: serum protein electrophoresis showing an M-protein in the g-globulin region and reduced levels of background β- and α-globulins. This "spike" and deficiency pattern is typical of patients with myeloma. (Total protein, 99 g/L; IgG M-protein component, 41 g/L.)

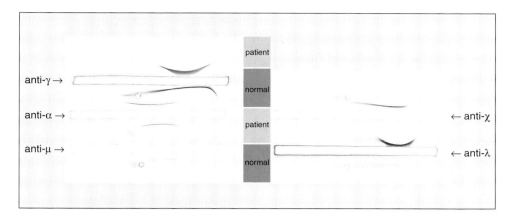

Fig. 22-14. Multiple myeloma: immunoelectrophoresis. Normal protein is recognized by characteristic arc patterns. In the reactions against anti-g and anti-l, the IgG-l M-protein maintains its electrophoretic position, but appears as a "bow" or thickened arc with a smaller than usual radius. Reduced levels of IgA and IgM are reflected in small or absent arcs in the reactions with anti-α and anti-μ.

Immunodiffusion or immunoturbidometry reveal which immunoglobulin fraction is increased, and the levels of the uninvolved classes of immunoglobulin are usually depressed. Immunoelectrophoretic techniques confirm the presence of an abnormal immunoglobulin and are able to establish the monoclonal nature of this protein (Fig. 22-14). In most cases whether or not a paraprotein is present, there is an excess in serum of kappa or lambda light chains (Fig. 22-15). In nonsecretory myeloma (3% of cases) there is absence of an M-protein but in up to two thirds there is elevation of a free light chain or abnormal free light chain ratio. Cytoplasmic Ig is present in the plasma cells in 85% of cases. There is a lower incidence of renal failure, hypercalcemia, and immune paresis.

In patients with complete monoclonal immunoglobulin in the serum, the synthesis of heavy and light chains in the neoplastic plasma cells is often imbalanced, with an excess production of light chains (see Fig. 22-15). The urine contains Bence-Jones protein in two thirds of cases; this consists of free light chains, either kappa or lambda, of the same type as the serum M-protein and the serum light chain in excess. Occasionally, patients have two or more M-proteins, and in less than 1% of patients no M-proteins are found in the serum or urine.

The advanced stage of this disease involves a normochromic normocytic anemia, often with an associated neutropenia and thrombocytopenia, reflecting the development of bone marrow failure. The increased globulin in the serum is frequently associated with an increased erythrocyte sedimentation rate, and the blood may show marked red cell rouleaux formation and increased background staining (Fig. 22-16). In some cases a leukoerythroblastic blood picture is

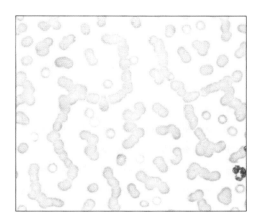

Fig. 22-16. Multiple myeloma: peripheral blood film shows marked rouleaux formation of red cells and increased background staining.

seen. Abnormal plasma cells appear in the blood film in about 15% of patients (Fig. 22-17). Sensitive gene rearrangement studies, however, reveal typical cells of the malignant clone in the peripheral blood in a higher proportion of patients.

Cytogenetic abormalities, detected by conventional cytogenetics or fluorescent in situ hybridization (FISH), are present in the marrow cells in 80% to 90% of cases. There are most frequently monosomy

Fig. 22-15. Multiple myleoma. There is usually an excess of either kappa or lambda light chains in the serum. Dotted lines indicate sensitivity of these tests. IFE, immunofixation electrophoresis; II, intact immunoglobulin; LC, light chain; MM, multiple myeloma; NS, nonsecretory; P, polyclonal; SPE, serum protein electrophoresis. (Courtesy of Professor A. R. Bradwell.)

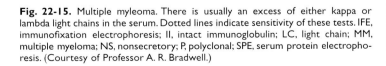
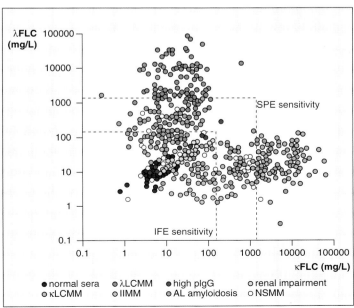

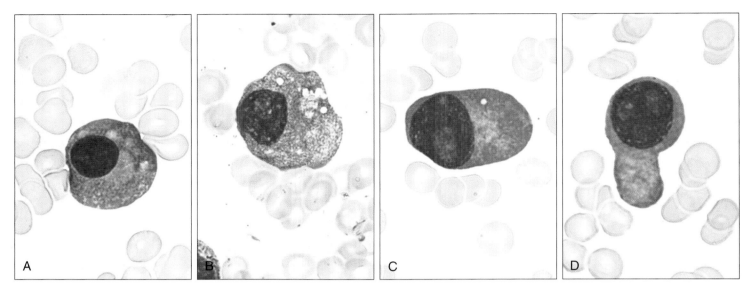

Fig. 22-17. Multiple myeloma: **(A–D)** isolated myeloma cells in peripheral blood films from two patients.

13, translocations into the switch regions of the IgH gene, and monosomy or trisomy of various other chromosomes (Table 22-2). Later changes involve RAS, MYC, or their oncogenes. There is usually overexpression of cyclin D1, D2, or D3 (Fig. 22-18). Gene expression studies can be used to assess prognosis (Fig. 22-19).

TABLE 22-2.   MULTIPLE MYELOMA: CYTOGENETICS.
THE ABNORMALITIES OFTEN LEAD
TO OVEREXPRESSION OF ONE CYCLIN

13q14 deletions; monoallelic monosomy 13 more frequent; interstitial deletions or translocations less frequent		
IgH translocations 14q32		
partner genes	**genes**	**cyclin involved/ over expressed**
11q13	CCNDI	D1
4p16	FGR3/MNSET MMSET	D2
16q23	MAF	D2
20q11	MAFB	D2
6p21	CCND3	D3
Monosomy, trisomy various chromosomes		
Later events		

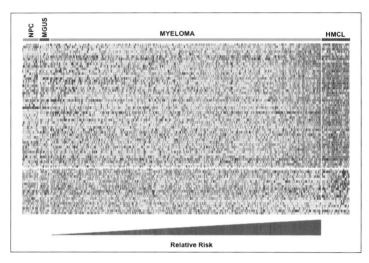

Fig. 22-19. Multiple myeloma: gene expression clustergram of 70 high-risk genes in plasma cells, of 22 healthy subjects (NPC), 14 with MGUS, 351 patients with newly diagnosed myeloma and 42 human myeloma cell lines. Red indicates above the median and blue below the median. (Adapted from Shaughnessy JD et al: *Blood* 109:2276-2284, 2007, Fig 2, p 2279.)

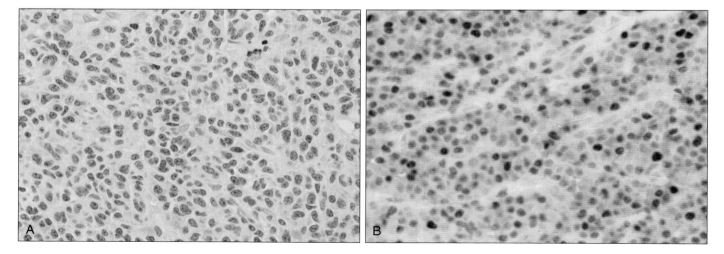

Fig. 22-18. Multiple myeloma: **(A)** the cells usually expressing cyclin D1 show a characteristic morphologic appearance of immature myeloma cells with eccentrically located nuclei and prominent central nucleoli. **(B)** in immunostaining positive for cyclin D1.

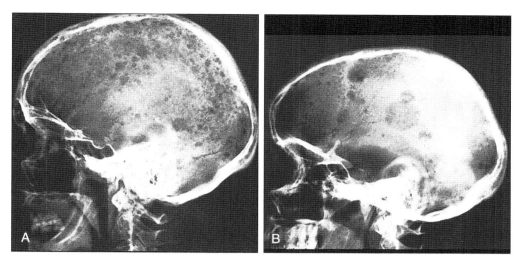

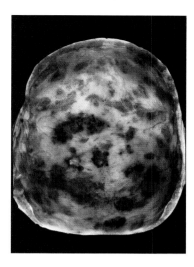

Fig. 22-20. Multiple myeloma: radiographs of skulls showing **(A)** typical multiple, small, "punched-out" osteolytic lesions; **(B)** a case in which the lesions vary much more in size.

Fig. 22-21. Multiple myeloma: inside of the skull shows characteristic "moth-eaten" osteolytic lesions.

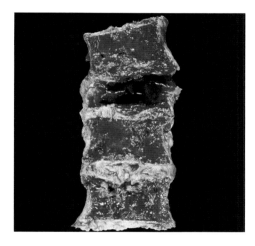

Fig. 22-22. Multiple myeloma: longitudinal section of lumbar spine shows a generalized replacement of normal medullary bone by vascular myeloma tissue. The body of L2 has collapsed and appears hemorrhagic.

Skeletal radiology shows osteolytic lesions in 60% of patients, and associated pain is characteristic. The lesions include the classic "punched-out" lesions of the skull (Figs. 22-20 and 22-21), lytic lesions and generalized bone rarefaction of the spine, ribs, and pelvis, and pathologic fractures (Figs. 22-22 to 22-25). Extensive bone resorption (Fig. 22-26), thought to be caused by excessive production of osteoclast activating factor (OAF), probably a combination of tumor necrosis factor and interleukin-1, results in elevation of serum calcium in half of the patients. In occasional patients, myeloma deposits may extend beyond the skeleton into surrounding soft tissues (Figs. 22-27 and 22-28). Magnetic resonance imaging (MRI) may be valuable in assessing sites of tumor invasion (Fig. 22-29). Rarely, osteosclerosis may occur. Osteosclerotic myeloma shows fibrosis and sclerosis of bone trabeculae (see Table 22-1, *A*). POEMS syndrome consists of polyneuropathy, osteosclerotic myeloma, and systems involvement (e.g., endocrinopathy, skin pigmentation, clubbing and arthropathy, hepatosplenomegaly, and lymphadenopathy; Figs. 22-30 and 22-31).

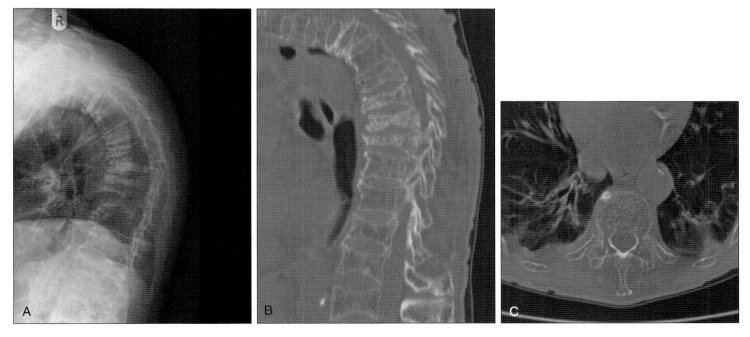

Fig. 22-23. Multiple myeloma. **A,** X-ray: thoracic vertebrae showing collapse, diffuse demineralization, and mottled appearance. **B,** CT scan: this shows wedge shaped, collapsed vertebrae in upper and mid-thoracic regions leading to hyper kyphosis. **C,** CT scan: cross-section of a thoracic vertebra showing demineralization of vertebra and ribs.

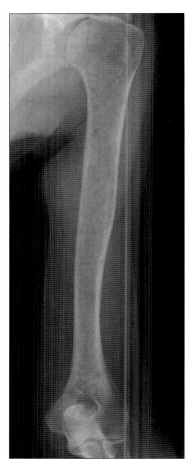

Fig. 22-24. Multiple myeloma: humerus showing punched out lesions and expanded mid-shaft.

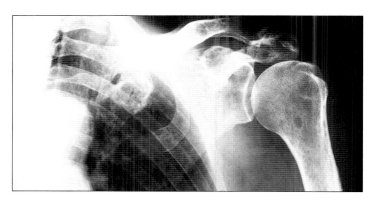

Fig. 22-25. Multiple myeloma: radiograph of left shoulder region shows a pathologic fracture of the acromial process of the scapula and osteolytic lesions in the humerus, clavicle, and ribs.

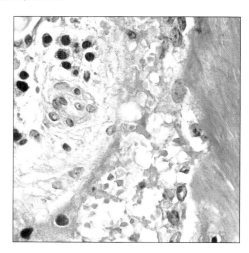

Fig. 22-26. Multiple myeloma: bone biopsy. Although plasma cells are seen in the upper left, osteoclasts (the multinucleate cells at the bone intertrabecular tissue interface) are the cells responsible for the bone absorption around the osteolytic lesion.

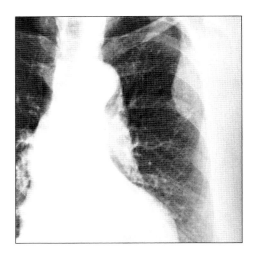

Fig. 22-27. Multiple myeloma: chest radiograph showing a prominent extrapleural soft tissue mass adjacent to the third left rib.

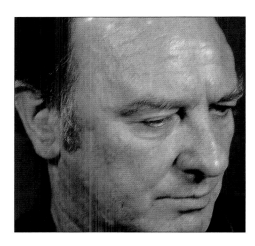

Fig. 22-28. Multiple myeloma: skull deposits have invaded the soft tissues and appear as lumps on the forehead. In this case, a proportion of marrow cells were positive for the surface antigen CD10 but negative for TdT. Such cells have been associated with aggressive disease.

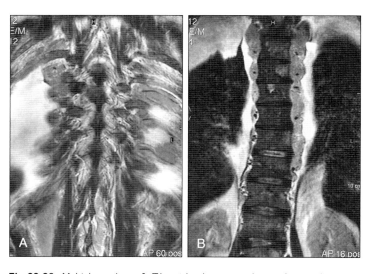

Fig. 22-29. Multiple myeloma. **A,** T1-weighted parasagittal image from a 60-year-old man. All bones are abnormal (patchy, heterogeneous signal). There is an extensive extradural tumor in the spinal canal behind the spinal cord, compressing it from D3 to D8, with absence of cerebrospinal fluid. Incidental hemangioma at D4 stains as a bright signal. **B,** T2-weighted coronal image of the thoracic spine in a 60-year-old man. The heterogeneous signal from the marrow is compatible with myeloma deposits with extraosseus soft tissue paraspinal masses of myeloma. (A, B, Courtesy of Dr. A. D. Platts.)

Renal complications have an important influence on the course of multiple myeloma. Patients with persistent renal failure and blood urea in excess of 14 mmol/l have a poor prognosis. Damage from heavy Bence-Jones proteinuria (Fig. 22-32), amyloid disease (Fig. 22-33), nephrocalcinosis (Fig. 22-34), and pyelonephritis (Fig. 22-35) may be important in the pathogenesis. A more generalized amyloid disease occurs in a small number of patients, and there may be macroglossia with tongue ulceration (Figs. 22-36 to 22-38), carpal tunnel syndrome (Fig. 22-39), skin deposits (Figs. 22-40 and 22-41), and cardiac involvement resulting in cardiomegaly and congestive heart failure (Fig. 22-42).

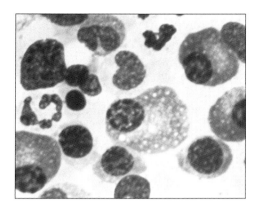

Fig. 22-30. Multiple myeloma: POEMS syndrome. The patient, a 39-year-old man, had lower limb weakness. Nerve conduction studies showed evidence of a peripheral neuropathy with demyelination. Endocrine screening was negative. Bone marrow shows excess plasma cells; serum IgG was raised (29.3 g/L) with Bence-Jones proteinuria. (Courtesy of Dr. R. Liang.)

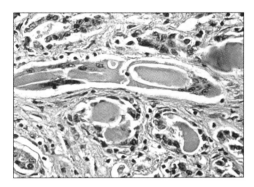

Fig. 22-32. Multiple myeloma: section of kidney showing acidophilic casts of myeloma protein blocking the renal tubules. There is surrounding giant cell reaction and interstitial fibrosis.

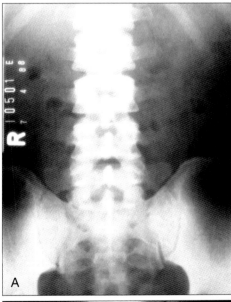

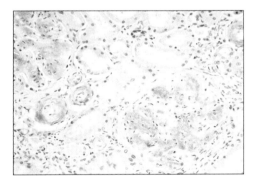

Fig. 22-33. Multiple myeloma: renal amyloid disease. Amyloid deposition in the glomeruli and associated arterioles is extensive. Congo red stain.

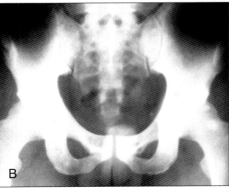

Fig. 22-31. Multiple myeloma: POEMS syndrome (same case as shown in Fig. 22-30). Radiographs of **(A)** lumbar spine, and **(B)** pelvis showing sclerosis and lytic areas with sclerotic rims. (A, B, Courtesy of Dr. R. Liang.)

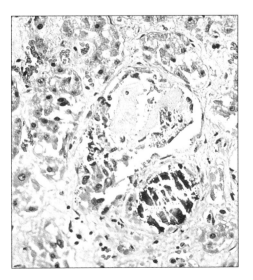

Fig. 22-34. Multiple myeloma: nephrocalcinosis. Irregular fractured hematoxylinophilic deposits of calcium are seen in the fibrotic renal tissue.

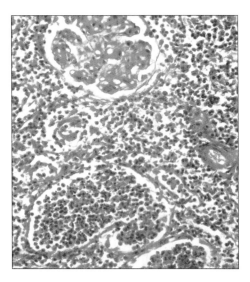

Fig. 22-35. Multiple myeloma: destruction of the renal parenchyma and acute inflammatory cellular infiltration of the interstitial tissues and tubular spaces in pyelonephritis.

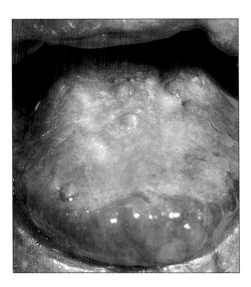

Fig. 22-38. Multiple myeloma: gross macroglossia. These nodular deposits of amyloid contrast with the diffuse enlargement in Fig. 22-36. Similar nodules are also evident in the lips.

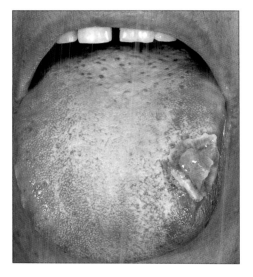

Fig. 22-36. Multiple myeloma: in amyloid disease, the tongue shows macroglossia and a deep ulcer on the upper and lateral anterior surfaces. The floor of the ulcer has the waxy appearance typical of amyloid deposition.

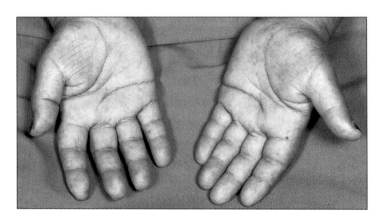

Fig. 22-39. Multiple myeloma: carpal tunnel syndrome caused by deposition of amyloid in the flexor retinaculum and resulting in compression of the median nerve. The thenar muscles are wasting. The patient complained of paresthesias and weakness of both hands.

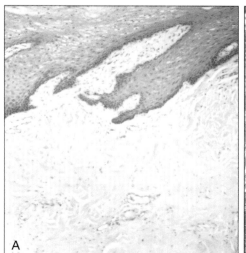
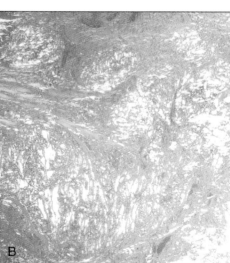

Fig. 22-37. Multiple myeloma. **A,** Biopsy of the ulcer seen in Fig. 22-36 shows extensive deposition of pale-staining acidophilic material. **B,** Stained with Congo red, this material shows the characteristic green birefringence of amyloid, when viewed with polarized light.

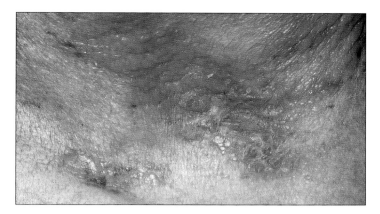

Fig. 22-40. Multiple myeloma: amyloid disease of the skin. There are plaque-like hyaline infiltrations of the skin folds in the supraclavicular area.

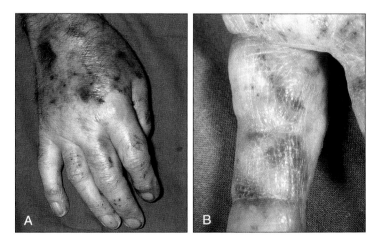

Fig. 22-41. Multiple myeloma. **A,** Amyloid disease on the back of the hand. Extensive diffuse and nodular deposits in the skin, subcutaneous tissues, and tendon sheaths have resulted in irregular swelling over the metacarpal heads; the skin surface appears hard, tense, and waxy. **B,** Extensive purpura, a characteristic feature, probably results from involvement of small cutaneous blood vessels.

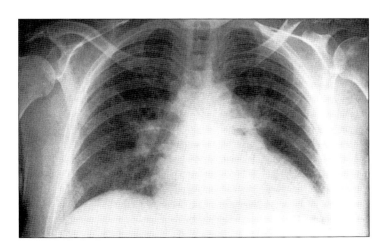

Fig. 22-42. Multiple myeloma: amyloid disease of the heart. This radiograph shows cardiomegaly and pulmonary congestion. Evidence of myeloma includes osteolytic lesions in the right humerus and ribs, as well as pathologic fractures of the left clavicle and the eighth right rib.

PLASMA CELL LEUKEMIA

At presentation, patients may have large numbers of circulating plasma cells, or this blood picture may arise during the course of the disease (Figs. 22-43 to 22-46). There are greater than $2 \times 10^9/L$ plasma cells in the peripheral blood and sometimes greater than $100 \times 10^9/L$. The circulating cells may have features of lymphoplasmacytic cells, typical plasma cells, or plasma blasts. The immunophenotyping is similar to myeloma. The prognosis is poor.

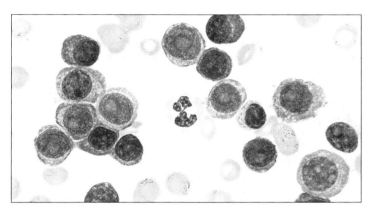

Fig. 22-43. Plasma cell leukemia: peripheral blood film showing large numbers of plasma cells and/or plasmablasts. (WBC, $100 \times 10^9/L$.) (Courtesy of Dr. D. M. Swirsky.)

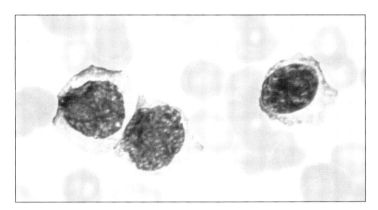

Fig. 22-44. Plasma cell leukemia: peripheral blood film showing lymphocytoid plasma cells. The patient, a 44-year-old man, had been treated 1 year earlier for myeloma with six courses of intensive therapy (vincristine, doxorubicin [adriamycin], and methylprednisolone [VAMP]). He relapsed with widespread lytic lesions and many circulating plasma cells. (Hb, 6.3 g/dl; WBC, $22.1 \times 10^9/L$; plasma cells, $18. \times 3\ 10^9/L$; platelets, $64 \times 10^9/L$.)

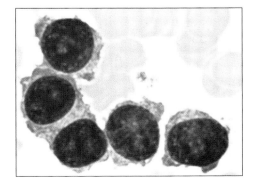

Fig. 22-45. Plasma cell leukemia: bone marrow of same case as shown in Fig. 22-44.

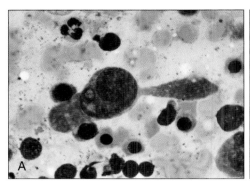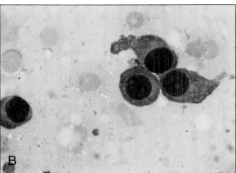

Fig. 22-46. Multiple myeloma with plasma cell leukemia: **(A, B)** bone marrow showing cells with motility-associated features (pseudopods and long extensions). (Reproduced with permission from Berneman ZN, Chen ZZ, Peetermans ME: Morphological evidence for a motile behavior by plasma cells, *Leukemia* 4:53-59, 1990.)

PROGNOSIS

A number of staging (Table 22-3) and prognostic systems (Table 22-4) have been used. 13q loss implies a poor prognosis, and gene expression can also be used to predict outcome. *Smoldering myeloma* has been defined to include a serum paraprotein at myeloma levels, 10% or more plasma cells in the bone marrow, but no end-organ damage (hypercalcemia, renal failure, anemia, bone lesions, or recurrent bacterial infections) (see Table 22-1).

TABLE 22-3. MULTIPLE MYELOMA: STAGING SYSTEM DURIE-SALMON

I All of the following

Hemoglobin > 10.5 g/dl
Serum calcium normal
X-rays show normal structure or solitary bone plasmocytoma only
Low paraprotein levels
    IgG < 50 g/L
    IgA < 30 g/L
Urinary light chain < 4 g per 24 h

II Fitting neither stage I nor stage III
III One or more of the following

Hemoglobin < 8.5 g/dl
Serum calcium > 3 mmol/L
Advanced lytic bone lesion (> 3 lytic lesions)
High paraprotein levels
    IgG > 70 g/L
    IgA > 50 g/L
Urinary light chain > 12 g per 24 h

Subclassification
A Serum creatinine < 170 µmol/L B Serum creatinine ≥ 170 µmol/L

TABLE 22-4. MULTIPLE MYELOMA: INTERNATIONAL PROGNOSTIC INDEX

Staging	Parameters	Number of patients	Median survival (months)
Stage 1	β_2-m < 3.5 ALB ≥ 35	2401	62
Stage 2	β_2-m < 3.5 ALB < 35 or β_2-m 3.5–5.5	3278	44
Stage 3	β_2-m > 5.5	2770	29

TABLE 22-5. CAUSES OF THE HYPERVISCOSITY SYNDROME: M-PROTEINS ARE THE DOMINANT CAUSE, BUT OTHERS OF IMPORTANCE ARE POLYCYTHEMIA, LEUKOSTASIS, AND HYPERFIBRINOGENEMIA

Causes	Diseases
M-proteins	Waldenström's macroglobulinemia Multiple myeloma
Polycythemia	Polycythemia vera Severe secondary polycythemia
Leucostasis	Chronic myeloid leukemia Other leukemias with very high white cell counts
Hyperfibrinogenemia	Following factor VIII replacement therapy with large amounts of cryoprecipitate

TREATMENT

Urgent initial therapy may be required to deal with hypercalcemia, hyperviscosity (Table 22-5), or renal failure. There are a number of different approaches to chemotherapy of the underlying disease. In older patients, alkylating agents such as melphalan and prednisone with thalidomide are now the preferred treatment. In younger subjects, repeated courses of cyclophosphamide, dexamethasone, and thalidomide are often used initially although idarubicin and dexamethasone, vincristine, doxorubin, and methylprednisolone with cyclophosphamides are still used. Bortezomib is used in late-stage disease but is also used in combinations as initial therapy; high-dose melphalan, with autologous peripheral blood stem cell transplantation, prolongs remission in some patients. New agents include lenalidomide, newer proteosome inhibitors (e.g., carfilzomib), cyclin D1 inhibitors, and other drugs aimed at "intercepting" growth factors for myeloma cells. Therapy can be assessed by reduction of plasma cells in the bone marrow (Fig. 22-47), as well as by reduction in plasma protein and light chain

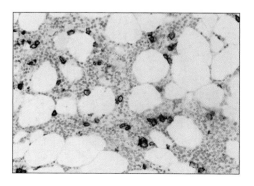

Fig. 22-47. Multiple myeloma: after therapy. Immunostaining for CD138 shows less than 10% plasma cells.

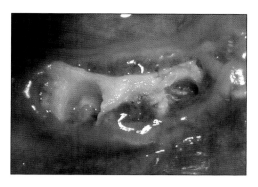

Fig. 22-48. Multiple myeloma: jaw necrosis in a patient treated with bisphosphonates. (Courtesy of Professor C. Mussolino.) (Nastro E, et al: Bisphosphonate-associated osteonecrosis of the jaw in patients with multiple myeloma and breast cancer. Acta Haematologica 117:181-187, 2007.)

levels. Biphosphonates may be of value in prolonging remission, and biphosphonates may also reduce bone damage. An unusual complication is necrosis of jaw bones (Fig. 22-48).

MONOCLONAL IMMUNOGLOBULIN DEPOSITION DISEASES (MIDDs)

MIDDs are characterized by visceral and soft tissue deposits of immunoglobulin resulting in compromised organ function. The immunoglobulin molecules accumulates in tissues before there is a large tumor burden. There are two main categories of MIDDs, primary amyloid (discussed later) and light chain deposition diseases (LCDDs), and more rarely light and heavy chain deposition diseases (LHCDDs) or heavy chain deposition diseases (HCDDs). LCDD (Randall disease), LHCDD, and HCDD occur with myeloma or MGUS and involve many organs, especially the kidneys, liver, heart, nerves, blood vessels, lungs, and joints with deposition of aberrant Ig on basement membranes, elastic and collagen fibers. Pale amorphous eosinophilic material is deposited in affected tissues, negative for Congo red but positive with fluorescent anti-light chain antibodies (e.g., on renal biopsy).

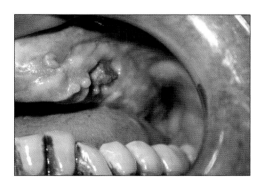

Fig. 22-49. Multiple myeloma: jaw necrosis in another patient treated with bisphosphonates.

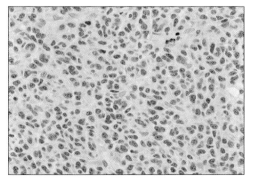

Fig. 22-50. Primary amyloid: the bone marrow shows less than 10% plasma cells.

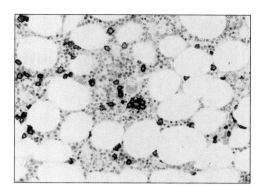

Fig. 22-51. Primary amyloid: immunostaining for CD138 confirms less than 10% plasma cells in the bone marrow.

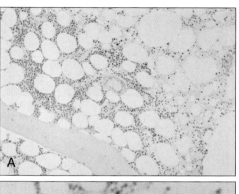

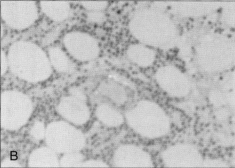

Fig. 22-52. Primary amyloid: **A** and **B,** Congo red staining and polarized light examination shows amyloid in the wall of a blood vessel.

PRIMARY AMYLOIDOSIS

Primary amyloidosis syndrome is dominated by clinical features caused by amyloid deposition in the tongue (Fig. 22-49), heart, tendon sheaths (Fig. 22-50), and skin. There may also be purpura, the nephrotic syndrome, peripheral neuropathy, orthostatic hypotension, and massive hepatomegaly. The disease can be assessed by serum amyloid P component scintigraphy (Fig. 27-55).[99] Tc-aprotinin scintigraphy is another sensitive test for detection of cardiac amyloid. There are usually less than 10% plasma cells in the bone marrow (Fig. 22-51), 6% of patients having 20% or more. The serum paraprotein is less than 30 g/L and present in 50% to 60% of patients. Patients with hereditary amyloidosis may also show a monoclonal paraprotein. Serum light chains are useful for diagnosis and essential for follow-up (see Fig. 22-15 and Fig. 27-55). Amyloid may be detected in the bone marrow by Congo red staining and polarized light microscopy (Fig. 22-52 and see page 494). Fine-needle abdominal fat aspiration may give sufficient material for Congo red staining (Fig. 22-53) and for protein studies to determine the exact type of amyloid. The prognosis depends largely on the degree of cardiac involvement.

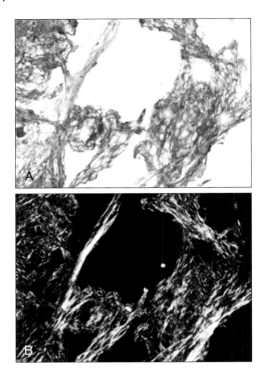

Fig. 22-53. Primary amyloid: diagnosis can be made by percutaneous abdominal wall fat biopsy. **A,** Congo red. **B,** polarized light. (Courtesy of Professor G. Merlini.)

OTHER PLASMA CELL TUMORS

Solitary and soft tissue plasmacytomas each make up half of the 6% of plasma cell tumors that are not multiple myeloma.

SOLITARY PLASMACYTOMA OF BONE

In solitary plasmacytoma of bone (Figs. 22-54 to 22-59), no plasma cell proliferation occurs in parts of the skeleton beyond the primary lesion; marrow aspirates distant from the primary tumor are usually normal. Associated M-proteins disappear following radiotherapy to the primary lesion.

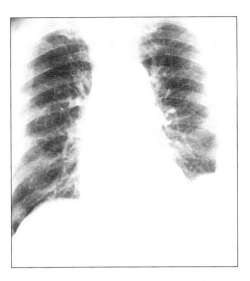

Fig. 22-55. Solitary plasmacytoma of bone: radiograph of the case in Fig. 22-54 shows a well-defined mass approximately 5 cm in diameter, in the lower left chest, pleural in position and arising from the ninth rib.

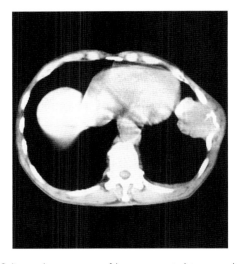

Fig. 22-56. Solitary plasmacytoma of bone: computed tomography scan of the case shown in Fig. 22-54, showing erosion of the rib, with soft tissue extension into both the pleural space and external soft tissues.

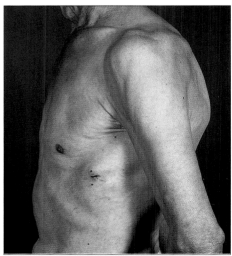

Fig. 22-54. Solitary plasmacytoma of bone: a firm ovoid mass, 9 cm in diameter, over the lower lateral aspect of the left chest wall. Protein studies, blood count, and bone marrow were normal. No other skeletal lesions were detected by a radiologic survey. (Courtesy of Dr. S. Knowles.)

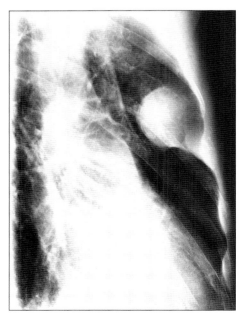

Fig. 22-57. Solitary plasmacytoma of bone: oblique radiograph of the left chest. There is expansion and destruction of the left fourth rib with an overlying soft tissue mass (the tumor).

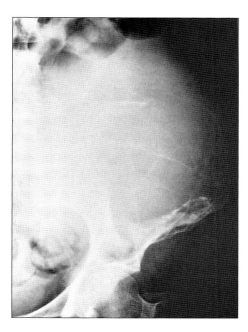

Fig. 22-58. Solitary plasmacytoma of bone: radiograph of left pelvic area shows massive destruction of the iliac bone and the tumor extending into the pelvis and abdomen. Linear residual streaks of bone produce the "soap bubble" appearance seen in this type of tumor.

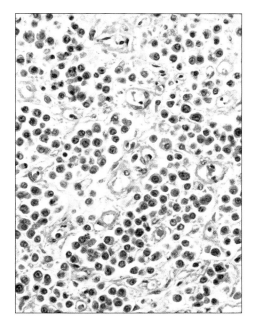

Fig. 22-59. Solitary plasmacytoma of bone: biopsy shows dense collections of plasma cells supported by a vascular stroma.

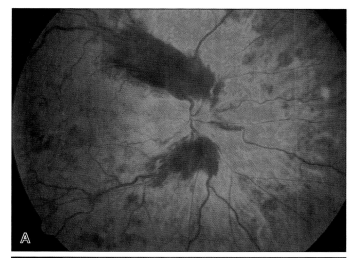

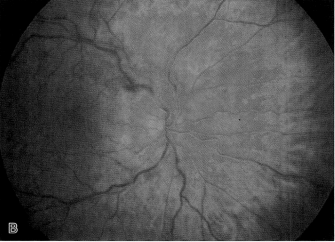

Fig. 22-60. Multiple myeloma: **(A)** distention of retinal veins and widespread hemorrhage in the hyperviscosity syndrome; **(B)** 2 months after plasmapheresis and chemotherapy the vessels are normal and almost all hemorrhage has cleared. The patient had some loss of vision and headache. (A, B, Courtesy of Professor J. C. Parr.)

in coma. The retina may show a variety of changes including engorged veins, hemorrhages, exudates, and a blurred optic disc (Fig. 22-60; see also Fig. 19-29).

The hyperviscosity syndrome may occur with multiple myeloma (see Fig. 22-60) when there is polymerization of the abnormal immunoglobulin; a similar syndrome is occasionally caused by increased levels of blood components other than M-proteins (Table 22-6). IgM M-protein increases blood viscosity more than equivalent concentrations of IgG or IgA.

EXTRAOSSEOUS (EXTRAMEDULLARY) PLASMACYTOMA

Soft tissue plasmacytomas are found most frequently in the submucosa of the upper respiratory and gastrointestinal tracts, in the cervical lymph nodes, and in the skin. They tend to remain localized and the majority are well controlled by excision or local irradiation.

HYPERVISCOSITY SYNDROME

Clinically, the hyperviscosity syndrome is characterized by loss of vision, symptoms involving the central nervous system, hemorrhagic diathesis, and heart failure; the most severely affected patients may be

TABLE 22-6. DIAGNOSTIC CRITERIA FOR MONOCLONAL GAMMOPATHY OF UNDETERMINED SIGNIFICANCE (MGUS) (WHO, 2008)

M-protein in serum <30 g/L
Bone marrow clonal plasma cells <10% and low level of plasma cell infiltration in a trephine biopsy
No lytic bone lesions
No myeloma-related organ or tissue impairment (CRAB: hypercalcemia, renial insufficiency, anemia, bone lesions)
No evidence of other B-cell proliferative disorder

Patients with acute hyperviscosity syndrome due to a paraproteinemia benefit from plasmapheresis. Cyclophosphamide and chlorambucil, plus corticosteroids, have been used to reduce the tumor mass. Fludarabine and 2-chlorodeoxadenosine and Rituximab are valuable newer agents. Thalidomide and bortezomib are also useful in some cases.

OTHER CAUSES OF SERUM M-PROTEINS

The appearance of an M-protein spike during serum electrophoresis is usually associated with more than 5 g/L of that protein. Uncontrolled proliferation of an M-protein–producing clone, as in multiple myeloma or Waldenström's disease, is distinguished by a progressive increase in the serum M-protein concentration. Production of M-protein is controlled or stable in benign monoclonal gammopathy and chronic cold agglutinin disease (cold autoimmune hemolytic anemia). Occasionally, production of M-protein is transient—for example, following recovery from infection or during a reaction to drug (Table 22-7).

MONOCLONAL GAMMOPATHY OF UNCERTAIN SIGNIFICANCE (MGUS)

Monoclonal gammopathy of uncertain significance is the most common cause of a serum M-protein. Its benign nature is distinguished by the fact that the level of M-protein in the serum is stable over many years. It is not associated with Bence-Jones proteinuria, bone lesions, or soft tissue plasma cell tumors. The bone marrow may have up to 10% plasma cells, but patients are generally asymptomatic, with no evidence of bone marrow failure (Table 22-6). When affected patients are followed, about 1% each year (30% in 25 years) develop myeloma or malignant lymphoma. Transformation is more likely in those with IgA or IgM compared to IgG paraproteins, those with greater than 5% plasma cells in the marrow, unbalanced serum light chains, and possibly in those with few (less than 3%) polyclonal plasma cells (CD38+, CD56−, CD19+) compared with malignant plasma cells (CD38+, CD56+, CD19−) in the marrow.

Although benign paraproteinemia is usually symptomless, clinical features that may be associated include peripheral neuropathy,

TABLE 22-7. M-PROTEINS: UNCONTROLLED PRODUCTION OF M-PROTEIN OCCURS WITH PLASMA CELL DYSCRASIAS, LYMPHOPROLIFERATIVE DISORDERS, AND PRIMARY AMYLOID

Malignant or uncontrolled production
Multiple myeloma
Plasma cell leukemia
Lymphoplasmacytic lymphoma/Waldenström's macroglobulinemia
Malignant lymphoma
Chronic lymphocytic leukemia
Primary amyloidosis
Heavy chain disease (λ, α, and μ)
Benign or stable production
Monoclonal gammopathy of uncertain significance
Chronic cold hemagglutinin disease
Transient M-proteins
Solitary plasmacytoma
Extramedullary plasmacytoma
Gaucher's disease
Acquired immunodeficiency syndrome (AIDS)
Occasional association with carcinoma, connective tissue and skin disorders, and many other conditions

The most common cause is benign monoclonal gammopathy with no apparent disease association. Benign controlled M-protein production has a number of causes, including human immunodeficiency virus and other infections, carcinoma, and other tumors; "benign" refers to the limited clone of M-protein–producing cells.

TABLE 22-8. BENIGN AND MALIGNANT PARAPROTEINEMIA: DISTINGUISHING FEATURES

	Benign	**Malignant**
Serum paraprotein	IgG <30 g/L IgA <20 g/L	IgG >30 g/L IgA >20 g/L and rising
Serum light chains	Balanced	Unbalanced*
Bence–Jones proteinuria	Absent	May be present (>1 g per 24 h of κ or λ chains)
Immuneparesis	Absent	Present
Bone marrow plasma cells	<10% without cytological abnormalities	>10% (myeloma)
Underlying lymphoproliferative disease or myeloma	Absent	Present

*Normal light chain ratios 0.26–1.65
Excess λ chains gives a ratio < 0.26,
excess κ chains > 1.65

acquired von Willebrand's syndrome, papular mucinosis, cold hemagglutinin disease (see Chapter 8), amyloid (see Chapter 27), and cryoglobulinemia. These syndromes may also occur, however, when the disease that causes the paraprotein is clearly malignant—for example, in lymphoma, myeloma, or macroglobulinemia (Table 22-7).

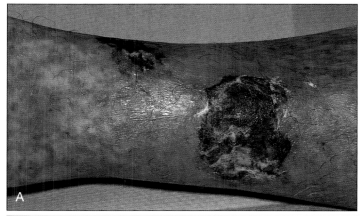

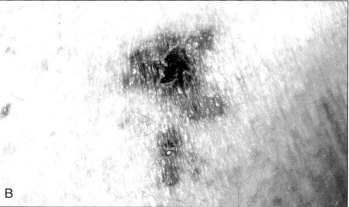

Fig. 22-61. Cryoglobulinemia. **A,** Discoloration of the leg with pigment deposition in a reticulated pattern because of vascular distention and hemorrhage. Areas of superficial necrosis and ulceration are seen. The patient showed a serum IgM paraprotein but no other evidence of myeloma or lymphoma. **B,** Ulceration and vascular distention in a 78-year-old man with chronic lymphocytic leukemia.

CRYOGLOBULINEMIA

Globulins that precipitate in the cold may occur in a primary disease (which may be monoclonal or oligoclonal; Figs. 22-61 and Fig. 22-62) or in association with abnormal globulin production in myeloma (Fig. 22-63), macroglobulinemia, or non-Hodgkin lymphoma.

HEAVY CHAIN DISEASES

In the heavy chain diseases (HCDs), a rare group of disorders, the neoplastic cells secrete immunoglobulin heavy chains (γ, α, or μ) without light chains attached to them. The secreted heavy chains in all types of HCD are usually incomplete.

Clinically, γ-HCD resembles a lymphoma. The disease is slightly more frequent in males, with a peak incidence in the seventh decade of life, with lymphadenopathy, hepatosplenomegaly, fever, and anemia as usual clinical features. Autoimmune diseases (e.g., rheumatoid arthritis and hemolytic anemia) occur in 25% of cases. They lymph nodes and marrow show a mixture of lymphocytes, immunoblasts, histiocytes, and plasma cells, often with eosinophilia, and the serum shows a monoclonal spike in the γ, α, or β region. The protein usually consists of two γ heavy chains linked together. The variable region and part of the first domain of the constant region are sometimes deleted.

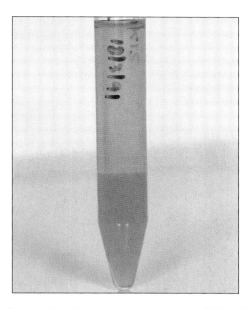

Fig. 22-62. Cryoglobulinemia: same case as shown in Fig. 22-61A. Serum from a patient with primary disorder, prepared from whole blood at 37° C, showing protein precipitation on cooling to room temperature. In this case the protein was monoclonal IgM.

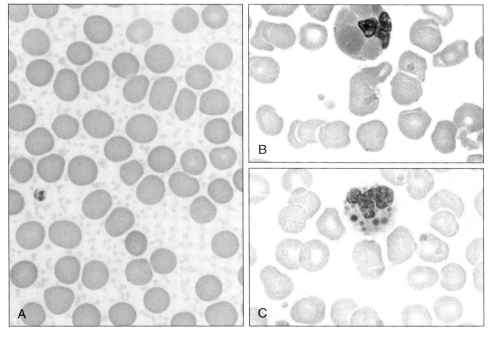

Fig. 22-63. Multiple myeloma: **(A)** cryoglobulin IgM protein—peripheral blood film showing pink staining aggregates of immunoglobulins between red cells; **(B, C)** neutrophils with multiple blue-staining inclusion bodies from ingested cryoglobulin. (B, C, From Bain BJ: *Blood cells: a practical guide,* London, 1989, Gower.)

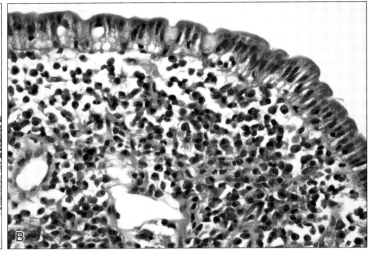

Fig. 22-64. Alpha-heavy chain disease: this 25-year-old Algerian man was treated in 1983 for a malabsorption syndrome, consisting of weight loss, chronic diarrhea, steatorrhea, and hypocalcemia, that responded to broad-spectrum antibiotics. **A,** At this stage, small intestinal biopsy showed a diffuse infiltration of the lamina propria. **B,** The cells were a mixture of lymphocytes, plasma cells, and plasmacytoid cells. Immunocytochemical staining showed that a vast majority of these cells contained α heavy chains without κ or γ light chains. Serum and urine samples revealed a broad band in the α2 globulin region, which precipitated with anti-IgA but showed no reactivity to anti-k or anti-γ. (A, B, Courtesy of Dr. J. E. McLaughlin.)

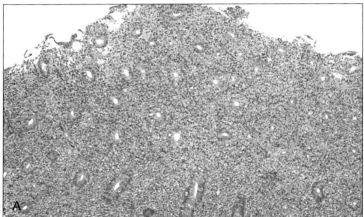
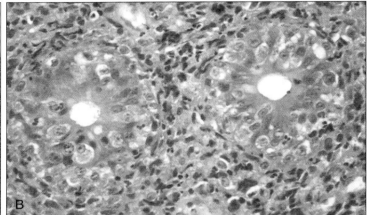

Fig. 22-65. Alpha-heavy chain disease (same case as shown in Fig. 22-64): 2 years after treatment the patient developed small intestinal obstruction; intestinal resection revealed the small bowel to be heavily infiltrated by a large cell "immunoblastic lymphoma" with an additional mixed infiltrate of neutrophils, plasma cells, and macrophages. Despite intensive chemotherapy, the tumor relapsed, involving the large and small bowel, and intraabdominal lymph nodes showed similar histologic findings. The appearances of the rectal mucosa at **(A)** low and **(B)** high power show complete loss of normal architecture, with remaining crypt cells surrounded by the diffuse infiltrate consisting of immunoblasts and mixed inflammatory cells. The α heavy chain could still be detected in serum, but not in urine at this relapse. (A, B, Courtesy of Dr. J. E. McLaughlin.)

The most common form of HCD, α-HCD, is now classified as a form of MALT lymphoma. It occurs largely in the Mediterranean area and Africa, often in young adult patients with an Arabic genetic background, and in areas where intestinal parasites (e.g., Campylobacter jejuni) are common. It commences as a relatively benign plasma cell proliferation in the gastrointestinal tract (Fig. 22-64); subsequently, a poorly differentiated lymphoma of the small bowel develops and may spread, although usually within the abdominal cavity (Fig. 22-65). The serum shows a monoclonal protein in the α2 or β region in 50% of cases, and the protein may also be found in the urine. It consists of a heavy chain with an internal deletion. The disease is a variant of extranodal marginal zone lymphoma of mucosa associated lymphoid tissue (MALT).

A rare form of α-HCD occurs sporadically outside the areas in which intestinal infection is common and is characterized by a lymphoplasmacytoid infiltrate of the respiratory tract.

The rarest form is μ-HCD; the patients are usually African, particularly from parasite-infected zones (as for α-HCD). However, μ-HCD manifests with a clinical picture that resembles chronic lymphocytic leukemia or lymphoma, with enlargement of the liver and spleen and infiltration of the marrow with vacuolated plasma cells admixed with small lymphocytes. Light chains of one type may also be found in urine, but these remain separate from the μ heavy chain.

TISSUE TYPING AND STEM CELL TRANSPLANTATION

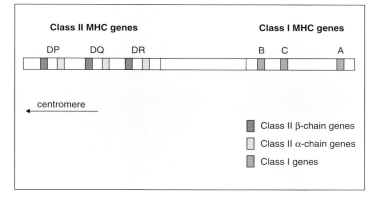

Fig. 23-1. Major histocompatibility complex polymorphism: the main genes that encode MHC Class I and MHC Class II molecules. In practice, the genes that encode most of the three main types of the Class IIα and β chains are located at more than one locus and there are additional Class I MHC loci. (Prepared by Steven G. E. Marsh.)

HUMAN LEUKOCYTE ANTIGEN SYSTEM

The short arm of chromosome 6 contains a cluster of genes known as the major histocompatibility complex (MHC) or the human leukocyte antigen (HLA) region (Fig. 23-1). Among the genes in this region are those that code for the proteins of the HLAs that are present on the cell membranes of many nucleated cells. As well as playing a major role in transplant rejection, these antigens are involved in many aspects of immunologic recognition and reaction.

The MHC proteins are classified into three types. Class I proteins comprise two polypeptides, the larger of which is encoded by the MHC. The small component, a β_2-microglobulin, is encoded outside the MHC. Class II proteins comprise an α and a β chain, both of which are encoded by the MHC (Fig. 23-2). Class III proteins are the complement components encoded by the MHC region.

In humans, the main regions of the MHC gene complex are A, B, C, and D. The Class I proteins encoded by the A, B, and C regions act as surface recognition antigens, which can be identified by cytotoxic CD8+ T lymphocytes. The D region genes encode Class II

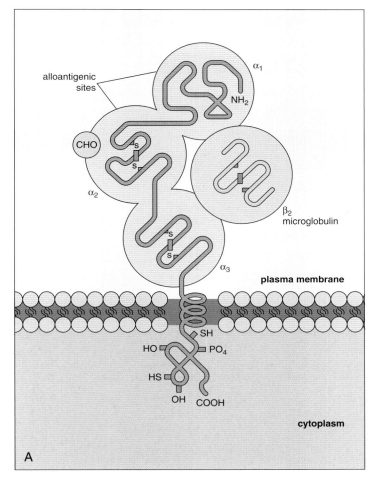

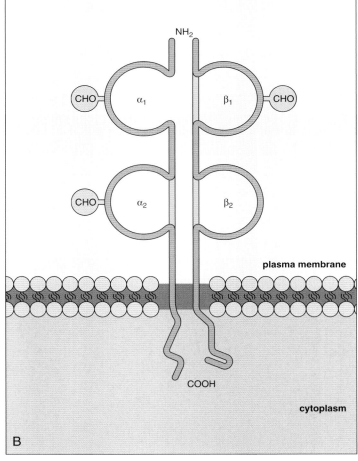

Fig. 23-2. Structure in the plasma membrane: **(A)** Class I and **(B)** Class II HLAs. The Class I MHC-encoded chain has three globular domains α1, α2, and α3. A non-MHC-encoded peptide, β2-microglobulin, is closely associated with the α3 domain. Alloantigens occur on the α1 and α2 domains. The HLA-DR antigen consists of an α and a β peptide, noncovalently bound together. Each peptide has two globular domains, which are structurally related to immunoglobulin (Ig) domains.

413

proteins, which are involved in cooperation and interaction between T helper CD4+ lymphocytes and antigen-presenting cells. HLA-A, HLA-B, and HLA-C antigens are present on all nucleated cells and platelets, and those encoded by the D region are present only on B lymphocytes, monocytes, macrophages, and some activated T cells. The D region is divided serologically into three groups: DR, DP, and DQ.

HUMAN LEUKOCYTE ANTIGEN NOMENCLATURE

The World Health Organization (WHO) Nomenclature Committee names HLA genes, alleles, and serologically defined antigenic specificities. The naming of antigens or types involves a letter to denote the locus and a number (given in chronologic order of discovery) to denote a particular specificity at that locus, determined originally by serologic or cellular techniques (e.g., HLA-A1, HLA-B8, HLA-Cw3, HLA-DR1). The lower case "w" is used to indicate a provisional specificity. Bw4 and Bw6 are public antigens, and for C antigens "w" is used to distinguish them from complement antigens. Some HLA types were subsequently divided into two or more subtypes; for example, DR13 and DR14 are splits of DR6, denoted DR13(6) and DR14(6).

Molecular typing has now produced definition of alleles by deoxyribonucleic acid (DNA) sequencing. Alleles are numbered using the letter that defines the locus and up to eight digits. The first two digits indicate the allele group, the third and fourth list subtypes, and the number is assigned in the order in which the DNA sequences have been determined. The fifth and sixth digits are used to name alleles that differ only by synonymous nucleotide substitutions ("silent" or "noncoding"). The seventh and eighth digits name alleles that differ in either intron or 3′ or 5′ regions of the gene. Finally, an allele may have a suffix indicating aberrant expression, for example, N for a null allele with no proteins expressed, L for low cell surface expression, and S for an allele only expressed in soluble form.

The most recent advances in HLA nomenclature can be found by accessing the IMGT/HLA Sequence Database (www.ebi.ac.uk/imgt/hla).

The asterisk after the gene name indicates a particular allele. For Class II, the gene name includes a reference to the specific heavy or light chain locus (e.g., HLA-DQA1* or HLA-DQA2* for the first two DQA chain loci). The DRB1 gene codes for the HLA-DR(1–18) antigens recognized serologically. DRB3 codes for the DR52 antigens, DRB4 for the DR53 antigens, and DRB5 for the DR51 antigens (Fig. 23-3).

TYPING OF HUMAN LEUKOCYTE ANTIGENS

HLA-A, HLA-B, and HLA-C typing is usually carried out on peripheral blood lymphocytes. Originally, antigens of the D system were identified by nonreactivity in mixed lymphocyte culture (a lymphocyte reaction proliferation assay) against rare homozygous D-locus cells. More than 30 genes code for the antigens in this region (Table 23-1), with multiple alleles at each locus (Table 23-2). It is now possible to detect HLA-D region antigens serologically or by molecular biologic techniques, including the following:

- Sequence-specific primer amplification (PCR-SSP)
- Sequence-specific oligonucleotide probe (PCR-SSO)
- Heteroduplex analysis
- Direct nucleotide sequencing (Fig. 23-4)
- Single-strand conformational polymorphism analysis (SSCPA)
- Double-stranded conformational analysis (DSCA; Figs. 23-5 and 23-6)

A current list of HLAs is given in Table 23-3.

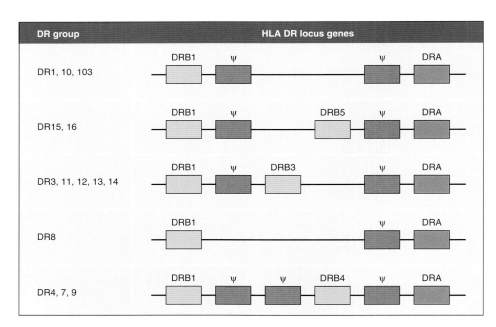

Fig. 23-3. Variable expression of genes according to HLA haplotype. *Yellow boxes,* DRB genes; *orange boxes,* nonpolymorphic DRA genes; *purple boxes,* pseudo-genes. (Adapted with permission from Mickelson E, Petersdorf EW: *Hematopoietic cell transplantation,* ed 2, Oxford, 1999, Blackwell Science.)

TABLE 23-1.   HUMAN MAJOR HISTOCOMPATIBILITY COMPLEX: GENES

Name	Molecular characteristics	Name	Molecular characteristics
HLA-A	Class I α-chain	HLA-DQB1	DQA β chain as expressed
HLA-B	Class I α-chain	HLA-DQA2	DQ α-chain-related sequence, not known to be expressed
HLA-C	Class I α-chain	HLA-DQB2	DQ β-chain-related sequence, not known to be expressed
HLA-E	Associated with class I 6.2 kb Hind III fragment	HLA-DQB3	DQ β-chain-related sequence, not known to be expressed
HLA-F	Associated with class I 5.4 kb Hind III fragment	HLA-DOA	DO α chain
HLA-G	Associated with class I 6.0 kb Hind III fragment	HLA-DOB	DO β chain
HLA-H	Class I pseudogene associated with 5.4 kb Hind III fragment	HLA-DMA	DM α chain
HLA-J	Class I pseudogene associated with 5.9 kb Hind III fragment	HLA-DMB	DM β chain
HLA-K	Class I pseudogene associated with 7.0 kb Hind III fragment	HLA-DPA1	DP α chain as expressed
HLA-L	Class I pseudogene associated with 9.2 kb Hind III fragment	HLA-DPB1	DP β chain as expressed
HLA-DRA	DR α chain	HLA-DPA2	DP α-chain-related pseudogene
HLA-DRB1	DR βI chain determining specificities DR1, DR2, DR3, DR4, DR5, etc.	HLA-DPB2	DP β-chain-related pseudogene
HLA-DRB2	Pseudogene with DR β-like sequences	TAP1	ABC (ATP binding cassette) transporter
HLA-DRB3	DR β3 chain determining DR52 and Dw24, Dw25, Dw26 specificities	TAP2	ABC (ATP binding cassette) transporter
HLA-DRB4	DR β4 chain determining DR53	LMP2	Proteasome-related sequence
HLA-DRB5	DR β5 chain determining DR51	LMP7	Proteasome-related sequence
HLA-DRB6	DRB pseudogene found on DR1, DR2, and DR10 haplotypes	MICA	Class I chain-related gene
HLA-DRB7	DRB pseudogene found on DR4, DR7, and DR9 haplotypes	MICB	Class I chain-related gene
HLA-DRB8	DRB pseudogene found on DR4, DR7, and DR9 haplotypes	MICC	Class I chain-related pseudogene
HLA-DRB9	DRB pseudogene, isolated fragment	MICD	Class I chain-related pseudogene
HLA-DQA1	DQA α chain as expressed	MICE	Class I chain-related pseudogene

(Adapted with permission from Bodmer JG, Marsh SGE, Albert ED, et al: Nomenclature for factors of the HLA system, 1998, *Hum Immunol* 60:361-395, 1999.)

TABLE 23-2.   ALLELES: NUMBER AT EACH HLA LOCUS, AS ASSIGNED BY THE WHO NOMENCLATURE COMMITTEE FOR FACTORS OF THE HLA SYSTEM, JANUARY 2009

	HLA gene	No of alleles	No of antigens
Class I	A	740	24
	B	1141	50
	C	400	9
Class II	DRB1	610	20
	DRB3	50	1
	DRB4	13	1
	DRB5	18	1
	DQA1	34	–
	DQB1	96	7
	DPA1	27	–
	DPB1	133	–

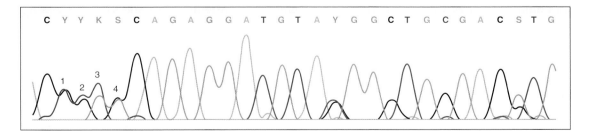

Fig. 23-4. Electropherogram of sequencing results from analysis of a heterozygous locus. The sequence is read from left to right. For this short stretch of nucleotides, many different results are possible. Heterozygous positions are given appropriate IUB codes. First heterozygous position (marked I): CC or CT, continuing to second heterozygous position (marked 2): CCC or CCT or CTC or CTT, continuing to third heterozygous position (marked 3): CCCG or CCCT or CCTG or CCTT or CTCT or CTCG or CTTT or CTTG, continuing to fourth heterozygous position (marked 4): CCCGG or CCCGC or CCCTG or CCCTC or CCTGG or CCTGC or CCTTG or CCTTC or CTCTG or CTCTC or CTCGG or CTCGC or CTTTG or CTTTC or CTTGG or CTTGC, etc. (Courtesy of Steven T. Cox, the Anthony Nolan Trust.)

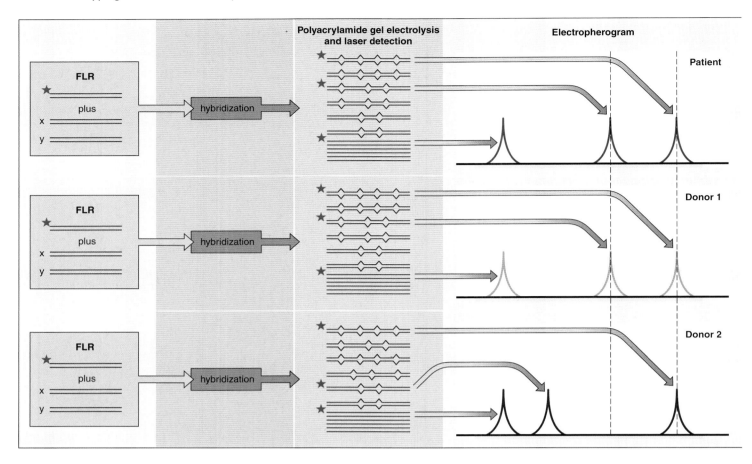

Fig. 23-5. Allogeneic bone marrow transplantation: reference-strand conformation analysis (RSCA) method. The locus-specific fluorescein-labeled reference (FLR) polymerase chain reaction (PCR) product contains a fluorescent Cy5 label on its sense strand (indicated by a star). The FLR is hybridized with the locus-specific PCR product from the sample to be tested. For heterozygous loci, two alleles are present (indicated as "x" and "y"). During hybridization the sense and antisense strands of the DNA strands present are initially separated by denaturation followed by reannealing, whereby the sense and antisense strands can cross-hybridize to generate, in addition to the starting homoduplexes, heteroduplexes, two of which possess the Cy5-labeled sense strand of the FLR. The duplexes formed are separated by polyacrylamide gel electrophoresis, and those duplexes that possess a Cy5 label are detected with the laser. In this example, the patient and donor 1 have alleles with identical mobility, whereas donor 2 has one allele that differs. (Redrawn with permission from Arguello JR, Little AM, Pay AL, et al: Mutation detection and typing of polymorphic loci through double-strand conformational analysis, *Nat Genet* 18:192-194, 1998; courtesy of Professor J.A. Madrigal.)

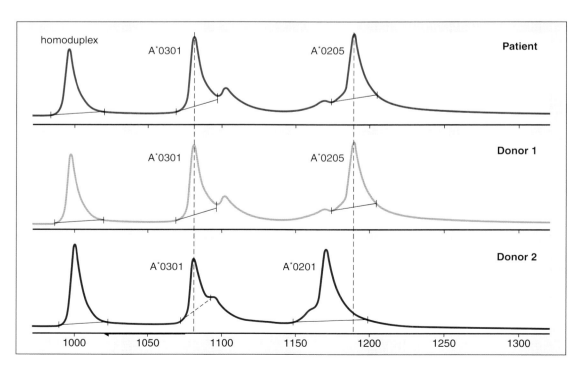

Fig. 23-6. Allogeneic bone marrow transplantation: electropherogram with results for HLA-A locus matching for a patient and two unrelated bone marrow donors. After electrophoresis the homoduplex peak is assigned an arbitrary value of 1000 on the horizontal scale. The vertical scale represents the homoduplex and heteroduplex peaks detected by laser. The patient and two potential donors were matched by serology for HLA-A2 and HLA-A3. By RSCA analysis, the patient shares allele A*0301 with both potential donors, but only shares the second allele, A*0205, with donor 1. (Courtesy of Professor J.A. Madrigal.)

TABLE 23-3.   RECOGNIZED (BY SEROLOGIC AND CELLULAR TECHNIQUES) HLA SPECIFICITIES

A	B	C	D	DR	DQ	DP
A1	B5	Cw1	Dw1	DR1	DQ1	DPw1
A2	B7	Cw2	Dw2	DR103	DQ2	DPw2
A203	B703	Cw3	Dw3	DR2	DQ3	DPw3
A210	B8	Cw4	Dw4	DR3	DQ4	DPw4
A3	B12	Cw5	Dw5	DR4	DQ5(1)	DPw5
A9	B13	Cw6	Dw6	DR5	DQ6(1)	DPw6
A10	B14	Cw7	Dw7	DR6	DQ7(3)	
A11	B15	Cw8	Dw8	DR7	DQ8(3)	
A19	B16	Cw9(w3)	Dw9	DR8	DQ9(3)	
A23(9)	B17	Cw10(w3)	Dw10	DR9		
A24(9)	B18		Dw11(w7)	DR10		
A2403	B21		Dw12	DR11(5)		
A25(10)	B22		Dw13	DR12(5)		
A26(10)	B27		Dw14	DR13(6)		
A28	B2708		Dw15	DR14(6)		
A29(19)	B35		Dw16	DR1403		
A30(19)	B37		Dw17(w7)	DR1404		
A31(19)	B38(16)		Dw18(w6)	DR15(2)		
A32(19)	B39(16)		Dw19(w6)	DR16(2)		
A33(19)	B3901		Dw20	DR17(3)		
A34(10)	B3902		Dw21	DR18(3)		
A36	B40		Dw22			
A43	B4005		Dw23	DR51		
A66(10)	B41					
A68(28)	B42		Dw24	DR52		
A69(28)	B44(12)		Dw25			
A74(19)	B45(12)		Dw26	DR53		
A80	B46					
	B47					
	B48					
	B49(21)					
	B50(21)					
	B51(5)					
	B5102					
	B5103					
	B52(5)					
	B53					
	B54(22)					
	B55(22)					
	B56(22)					
	B57(17)					
	B58(17)					
	B59					
	B60(40)					
	B61(40)					
	B62(15)					
	B63(15)					
	B64(14)					
	B65(14)					
	B67					
	B70					
	B71(70)					
	B72(70)					
	B73					
	B75(15)					
	B76(15)					
	B77(15)					
	B78					
	B81					
	Bw4					
	Bw6					

Established specificities are denoted by a number; those not fully confirmed are prefixed by a "w" (workshop). More restricted specificities are included in a broader group ("splits") shown in parentheses following the firmer specificity. Antigens Bw4 and Bw6 are very broad ("public") and include splits that have been further subdivided. Molecular typing nomenclature is described in the text.

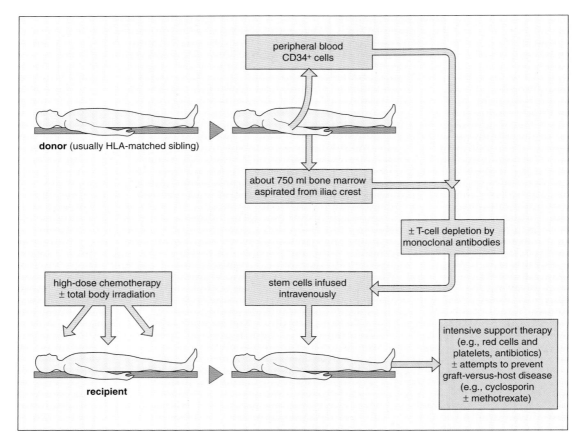

Fig. 23-7. Allogeneic stem cell transplantation: stem cells may be harvested from peripheral blood or bone marrow.

OTHER HUMAN LEUKOCYTE ANTIGENS

Human leukocytes carry a variety of antigens (CD) (currently numbering 247) that are recognized by monoclonal antibodies. These various CD antigens are listed electronically including cellular expression, molecular weight, and functions, together with examples of antibodies that detect them. The use of these antibodies to define normal and malignant hematopoietic cell subpopulations is described in other chapters.

STEM CELL TRANSPLANTATION

Stem cell transplantation may be carried out between siblings (allogeneic transplantation; Fig. 23-7) who are HLA identical or can be shown to be matching by a number of different techniques of DNA analysis. Syngeneic (identical twin), haploidentical, HLA-matched but unrelated donors, and placental (cord) blood may also be used in appropriate cases (Table 23-4).

The recipient has a malignant marrow disorder (e.g., poor-prognosis acute leukemia, myelodysplasia, chronic myeloid leukemia failing imatinib therapy); myeloma or lymphoma failing initial therapy; aplastic anemia; or a genetic abnormality (e.g., thalassemia major) (Table 23-5).

In autologous transplantation, the patient's own stem cells are used to rescue the patient from profound marrow ablation caused by high-dose chemotherapy, with or without total body irradiation, for malignant disease (Fig. 23-8).

Peripheral blood stem cells (PBSCs) may be harvested using a cell separator (Fig. 23-9) and used instead of bone marrow both for allogeneic and autologous transplantation. Usually the patient is given cyclophosphamide and a 4- to 6-day course of granulocyte colony-stimulating factor (G-CSF) to mobilize PBSCs. Normal donors receive G-CSF but not cyclophosphamide. A collection of greater than 2.5×10^6/kg CD34+ cells is regarded as adequate (see Fig. 23-9). Stem cells appear similar to small or medium-sized lymphocytes (Fig. 23-10) and are contained in a CD34-enriched cell population

TABLE 23-4.	STEM CELL (BONE MARROW OR PERIPHERAL BLOOD) TRANSPLANTATION: DONORS
Stem cell transplantation – donors	
Type	**Donor**
Syngeneic	Identical twin
Allogeneic	HLA-matching brother or sister HLA-matching other family member (e.g., parent, cousin) HLA-matching unrelated volunteer donor (VUD or MUD)
Cord (placental) blood	
Autologous	

TABLE 23-5.   STEM CELL (BONE MARROW OR PERIPHERAL BLOOD)
              TRANSPLANTATION: INDICATIONS

Stem cell transplantation: indications	
Allogeneic (or syngeneic)	
Malignant	**Immunodeficiency**
Acute myeloid leukemia (some cases)	Severe combined Immunodeficiency
Acute lymphoblastic leukemia:	Wiscott–Aldrich syndrome
poor prognosis: first remission	
second remission or subsequently	**Metabolic storage diseases**
Chronic myeloid leukemia (imatinib failures)	
Other severe acquired disorders of the marrow,	Gaucher's disease (type II)
selected cases, e.g., Hodgkin's disease, non-Hodgkin's	Mucopolysaccharidosis
lymphoma, myeloma, myelodysplasia, myelofibrosis,	
chronic lymphocytic leukemia	
Bone marrow disorders	
Aplastic anemia	
Paroxysmal nocturnal hemoglobinuria	
Thalassemia major	
Sickle cell anemia	
Kostmann's syndrome	**Autologous**
Chronic granulomatous disease	
Chediak–Higashi syndrome	Malignant lymphoma (Hodgkin's or
Adhesion molecule deficiency	non-Hodgkin's) usually post first relapse
Glanzmann's disease	
Bernard–Soulier disease	Myeloma
Osteoporosis	Gene therapy, e.g., adenosine
Congenital hemophagocytic syndrome	deaminase deficiency

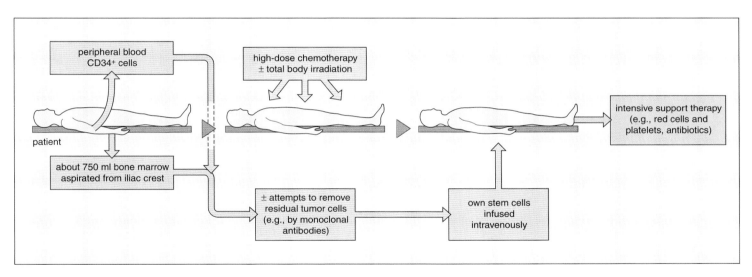

Fig. 23-8. Autologous stem cell transplantation: stem cells may be harvested from peripheral blood or bone marrow.

Fig. 23-9. Peripheral blood stem cell collection: blood is circulated from one arm to a cell separator and the buffy coat harvested, the red cells and plasma being returned to the donor.

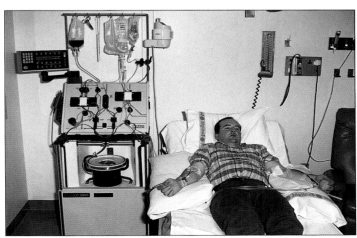

(Fig. 23-11). Recovery of platelets after PBSC transplantation is enhanced compared to the recovery of platelets after bone marrow (BM) transplantation.

A typical hematologic chart of a patient having allogeneic stem cell transplantation (SCT) for aplastic anemia is shown in Fig. 23-12.

Immediately following SCT, the recipient's blood shows chimerism, the presence of both recipient and donor cells. The degree of chimerism can be determined by DNA analysis at subsequent time points and in different cell lineages (Fig. 23-13, *A*). If there is a sex mismatch between donor and recipient, fluorescent in situ hybridization (FISH) analysis of the proportion of circulating Y-chromosome–containing cells can also be used (Fig. 23-13, *B*).

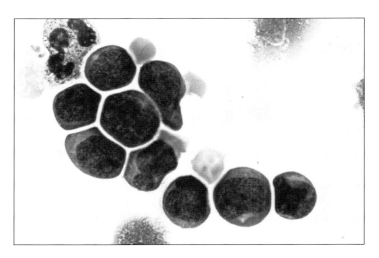

Fig. 23-10. Peripheral blood stem cell collection: enriched CD34+ cells stained by May-Grunwald Giemsa. The cells have the appearance of small- and medium-sized lymphocytes. (Courtesy of Dr. M. Potter.)

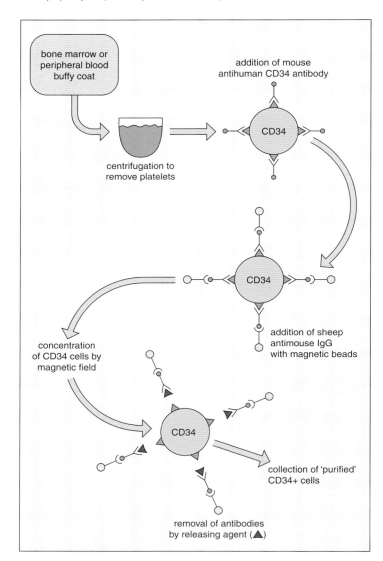

Fig. 23-11. Peripheral blood stem cell collection: steps in the Baxter system of purification of CD34+ cells. Many different techniques are now available.

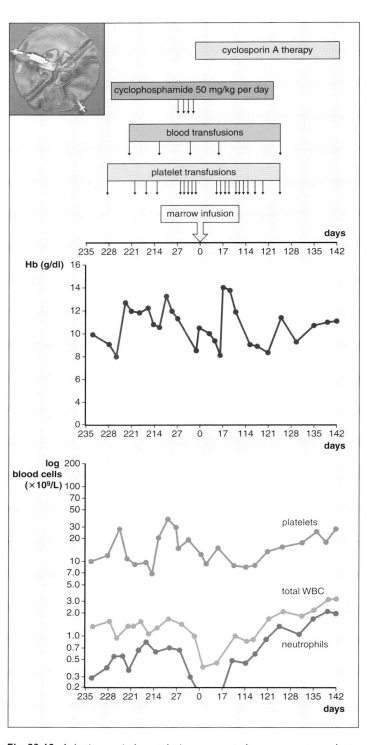

Fig. 23-12. Aplastic anemia: hematologic response to bone marrow transplantation. Marrow (500 to 1000 ml) is harvested from the pelvis of the donor. Red cells are removed and in some circumstances T lymphocytes are also eliminated (e.g., by monoclonal antibodies) to prevent graft-versus-host disease (GVHD). Cyclosporin A is used to ameliorate GVHD and to enhance engraftment in aplastic anemia. When the recipient has leukemia, total body irradiation is usually used in addition to chemotherapy in the conditioning. The inset shows donor marrow depleted of red cells and T lymphocytes before infusion into the recipient. (Courtesy of M. Gilmore.)

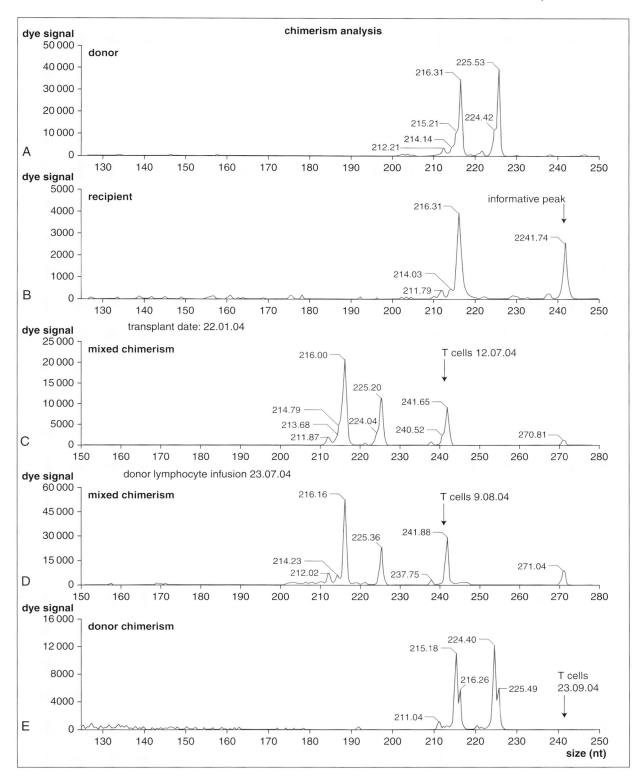

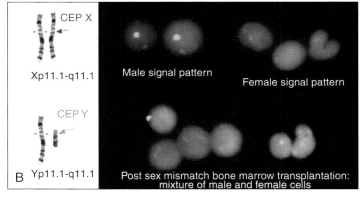

Fig. 23-13. A, Chimerism analysis after stem cell transplantation. Fluorescent polymerase chain reaction (PCR) products are electrophoresed through a capillary matrix and are detected following excitation with a laser. The results are displayed in an electrophoretogram as shown. *Panel* **(A)** shows the donor profile and *panel* **(B)** shows the pretransplant recipient profile. Using a microsatellite marker, the donor and recipient are both heterozygous with one common allele. The *red arrow* highlights the informative peak—the presence of which in a posttransplant sample would indicate a mixed chimera. *Panel* **(C)** shows the presence of mixed chimerism in the T-cell lineage. A donor lymphocyte infusion (DLI) was administered, and *panel* **(D)** shows the persistence of mixed chimerism. Within 2 months after DLI the T cells are showing a full donor chimerism *(panel* **[E]**). More than 2 years after the DLI, the patient remained fully donor in the following lineages: T cells, B cells, granulocytes, and peripheral blood mononuclear cells. **B,** Chimerism analysis after sex-mismatched stem cell transplantation using FISH analysis of peripheral blood leukocytes with probes specific for the centromere regions (CEP) of the X *(red)* and Y *(green)* chromosomes: The upper panel shows normal male signal pattern *(left)* and normal female pattern *(right)*. The lower panel shows a mixture of male and female cells in a patient following sex-mismatched stem cell transplantation. (A, Courtesy Professor S. Mackinnon)

Failure of engraftment is unusual in well-matched transplants for leukemia but is more common when the recipient has aplastic anemia or when donor and recipient are not fully matched or when T-cell depletion has been carried out.

NONMYELOABLATIVE ("MINI") TRANSPLANTS

In "mini"-transplant procedures, the donor is treated with drugs and/or radiotherapy at a less intensive level than used for standard stem cell transplantation. The aim is to achieve immunosuppression sufficient for donor stem cells to be accepted into the marrow microenvironment, and to establish a durable graft without total marrow ablation by the conditioning treatment. Drugs used in different regimens include fludarabine, cyclophosphamide, antilymphocytic globulin, alemtuzemab (anti-CD52, Campath), and busulphan. The aim is to establish chimerism between recipient and donor cells (see Fig. 23-13) and for the donor immune-competent cells to effect a cure by a graft versus leukemia, myelodysplasia, myeloma, or lymphoma effect.

DONOR LEUKOCYTES

Donor leukocytes may be given after allogeneic stem cell transplantation if residual disease or recurrence of disease is evident. The best results are obtained if only minimal disease is present (e.g., chronic myeloid leukemia detected by molecular methods or cytogenetics only, rather than from hematologic relapse of the disease) (Fig. 23-14). Also, it is important that chimerism is still present (i.e., there is evidence of donor as well as recipient cells in the blood or bone marrow of the recipient).

COMPLICATIONS OF STEM CELL TRANSPLANTS

Allogeneic transplantation is not usually carried out for patients older than 65 years because of the increased incidence of complications (Table 23-6), but autologous transplantation is carried out for patients up to age 70 years. In full intensity transplants, the recipient's marrow is first eliminated by intensive chemotherapy, which is usually combined in the case of leukemia with total body irradiation. At least 2 weeks of pancytopenia follows before the infused donor pluripotent stem cells, having seeded the recipient's bone marrow, proliferate and differentiate sufficiently to produce new mature red cells, leukocytes, and platelets.

Infections are a major hazard during the posttransplant period. Attempts at prevention include reverse-barrier or laminar-flow nursing,

TABLE 23-6. ALLOGENEIC STEM CELL TRANSPLANTATION: COMPLICATIONS

Early (<100 days)
Acute graft-versus-host disease
Skin
Liver
Gut
Infections
Bacterial
Fungal
Herpes simplex
Cytomegalovirus
Graft failure
Hemorrhagic cystitis
Interstitial pneumonitis
Veno-occlusive disease
Late (>100 days)
Chronic graft-versus-host disease
Scleroderma
Sicca syndrome
Arthritis
Hepatitis
Malabsorption
Pulmonary lesions
Chronic pulmonary disease
Autoimmune disorders
Cataracts
Infertility
Leukoencephalopathy
Secondary malignancy

prophylactic nonabsorbable antibiotics and antifungal agents, and early use of systemic antibiotics for febrile episodes. Prolonged antibiotic therapy, however, increases the likelihood of fungal infections (Figs. 23-15 and 23-16). Hematopoietic growth factors (e.g., G-CSF) may be used to enhance granulocyte recovery.

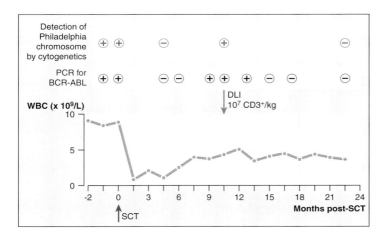

Fig. 23-14. Example of donor leukocyte infusion (DLI) in the treatment of chronic myeloid leukemia (CML) that relapsed following allogeneic stem cell transplantation (SCT). Polymerase chain reaction (PCR) analysis of the blood for the BCR-ABL transcript shows that there was transient loss of the transcript, but molecular and cytogenetic relapse occurred at 10 months. One infusion of donor leukocytes led to re-establishment of a durable complete remission.

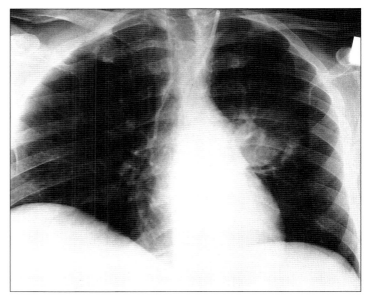

Fig. 23-15. Stem cell transplantation: chest radiograph showing an opacity in the upper left zone, with a cystic center that contains a dense central zone, caused by aspergillosis.

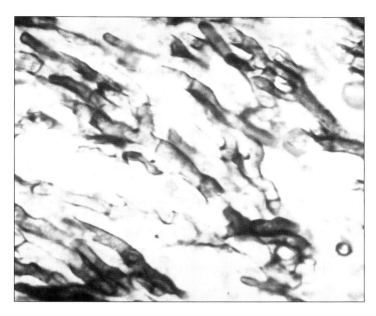

Fig. 23-16. Stem cell transplantation: cytology of sputum from the case shown in Fig. 23-15 illustrates the typical branching septate hyphae of aspergilli. (Methenamine silver stain.)

Cytomegalovirus (CMV) infection may result from reactivation of a previous latent infection or from transmission of the virus in blood products, and may result in severe pneumonitis and marrow suppression. Treatment is with ganciclovir alone or along with foscarnet (Figs. 23-17 and 23-18).

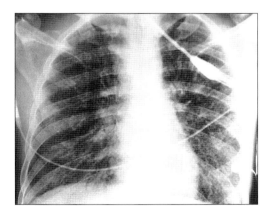

Fig. 23-17. Stem cell transplantation: chest radiograph showing widespread interstitial pneumonia. Sputum cultures and indirect immunofluorescence showed the presence of cytomegalovirus.

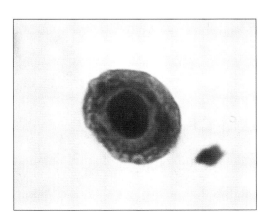

Fig. 23-18. Stem cell transplantation: sputum cytology shows a pulmonary cell with degenerative changes and a large intranuclear inclusion body typical of cytomegalovirus infection. (Papanicolaou stain.) (Courtesy of Professor Y. S. Erozan.)

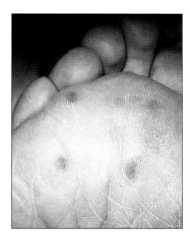

Fig. 23-19. Stem cell transplantation: herpes simplex virus infection with multiple widespread lesions on the skin of the sole of the foot. (Courtesy of Professor H. G. Prentice.)

Herpes simplex virus (e.g., HHV6) infection is a frequent complication that tends to become generalized and may cause pneumonia, encephalitis, skin lesions (Fig. 23-19), or marrow suppression. Infection can be prevented by the use of prophylactic intravenous aciclovir. Treatment is with ganciclovir and foscarnet. Pneumonia caused by *Pneumocystis carinii* is another frequent complication of the immunosuppression and neutropenia (Figs. 23-20 and 23-21).

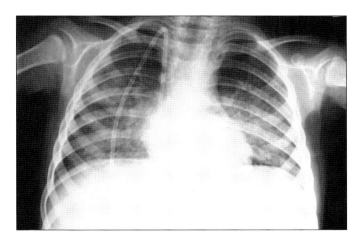

Fig. 23-20. Stem cell transplantation: chest radiograph showing typical "bat wing" shadowing of both lung fields caused by *P. carinii* infection.

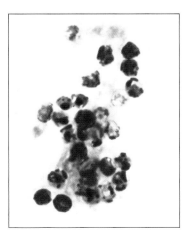

Fig. 23-21. Stem cell transplantation: high-power view of concentrated bronchial washings showing typical appearance of *P. carinii*. (Gram-Weigert stain.) (Courtesy of Professor Y. S. Erozan.)

Total body irradiation itself may cause side effects that involve epithelial structures; damage to the nails and nail beds (Fig. 23-22) and temporary complete alopecia (Fig. 23-23) occur. Veno-occlusive disease (VOD) of the liver (Fig. 23-24) is an acute complication caused by chemotherapy and radiotherapy. Preceding chemotherapy

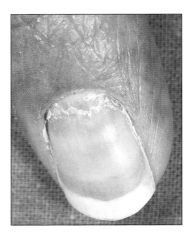

Fig. 23-22. Stem cell transplantation: this nail shows horizontal ridges and atrophy of the nail bed as a result of total body irradiation. (Courtesy of Professor H. G. Prentice.)

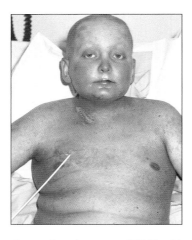

Fig. 23-23. Stem cell transplantation—acute GVHD: widespread erythematus skin rash. An indwelling central Hickman catheter is in place. (Courtesy of Professor H. G. Prentice.)

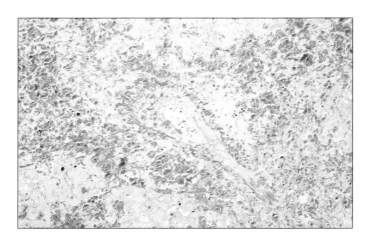

Fig. 23-24. Stem cell transplantation: VOD. Section showing a terminal hepatic venule with marked narrowing of its lumen. The deep-blue staining identifies the collagen of the original venule wall, while the inner paler blue area represents new collagen obstructing the lumen. Note the loss of hepatocytes in the perivenular area and the intense congestion of the sinusoids. (Chromotrope Aniline Blue × 40 stain.) (Courtesy of Dr. M. Jarmulowicz.)

and abnormal liver function may also predispose to VOD. Hemorrhagic cystitis may result from cyclophosphamide metabolites (mesna is given to try to prevent this) or from viral infection (e.g., adenovirus, CMV, or polyoma virus).

GRAFT-VERSUS-HOST DISEASE

Another major posttransplant complication is reaction of the immunocompetent cells in the graft against the tissues of the host, which causes graft-versus-host disease (GVHD) that may be acute (occurring in the first 100 days posttransplant) or chronic. The risk factors for acute GVHD are given in Table 23-7. The triad of skin, mucus membrane and gut, and liver involvement is classified according to severity into grades I, II, III, and IV.

In acute cases of GVHD an erythematus itchy skin rash is widespread (see Fig. 23-23) and tends to be particularly severe on the hands and feet. In severe cases a bullous eruption and subsequent widespread exfoliation may occur (Fig. 23-25).

In chronic cases the lesions tend to be firm, red, and plaque-like (Fig. 23-26) and ultimately may, in some patients, form a scleroderma-like picture with contractures and ulceration (Fig. 23-27). The hands and feet may continue to exfoliate (Fig. 23-28).

The mucus membranes may also be affected, with formation of lichen planus-like lesions in the mouth and pharynx (Fig. 23-29).

TABLE 23-7.	STEM CELL TRANSPLANTATION: RISK FACTORS FOR THE DEVELOPMENT OF ACUTE GVHD

Histocompatibility

Allosensitization of donor

Older donor

Older recipient

Sex mismatch

Lack of prophylaxis for graft-versus-host disease

Infusion of viable donor leukocytes

Intensity of conditioning regimen

Adapted with permission from Atkinson K: *The BMT data book,* Cambridge, 1998, Cambridge University Press, p 464.

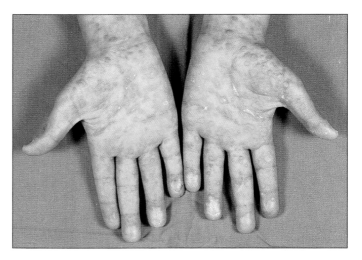

Fig. 23-25. Stem cell transplantation—acute GVHD: the palmar surfaces of these hands show an erythematus maculopapular eruption with bullous ulceration and denudation. (Courtesy of Professor H. G. Prentice.)

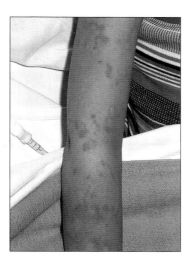

Fig. 23-26. Stem cell transplantation—chronic GVHD: these patchy raised erythematous skin lesions are characteristic. (Courtesy of Professor H. G. Prentice.)

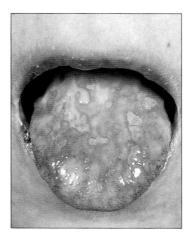

Fig. 23-29. Stem cell transplantation—chronic GVHD: lesions of the tongue and lips similar to those of lichen planus. (Courtesy of Professor H. G. Prentice.)

The histologic appearances of GVHD are normally seen after skin or rectal biopsy. In acute GVHD the skin shows inflammatory changes with death of epidermal cells and a lymphoid infiltrate (Fig. 23-30) leading, in severe cases, to denudation.

The rectal mucosa also shows death of epithelial (crypt) cells and inflammatory changes (Fig. 23-31). When severe, there is loss of small and large intestinal mucosa (Fig. 23-32).

Liver function is abnormal in acute and chronic GVHD, except in mild cases. The histologic appearances include damage to bile duct epithelial cells, inflammatory changes, and cholestasis (Fig. 23-33).

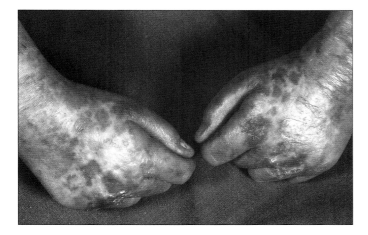

Fig. 23-27. Stem cell transplantation—chronic GVHD: scleroderma-like contractions of the hands with thickening of the skin and marked pigmentation. (Courtesy of Professor H. G. Prentice.)

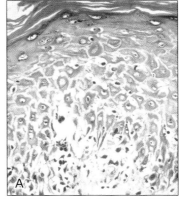

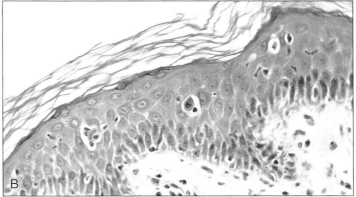

Fig. 23-30. Stem cell transplantation—acute GVHD: histologic sections of skin in moderately severe (Grade II) acute GVHD, showing **(A)** vacuolation of the basal epidermal cells with inflammatory changes in the superficial dermis; **(B)** prominent vacuoles containing necrotic epidermal cells and lymphocytes, from an African patient.

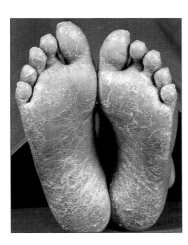

Fig. 23-28. Stem cell transplantation—chronic GVHD: erythema and exfoliation of the epidermis of the soles of the feet. (Courtesy of Professor H. G. Prentice.)

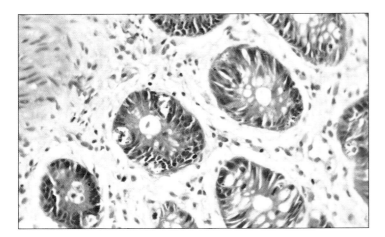

Fig. 23-31. Stem cell transplantation—acute GVHD: high-power view of rectal biopsy in Grade I acute GVHD showing individual crypt cell necrosis and edema of the lamina propria.

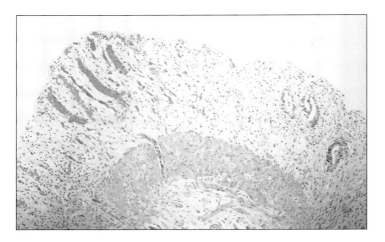

Fig. 23-32. Stem cell transplantation—acute GVHD: postmortem section of colon in Grade IV acute GVHD showing almost complete denudation of the epithelium, with edema and lymphocytic infiltration of the submucosa.

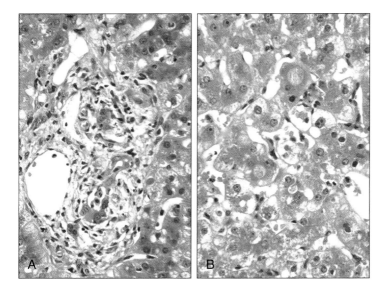

Fig. 23-33. Stem cell transplantation—acute GVHD: high-power views of liver biopsy showing (**A**) damaged, irregular, and elongated bile duct epithelial cells with occasional pyknotic nuclei in the portal tract (there is a moderate infiltration of lymphocytes and neutrophils). **B,** Cholestatic changes include dilated bile canaliculi and pigmented hepatocytes. (*A, B,* Courtesy of Professor P. J. Scheuer.)

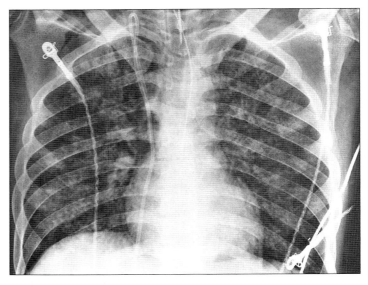

Fig. 23-34. Stem cell transplantation: chest radiograph of interstitial pneumonitis showing widespread diffuse mottling. The patient had received total body irradiation and had Grade III GVHD. No infective cause of the pneumonitis was identified in this case.

GVHD can be prevented in HLA-matched allogeneic transplantation if T lymphocytes (or selected T cell subsets) are completely removed in vitro from donor bone marrow, but this may increase the risk of graft failure or of leukemic relapse in some situations. Prevention of GVHD is usually carried out with cyclosporin with or without methotrexate; tacrolimus, mycophenolate mofetil, and thalidomide and its derivatives are drugs used for prevention and treatment of GVHD.

A frequent posttransplantation complication is an interstitial pneumonia (Fig. 23-34), which is more common in GVHD but may also be related to lung irradiation and to infection, particularly with CMV.

POST-TRANSPLANT LYMPHOPROLIFERATIVE DISORDERS

Post-transplant lymphoproliferative disorders (PTLDs) are polyclonal or monoclonal lymphoid proliferations or lymphomas that occur in recipients of stem cell or more frequently solid organ allografts, as a result of the immunosuppression. There may be polyclonal Epstein-Barr virus (EBV)–driven lymphocytosis and lymphadenopathy resembling infectious mononucleosis or EBV-positive or EBV-negative

TABLE 23-8.   POSTTRANSPLANT LYMPHOPROLIFERATIVE DISORDERS (PTLDs):WHO (2008) CATEGORIES OF PTLDs

1. Early lesions
Plasmacytic hyperplasia Infectious mononucleosis-like lesion
2. Polymorphic PTLD
3. Monomorphic PTLD (classify according to lymphoma classification)

B-cell neoplasms
    Diffuse large B-cell lymphoma
    Burkitt lymphoma
    Plasma cell myeloma
    Plasmacytoma-like lesions
    Other*
T-cell neoplasma
    Peripheral T-cell lymphoma, not otherwise specified
    Other types

4. Hodgkin lymphoma-like PTLD

*Indolent small B-cell lymphomas arising in transplant recipients are not included among the PTLD.

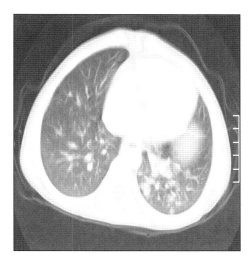

Fig. 23-35. Post-transplant lymphoproliferative disease. Lung nodules after liver transplant: a 5-year-old boy 23 months after orthotopic liver transplant had adeno-tonsillar hypertrophy, pulmonary nodules, and mediastinal adenopathy. Biopsy showed polymorphic, polyclonal hyperplasia with CD20+ EBER+ B cells. He was treated with rituximab with a complete response. (Courtesy of Dr. H. E. Heslop.)

lymphomas, most frequently B cell but occasionally T cell. They are classified by WHO as shown in Table 23-8. Figures 23-35 and 23-36 show an examples of polymorphic, hyperplasia with CD20+, EBER+ B cells. Figures 23-37 to 23-40 are examples of monomorphic, monoclonal B-cell lymphomas.

Treatment of these disorders can be with rituximab (anti-CD20), chemotherapy, or specific anti-EBV cytotoxic T lymphocytes (Fig. 23-41). Withdrawal of immunosuppressive therapy is also helpful, particularly when the proliferation is polyclonal.

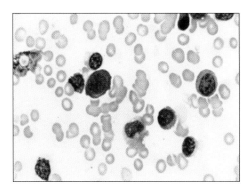

Fig. 23-37. Post-transplant lymphoproliferative disease: blood film with circulating EBV-transformed lymphoid cells. A 3-year-old girl 64 days following a T-cell–depleted unrelated stem cell transplant had fevers and an EBV DNA greater than 100,000 copies/μL peripheral blood. On examination of a blood film she had circulating B lymphoblasts, which were LMP1 (EBV viral antigen) positive by immunostaining. (Courtesy of Dr. H. E. Heslop.)

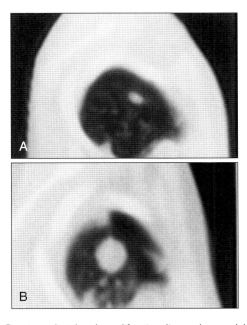

Fig. 23-38. Post-transplant lymphoproliferative disease: lung nodule after bone marrow transplant (BMT). A 3-year-old boy 8 months after a T-cell–depleted transplant from a mismatch family member had fevers and lymphadenopathy. A computed tomography (CT) scan showed pulmonary nodules, and biopsy confirmed diffuse large B-cell lymphoma, and EBV was detected in the tumor by amplification of viral DNA with the polymerase chain reaction and by immunofluorescence staining for the viral antigen LMP-1. He attained complete remission after infusion of donor cells. (Courtesy of Dr. H. E. Heslop.)

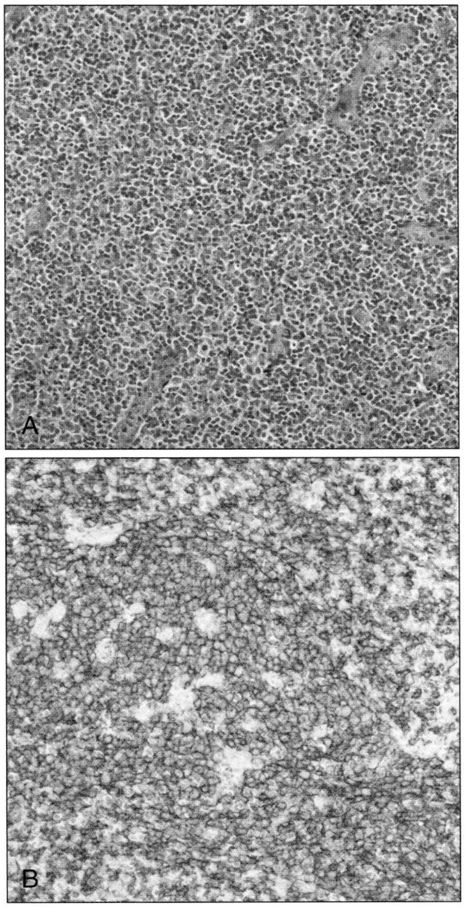

Fig. 23-36. Post-transplant lymphoproliferative disease (PTLD): a 2-year-old girl with tonsillar and pulmonary PTLD 18 months following cardiac transplantation for congenital dilated cardiomyopathy. The cells were EBV positive but polymorphic. (*A,* H&E stain; *B,* CD20 stain.) (Courtesy of Dr. P. Amrolia and Dr. N. Sabire.)

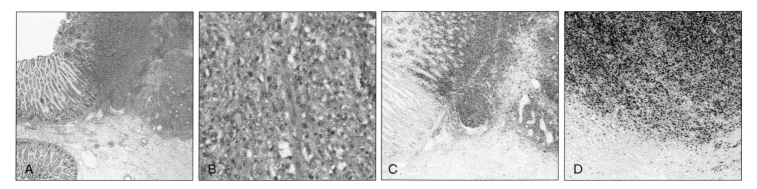

Fig. 23-39. Posttransplant lymphoproliferative disease: male 17-year-old 5 months after renal transplantation had small bowel perforation caused by diffuse large B-cell lymphoma. **A,** Low-power view of lymphoid mass invading small bowel. **B,** High-power view of lymphoid mass. **C,** Immunostaining for CD20. **D,** EBV-ISH (in situ hybridization) stain showing the tumor cells are positive for EBV. (Courtesy of Dr. P. Amrolia and Dr. N. Sebire.)

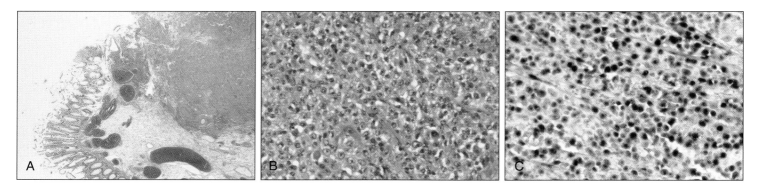

Fig. 23-40. Posttransplant lymphoproliferative disease: 12-year-old boy 8 months after bilateral lung transplantation for cystic fibrosis had colonic perforation. **A,** Low-power view of tumor invading large bowel. **B,** High-power view of tumor showing diffuse, large cell lymphoblast replacement. **C,** EBV-ISH stain showing the tumor cells are positive for EBV. (Courtesy of Dr. P. Amrolia and Dr. N. Sebire.)

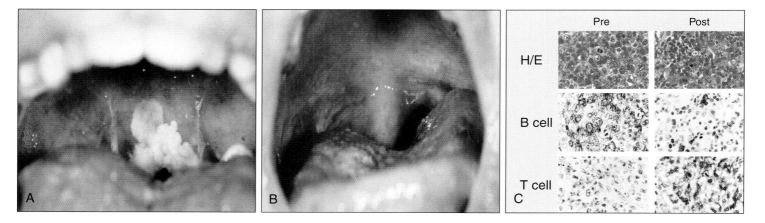

Fig. 23-41. Posttransplant lymphoproliferative disease. **A,** A 12-year-old boy 7 months after HLA-matched unrelated bone marrow transplantation had massive lymphadenopathy and respiratory obstruction. **B,** He was treated with EBV-specific cytotoxic T lymphocytes (CTLs). All symptoms resolved and he remained in remission 4 years later. **C,** Tumor biopsies before and after CTL therapy. (Courtesy of Dr. H. E. Heslop, with permission, Rooney CM, et al. *Blood* 92:1549–1555, 1998.)

VASCULAR AND PLATELET BLEEDING DISORDERS

The mechanism of normal hemostasis involves the interaction of blood vessels, platelets, and coagulation factors (Fig. 24-1). The initial arrest of hemorrhage is the result of vasoconstriction and the elastic recoil of severed blood vessels, together with the formation of platelet plugs. This is followed by activation of blood coagulation factors, which convert the fluid blood into an insoluble fibrin clot, reinforcing the sealing effect (Fig. 24-2). The coagulation cascade is detailed in Chapter 25.

The main function of the intact vessel wall is to prevent hemostasis and platelet aggregation (Fig. 24-3). A number of substances produced by the endothelium cause vasodilatation (e.g., nitric oxide), inhibit platelet aggregation (e.g., prostacyclin or epoprostenol) or blood

coagulation (e.g., antithrombin and protein C activator), or activate fibrinolysis (e.g., tissue plasminogen activator). Von Willebrand's factor (VWF), necessary for platelet–cell wall interaction, is also produced. VWF is expressed in endothelial cells, stored in Weibel-Palade bodies (Fig. 24-4). When the cells are activated, the VWF multimers form a long "string" to which platelets attach (Fig. 24-5). The change of

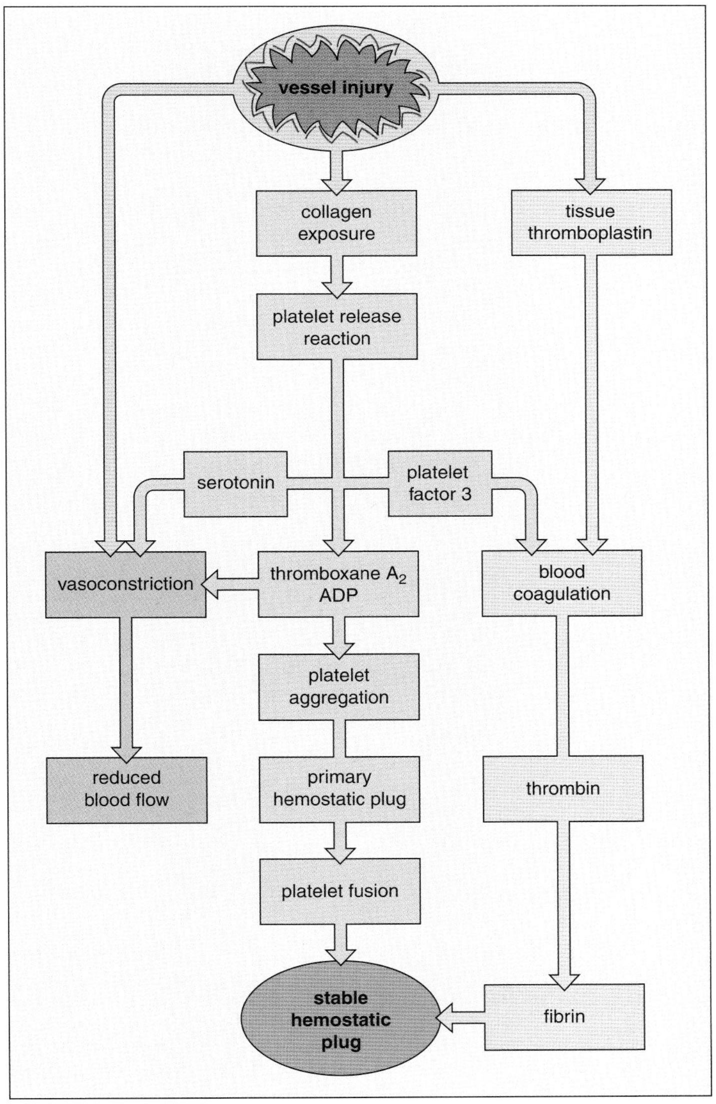

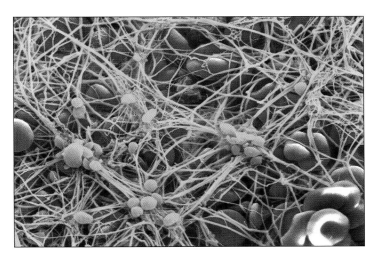

Fig. 24-2. Colorized scanning electron micrograph of a whole blood clot formed in vitro. Platelets are violet, fibrin fibers are light blue, and erythrocytes are red. (Image courtesy of Dr. Yuri I. Veklich and Dr. John W. Weisel, Department of Cell and Developmental Biology, University of Pennsylvania School of Medicine, Philadelphia.)

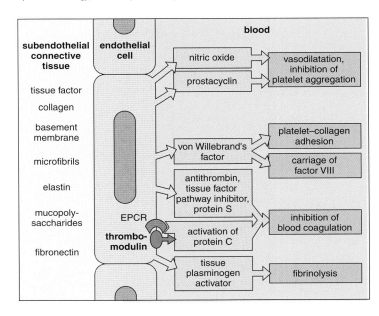

Fig. 24-3. Function of intact vessel wall: the endothelial cell forms a barrier between platelet and plasma clotting factors, and subendothelial connective tissues. Endothelial cells produce a variety of substances that cause vasodilation, inhibit hemostasis or platelet aggregation, or activate fibrinolysis. EPCR, endothelial protein C receptor.

Fig. 24-1. Normal hemostasis: mechanisms.

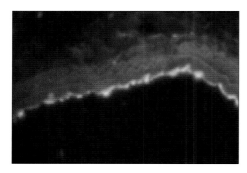

Fig. 24-4. Immunofluorescent staining with polyclonal anti-VWF antibodies of a cross section of mouse carotid artery. VWF is expressed only in endothelial cells, and stored in Weibel-Palade bodies; it exhibits a granular distribution. (Courtesy of Professor M. Hoylaerts.)

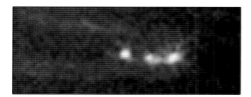

Fig. 24-5. Platelet–von Willebrand's factor adherence. Endothelial cells have been activated by the calcium ionophore A23187 and superfused with platelets. The strings of platelets adhere to the long VWF multimers retained on endothelial cells. The shear forces on the platelets caused by flowing blood stretch VWF threads. (Courtesy of Professor M. Hoylaerts.)

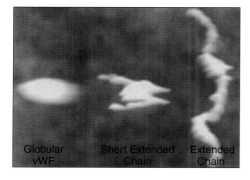

Fig. 24-6. Von Willebrand's factor atomic force microscopy (AFM) shows a globular structure under negligible shear; shear forces applied by the AFM probe tip cause protein unfolding, giving VWF a short extended chain information. With a more extended and severe shear stress, VWF has an extended conformation. (Courtesy of Siedlecki CA et al: Shear-dependent changes in the three-dimensional structure of human von Willebrand factor, *Blood* 88:2939-2950, 1996.)

VWF from a globular to unfolded protein in an extended chain under shear strain is visualized in Fig. 24-6. A break in the vessel wall exposes clotting factors and platelets to the subendothelial connective tissue.

The platelet has a trilamellar surface membrane that invaginates into the cytoplasm to form an open canalicular system, giving a large surface (platelet factor 3) to which clotting factors may adsorb (Fig. 24-7). A mucopolysaccharide coat outside the membrane is important in platelet adhesion to the vessel wall and in aggregation and adsorption of clotting factors, especially fibrinogen and factor VIII. Glycoproteins (GPs) on the platelet surface include GP Ib (defective in Bernard-Soulier syndrome) and GP IIb–IIIa (defective in thrombasthenia). Both sites are important in the attachment of platelets to VWF and, hence, to vascular endothelium (Fig. 24-8). The binding site for GP IIb–IIIa is also the receptor for fibrinogen and, after conformational change, leads to platelet-platelet aggregation.

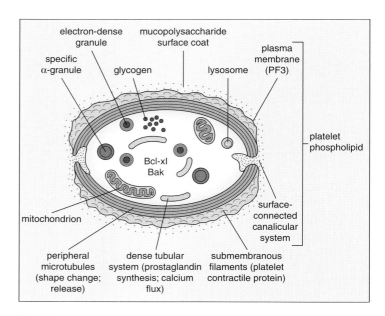

Fig. 24-7. Ultrastructure of a platelet: electron-dense granules contain adenine nucleotides, calcium, and serotonin; specific α-granules contain growth factors, for example, PDGF, fibrinogen, factors V and VIII and von Willebrand's factor, fibronectin, β-thromboglobulin (TGF-β), plasminogen, thrombospondin, vascular endothelial growth factor (VEGF) A and C, and chemokines and proteases; lysosomes contain acid hydrolases; the plasma membrane is the site of receptors for clotting factors and aggregating agents. The ratio of BCL-XL to BAK determines the platelet life span (see text).

A submembranous microtubular system maintains the platelet shape; microfilaments distributed throughout the cytoplasm (including a complex mixture of muscle proteins) are involved in changes in platelet contraction and secretion, and clot retraction. The platelets also contain a number of organelles, including α-granules, which contain a variety of proteins (see Fig. 24-7): dense bodies (δ-granules), which contain calcium, adenine nucleotides, and serotonin; lysosomes, which contain acid hydrolases; peroxisomes, which contain catalase; mitochondria; and a dense tubular system that contains substantial quantities of calcium and may be a site of synthesis of prostaglandins and thromboxane A2.

The life span of the platelet is determined by the relative activity of pro-apoptotic and anti-apoptotic BCL-2 proteins, principally by the ratio of BAK (pro-apoptotic) and the pro-survival protein BCL-xl. In young platelets BAK is held in check by BCL-xl, but as the platelet

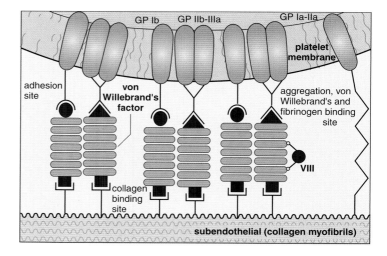

Fig. 24-8. Adhesion of platelets to vascular endothelium: this is mediated by von Willebrand's factor, which also carries factor VIII coagulation factor (VIII:C). There are two binding sites on the platelet membrane for von Willebrand's factor: GP Ib and GP IIb–IIIa complex (see also Fig. 25-32). The GP Ia-IIa complex attaches directly to subendothelial collagen.

ages in the circulation, there is loss of the less stable Bcl-xl protein and Bak initiates cell death by apoptosis.

The platelet attaches to subendothelial structures of damaged vessels, initially via attachment to VWF (see Fig. 24-5), which has binding sites for collagen microfibrils in the exposed subendothelium. The GP Ia-IIa complex attaches to collagen.

Bleeding disorders may be the result of abnormalities in blood vessels, qualitative or quantitative defects of blood platelets (discussed in this chapter), or deficiencies of blood coagulation factors (discussed in Chapter 25).

Disorders of platelets and small blood vessels manifest as purpuras with pronounced cutaneous and mucosal bleeding, either petechial or multiple small ecchymoses. Prolonged bleeding from superficial cuts and abrasions is a feature of thrombocytopenia and disorders of platelet function. Gastrointestinal bleeding may occur. Menorrhagia is often the dominant clinical problem of women with severe thrombocytopenia or von Willebrand's disease. Deep hematomas and hemarthroses are rare. Repeated hemarthroses, deep dissecting hematomas, and serious delayed excessive post-traumatic bleeding are characteristic of severe deficiencies of blood coagulation factors (see Chapter 25). Initial hemostasis, in these cases, may be accomplished by vascular reaction and platelet plugs.

VASCULAR BLEEDING DISORDERS

Disorders associated with vascular bleeding are listed in Table 24-1.

TABLE 24-1. ABNORMAL VASCULAR BLEEDING: ASSOCIATED DISORDERS.

Hereditary
Hereditary hemorrhagic telangiectasia
Ehlers–Danlos syndrome
Marfan's syndrome
Osteogenesis imperfecta
Fabry's syndrome
Infections
Bacterial
Viral
Rickettsial
Allergic
Henoch–Schönlein syndrome
Systemic lupus erythematosus
Drugs
Food
Atrophic
Senile purpura
Cushing's syndrome and corticosteroid therapy
Scurvy purpura
Dysproteinemia
Amyloid
Miscellaneous
Simple easy bruising
Factitious
Autoerythrocyte sensitization
Fat embolism

HEREDITARY HEMORRHAGIC TELANGIECTASIA (OSLER-WEBER-RENDU SYNDROME)

The small vascular malformations that are the essential lesion in hereditary hemorrhagic telangiectasia may be confused with petechiae. These bright red or purple spots are permanent and most noticeable on the face, nose, lips, and tongue, and on plantar and palmar surfaces (Figs. 24-9 to 24-11). Usually the lesions do not appear until adulthood, becoming more numerous with advancing age. Bleeding from the telangiectasia of the gastrointestinal mucosa produces a state of chronic severe iron deficiency.

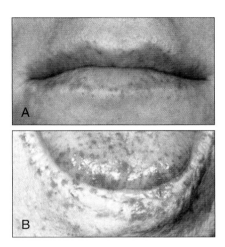

Fig. 24-9. Hereditary hemorrhagic telangiectasia: the characteristic small vascular lesions are obvious on **(A)** lips and **(B)** tongue.

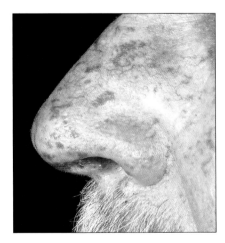

Fig. 24-10. Hereditary hemorrhagic telangiectasia: characteristic vascular malformations in the skin of the nose.

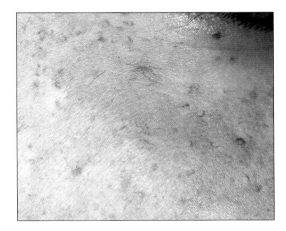

Fig. 24-11. Hereditary hemorrhagic telangiectasia: close-up view of the linear and punctate vascular lesions.

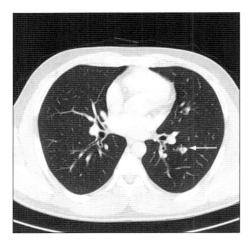

Fig. 24-12. Hereditary hemorrhagic telangiectasia: arteriovenous fistula in the lung (arrow).

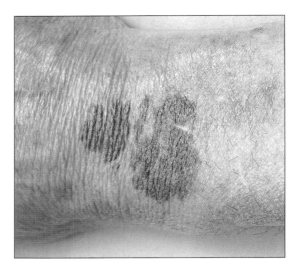

Fig. 24-14. Senile purpura: typical ecchymoses on the extensor surface of the wrist of an elderly man.

Hepatic and splenic arteriovenous shunts, as well as intracranial, aortic, and splenic aneurysms, may develop; pulmonary arteriovenous fistulas (see Fig. 24-12) are associated with oxygen desaturation, hemoptysis, and paradoxic emboli to the brain. This form of the disease is due to an abnormality of the endothelial protein endoglin, the gene being on chromosome 9. Other faults include defects of the gene on chromosome 12q 12 coding for the activin receptor-like kinase, a receptor for TGF-β ligands.

EHLERS-DANLOS SYNDROME

In Ehlers-Danlos syndrome the purpura arises from defective platelet aggregation because of an inherited abnormality of skin collagen. It is most marked in Type IV Ehlers-Danlos syndrome (Fig. 24-13), in which deficiency of Type III collagen occurs.

SENILE PURPURA

Relative indolent purpuric ecchymoses are found frequently in the elderly, particularly on areas of skin exposed to sunlight—for example, on the backs of the hands and wrists (Fig. 24-14), the extensor surfaces of the forearms, and the back of the neck. This condition

may be caused by atrophy of dermal collagen and loss of subcutaneous fat, weakening the supporting tissue of the small blood vessels of the skin, which then become more susceptible to shear strain.

SCURVY

Petechiae of perifollicular distribution (Fig. 24-15) are a feature of scurvy, probably because of a defect in the microvascular supporting tissue. Disordered platelet function may also be present.

PURPURA ASSOCIATED WITH ABNORMAL PROTEINS

Petechiae and ecchymoses may be seen in patients with multiple myeloma (Fig. 24-16), Waldenström's macroglobulinemia, benign monoclonal gammopathy, cryoglobulinemia, or cryofibrinogenemia. Many of the proteins involved in these conditions interfere with platelet function and fibrin formation.

Small vessel hemorrhages may also result from hyperviscosity of blood or from damage to the vessel on precipitation of these proteins in the cooler parts of the skin. Similarly, patients with amyloidosis may show purpura caused by deposition of amyloid in the microcirculation (Fig. 24-17).

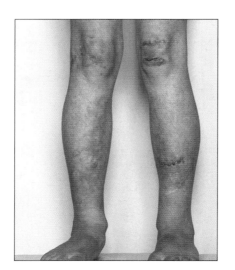

Fig. 24-13. Ehlers-Danlos syndrome: purpura into scars of the skin, especially around the knees, of a 16-year-old boy who also displayed hyperextensible joints, thin, easily torn skin, and poor healing. The scars are raised into folds by the underlying bulging subcutaneous tissues. (Courtesy of Dr. I. Sarkany.)

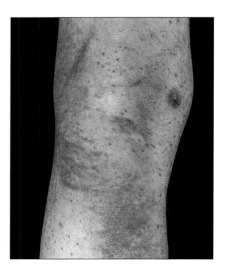

Fig. 24-15. Scurvy: widespread petechial perifollicular hemorrhages becoming confluent. Deeper hematomas were also present.

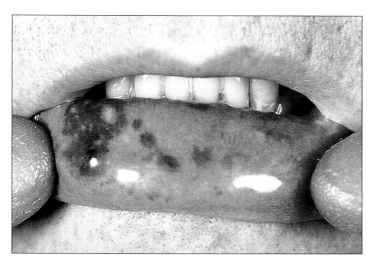

Fig. 24-16. Multiple myeloma: purpuric hemorrhages in the mucosal surface of the lower lip.

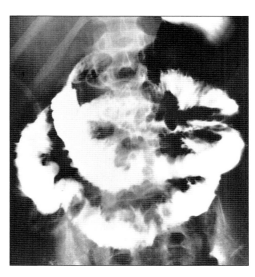

Fig. 24-19. Allergic purpura: radiograph of Henoch-Schönlein syndrome with mucosal bleeding in the small intestine, indicated by the characteristic "thumbprint" appearance of the barium pattern.

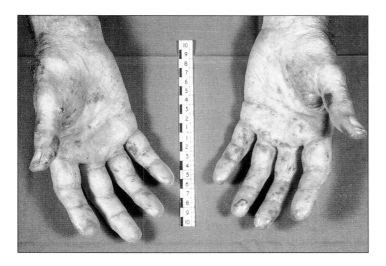

Fig. 24-17. Amyloidosis: purpura of the skin with characteristic smooth yellowish deposits secondary to multiple myeloma.

ALLERGIC PURPURAS

The skin lesions in the allergic purpuras are more variable. Petechiae and ecchymoses associated with the Henoch-Schönlein syndrome may be accompanied by itching, tingling sensations, erythema, and urticarial swelling. The lesions occur most commonly on the buttocks and legs (Fig. 24-18). In this syndrome there may be associated submucosal hemorrhage in the intestine (Fig. 24-19), hematuria, and joint pain.

Some allergic drug reactions manifest as erythematous and purpuric skin eruptions (Fig. 24-20). The lesions may be generalized or may have a symmetric proximal distribution. Extensive purpuric bleeding may also accompany severe vasculitis, as in systemic lupus erythematosus (SLE; Figs. 24-21 and 24-22) and other connective tissue disorders.

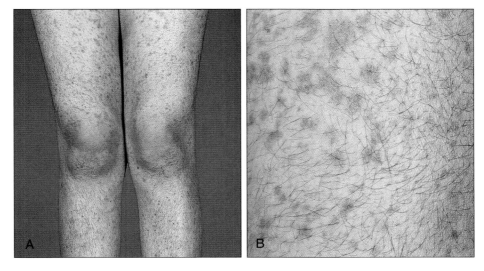

Fig. 24-18. Allergic purpura: **(A)** extensive purpura of the skin of the legs in Henoch-Schönlein syndrome; **(B)** the early lesions are more an urticarial erythema than true petechial hemorrhage.

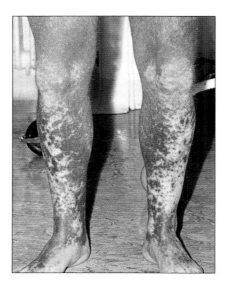

Fig. 24-20. Allergic purpura: symmetric widespread erythematous and purpuric eruption as a hypersensitivity reaction to allopurinol.

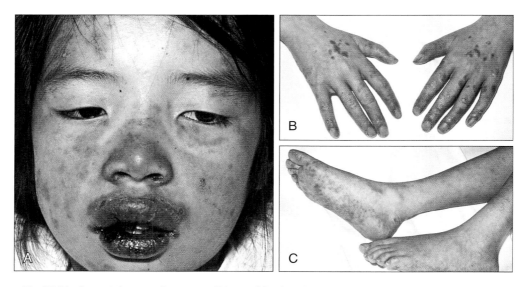

Fig. 24-21. Systemic lupus erythematosus: **(A)** typical fixed erythematous reaction over the "butterfly" area of the face, and mucosal hemorrhage from the petechial lesions of the nasal and oral mucous membranes; skin of **(B)** the hands and **(C)** feet of the same patient shows erythematous and purpuric lesions. (A, B, Courtesy of Dr. M. D. Holdaway.)

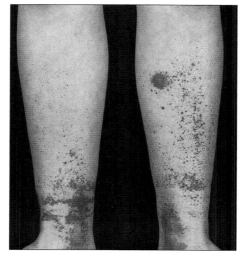

Fig. 24-22. Systemic lupus erythematosus: purpuric lesions over the shins of a 17-year-old girl (platelet count normal).

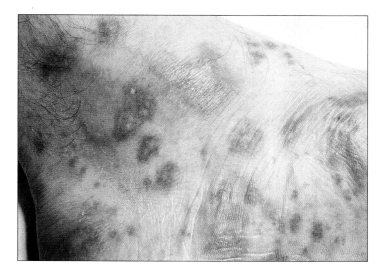

Fig. 24-23. Meningococcal septicemia: typical purpuric skin lesions around the ankle in acute fulminating disease with disseminated intravascular coagulation.

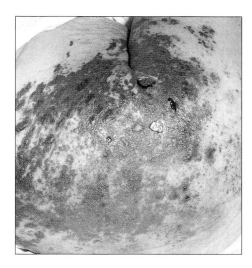

Fig. 24-24. Herpes zoster: hemorrhagic herpetic skin eruption over the lower back and upper thigh (lateral view) in a patient with acute leukemia.

PURPURA ASSOCIATED WITH INFECTION

Purpura associated with infection may be the result of toxic damage to the endothelium or of immune complex–type hypersensitivity. In some conditions, for example, meningococcal septicemia (Fig. 24-23), disseminated intravascular coagulation (DIC) is often associated. There may be extensive bleeding into the vesicular lesions of herpes zoster in patients with leukemia (Fig. 24-24), and petechial hemorrhage of the palate in infectious mononucleosis (Fig. 24-25).

The rare condition known as purpura fulminans is characterized by the widespread development of painful, large, confluent, and necrotic ecchymoses (Fig. 24-26). Almost any area of skin may be involved, but the face, extremities, buttocks, and lower back are often the worst affected. Its occurrence is usually in children who are recovering from scarlet fever, varicella, or other infections; in such cases it may result from the development of antibodies to protein C or protein S, or from excess consumption of them. Congenital deficiencies of protein C, protein S, or antithrombin in humans also underlie these conditions. Some patients have shown evidence of associated DIC with thrombocytopenia and coagulation factor deficiencies.

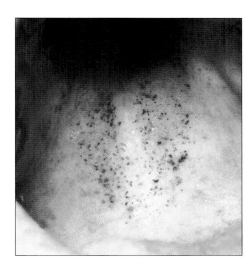

Fig. 24-25. Infectious mononucleosis: extensive petechiae in the mucosa of the palate.

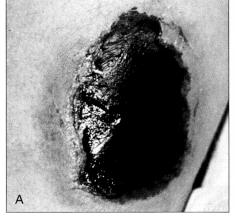
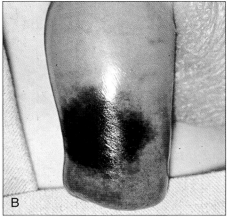

Fig. 24-26. Purpura fulminans: large necrotic ecchymoses of skin of **(A)** the leg and **(B)** penis of an infant, following varicella infection. (A, B, Courtesy of Dr. M. D. Holdaway.)

TABLE 24-2. THROMBOCYTOPENIA: CAUSES—
(A) INHERITED

Syndrome	Gene mutation	Chromosomal location inheritance
MYH9-related diseases May–Hegglin anomaly, Fechtner, Epstein and Sebastian syndromes	MYH9	22q11 (AD)
Mediterranean macrothrombocytopenia	*GPIBA*, possibly others	17per-p12 (AD)
Bernard–Soulier syndrome	*GPIBA*, *GP1BB, GP9*	22q11.2, 3q21, 17, 22, and 3 (AR)
DiGeorge/Velocardiofacial syndrome	Hemizygous microdeletion including *GP1BB*	22q11 (AD)
Familial platelet disorder/acute myeloid leukemia	*RUNX1 (CBFA2, AML1)*	21q22.2 (AD)
Chromosome10/THC2	*FLI14813*	10p12-11.2 (AD)
Paris–Trousseau/Jacobsen syndromes	Hemizygous deletion including FLI1	11q23 (AD)
Gray platelet syndrome	Unknown	Unknown Mostly recessive
Congenital amegakaryocytic thrombocytopenia	*c-MPL*	z1p34 (AR)
Thrombocytopenia and absent radii (TAR)	Unknown, c-Mpl signaling	Unknown (AR)
Thrombocytopenia with radio-ulnar synostosis	*HOXA11*	7p15-p14.2 (AD)
Wiskott–Aldrich syndrome	*WAS*	Xp11.23-p11.22 X-linked
X-linked thrombo-cytopenia (XLT)	*WAS*	Xp11.23-p11.22
GATA-1-related thrombo-cytopenia with dyserythropoiesis	*GATA1*	Xp11.23 X-linked

AD = autosomal dominant AR = autosomal recessive

A

TABLE 24-2. (B) ACQUIRED

Failure of platelet production

Generalized bone marrow failure
  Leukemia; myelodysplasia; aplastic anemia; human immunodeficiency virus (HIV) infection; myelofibrosis; megaloblastic anemia; uremia; multiple myeloma; marrow infiltration (e.g., carcinoma, lymphoma), cytotoxic chemotherapy

Selective megakaryocyte depression
  Drugs; alcohol; chemicals; viral infections

Hereditary thrombocytopenias

Abnormal distribution of platelets

Splenomegaly

Increased destruction of platelets

Immune
  Alloantibodies – neonatal; post-transfusion
  Autoantibodies – primary; secondary (e.g., systemic lupus erythematosus, chronic lymphocytic leukemia, post-infection, HIV infection, post-stem cell transplantation

Drug induced
  Immune or because of platelet aggregation

Disseminated intravascular coagulation

Microangiopathic processes
  Hemolytic–uremic syndrome; thrombotic thrombocytopenic purpura; extracorporeal circulation; HELPP (hemolysis, elevated liver enzymes and low platelet count in association with pre-eclampsia) syndrome; post-stem cell transplantation
Giant hemangioma (Kasabach–Merritt syndrome)

Dilutional loss

Massive transfusion of stored blood

B

TABLE 24-3. ABNORMAL PLATELET FUNCTION: CAUSES

Inherited

Plasma membrane defects
  Thrombasthenia (Glanzmann's)
  Bernard–Soulier syndrome
  Scott syndrome

Disorders of platelet granules
  Idiopathic dense granule disorders (δ-storage pool disease)
  Hermansky–Pudlak syndrome
  Wiskott–Aldrich and Chediak–Higashki syndrome
  α-granule disorders
    gray platelet syndrome
    Paris–Trousseau or Jacobsen syndrome
    Quebec platelet syndrome
    arthrogryposis–renal dysfunction–cholestasis (ARC) syndrome
  α- and dense-granule disorders

Disorders of receptors and signal transduction
  Cyclo-oxygenase deficiency
  Thromboxane synthase deficiency
  Thromboxane A2 receptor defect
  ADP receptor defect (P2 Y12)

A

Acquired

Myeloproliferative disorders

Myelodysplastic syndromes

Acute myeloid leukemia

Dysproteinemias

Uremia

Acquired storage pool deficiency
  Disseminated intravascular coagulation; hemolytic-uremic syndrome; thrombotic, thrombocytopenic purpura; disseminated autoimmune disease
  Acquired von Willebrand's disease

Drugs
  e.g., aspirin; dipyridamole; sulfinpyrazone; prostacyclin; imipramine; non-steroidal anti-inflammatory

B

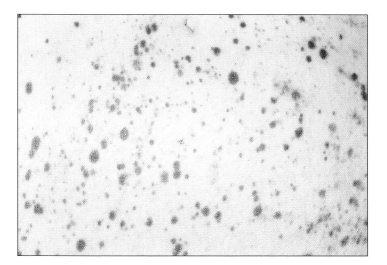

Fig. 24-27. Thrombocytopenia: abdominal skin purpura in myelodysplastic syndrome. The platelets are often functionally abnormal, as well as reduced in number.

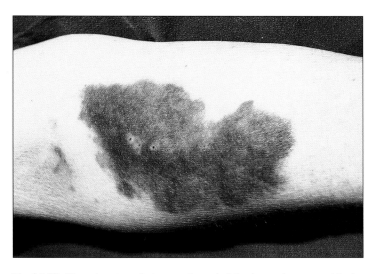

Fig. 24-28. Thrombocytopenia: large ecchymosis following performance of the Ivy bleeding-time test. The puncture marks of the stylet cutter are clearly seen.

PLATELET BLEEDING DISORDERS

The most common cause of abnormal bleeding is a platelet disorder caused by either reduced numbers of platelets (thrombocytopenia; Table 24-2) or defective platelet function (Table 24-3). It is characterized by spontaneous skin purpura (Fig. 24-27), mucosal hemorrhage, and prolonged bleeding after trauma (Fig. 24-28).

THROMBOCYTOPENIA

Failure to produce platelets is the most common cause of thrombocytopenia. Drug toxicity or viral infections may result in selective megakaryocyte depression, whereas in aplastic anemia, leukemia, myelofibrosis, cytotoxic chemotherapy, or marrow infiltrations, decreased numbers of megakaryocytes may be part of a generalized bone marrow failure. Congenital deficiency of megakaryocytes can occur, in many cases with associated skeletal, renal, or cardiac malformations—bilateral aplasia of the radii being the most common associated abnormality (Fig. 24-29).

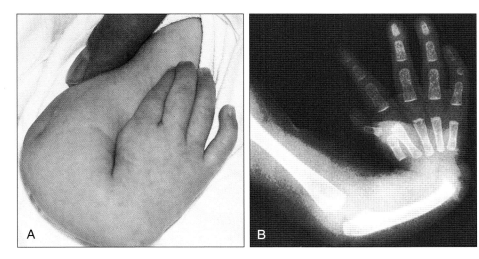

Fig. 24-29. Thrombocytopenia with absent radii syndrome: **(A)** the characteristic flexion deformity; **(B)** radiography shows complete absence of the radius.

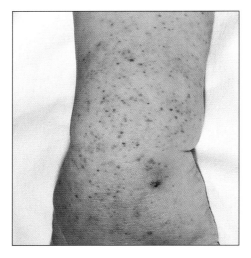

Fig. 24-30. Wiskott-Aldrich syndrome: eczema and skin purpura in an infant. (Courtesy of Dr. U. O'Callaghan.)

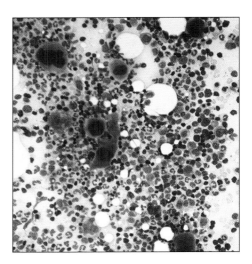

Fig. 24-32. Immune thrombocytopenia: bone marrow aspirate showing increased numbers of megakaryocytes.

Neonatal thrombocytopenia occurs in newborn infants as a result of intrauterine rubella or other infections, platelet antibodies, DIC, hereditary thrombocytopenias, giant hemangioma, or congenital absence of megakaryocytes. Among the variety of hereditary thrombocytopenias, in the Wiskott-Aldrich syndrome there is associated immunodeficiency and eczema (Fig. 24-30); in some, such as the Bernard-Soulier syndrome, abnormalities of platelet morphology and function also occur (see Fig. 24-42), whereas other syndromes are better known for the associated abnormalities (e.g., May-Hegglin, Chédiak-Higashi; see Chapter 10).

IMMUNE THROMBOCYTOPENIC PURPURA

In immune thrombocytopenic purpura (ITP), a relatively common disorder, platelet sensitization with autoantibodies (usually immunoglobulin G [IgG]) leads to their premature removal from the circulation by cells of the reticuloendothelial system. Megakaryopoiesis may also be impaired; plasma levels of thrombopoietin (TPO) are normal or only slightly increased. Patients have petechial hemorrhage, easy bruising, or menorrhagia. The blood film shows reduced numbers of platelets, which are often large (Fig. 24-31), and the bone marrow has increased numbers of megakaryocytes (Fig. 24-32).

The disease may occur alone (primary) or be accompanied by autoimmune hemolytic anemia (Evans' syndrome). Also, ITP may occur in patients with other diseases, such as SLE (Fig. 24-33), human immunodeficiency virus infection, and chronic lymphocytic leukemia, and following stem cell transplantation.

Initial treatment is with high-dose corticosteroids; splenectomy may be performed in patients who do not respond to corticosteroids or who relapse when corticosteroids are withdrawn. Sections of splenic tissue show prominent collections of macrophages with lipid-laden cytoplasm (Fig. 24-34). High-dose intravenous immunoglobulin has produced substantial rises in platelets in about 75% of cases of chronic ITP (Fig. 24-35). This therapy is most useful during the later stages of pregnancy to control acute bleeding episodes or in preparation of the patient for surgery, since the improvement is usually only marked for about 4 weeks. It is often valuable in children and infants. The mechanism of action may be either blockage of Fc receptors on macrophages or inhibition of the antiplatelet antibody biosynthesis. Rituximab (anti-CD20), azathiopine and other immunosuppressive drugs are used in refractory cases.

A number of drugs (thrombomimetics) are now in clinical trials that bind to thrombopoietin receptors and stimulate platelet production (Fig. 24-36). These may reduce sensitization with antibody and so peripheral clearance.

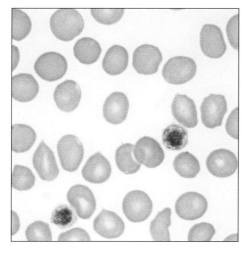

Fig. 24-31. Immune thrombocytopenia: blood film showing two large platelets.

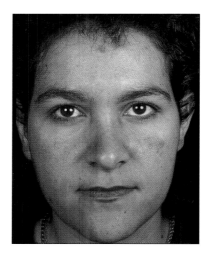

Fig. 24-33. Systemic lupus erythematosus: typical butterfly rash and frontal alopecia in a woman who also suffered from immune thrombocytopenia.

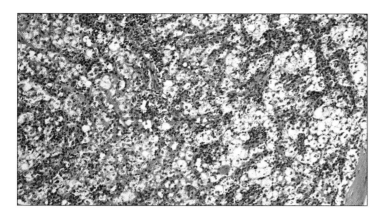

Fig. 24-34. Immune thrombocytopenic purpura: histologic section of spleen showing prominent collections of lipid-filled macrophages caused by excessive breakdown of platelets in the splenic pulp.

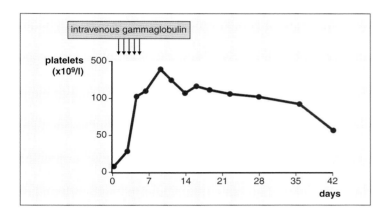

Fig. 24-35. Chronic immune thrombocytopenic purpura: typical response in platelet count to therapy with intravenous high-dose gammaglobulin (IVG) therapy (5-day course; 0.4 g/kg per day).

DRUG-INDUCED IMMUNE THROMBOCYTOPENIA

An allergic mechanism has been demonstrated to be the cause of many drug-induced thrombocytopenias. Rapid removal of platelets from the circulation may result in severe thrombocytopenia, and many patients have mucosal hemorrhage (Fig. 24-37) in addition to skin purpura. Heparin-induced thrombocytopenia (HIT), on the other hand, is associated with thrombosis. It is caused by platelet-activating IgG antibodies that recognize complexes of platelet factor 4 and heparin. There are markedly elevated thrombin/antithrombin complexes with in vivo platelet activation of endothelium and monocytes.

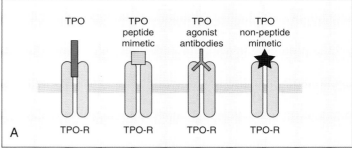
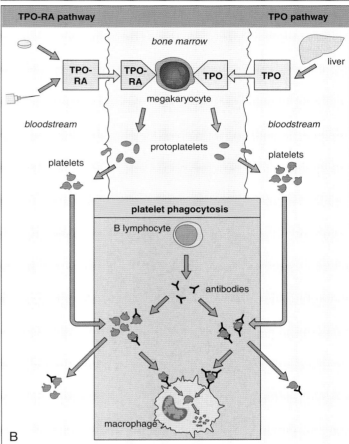

Fig. 24-36. A, Thrombomimetics: pharmaceuticals that activate the thrombopoietin (TPO) receptor by different mechanisms. **B,** Role of thrombopoietin receptor agonists (RAs) in ITP. Stimulation of megakaryocytes with TPO receptor agonists generates larger numbers of platelets and may overcome antibody destruction of megakaryocytes and reduce peripheral destruction of platelets. (Adapted from Cines DB: *Blood* 109:4591, 2007.)

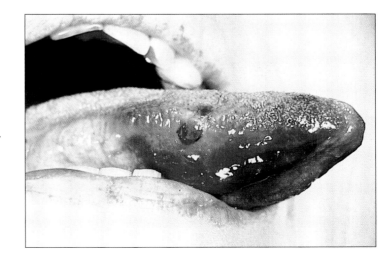

Fig. 24-37. Drug-induced thrombocytopenia: sublingual mucosal hemorrhage.

DISSEMINATED INTRAVASCULAR COAGULATION, THROMBOTIC THROMBOCYTOPENIC PURPURA, AND HEMOLYTIC-UREMIC SYNDROME

In these conditions, thrombocytopenia is the result of increased consumption of platelets. In thrombotic thrombocytopenic purpura (TTP), platelet aggregation and accretion in small blood vessels is widespread (Fig. 24-38), but plasma levels of coagulation factors are normal. The clinical course may be fulminant and fatal, with confluent purpura and ischemic damage to many organs, such as the brain, kidneys, and skin (Figs. 24-39 and 24-40); serum lactate dehydrogenase (LDH) activity is raised, and the majority of patients have an associated microangiopathic hemolytic anemia (see Chapter 8). The acquired form may have no obvious precipitating cause, but some cases follow an infection, occur in pregnancy, or follow allogeneic stem cell transplantation, particularly with cyclosporin use. Inhibitory antibodies against ADAMTS-13 (a disintegrin and metalloprotease with thrombospondin type 1 repeats), a protease that cleaves VWF (Fig. 25-33), occur in the plasma of patients with acute TTP (Fig. 24-41). A familial form of TTP, the Schulman-Lipshaw syndrome, results from mutations of the ADAMTS-13 gene situated on chromosome 9q34. It is characterized by TTP of neonatal onset with response to fresh plasma infusion. An unusual preponderance of large multimers of von Willebrand's factor occurs in the plasma of patients with TTP and of those with hemolytic-uremic syndrome (HUS). It is likely that the unusual large multimers of von Willebrand's factor cause platelet aggregation in the microcirculation in TTP. Treatment is with plasma exchanges, which remove autoantibodies and multimers of von Willebrand's factor, and provide the necessary ADAMTS-13 protease. Antiplatelet drugs, corticosteroids, vincristine, Rituximab, and splenectomy have also been used with varying success.

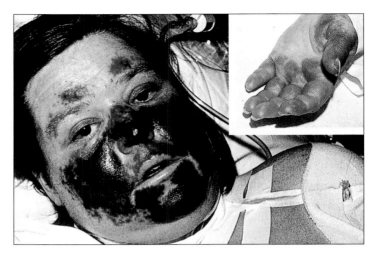

Fig. 24-40. Thrombotic thrombocytopenic purpura: massive area of hemorrhagic necrosis of the facial skin and extensive confluent ecchymoses on the hand (inset).

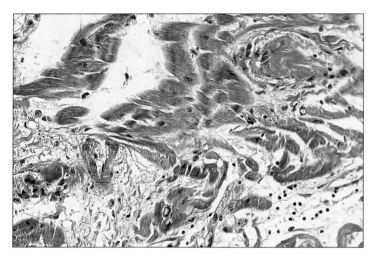

Fig. 24-38. Thrombotic thrombocytopenic purpura: fibrin thrombus (red) in an arteriole of the heart and microthrombi (purple) of von Willebrand's factor aggregate in another vessel. (Martius scarlet blue; courtesy of Professor S. Lucas.)

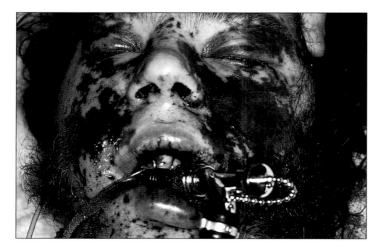

Fig. 24-39. Thrombotic thrombocytopenic purpura: widespread confluent and necrotic ecchymoses of the facial skin.

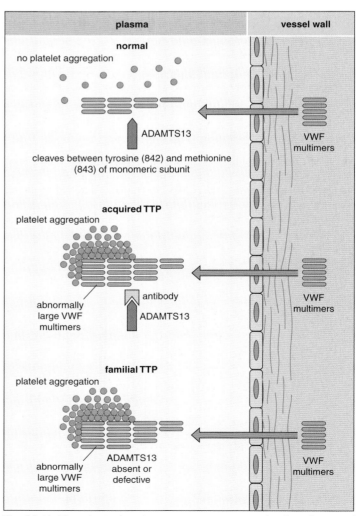

Fig. 24-41. Thrombotic thrombocytopenic purpura: postulated mechanism of how large von Willebrand's factor (VWF) multimers accumulate in plasma because of the lack of protease ADMTS13 as a result of an immune mechanism or a congenital deficiency.

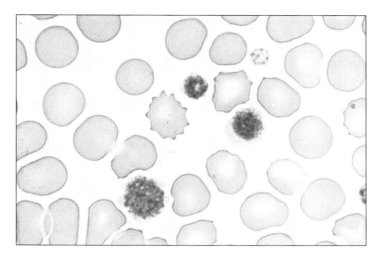

Fig. 24-42. Bernard-Soulier syndrome: blood film showing abnormally large platelets.

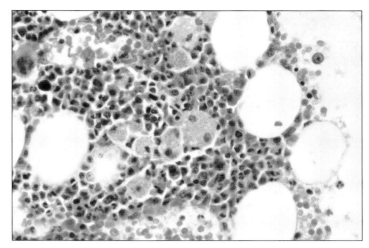

Fig. 24-43. Hermansky-Pudlak syndrome: bone marrow trephine biopsy showing prominent macrophages with ceroid-like pigment-laden cytoplasm. There is a defective platelet function resulting from a storage pool defect caused by dense body deficiency. (Courtesy of Professor E. G. D. Tuddenham.)

Although HUS resembles TTP, it occurs mainly in infants and young children and is characterized by acute anemia, thrombocytopenia, and renal failure. Gastrointestinal symptoms include bloody diarrhea and hypotension, and fits may occur. There is an association with infection by verotoxin-producing organisms, especially *Escherichia coli* O157:H57 strain and *Shigella dysenteriae* types 1 and 24. The protease that cleaves VWF is present.

The HELPP syndrome occurs in late pregnancy and consists of hemolysis, elevated liver enzymes, and low platelet count in association with preeclampsia; DIC may be present.

DISORDERS OF PLATELET FUNCTION

Many of the conditions associated with abnormal platelet function are listed in Table 24-3.

HEREDITARY DISORDERS

The rare inherited disorders of platelet function may, at different phases of the reactions, produce defects in the formation of the hemostatic plug. In thrombasthenia (Glanzmann's disease), primary platelet aggregation fails with all agonists, but platelet count, size, and morphology are normal. There is deficiency of membrane GP IIb/IIIa (gene 17q 21.32), on which receptors for fibrinogen and VWF are normally exposed during aggregation (see Fig. 24-8).

In Bernard-Soulier syndrome the platelets are large (Fig. 24-42) and are deficient in a surface GP (Ib) necessary for interaction between platelets and VWF (see Fig. 24-8); there is defective adhesion and diminished availability of platelet phospholipid.

In the Hermansky-Pudlak syndrome (HPS), defective platelet aggregation is associated with oculocutaneous albinism and the accumulation of ceroid-like pigment in bone marrow, intestinal, and pulmonary macrophages, which may lead to pulmonary fibrosis (Fig. 24-43). It is a genetically heterogeneous autosomal recessive disease of proteins involved in vesicle formation and trafficking. Mutations in at least eight genes have been described: HPS1, AP3B1 (HPS2), HPS3, HPS4, HPS5, HPS6, DTNBP1 (HPS7), and BLOC1S3 (HPS8). In the HPS2 variety, which is associated with neutropenia, there are genetic defects of the protein AP3B1, which encodes the β-subunit of the heterotetrameric AP3 adapter protein complex. AP3 directs posttranslational trafficking of the intraluminal "cargo" proteins from the trans Golgi network to lysosomes. There is defective platelet granule formation and defective platelet aggregation with collagen, ristocetin, and arachidonic acid. There is storage pool deficiency due to dense body deficiency.

In storage pool disorders (SPDs), defective platelet aggregation (Fig. 24-44) results from an intrinsic deficiency in the number of dense granules (δ-SPD). One type of SPD, the gray platelet syndrome, is characterized by variable thrombocytopenia and large platelets that have a specific deficiency of α-granules (α-SPD) (Fig. 24-45).

Fig. 24-44. Storage pool disease: platelet aggregation studies show defective primary and secondary aggregation with adenosine diphosphate, adrenaline, and collagen. (Courtesy of Dr. R. A. Hutton.)

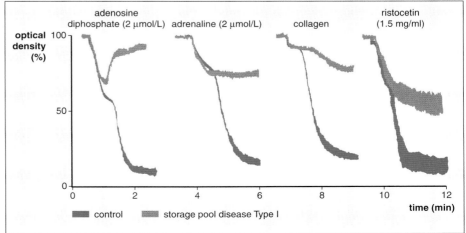

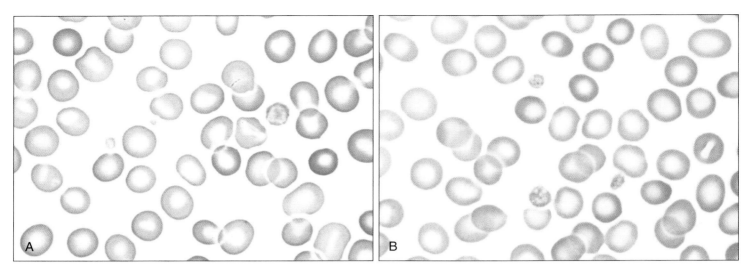

Fig. 24-45. Gray platelet syndrome. **A, B,** Typical large platelets that lack normal α-granules. (*A, B,* Courtesy of Dr. P. C. Shrivastava.)

In the ARC syndrome (Fig. 24-46), there is defective platelet aggregation with arachidonate and ADP. Mutations of VPS33B a Secl/Munc 18 protein involved in intracellular vesicle trafficking underlie the syndrome. Platelet α-granules are absent.

Von Willebrand's disease is due to an inherited quantitative deficiency or functional abnormality of Von Willebrand's factor (see Fig. 25-32). This results in defective platelet adhesion and defective in vitro aggregation activity with, for example, ristocetin (Fig. 24-47).

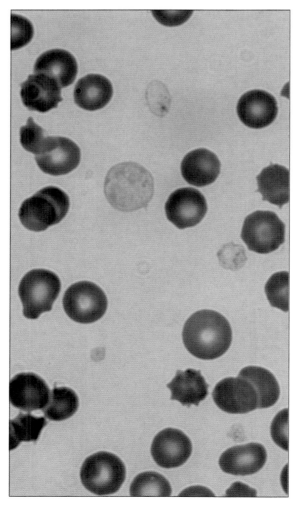

Fig. 24-46. ARC (arthrogryposis, renal dysfunction, and cholestasis) syndrome: platelets appear large and pale, with aberrant α-granules. (Courtesy of Professor W. H. A. Kahr.)

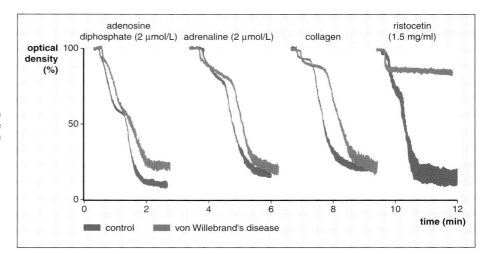

Fig. 24-47. Von Willebrand's disease: platelet aggregation studies show normal aggregation patterns with adenosine diphosphate, adrenaline, and collagen, but no aggregation with ristocetin. (Courtesy of Dr. R. A. Hutton.)

ACQUIRED DISORDERS

Intrinsic abnormalities of platelet function are found in many patients with essential thrombocythemia and other myeloproliferative diseases, uremia, liver disease, and hyperglobulinemia. Aspirin and other nonsteroidal antiinflammatory drugs produce a platelet functional defect (Fig. 24-48), which often manifests as abnormal bleeding time; however, spontaneous hemorrhage during therapy, except for gastric mucosal bleeding caused by erosions, is not common. Antiplatelet drugs (usually aspirin or clopidogel) are used in the prevention of thrombosis, which reduces the risk of recurrence of myocardial infarct or of stroke in patients with transient ischemic attacks.

Antiplatelet drugs that block the GP IIa–IIIb receptor (Fig. 24-49)—one of the integrin adhesion molecule receptors—are used in the setting of percutaneous coronary intervention or acute coronary syndrome in patients on aspirin.

Fig. 24-48. Sites of action of antiplatelet drugs: aspirin acetylates the enzyme cyclo-oxygenase irreversibly. Sulfinpyrazone inhibits cyclo-oxygenase reversibly. Dipyridamole inhibits phosphodiesterase, increases cyclic adenosine monophosphate levels, and inhibits aggregation. Inhibition of adenosine uptake by red cells allows adenosine accumulation in plasma, which stimulates platelet adenylate cyclase. Prostacyclin stimulates adenylate cyclase. Clopidogrel inhibits conformational activation of GP IIb–IIIa needed for platelet aggregation. Three GP IIb–IIIa blockers are licensed for human use—abciximab, eptifibatide, and tirofiban. The lipid-soluble β-blockers inhibit phospholipase. Calcium channel antagonists block the influx of free calcium ions across the platelet membrane. Dextrans coat the surface, interfering with adhesion and aggregation. (*ATP*, adenosine triphosphate; *ADP*, adenosine diphosphate; *c-AMP*, cyclic adenosine monophosphate; *PG*, prostaglandin.) (Modified from Hoffbrand AV, Pettit JE: *Essential hematology*, ed 3, Oxford, 1993, Blackwell Scientific.)

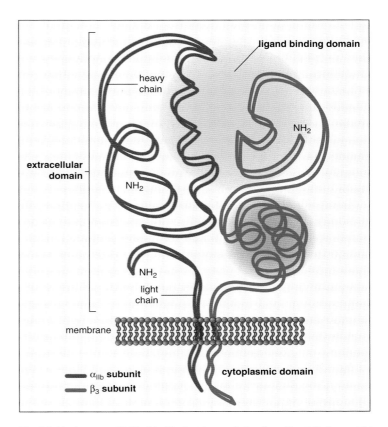

Fig. 24-49. Integrin αIIbβ3. (Modified with permission from Topol EJ, Byzova TV, Plow EF: Platelet GPIIb–GPIIIa blockers, *Lancet* 353:227-231, 1999.)

THE INHERITED AND ACQUIRED COAGULATION DISORDERS

THE COAGULATION PATHWAY

The components of the blood coagulation cascade are proenzymes, procofactors, and regulatory factors (Fig. 25-1). Following the initiation of blood coagulation, the coagulation factor enzymes are activated sequentially. The likely sequence in vivo is depicted in Fig. 25-2. The final steps involve the conversion of soluble plasma fibrinogen into fibrin by thrombin (see Fig. 25-2). In vitro, the cascade has been divided into intrinsic and extrinsic pathways, which are useful for understanding the results of laboratory tests of coagulation. Figure 25-3 shows the three-dimensional nature of the complexes formed on the surface of the vascular endothelium or platelet. The structure of the clot formed is shown in Fig. 24-2. Physiologic inhibitors of various components in the coagulation sequence include antithrombin, plasminogen activators, tissue factor pathway inhibition, and proteins C and S (see Chapter 24).

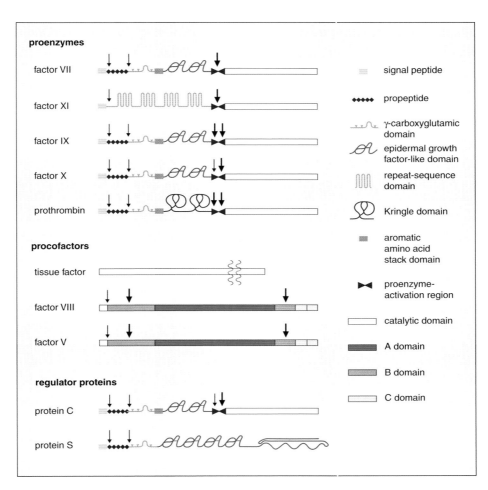

Fig. 25-1. Domains of the enzymes, receptors, and cofactors involved in blood coagulation and regulation: the components are proenzymes, procofactors, and regulatory proteins. The proenzymes, including protein C, contain a catalytic domain, an activation region, and a signal peptide. The vitamin K–dependent proteins include a propeptide and a γ-carboxyglutamic acid domain. Other important domains include the epidermal growth factor–like domain, the Kringle domain, and the repeat-sequence domain. Tissue factor is an integral membrane protein unrelated to other known proteins. Factors V and VIII have marked similarities in structure. Sites of intracellular peptide bonds cleaved during synthesis are indicated by thin arrows, and sites of peptide bonds cleaved during protein activation are indicated by thick arrows. The transmembrane domain of tissue factor is shown within the phospholipid bilayer. (Modified with permission from Furie B, Furie BC: Molecular and cell biology of blood coagulation, *N Engl J Med* 326: 800-806, 1992.)

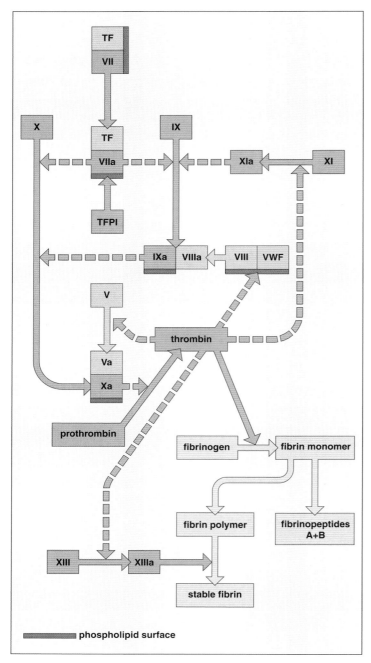

Fig. 25-2. Physiologic pathways of blood coagulation: blood coagulation is initiated by tissue factor (TF) expressed on the cell surface. When plasma comes in contact with tissue factor, factor VII (VII) binds to this receptor. The complex of TF and activated VII (VIIa) activates factors IX (IXa) and X (Xa). Tissue factor pathway inhibitor (TFPI) is an important inhibitor of TF–VIIa activity. The VIIIa–IXa complex greatly amplifies Xa production from X. The generation of thrombin from prothrombin (factor II) by the action of the Xa–Va complex leads to fibrin formation. Thrombin also activates factor XI, which increases IXa production; cleaves factor VIII from its carrier molecule, von Willebrand's factor (VWF), so activating factor VIII and greatly augmenting Xa production by the VIIIa–IXa complex; activates factor V to Va; activates factor XIII to XIIIa, which stabilizes the fibrin clot; and activates thrombin activatable fibrinolysis inhibitor (TAFI) (see Fig. 26-8). (*Blue,* enzymes in coagulation sequence; *yellow,* cofactors; *orange,* von Willebrand's factor; *green,* fibrinogen to fibrin pathway; *dotted lines,* activation or inhibition; *solid lines,* conversion of factor into a different form.)

HEREDITARY COAGULATION DISORDERS

Most inherited coagulation disorders involve deficiency of a single factor, with deficiencies of factor VIII (hemophilia A) von Willebrand's disease and factor IX (hemophilia B) being the most frequent. All other hereditary disorders are rare (Table 25-1).

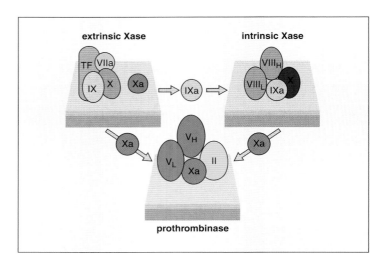

Fig. 25-3. The three vitamin K–dependent procoagulation complexes bound to membrane platelet or vascular endothelium. The factor IXa generated by the factor VIIa–tissue factor complex combines with factor VIIIa on the activated platelet membrane to form the intrinsic Xase complex, which is the major activator of factor X and is at least 50 times more powerful than the extrinsic Xase complex. H, heavy; L, light. (Adapted from Mann JG, Butenas S, Brummel K: Arteriosclerosis and thrombosis, *Vascular Biology* 23:17-25, 2003.)

HEMOPHILIA

In hemophilia A, plasma factor VIII activity is absent or at a low level (less than 2% in severe cases and 2% to 10% in moderately severe cases), because of either defective synthesis of the factor VIII molecule or synthesis of a structurally abnormal molecule (Fig. 25-4). The protein consists of three homologous regions, A1, A2, and A3, separated by a long B domain, rich in glycosylation sites and followed by two homologous C regions (Fig. 25-5). The A regions show homology with the copper-binding protein ceruloplasmin. Although the single-chain mature polypeptide has a molecular weight (MW) of about 267 kDa, it is cleaved by thrombin into two calcium-linked polypeptides of MW 90 kDa and 80 kDa, and it is in this activated form that it activates factor X. The gene maps to the distal band of

TABLE 25-1.   NUMBER OF PATIENTS AND RELATIVE FREQUENCY (IN PARENTHESES) OF INHERITED COAGULATION DEFICIENCIES IN THE UK (EXCLUDING VON WILLEBRAND'S DISEASE)

Defect	Number (%)	Gene location
X-linked		
Factor VIII (hemophilia A)	3554 (76.8)	X
Factor IX (hemophilia B)	762 (16.1)	X
Autosomal recessive		
Fibrinogen	11 (0.2)	4
Prothrombin	1 (0.02)	11
Factor V	28 (0.6)	1
Factor VIII	62 (1.3)	13
Factor VII + VIII	18 (0.3)	18 (LMAN1)*
		2 (MCFD2)*
Factor X	25 (0.5)	13
Factor XI	150 (3.3)	
Factor XIII	26 (0.5)	6 subunit A
		1 subunit B

*LMAN1s act as chaperone for factor VII and factor VIII; MCFD2 is a cofactor for LMAN1

Adapted from Peyvandi F, Mannucci PM: In Hoffbrand AV, Catovsky D, Tuddenham EGD, editors: *Postgraduate haematology,* ed 5, Oxford, 2005, Blackwell's, Table 50.2.

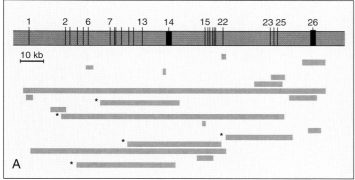

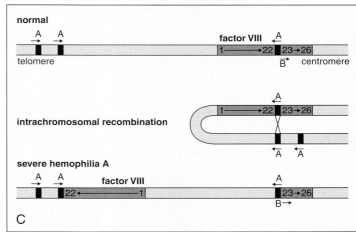

Fig. 25-4. Some of the mutations in the factor VIII gene and the region of chromosome X that contains it. **A,** Examples of deletion mutations. Bars beneath the representation of the factor VIII gene show the approximate size of DNA deletions that lead to hemophilia. The deletion in pink corresponds to a case of mild hemophilia; all other patients have severe disease. The asterisks correspond to gene deletion in hemophiliacs who have developed inhibitor antibodies. **B,** Examples of point mutations. Nonsense (red) and missense (yellow and green) mutations have been discovered in parts of the factor VIII gene that normally encode the amino acid arginine. Many other examples of point mutations and deletions exist (see Anatorakis SE, Kazazian HH, Tuddenham EG: *Hum Mutat* 5: 1-22, 1995). **C,** The region of chromosome X q28 that contains the factor VIII gene. Inversion model of the recombination that accounts for approximately 45% of severe hemophilia A. (*A,* Homologous promoter that is repeated; *B,* second promoter near *A* that is only in intron 22 and when active transcribes exons 23 to 26—the opposing orientation of *A* sequences allows intrachromosomal homologous recombination.) (*A, B,* Modified with permission from Hoffman R, Benz EJ, Shattil SJ, editors: *Hematology: basic principles and practice,* New York, 1991, Churchill Livingstone, p 1286. *C,* Courtesy of Professor K. J. Pasi.)

the long arm of chromosome X (Xq28). Over 100 different large deletions and unique small deletions (less than 100 bp) have been described, as well as >100 different sequence insertions (all associated with severe disease). Also, >1000 different point mutations have been identified and these may be associated with severe or mild disease. In some of the cases with single-point mutations and with deletions, the patients develop a factor VIII inhibitor in plasma. Intrachromosomal rearrangement accounts for 45% of cases (see Fig. 25-4). Von Willebrand's factor (VWF) activity is normal and VWF is present in normal amounts.

In hemophilia B (Christmas disease), either factor IX is absent or the factor IX molecule is structurally abnormal. The inheritance of both hemophilias is sex linked (Fig. 25-6).

Major hemorrhage of the joints is the dominant problem in severe hemophilia A or B and most frequently affects the knees, elbows, ankles, and wrists, although other synovial joints may be involved. Usually severe pain is present and the affected joint is tender, warm, and may be grossly distended (Figs. 25-7 and 25-8). Chronic joint hemorrhage results in degenerative joint changes and mechanical derangement of articular surfaces (Figs. 25-9 and 25-10).

Demineralization, loss of articular cartilage, bone lipping, and osteophyte formation produce deformity and crippling (Figs. 25-11 to 25-13). The end result in poorly treated patients is permanent fixation of the affected joint or flexion deformities (Figs. 25-14 and 25-15).

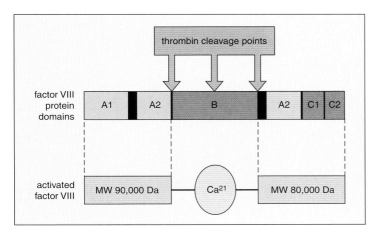

Fig. 25-5. Factor VIII clotting factor: structure.

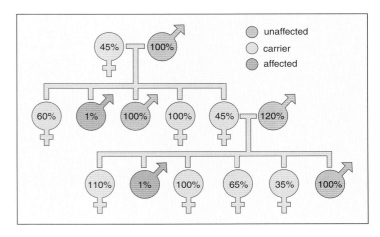

Fig. 25-6. Hemophilia: pattern of inheritance (family tree).

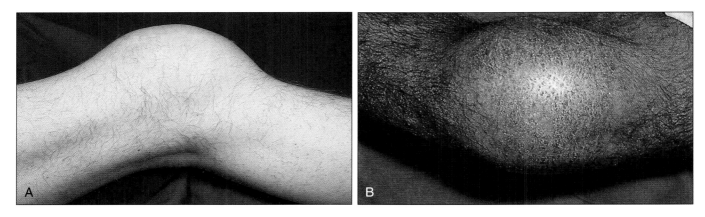

Fig. 25-7. Hemophilia A. **A, B,** Gross swelling from acute hemarthroses of the knee joints.

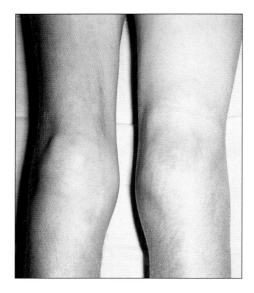

Fig. 25-8. Hemophilia A: acute hemarthrosis of the left knee joint, with swelling of the suprapatellar area. The quadriceps muscles are wasted, particularly on the patient's right thigh.

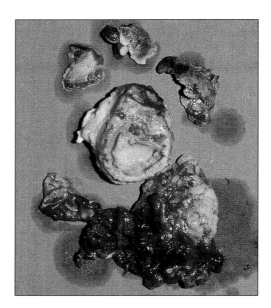

Fig. 25-10. Hemophilia A: resected material from the knee in Fig. 25-9 included (from top to bottom) osteophytes from the arthritic femoral condyles; the patella, which shows hemosiderin-stained articular cartilage and secondary arthritic changes; and a portion of grossly hemosiderin-stained synovium of the suprapatellar pouch.

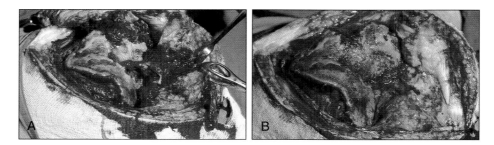

Fig. 25-9. Hemophilia A. **A,** Opened knee joint showing the femoral condyles and hypertrophied hemosiderin-stained synovium. Widespread erosion of the articular cartilage has exposed large areas of hemosiderin-stained bone. **B,** Removal of the synovium of the suprapatellar pouch and of the patella exposes the grossly damaged femoral articular surface.

Fig. 25-11. Hemophilia A. **A,** Radiograph of the knee joint, showing marked narrowing of the joint space (particularly medially), a widened intercondylar notch, prominent osteo-arthritic changes, and subchondral cyst formation, with erosion of the upper lateral border of the tibial plateau. **B,** Radiograph of the elbow joint, showing marked joint space narrowing, enlargement of the radial head, secondary osteoarthritic features, and subchondral cyst formation.

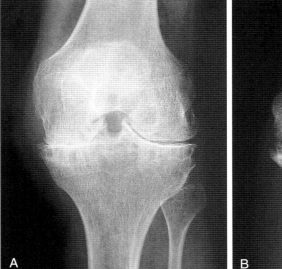
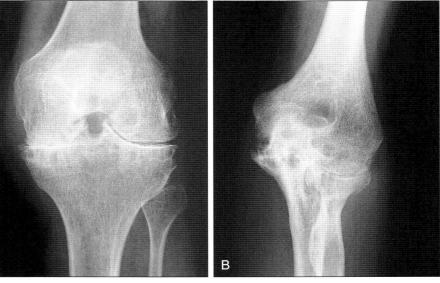

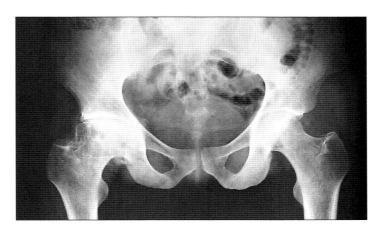

Fig. 25-12. Hemophilia A: radiograph of the pelvis, showing marked destruction and deformation of the right acetabulum and femoral head. Numerous subchondral cysts are present, and the right femoral neck is shortened and widened.

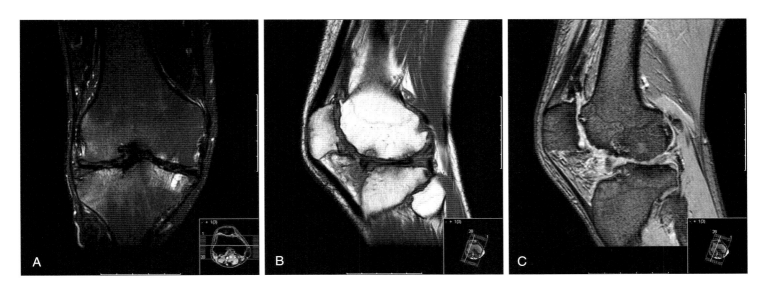

Fig. 25-13. Hemophilia A. **A–C,** Magnetic resonance imaging (MRI) of knee joint: gross arthritic changes affecting all three compartments of the knee joint with severe articular cartilage thinning and irregularity, prominent subarticular cysts, and flattening and tears of the posterior horns of both medial menisci.

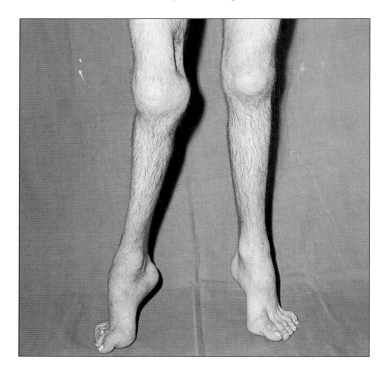

Fig. 25-14. Hemophilia A: gross crippling. The right knee is swollen, with posterior subluxation of the tibia on the femur. The ankles and feet show residual deformities of talipes equinus and some degree of cavus and associated toe clawing. Generalized muscle wasting is most marked on the right. The scar on the medial side of the right lower thigh is the site of a previously excised "pseudotumor."

Traumatic and spontaneous soft-tissue hemorrhage is another feature of hemophilia (Figs. 25-16 to 25-19). Dissecting hematomas may involve large areas of muscle or deep fascial layers (Fig. 25-20). Hemorrhage into retroperitoneal fascial spaces or into the psoas muscle may produce considerable problems in differential diagnosis (Figs. 25-21 to 25-23), since associated pain, tenderness, and fever may suggest other causes of the acute abdomen.

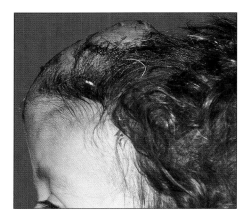

Fig. 25-16. Hemophilia A: extensive posttraumatic hematoma of the forehead in an infant.

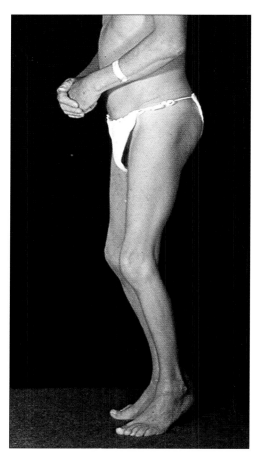

Fig. 25-15. Hemophilia A: flexion deformities of the elbow, hip, knee, and ankle joints following a 35-year history of multiple hemarthroses.

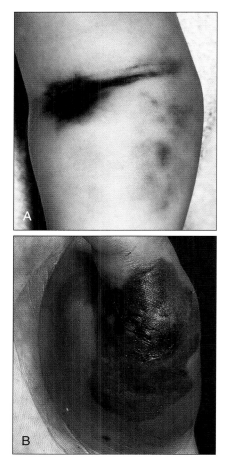

Fig. 25-17. Hemophilia B. **A,** Extensive subcutaneous hemorrhage about the elbow joint of an infant following venipuncture. **B,** Extensive bleeding into the thenar muscles and overlying subcutaneous tissue.

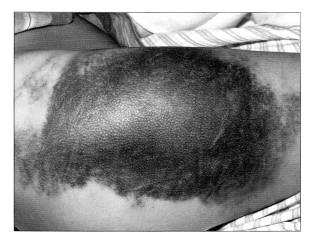

Fig. 25-18. Hemophilia A: massive hemorrhage in the area of the right buttock, following an intramuscular injection.

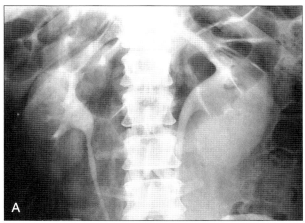

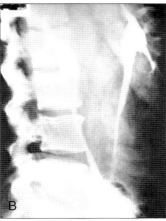

Fig. 25-21. Hemophilia A: intravenous pyelogram showing acute retroperitoneal hemorrhage. **A,** A soft-tissue mass in the left flank has caused medial rotation of the left kidney and anteromedial displacement of the ureter. **B,** The lateral view confirms the anterior displacement of both the kidney and ureter.

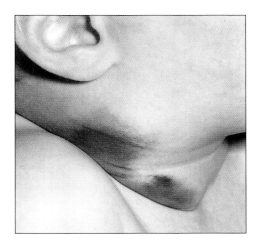

Fig. 25-19. Hemophilia B: extensive hemorrhage into the soft tissues of the neck following venipuncture of the external jugular vein.

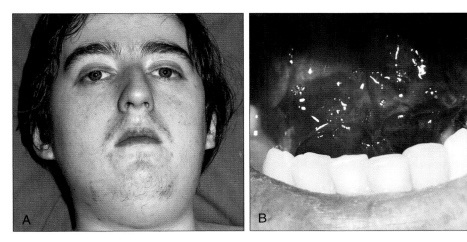

Fig. 25-20. Hemophilia A. **A,** Marked submandibular swelling resulting from a large hemorrhage in the sublingual tissues. **B,** The most superficial part of the sublingual hemorrhage is clearly visible beneath the mucosa of the floor of the mouth.

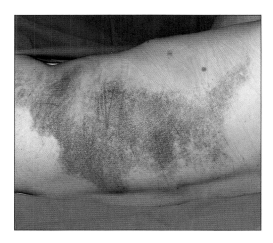

Fig. 25-22. Hemophilia A: acute retroperitoneal hemorrhage (same patient as shown in Fig. 25-21). The extensive subcutaneous bruising of the left flank appeared 24 hours after presentation.

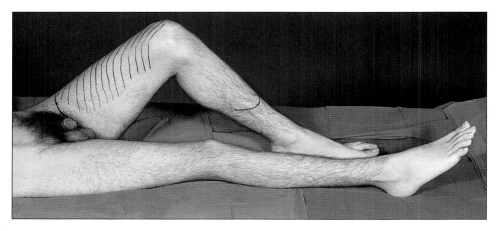

Fig. 25-23. Hemophilia A: acute retroperitoneal hemorrhage into the left psoas muscle. The lines indicate an area of anesthesia over the distribution of the femoral nerve. There was also weakness of the quadriceps muscle and a flexion contracture at the left hip.

Hemophilic "pseudotumors" are a serious complication of extensive fascial or subperiosteal hemorrhage. These blood-filled multiloculated cysts may cause extensive destruction of both soft tissue (Fig. 25-24) and bone (Figs. 25-25 and 25-26) as they increase in size.

Ischemic contractures may follow extensive hemorrhage into the muscles of the limbs (Fig. 25-27), for example, Volkmann's contracture of the forearm (Fig. 25-28). Prolonged bleeding occurs after dental extractions, and operative hemorrhage is life-threatening in both severely and mildly affected patients.

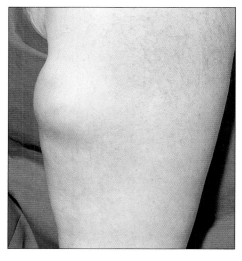

Fig. 25-24. Hemophilia A: "pseudotumor" of the biceps, in fact a hard residual encapsulated swelling following incomplete resolution and repair of previous muscle hemorrhage.

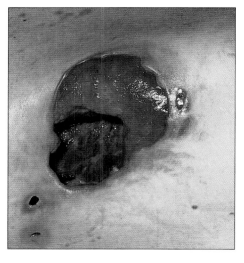

Fig. 25-25. Hemophilia A: large ulcer overlying the entrance to a multiloculated and cavernous pseudotumor of the right iliac bone and overlying soft tissues.

Fig. 25-26. Hemophilia A: pelvic radiograph (same patient as shown in Fig. 25-25). The pseudotumor destroyed a large area of the wing of the right iliac bone, including the anterior crest. The hip joint space on the right is obliterated and the femoral neck has a disunited fracture, with resultant pseudoarthrosis, gross deformity, and shortening.

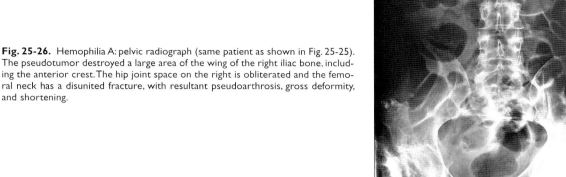

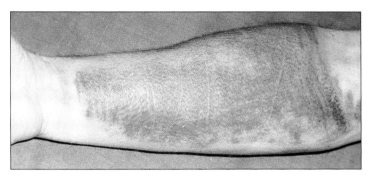

Fig. 25-27. Hemophilia A: subcutaneous bruising and extensive hemorrhage into the flexor muscles and associated soft tissues of the right forearm.

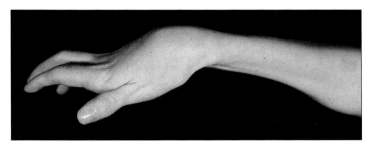

Fig. 25-28. Hemophilia A: Volkmann's contracture. The wasting and flexion deformities are a result of extensive repair and stricture formation in muscles damaged by repeated hematomas.

Spontaneous intracranial hemorrhage (Fig. 25-29), although an infrequent cause of bleeding in individuals, remains the most common cause of death in severe hemophilia.

The management of the hemophilias has been greatly improved by therapy with coagulation factor concentrates (factor VIII concentrates in hemophilia A and factor IX concentrates in hemophilia B) or factors made by recombinant deoxyribonucleic acid (DNA) techniques. Prophylactic therapy and early treatment of bleeding episodes have reduced the occurrence of repeated and crippling hemarthroses and soft-tissue hemorrhage. With regular therapy even severely affected patients reach adult life without significant degenerative arthritis. In the majority of patients, replacement therapy with the appropriate coagulation factor concentrates has allowed even major surgical procedures to be undertaken without excessive risk.

Carrier Detection and Antenatal Diagnosis

DNA analysis has improved carrier detection and prenatal diagnosis compared with the measurement of factor VIII or factor IX antigenic and coagulation activity in plasma. Direct detection of the defect is possible using DNA sequencing providing an index case is available to establish the particular mutation present in the family (Figs. 25-30 and 25-31).

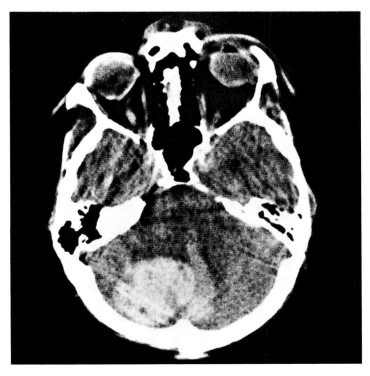

Fig. 25-29. Hemophilia A: computed tomography (CT) scan showing a large hematoma of the cerebellum.

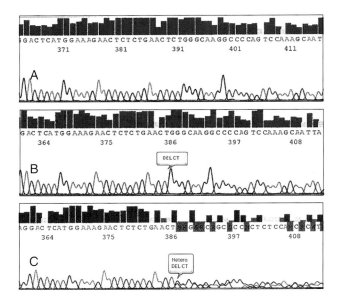

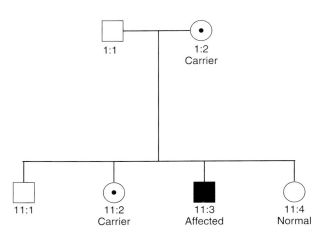

Fig. 25-30. Family 1 Hemophilia A: carrier detection by DNA analysis of peripheral blood leucocytes. **A,** Normal reference sequence. **B,** Automated dideoxy sequencing of the factor VIII gene has shown the affected son in this family (II-3) to have a 2 basepair (CT) deletion in exon 14, resulting in a frameshift causing the introduction of a premature stop codon. **C,** His mother is shown to be a carrier illustrated by one allele showing normal sequence and the second carrying the 2 basepair deletion. His older sister (II-2) was also a carrier, whereas his younger sister (II-4) was normal. (Courtesy of Haemophilia Centre, Royal Free Hospital.)

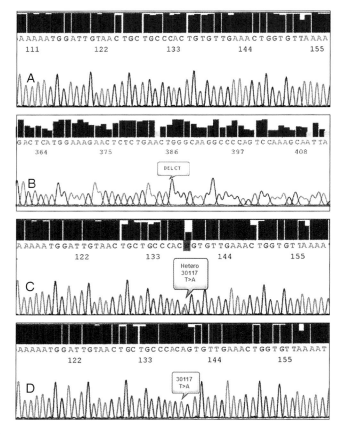

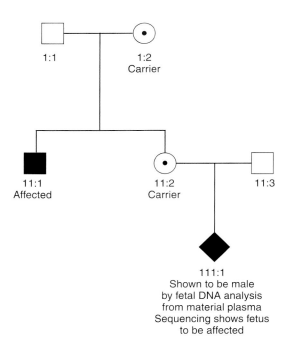

Fig. 25-31. Factor IX deficiency: antenatal diagnosis. Hemophilia B: prenatal diagnosis by chorion villus biopsy and direct sequencing. **A,** Normal reference sequence. **B,** Automated dideoxy sequencing of the factor IX gene has shown the affected son in this family (II-1) to have a T>A substitution at nucleotide 30117 in exon 7. This results in a cysteine to serine change at codon 222. **C,** His sister is shown to be a carrier, illustrated by the heterozygous peak at 30117 showing both the T and the A nucleotides. **D,** Direct sequencing shows that her male fetus is affected as he has only the abnormal A at position 30117. (Courtesy of Haemophilia Centre, Royal Free Hospital.)

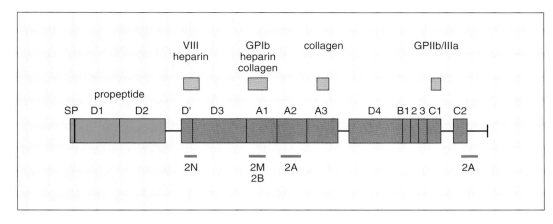

Fig. 25-32. Von Willebrand's disease: the mature VWF protein with the various domains. The portions that have been shown to interact with factor VIII, heparin, collagen, and platelet glycoproteins GP Ib and GP IIb–IIIa are shown by square brackets. The regions in which mutations identified in patients with type II von Willebrand's disease cluster are shown. The propeptide is cleaved off the mature protein.

VON WILLEBRAND'S DISEASE

Von Willebrand's disease is a bleeding disorder caused by inherited defects in the concentration, structure, or function of VWF due to mutations at the VWF locus and possibly other mutations (Fig. 25-32). This protein is an oligomer of units, each of MW 210,000. It carries factor VIII coagulation factor and is itself essential for the adhesion of platelets to damaged vessel walls (see Fig. 24-8). The subunits dimerize "tail to tail" in the endoplasmic reticulum and then form multimers through "head to head" disulfide bonds in the D domains. The multimers may be secreted or stored in the Weibel-Palade bodies (see Fig. 24-4) or in platelets. The fate of secreted VWF multimers depends on their size, interactions with platelets, susceptibility to proteolysis by ADAMTS13 (see Fig. 24-41), and rate of clearance from the circulation (Fig. 25-33). Under high fluid shear stress, multimers are stretched (see Fig. 24-6) may bind platelets (see Fig. 24-5) and are exposed to cleavage by ADAMT513. Normal blood contains multimers of different sizes with characteristic cleavage products, not found in endothelial VWF. In normal plasma, the largest VWF multimers are smaller than those assembled initially in the endothelial cell (see Fig. 25-33). In thrombocyte thrombocytopenic purpura, ultralarge multimers are present in plasma (see Fig. 24-41). The pattern of VWF multimer distribution differs in the different types of VW disease.

The inheritance pattern of von Willebrand's disease found in most patients is autosomal dominant. The disorder is characterized by operative and posttraumatic hemorrhage, mucous membrane bleeding, and excessive blood loss from both superficial cuts and abrasions (Fig. 25-34). Spontaneous hemarthroses and arthritic changes are particularly rare, and occur only in homozygous patients (Fig. 25-35).

The molecular defects include point mutations or deletions (see Fig. 25-32). The disease is divided into three types based on laboratory findings and type 2 is further divided into four subtypes. The results of hemostasis tests in von Willebrand's disease and the hemophilias are given in Table 25-3.

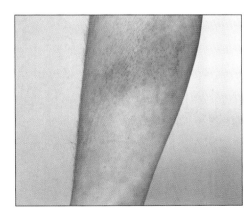

Fig. 25-34. Von Willebrand's disease: subcutaneous bruising overlying hemorrhage into the muscles and soft tissues of the left forearm.

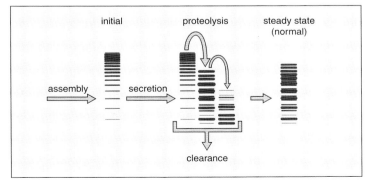

Fig. 25-33. Synthesis and catabolism of VWF multimers. In plasma VWF is cleaved by ADAMTS13 metalloprotease so that the largest multimers are smaller than those assembled initially. Faint satellite bands flank the smallest bands, reflecting proteolytic remodeling. (Adapted from Sadler et al: *Journal of Thrombosis and Haemostasis* 4:2103-2114, 2006.)

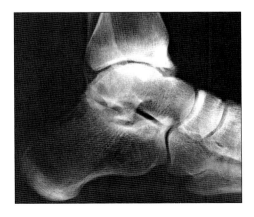

Fig. 25-35. Von Willebrand's disease: lateral radiograph of ankle joint showing loss of joint space, marginal sclerosis, and a small subchondral cyst in the tibial epiphysis.

TABLE 25-2. PATHOPHYSIOLOGY AND CLASSIFICATION OF VON WILLEBRAND'S DISEASE

Type	Description	FVIII:C	VWF:Ag	VWF:RCo	VWF:CB	VWF: FVIIIB	VWF: Multimers	RIPA
1	Partial quantitative deficiency of VWF	Decreased	Decreased	Decreased (concordant)	Decreased (concordant)	Normal	May or may not contain mutant VWF subunits	Reduced
2	Qualitative VWF defects	Decreased	Decreased	Decreased (discordant)	Decreased (discordant)	Normal		Reduced
2A	Decreased VWF-dependent platelet adhesion and a selective deficiency of HMW VWF multimers	Decreased or normal	Decreased or normal	Decreased (discordant)	Decreased (discordant)	Normal	Absent HMW Medium MW multimers	Reduced
2B	Increased affinity for platelet glycoprotein Ib	Decreased or normal	Decreased or normal	Decreased (discordant)	Decreased (discordant)	Normal	Absent HMW multimers 2B Malmo or New York (normal pattern)	Increased with low dose Ristocetin (0.5 mg/ml)
2M	Decreased VWF-dependent platelet adhesion without a selective deficiency of HMW VWF multimers	Decreased or normal	Decreased or normal	Decreased (discordant)	Decreased (concordant)	Normal	Normal pattern	Reduced
2N	Markedly decreased binding affinity for FVIII:C	Markedly decreased	Normal	Normal	Normal	Decreased	Normal pattern	Normal
3	Virtually complete deficiency of VWF	Markedly decreased	Markedly decreased	Markedly decreased (concordant)	Markedly decreased (concordant)	Normal	Markedly decreased	Reduced

VWF = von Willebrand factor, VWF:Ag = VWF antigen, VWF:CB = VWF collagen binding, VWF:RCo = VWF Ristocetin cofactor, VWF:FVIII:B = VWF factor VIII binding, HMW = high molecular weight. Concordant/discordant refers to a reduction in relation to VWF:Ag, RIPA = Ristocetin-induced platelet agglutination

OTHER HEREDITARY COAGULATION DISORDERS

Patients with inherited defects of coagulation factors other than VIII or IX (e.g. Factor XI) often show easy bruising and spontaneous and excessive posttraumatic bleeding. Spontaneous hemarthroses and soft-tissue hematomas are, however, most unusual.

ACQUIRED COAGULATION DISORDERS

In clinical practice the acquired coagulation disorders (Table 25-4) are seen more often than the inherited disorders. Unlike the inherited diseases, there are usually multiple clotting factor deficiencies. Bleeding episodes that result from vitamin K deficiency, overdosage with oral anticoagulants, or in association with liver disease and with disseminated intravascular coagulation (DIC) are seen most frequently.

TABLE 25-3. HEMOSTASIS TESTS: TYPICAL RESULTS IN THE HEMOPHILIAS A AND B AND VON WILLEBRAND'S DISEASE

	Hemophilia A	Hemophilia B	von Willebrand's disease
Bleeding time or PFA-100 test	Normal	Normal	Prolonged
Prothrombin time	Normal	Normal	Normal
Activated partial thromboplastin time	Prolonged	Prolonged	Prolonged
Thrombin clotting time	Normal	Normal	Normal
Factor VIII	Low	Normal	Low or normal
VWF:antigen	Normal	Normal	Low or normal (rarely raised)
VWF: ristocetin cofactor activity	Normal	Normal	Low (or rarely raised)
Factor IX	Normal	Low	Normal

TABLE 25-4. THE ACQUIRED COAGULATION DISORDERS

Liver disease

Deficiency of vitamin K-dependent factors
  Hemorrhagic disease of the new-born
  Biliary obstruction
  Malabsorption of vitamin K, e.g., sprue, celiac disease
  Vitamin K-antagonist therapy, e.g., coumarins, indanediones

Disseminated intravascular coagulation

Inhibition of coagulation
  Specific inhibitors, e.g., antibodies against factor VIII components
  Non-specific inhibitors, e.g., antibodies found in systemic lupus erythematosus, rheumatoid arthritis

Miscellaneous
  Diseases with M-protein production
  L-Asparaginase
  Therapy with heparin, defibrinating agents or thrombolytics
  Massive transfusion syndrome

LIVER DISEASE

Liver cell immaturity and lack of vitamin K synthesis in the gut are principal causes of hemorrhagic disease of the newborn. In adults, vitamin K deficiency may be the result of obstructive jaundice or pancreatic or small bowel disease. Multiple hemostatic abnormalities contribute to increased surgical bleeding and may exacerbate hemorrhage from esophageal varices. Biliary obstruction results in impaired absorption of vitamin K and decreased synthesis of factors II, VII, IX, and X by the liver parenchymal cells. The hypersplenism associated with portal hypertension frequently results in thrombocytopenia. Patients in liver failure have deficiency of factor V and variable abnormalities of platelet function, and often produce functionally abnormal fibrinogen. As well as variceal bleeding and increased loss of blood during surgery, patients with severe liver disease may also suffer from spontaneous superficial hemorrhage (Figs. 25-36 and 25-37).

OVERDOSAGE WITH ANTICOAGULANTS

Overdosage with oral anticoagulants that are vitamin K antagonists results in severe deficiencies of coagulation factors II, VII, IX, and X. Patients may have extensive skin bruising (Fig. 25-38) or severe internal bleeding (Fig. 25-39).

Similar skin lesions to those seen in homozygous protein C deficiency (see Fig. 26-9) may occur in patients commencing anticoagulant therapy with coumarin drugs (Fig. 25-40). Selective severe protein C deficiency may occur temporarily before the levels of the vitamin K–dependent clotting factors fall (Fig. 25-40).

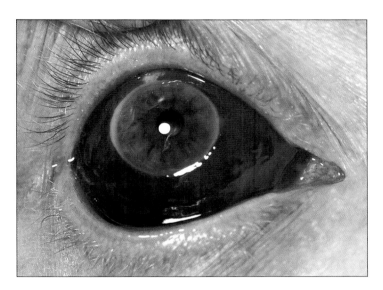

Fig. 25-36. Liver failure: extensive subconjunctival hemorrhage.

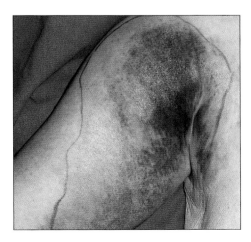

Fig. 25-37. Liver failure: subcutaneous hemorrhage of the upper arm following minor trauma. Laboratory tests revealed deficiencies of factors II, VII, IX, and X, as well as dysfibrinogenemia.

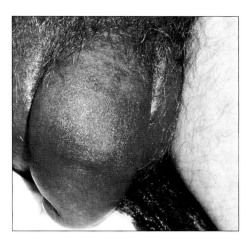

Fig. 25-38. Warfarin overdose: massive subcutaneous hemorrhage over the penis, scrotal, and pubic areas following sexual intercourse.

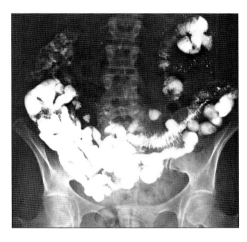

Fig. 25-39. Warfarin overdose: radiograph shows intramural bleeding in the small intestine with the characteristic "stacked coin" pattern of barium distribution. (Courtesy of Dr. D. Nag.)

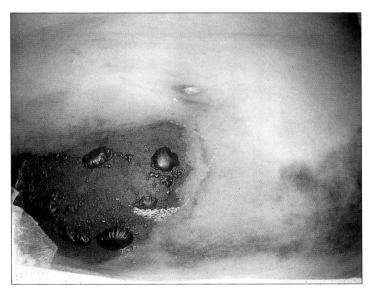

Fig. 25-40. Warfarin skin necrosis: these lesions over the abdomen developed in the first few days of warfarin therapy in a 40-year-old woman. Her protein C level was not measured but, in more recent examples of coumarin-induced skin necrosis, patients have been found to have reduced plasma levels of protein C. (Courtesy of Profesor S. J. Machin.)

TABLE 25-5. DISSEMINATED INTRAVASCULAR
COAGULATION: CAUSES

Infections	Hypersensitivity reactions
Gram-negative and meningococcal septicemia	Anaphylaxis
	Incompatible blood transfusion
Septic abortion and *Clostridium welchii* septicemia	**Widespread tissue damage**
Severe falciparum malaria	Following surgery or trauma
Viral infection (purpura fulminans)	
	Miscellaneous
Malignancy	Liver failure
Widespread mucin-secreting adenocarcinoma	Snake and invertebrate venoms
	Severe burns
Acute promyelocytic leukemia (AML M₃)	Hypothermia
	Heat stroke
Obstetric complications	Hypoxia
Amniotic fluid embolism	Vascular malformations (e.g., Kasabach–Merritt syndrome)
Premature separation of placenta	
Eclampsia; retained placenta	

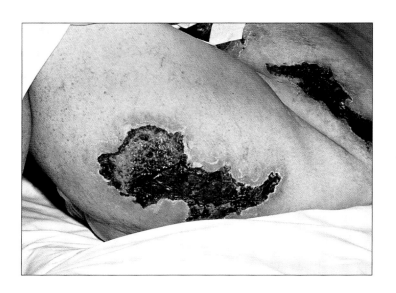

Fig. 25-41. Disseminated intravascular coagulation: pathogenesis.

DISSEMINATED INTRAVASCULAR COAGULATION

A consequence of many disorders, DIC causes widespread endothelial damage, platelet aggregation, or release of procoagulant material into the circulation (Table 25-5). It is associated with widespread intravascular deposition of fibrin and consumption of coagulation factors and platelets (Fig. 25-41). This may lead to both abnormal bleeding and widespread thrombosis, which is often fulminant (Figs. 25-42 to 25-45), although it can run a less severe, chronic course.

In the Kasabach-Merritt syndrome, a congenital hemangioma is associated with DIC (Fig. 25-46). The stimulus to intravascular coagulation is local, but the enhanced proteolytic activity of both coagulation and fibrinolytic systems probably becomes disseminated throughout the blood.

ACQUIRED COAGULATION FACTOR INHIBITOR

Occasionally patients have a bleeding syndrome (Fig. 25-47) caused by circulating antibodies to coagulation factor VIII or to other clotting factors. These antibodies usually occur postpartum, in systemic lupus erythematosus (SLE) associated with a malignancy, and in old age.

Patients with SLE, other autoimmune disorders, and, rarely, infections may also develop a less specific inhibitor, immunoglobulin G (IgG) or immunoglobulin M (IgM), which is directed against phospholipid and is associated with a prolongation of the partial thromboplastin time not corrected by normal plasma. Patients with this "lupus anticoagulant" may have no clinical symptoms, or may

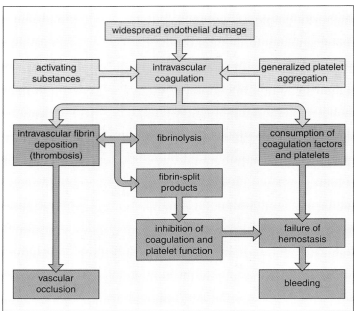

Fig. 25-42. Disseminated intravascular coagulation: later stages of skin necrosis (same patient as shown in Fig. 25-44). Loss of superficial necrotic tissue over the thigh and lateral abdominal wall has left large, deep, irregular ulcers with hemorrhagic areas of exposed tissue. (Courtesy of Dr. B. B. Berkeley.)

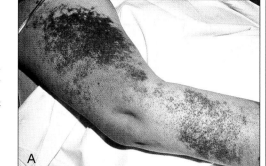
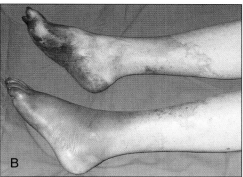

Fig. 25-43. Disseminated intravascular coagulation. **A,** Indurated and confluent purpura of the arm. **B,** Peripheral gangrene with swelling and discoloration of the skin of the feet in fulminant disease.

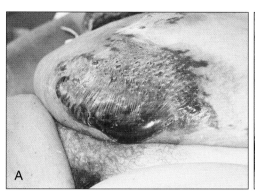
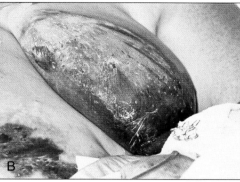

Fig. 25-44. Disseminated intravascular coagulation: extensive necrosis of the skin and subcutaneous tissues of **(A)** the lower abdominal wall and **(B)** breast in a grossly obese patient (same patient as shown in Fig. 25-42). (*A, B,* Courtesy of Dr. B. B. Berkeley.)

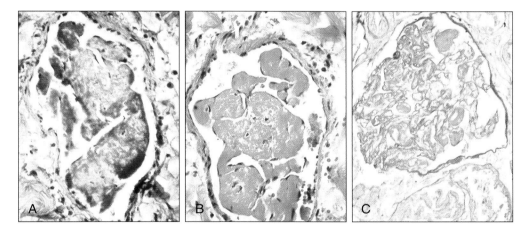

Fig. 25-45. Disseminated intravascular coagulation. **A, B,** Sections through a skin venule deep to an area of necrosis show occlusion by a thrombus composed mainly of fibrin. **C,** Necrosis of the glomerulus and the surrounding tubules with variable amounts of fibrinous material in the glomerular blood vessels. (*A,* Martius scarlet-blue; *B,* H & E; *C,* periodic acid–Schiff stains.)

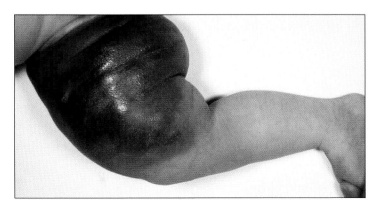
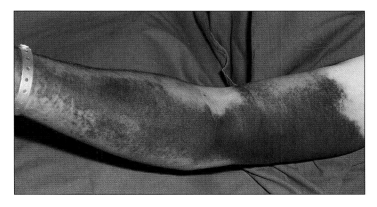

Fig. 25-46. Kasabach-Merritt syndrome: this giant congenital hemangioma of the thigh was associated with DIC.

Fig. 25-47. Acquired coagulation factor inhibitor: extensive subcutaneous and deep soft-tissue hemorrhage in the arm because of circulating autoantibody to factor VIII.

TABLE 25-6.   HEMOSTASIS TESTS: TYPICAL RESULTS IN ACQUIRED BLEEDING DISORDERS

	Platelet count	Prothrombin time	Activated partial thromboplastin time	Thrombin time
Liver disease	Low	Prolonged	Prolonged	Normal (rarely prolonged)
Disseminated intravascular coagulation	Low	Prolonged	Prolonged	Grossly prolonged
Massive transfusion	Low	Prolonged	Prolonged	Prolonged
Heparin	Normal (rarely low)	Mildly prolonged	Prolonged	Prolonged
Circulating anticoagulant	Normal	Normal or prolonged	Prolonged	Normal

thrombose arteries or veins or suffer recurrent spontaneous abortions (see Chapter 26). Results of hemostasis tests in the major acquired coagulation disorders are shown in Table 25-6.

THROMBOELASTOMETRY AND THROMBOELASTOGRAPHY

Thromboelastometry (TEM) or thromboelastography (TEG) may be used for a global assessment of hemostatic function. Freshly drawn blood is placed in a cuvette. In TEM rotational movement of a pin oscillated via an elastic string is detected by a light-sensitive sensor. The fibrin clot affects movement of the pin. Amplitude 0 mm means unobstructed rotation whereas amplitude 100 mm implies infinite firmness and choking the pin by the clot. The rate of initial fibrin formation, coagulation time, strength of fibrin clot, clot lysis index, or retraction is measured. Typical TEM results in different disorders are shown in Fig. 25-48.

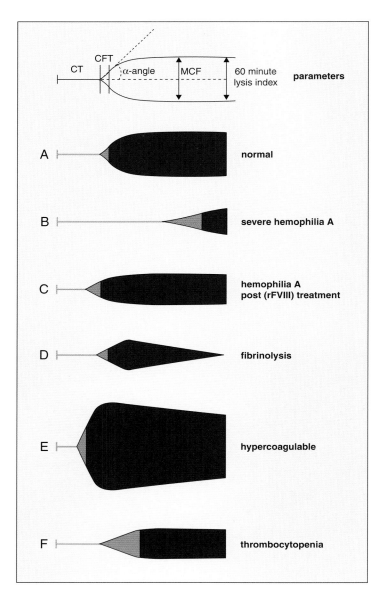

Fig. 25-48. Thromboelastometry (TEM); **(A)** normal trace and appearance, in hemophilia **(B)** before and **(C)** after factor VIII infusion, **(D)** fibrinolysis (as in disseminated intravascular coagulation), **(E)** hypercoaguable states, and **(F)** thrombocytopenia. Parameter definitions: clotting time (CT)—time until 2 mm clot firmness has been activated after the test has been started by the addition of a trigger; clot formation time (CFT)—the kinetics of the formation of a stable clot from activated platelets and fibrin and is defined as the time elapsed between 2 mm and 20 mm clot firmness; alpha angle (°)—alpha angle is a tangent to the clotting curve through the 2 mm point and describes the kinetics of clot formation. It is the angle between slope and baseline; clot formation rate (CFR)—the tangent at the maximum slope; maximum clot firmness (MCF)—the measure for the firmness of the clot and is measured at the maximum amplitude achieved during coagulation before fibrinolysis; lysis index (Ly60)—degree of lysis that takes place after 60 minutes of clot time and is calculated as the ratio of the amplitude and the maximum firmness (% remaining clot firmness).

THROMBOSIS

Intravascular thrombi have a basic structure of platelets and fibrin. Consequential ischemia from vascular obstruction or thrombotic embolism is of great clinical importance. Thrombi are involved in the pathogenesis of coronary artery disease and myocardial infarcts, cerebrovascular disease, peripheral arterial disease, deep vein occlusion, and pulmonary emboli.

ATHEROTHROMBOSIS

The pathogenesis of arterial atherosclerosis is illustrated in Fig. 26-1. Multiple factors contribute, including endothelial dysfunction, dyslipidemia and oxidation of low-density lipoprotein (LDL), intimal inflammation, platelet adhesion and aggregation, plaque rupture, and thrombosis. Increased endothelial permeability to lipoproteins is mediated by nitric oxide released by endothelial cells, prostacyclin, platelet-derived growth factor (PDGF), angiotensin II, and endothelin.

Oxidation of LDL in the subendothelial space stimulates monocyte chemotaxis, and phagocytosis of lipid by macrophages results in foam cells. Mitochondrial dysfunction, apoptosis, and necrosis of foam cells release cellular lysosomal proteases, inflammatory cytokines, tissue factor, and other prothrombotic factors. Migration of inflammatory cells into the intima is mediated by oxidized LDL, monocyte chemotactic protein I, interleukin 8, PDGF, and macrophage colony-stimulating factor (M-CSF). Following intimal migration and proliferation, smooth muscle cells become laden with lipid. Apoptosis of inflammatory cells and smooth muscle cells stimulates repair processes with increasing fibrous connective tissue contributing to the development of the fibrous cap and the atherosclerotic plaque.

With expansion, the intimal plaque develops its own microvascular network and plaque hemorrhage may increase the size of the lesion. Regrowth of endothelium and repair processes at the site of overlying thrombus and its subsequent incorporation into the arterial wall contribute further to arterial thickening and restriction of the

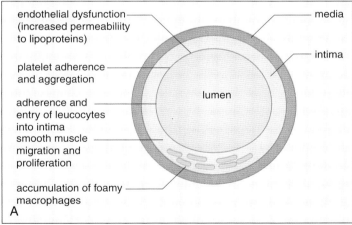

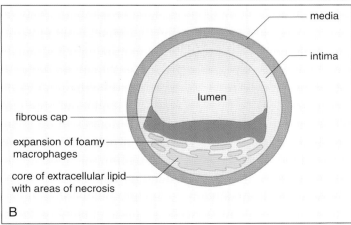

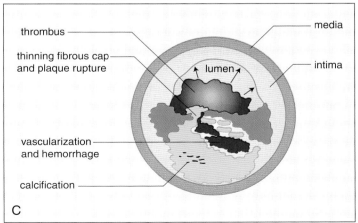

Fig. 26-1. Atherosclerosis: pathogenesis of arterial lesion. **A,** Fatty streak stage. **B,** Atherosclerotic plaque. **C,** Complicated lesion with thrombosis.

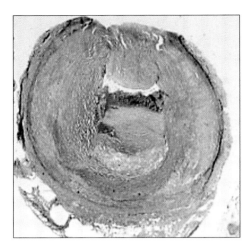

Fig. 26-2. Coronary artery atherosclerosis: left coronary artery of a 51-year-old man who died suddenly. The lesion is complicated with gross sclerosis and thickening of the intima, plaque hemorrhage, and rupture with overlying thrombus. The lumen is almost completely occluded. (Elastic Van Giesen stain.) (Courtesy of Dr. Ken Anderson.)

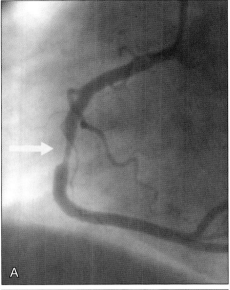

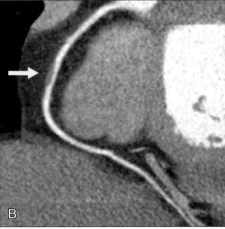

Fig. 26-3. Coronary artery atherosclerosis: a 43-year-old woman who had atypical chest pain and was at low risk for ischemic heart disease. Corresponding images of the right coronary artery from cardiac catheter **(A)** and computed tomography (CT) coronary angiography **(B)** demonstrate a noncalcified plaque resulting in 70% stenosis. (Courtesy of Dr. Sharyn MacDonald and Dr. Tony Young.)

arterial lumen. Thinning of the fibrous cap, plaque rupture, and associated thrombosis may lead to acute coronary occlusion, myocardial infarct, or stroke.

In addition to local arterial obstruction by the thrombus, emboli of platelet and fibrin thrombi may break from the primary thrombus and occlude distal arteries (e.g., emboli from carotid artery thrombi may cause cerebral thrombosis or transient ischemic attacks; heart valve and heart chamber thrombi may lead to systemic emboli and infarcts). Histology of a left coronary artery in a patient who died a sudden death is shown in Fig. 26-2.

Risk factors for arterial thrombosis and atherosclerosis are listed in Table 26-1. For coronary artery disease, risk profiles based on sex, age, family history, elevated blood pressure, cholesterol levels, glucose intolerance, cigarette smoking, and electrocardiogram (ECG) abnormalities have been useful in initiating therapeutic and lifestyle changes aimed at preventing or delaying the onset of clinical disease.

Arterial narrowing, thrombi, and emboli are readily identified by angiography (Figs. 26-3 to 26-5).

TABLE 26-1.	ARTERIAL THROMBOSIS RISK FACTORS
Positive family history
Male sex
Hyperlipidemia
Hypertension
Diabetes mellitus
Gout
Polycythemia
Hyperhomocysteinemia
Cigarette smoking
ECG abnormalities
Elevated factor VII
Elevated fibrinogen
Lupus anticoagulant
Collagen vascular diseases
Behçet's disease

VENOUS THROMBOSIS

Multiple factors contribute to the pathogenesis of venous and arterial thrombosis, including genetic predisposition and many acquired risk factors. Venous thrombosis occurs most frequently in the calf veins and/or femoral and iliac veins and may be complicated by pulmonary embolism.

In the nineteenth century, Virchow proposed an important triad of factors that were important for thrombosis: reduced blood flow, vessel wall damage, and blood hypercoagulability. In most patients with venous thrombosis, vascular stasis and increased blood coagulability are most important and vessel wall damage is less important than in arterial disease. However, vascular damage may be important in patients with sepsis, trauma, or malignancy or in those with indwelling catheters. Stasis allows completion of blood coagulation at sites where thrombus formation is initiated (e.g., behind valve pockets of the leg veins in immobile patients).

THROMBOPHILIA

Many factors may contribute to a genetic predisposition to thrombosis (Table 26-2). A hereditary risk factor should be suspected, particularly in young patients with spontaneous thrombosis, recurrent

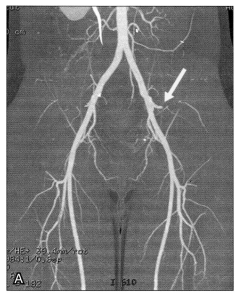

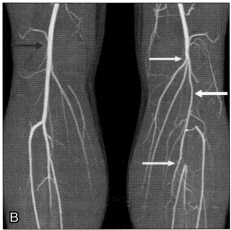

Fig. 26-4. Arterial thrombosis: computed tomography arteriography. **A,** Embolic occlusion of left superior gluteal artery in a patient with endocarditis. **B,** Thrombotic occlusion of left popliteal artery (between *yellow arrows*) with collateral blood flow in the geniculate artery *(white arrow)* Right popliteal artery is normal *(red arrow)*. (Courtesy of Professor Tim Buchenham.)

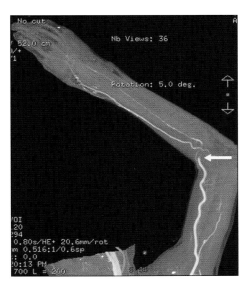

Fig. 26-5. Arterial thrombosis: computed tomography arteriography showing thrombotic occlusion of the right brachial artery *(yellow arrow)*. (Courtesy of Professor Tim Buchenham.)

TABLE 26-2.	INHERITED THROMBOPHILIA: CAUSES

Established
Activated protein C resistance (factor V:R506Q, V Leiden)
Protein C deficiency
Protein S deficiency
Antithrombin deficiency
Hyperhomocysteinemia
Elevated prothrombin levels (mutation G20210A)
Nonestablished as hereditary
Elevated factor VIII levels
Heparin cofactor II deficiency
Plasminogen deficiency
Elevated plasminogen inactivation inhibitor 1
Dysfibrinogenemia

deep vein thrombosis, or thrombosis at unusual sites (e.g., splanchnic veins, sagittal sinus). The hereditary predisposition is often referred to as thrombophilia.

FACTOR V LEIDEN

The factor V Leiden mutation *(FV R506Q)* is the most common cause of thrombophilia and is detected in about 30% of patients with venous thrombosis. The abnormal factor V is resistant to the action of activated protein C.

The mutation occurs at the site at which activated protein C normally cleaves factor Va (Fig. 26-6). Heterozygosity for this disorder is as high as 8% in some white populations. The global distribution is illustrated in Fig. 26-7. The risk of thrombosis in heterozygotes is 8 times greater than that of a control population; in the homozygous form of factor V Leiden the risk rises to at least fiftyfold. The risks are compounded in women taking the contraceptive pill.

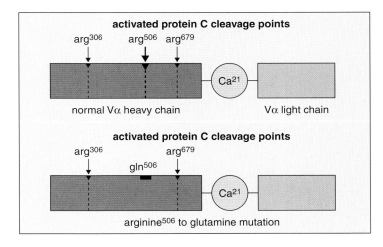

Fig. 26-6. Inactivation of factor Va. Activated protein C inactivates membrane-bound factor Va through proteolytic cleavage at three points in the Va heavy chain. In the factor V Leiden mutation, arginine at position 506 is replaced by glutamine, which renders this position resistant to activated protein C cleavage. The mutant factor V molecule can still be inactivated, but more slowly, at the remaining cleavage sites.

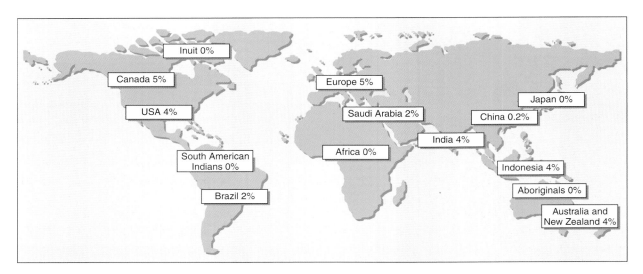

Fig. 26-7. Mutation *FV:R506Q*: distribution in the world population. (Modified with permission from Axelsson F, Rosén S: *Activated protein C resistance,* product monograph, Mölindal, Sweden, 1997, Chromogenix.)

PROTEIN C DEFICIENCY

Protein C is a vitamin K–dependent plasma protein synthesized by the liver. Its active form inhibits the active forms of coagulation factors V and VIII, and also increases lysis of clots by inactivating a protein that normally destroys tissue plasminogen activator. Activation of protein C occurs via thrombin bound to a protein, thrombomodulin, on the surface of the endothelial cell (Fig. 26-8).

Heterozygous protein C deficiency predisposes affected individuals to recurrent venous thromboses, which tend to manifest at an early age, usually less than 30 years. Homozygous protein C deficiency results in neonatal purpura fulminans, characterized by superficial thromboses. The skin lesions are initially swollen and red or purple; they become blue-black and may become necrotic (Fig. 26-9). The blood shows features of disseminated intravascular coagulation (DIC) with low levels of factors V and VIII, antithrombin, fibrinogen, and platelets.

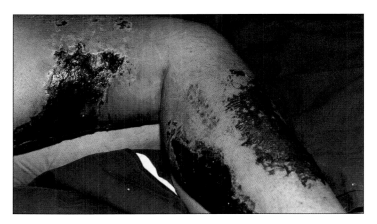

Fig. 26-9. Homozygous protein C deficiency. The patient, a 15-year-old girl, had skin necrosis and multiple venous thrombosis at 2 years of age.

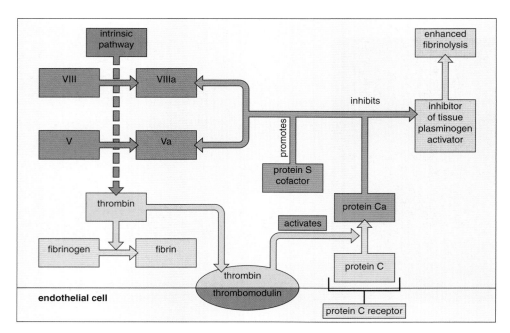

Fig. 26-8. Anticoagulant and fibrinolytic actions of protein C and protein S. *a,* activated.

PROTEIN S DEFICIENCY

The anticoagulant activity of protein C requires a cofactor protein S, which is also vitamin K dependent and exists in plasma as free and bound forms. Protein S deficiency, inherited probably as a dominant, causes recurrent venous thromboses.

ANTITHROMBIN DEFICIENCY

Antithrombin is a potent inhibitor of the activated serum protease factors XIa, Xa, IXa, IIa, and thrombin, forming high-molecular-weight inactive complexes with these proteins. Deficiency of antithrombin leads to recurrent venous thromboses that tend to be severe and manifest early in the homozygous form.

HYPERHOMOCYSTEINEMIA

The plasma concentration of homocysteine is an important contributing factor in thrombosis and vascular disease, including peripheral vascular disease, myocardial infarct, stroke, and venous thrombosis. Hyperhomocysteinemia is, in part, genetically determined—several alterations in enzymes involved in homocysteine metabolism (Fig. 26-10) have been described (e.g., the mutation *MTHFR C677T*). The mechanism of thrombosis is unclear, but endothelial cell damage may be important. Deficiencies of folate, vitamin B_{12}, and vitamin B_6 also cause hyperhomocysteinemia. The plasma level of homocysteinemia rises with age, is higher in men than in premenopausal women, and is raised after liver or renal transplantation.

HYPERPROTHROMBINEMIA

The *G20210A* mutation of prothrombin causes high levels of prothrombin and is thrombogenic.

OTHER DISORDERS

Although there are associations between thrombotic risk and high factor VIII levels, deficiency of heparin cofactor II and plasminogen, as well as other fibrinolytic defects, the evidence for familial thrombophilia as a result of these conditions is inconclusive. Dysfibrinogenemia is rarely a cause of thrombophilia.

ACQUIRED RISK FACTORS FOR VENOUS THROMBOSIS

Prominent acquired risk factors for venous thrombosis are listed in Table 26-3. These may be responsible for thrombosis in patients without another identifiable risk factor, but thrombosis is more likely if an inherited predisposition is also present.

Venous stasis and immobility are responsible for high rates of venous thrombosis in congestive heart failure, myocardial infarction, and varicose veins. In atrial fibrillation, thrombin generation from

---

TABLE 26-3.   VENOUS THROMBOSIS: ACQUIRED RISK FACTORS

Advanced age
Heart disease, myocardial infarct
Stroke
Immobility
Lupus anticoagulants
Malignancy
Obesity
Estrogen therapy (oral contraceptive and hormone replacement therapy)
Pregnancy and puerperium
Trauma and surgery
Varicose veins
Nephrotic syndrome
Hyperhomocysteinemia
Hyperviscosity states
Myeloproliferative diseases
Pelvic obstruction
Dehydration
Sepsis
Heparin-induced thrombocytopenia
Coagulation factor IX concentrates
Raised fibrinogen, factors VII, VIII, IX, and XI
Glucosylceremide deficiency
Paroxysmal nocturnal hemoglobinuria
Behçet's syndrome

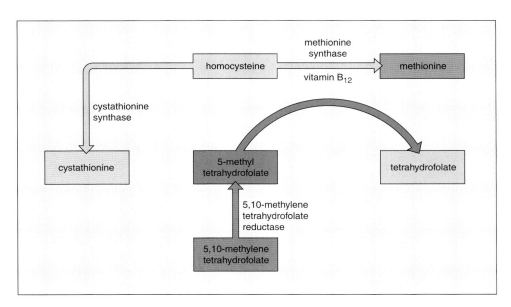

Fig. 26-10. Homocysteine metabolism: the roles of methionine synthase, cystathionine synthase, and 5,10-methylene tetrahydrofolate reductase (see also Fig. 7-10).

accumulated activated coagulation factors may lead to a high risk of systemic embolism. Venous stasis and immobility are also responsible for thrombosis associated with prolonged air, road, or rail travel.

Malignant tumors release tissue factors and a procoagulant that directly activates factor X. Deep vein thrombosis (DVT) is associated particularly with ovarian, pancreatic, and cerebral tumors.

Postoperative thrombosis is more likely in hip and abdominal surgery and in the obese, the elderly, or those with a previous history or family history of thrombosis.

Thrombosis in inflammation may be related to increased activity of procoagulant factors and is particularly associated with systemic tuberculosis, inflammatory bowel disease, systemic lupus erythematosus (SLE) and Behçet's disease.

Increased viscosity, thrombocytosis, and platelet function defects may all contribute to a high incidence of thrombosis in patients with myeloproliferative disorders.

Estrogen therapy (particularly high-dose contraceptive or hormone replacement therapy) is associated with increased thrombosis risk. These patients have elevated levels of coagulation factors II, VII, VIII, IX, and X and decreased plasma levels of antithrombin and tissue plasminogen activator.

Thrombosis occurring with coagulation factor IX concentrates is related to small quantities of activated coagulation factors in the preparations. Patients with liver disease who are unable to clear these activated factors promptly are particularly at risk.

Glucosylceramide is a modulator of the protein C pathway. Deficiency, especially in young males, has been linked to thrombosis.

ANTIPHOSPHOLIPID SYNDROME

In this syndrome, arterial or venous thrombosis or recurrent miscarriage is associated with laboratory evidence of persistent antiphospholipid antibodies. The "lupus anticoagulant" is identified when prolongation of the activated partial thromboplastin time (APTT) is not corrected by the addition of normal plasma. Other antibodies are anticardiolipin and antibodies to β_2-GPI. The reaction on the platelet surface is thrombogenic, even though coagulation tests such as the activated partial thromboplastin time (APTT) appear to show anticoagulation. These antibodies were first described in SLE and other autoimmune disorders. They also occur in lymphoproliferative disorders and with drugs such as phenothiazines, or they may be primary or idiopathic. Transient examples may follow viral or other infections. In addition to thrombosis and recurrent miscarriage, the antiphospholipid antibodies may be associated with persistent or relapsing thrombocytopenia and the skin condition livedo reticularis.

DIAGNOSIS OF VENOUS THROMBOSIS

CLINICAL PROBABILITY ASSESSMENT

DVT is suspected in patients with calf swelling or tenderness, unilateral pitting edema, and the presence of collateral superficial nonvaricose veins. Previous DVT, immobility, and cancer are important associations. A number of clinical probability assessments have been proposed. The Wells score (Table 26-4) has been used in numerous trials as a prediction of either the presence or absence of leg DVT confirmed by venography. In low-probability patients the median negative predictive value was 96%. Positive predictive values for high-probability patients were less than 75%.

D-DIMER ASSAY

After the stabilization of fibrin monomer by the action of activated factor XIII, covalent bonds between adjacent D-domains produce cross-linked fibrin. During fibrinolysis proteolytic cleavage of cross-linked fibrin by plasmin produces a heterogeneous group of degradation products, the smallest of which is D-dimer (Fig. 26-11). The

TABLE 26-4.   DEEP VEIN THROMBOSIS: CLINICAL ASSESSMENT: THE WELLS SCORE

	Points
Active cancer (treatment ongoing or within previous 6 months or palliative)	1
Paralysis, plaster	1
Bed more than 3 days, surgery within 4 weeks	1
Tenderness along veins	1
Entire leg swollen	1
Pitting edema	1
Collateral veins	1
Alternative diagnosis likely	−2
Low probability 0–1 *High probability 2 or more*	

From Wells PS et al: *N Engl J Med* 349:1227, 2003.

immunoassay for D-dimer is fibrin specific because D-dimer is not found in fibrinogen or in proteolytic fragments of fibrinogen. Elevated levels of D-dimer are almost invariably found when there is recent venous thrombosis or pulmonary embolism. The test has excellent negative predictive value and is most useful to exclude a diagnosis of DVT in patients with equivocal clinical features. In trials a negative D-dimer result in these patients was associated with a median negative predictive value of 99%. D-dimer testing in high-risk patients is not useful because most will have a positive result and will require radiologic imaging regardless of the result.

D-dimer elevation in trauma, postsurgery, postpartum, cancer, and inflammation limits its usefulness in hospital patients.

ULTRASOUND AND RADIOLOGIC IMAGING

Serial compression ultrasound is a reliable and practical method for detecting DVT in the thigh and other sites. The main signs are the absence of flow on color Doppler and an inability to compress the vein (Fig. 26-12). DVT in the popliteal and calf veins is detected more reliably by contrast computed tomography (CT) scanning (Fig. 26-13). Contrast venography (Figs. 26-14 and 26-15) has been largely replaced by contrast CT scanning but remains a very sensitive technique to demonstrate the site, size, and extent of the thrombus. It is often a painful technique and carries a risk of procedure-induced DVT. Both contrast venography and CT scanning have been used in diagnosis of venous thrombosis in other sites (e.g., hepatic) (Figs. 26-16 and 26-17).

A possible diagnostic approach for DVT is shown in Fig. 26-18.

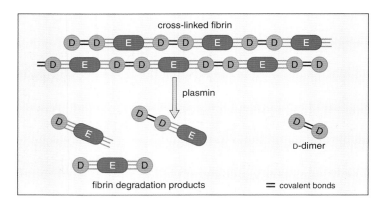

Fig. 26-11. Venous thrombosis: the formation of D-dimer.

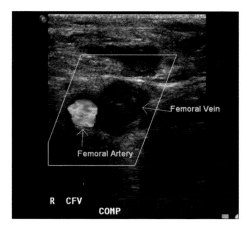

Fig. 26-12. Deep vein thrombosis: color power Doppler ultrasound of right femoral vessels with compression showing normal flow in the femoral artery but absent flow in the vein because of thrombosis. A normal vein would collapse with compression of the probe. (Courtesy of Dr. Tony Young.)

Fig. 26-13. Deep vein thrombosis: computed tomography scan of the popliteal region following intravenous injection of contrast. There is normal enhancement of veins on the *right (red arrow)*. The *left* image shows a peripheral rim of enhancement surrounding thrombus within the popliteal vein *(yellow arrow)*. (Courtesy of Dr. Sharyn MacDonald.)

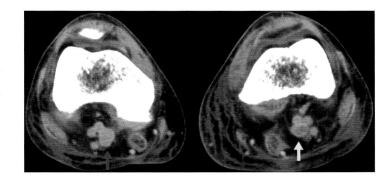

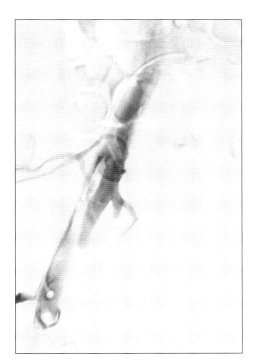

Fig. 26-14. Deep vein thrombosis: a femoral venogram demonstrating extensive thrombus within the right external iliac vein extending into the right common iliac vein. (Courtesy of Dr. I. S. Francis and Dr. A. F. Watkinson.)

Fig. 26-15. Deep vein thrombosis: a Gunther-Tulip filter positioned within the infrarenal inferior vena cava to prevent pulmonary embolism. Percutaneous access is via either the femoral or internal jugular vein. This particular device has a proximal hook, which permits its removal up to 2 weeks following placement. (Courtesy of Dr. I. S. Francis and Dr. A. F. Watkinson.)

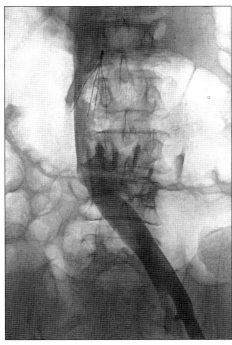

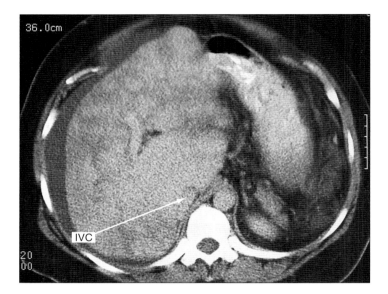

Fig. 26-16. Hepatic veno-occlusive disease (Budd–Chiari syndrome): dynamic contrast-enhanced computed tomography showing the reticulated mosaic pattern of hepatic parenchymal enhancement with poor visualization of the hepatic veins. Typically, the caudate lobe enhances normally and appears hyperdense relative to the remaining liver parenchyma. Ascites is present, and the inferior vena cava is narrowed. (Courtesy of Dr. I. S. Francis and Dr. J. Tibballs.)

DIAGNOSIS OF PULMONARY EMBOLUS

CLINICAL ASSESSMENT

A sudden onset of dyspnea is the usual presenting symptom. Oppressive substernal pain is a feature of massive embolism. Pleuritic chest pain and hemoptysis occur only after infarction has occurred. Physical examination may be deceptively normal. In massive embolism signs may include a palpable lift over the right ventricle at the left sternal edge and right ventricular gallop.

A pleural friction rub and signs of pleural effusion will not be present unless infarction has occurred. Electrocardiograms may show evidence of right-sided heart strain in relatively severe cases. Chest x-rays are often normal but may show evidence of pulmonary infarcts or pleural effusion.

CT pulmonary angiography is an accurate and rapid way to diagnose pulmonary embolism and has virtually replaced nuclear medicine ventilation-perfusion scans and conventional pulmonary angiography. The emboli are visualized as filling defects within the contrast-filled pulmonary arteries (Figs. 26-19 and 26-20). Gallium-enhanced magnetic resonance imaging (MRI) is a relatively new and expensive technique, but it is accurate.

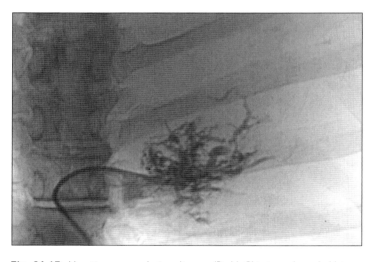

Fig. 26-17. Hepatic veno-occlusive disease (Budd–Chiari syndrome). Using a transjugular approach, a catheter was introduced into the right hepatic vein. Direct injection of contrast shows a characteristic interlacing network of intrahepatic, portal and hepatic veins, with no flow exiting via the hepatic veins. This "spider web" appearance is unique to Budd–Chiari syndrome. (Courtesy of Dr. I. S. Francis and Dr. J. Tibballs.)

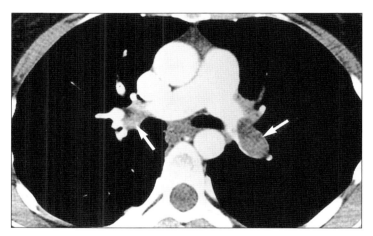

Fig. 26-19. Pulmonary embolus: contrast-enhanced spiral computed tomography that shows filling defects within both main pulmonary arteries (arrows). These represent large pulmonary emboli. (Courtesy of Professor D. M. Hansell.)

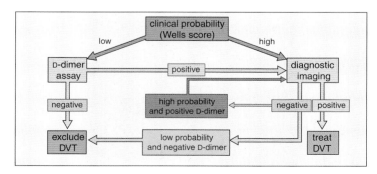

Fig. 26-18. Deep vein thrombosis (DVT): an approach to diagnosis.

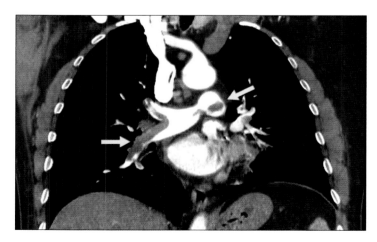

Fig. 26-20. Pulmonary embolus: computed tomography pulmonary angiography. A coronal image shows bilateral filling defects in the central pulmonary arteries indicating pulmonary emboli (yellow arrows). (Courtesy of Dr. Tony Young.)

ANTIPLATELET DRUGS

The action of antiplatelet drugs is depicted in Fig. 26-21.

ASPIRIN

Aspirin inhibits platelet cyclo-oxygenase irreversibly, thus reducing the production of platelet thromboxane A2. It has been suggested that vascular endothelial cyclo-oxygenase is less sensitive to aspirin than platelet cyclo-oxygenase. Low-dose therapy (e.g., 75 mg/day) is more effective than standard doses at enhancing the prostacyclin-to-thromboxane A2 ratio and may have a greater antithrombotic effect. Aspirin is now used widely in the prevention of coronary, cerebrovascular, and peripheral arterial disease, as well as in patients who have a history of these conditions. It may also be useful in preventing thrombosis in patients with thrombocytosis.

DIPYRIDAMOLE (PERSANTIN)

This drug is a phosphodiesterase inhibitor thought to elevate cyclic adenosine monophosphate (cAMP) levels in circulating platelets, which decreases their sensitivity to activating stimuli. Dipyridamole has been shown to reduce thromboembolic complications in patients with prosthetic heart valves and to improve the results in coronary bypass operations.

SULFINPYRAZONE

This drug is a competitive inhibitor of cyclo-oxygenase. It has been effective in reducing the frequency of blockage in arteriovenous shunts in chronic dialysis patients.

TICLOPIDINE

This antiplatelet drug was used following coronary angioplasty. Side effects include neutropenia and thrombocytopenia. It has been replaced by clopidogrel except in patients intolerant of clopidogrel.

CLOPIDOGREL

This adenosine diphosphate (ADP) receptor antagonist is an antiplatelet agent in use for reduction of ischemic events in patients with ischemic stroke, myocardial infarction, or peripheral vascular disease. It is used after coronary artery stenting or angioplasty and in patients requiring long-term antiplatelet therapy who are intolerant of or allergic to aspirin.

GLYCOPROTEIN IIb/IIIa INHIBITORS

Abciximab, eptifibatide, and tirofiban are monoclonal antibodies that inhibit the platelet GPIIb/IIIa complex, a member of the integrin family of receptors (Fig. 26-22). They are used in conjunction with heparin and aspirin for the prevention of ischemic complications in high-risk patients undergoing percutaneous transluminal coronary angioplasty and in those with an acute coronary syndrome. They can be used once only. A summary of antiplatelet therapy in acute coronary syndromes is tabulated in Table 26-5.

PROSTACYCLIN

Intravenous prostacyclin has been used in clinical trials in patients with peripheral vascular disease and thrombotic thrombocytopenic purpura. It has also reduced arteriovenous shunt blockage in hemodialysis patients.

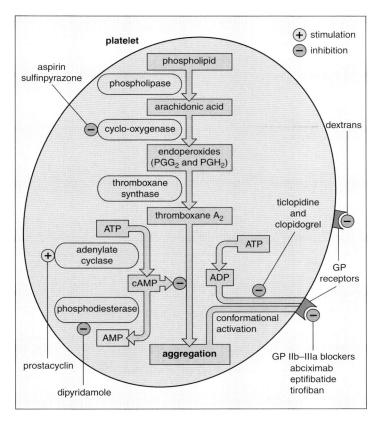

Fig. 26-21. Sites of action of antiplatelet drugs: aspirin acetylates the enzyme cyclo-oxygenase irreversibly. Sulfinpyrazone inhibits cyclo-oxygenase reversibly. Dipyridamole inhibits phosphodiesterase, increases cyclic adenosine monophosphate (cAMP) levels, and inhibits aggregation. Inhibition of adenosine uptake by red cells allows adenosine accumulation in plasma, which stimulates platelet adenylate cyclase. Prostacyclin stimulates adenylate cyclase. Ticlopidine and clopidogrel inhibit conformational activation of GP IIb/IIIa needed for platelet aggregation. Three GP IIb/IIIa blockers are licensed for human use: abciximab, eptifibatide, and tirofiban. The lipid-soluble β-blockers inhibit phospholipase. Calcium channel antagonists block the influx of free calcium ions across the platelet membrane. Dextrans coat the surface, interfering with adhesion and aggregation. ADP, Adenosine diphosphate; ATP, adenosine triphosphate; PG, prostaglandin. (Modified from Hoffbrand AV, Pettit JE: *Essential hematology,* ed 3, Oxford, 1993, Blackwell Scientific.)

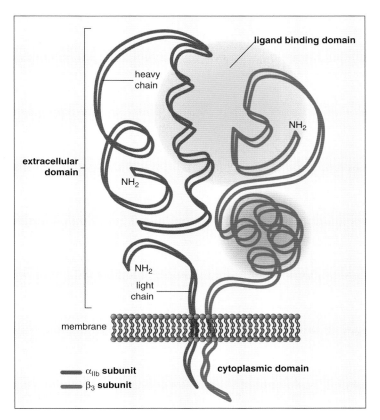

Fig. 26-22. The platelet GPIIb-GPIIIa complex. (Modified with permission from Topol EJ, Byzova TV, Plow EF: Platelet GPIIb–GPIIIa blockers, *Lancet* 353:227–231, 1999.).

TABLE 26-5. ANTIPLATELET THERAPY: ANTIPLATELET DRUGS USED IN PATIENTS WITH AN ACUTE CORONARY SYNDROME AND IN THOSE UNDERGOING PERCUTANEOUS CORONARY INTERVENTION

Drug	Target/patient group	Duration
Acute coronary syndrome		
Aspirin	All	Lifelong
Clopidogrel	All	9–12 months
Glycoprotein IIb/IIIa inhibitors		
Abciximab	None	–
Eptifibatide	High risk	48–72 hours
Tirofiban	High risk	48–72 hours
Patients undergoing PCI		
Aspirin	All	Lifelong
Clopidogrel	All	9–12 months
Abciximab	High risk	12 hours after PCI
Eptifibatide	High risk	18–24 hours after PCI

After Lange RA, Hillis LD: *N Engl J Med* 350:277–280, 2004.
PCI, Percutaneous coronary intervention.

TABLE 26-6. HEPARINS (UNFRACTIONATED AND OF LOW MOLECULAR WEIGHT): COMPARISON OF EFFECTS

	Unfractionated	Low molecular weight
Mean molecular weight (kDa)	15	4.5
Inhibits	Xa and thrombin equally	Xa ± thrombin (2:1–4:1)
Platelet function	Inhibits	No inhibition
Protein binding	Yes	Reduced
Bioavailability	50%	100%
Elimination	Hepatic and renal	Renal
Half-life of anti-Xa, intravenous	1 hr	2 hr
Half-life of anti-Xa, subcutaneous	2 hr	4 hr
Frequency of heparin-induced thrombosis	High	Low
Osteoporosis	More frequent	Less frequent

ANTICOAGULANT THERAPY

HEPARIN

Heparin is an acid polysaccharide that potentiates (with antithrombin and heparin cofactor) inactivation of the serine protease coagulation factors (Fig. 26-23). Preparations are either unfractionated (standard heparin, molecular weight [MW] 15 to 18 kDa) or fractionated (low-molecular-weight heparin [LMWH], MW 4.8 kDa). Lower-molecular-weight preparations (e.g., dalteparin, enoxaparin) are better able to inhibit factor Xa than thrombin (Fig. 26-24), interact less with platelets, and cause less bleeding (Table 26-6). Side effects of heparin include bleeding and thrombocytopenia, either type I within 1 or 2 days because of agglutinates or type II after 5 days or more because of platelet-activating autoantibodies directed against platelet factor 4 complexes. Type II is associated with thrombosis. Rarely, skin necrosis may occur at sites of injection (Fig. 26-25), and osteoporosis is a late complication.

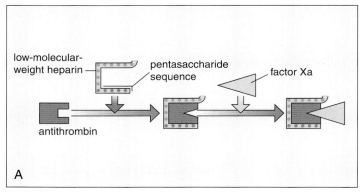

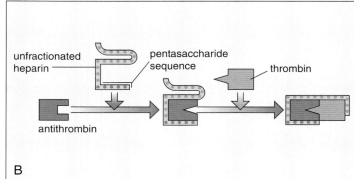

Fig. 26-24. Heparins (unfractionated and of low molecular weight): catalysis of antithrombin-mediated inactivation of thrombin or factor Xa. **A,** The pentasaccharide sequence of both types of heparin causes a conformational change at the reactive center of antithrombin when bound to it, which accelerates its reaction with factor Xa. **B,** Catalysis of antithrombin-mediated inactivation of thrombin requires the formation of a ternary heparin-antithrombin-thrombin complex, which can be formed only by chains at least 18 saccharide units long. This explains why heparins of low molecular weight have less inhibitory activity against thrombin than unfractionated heparin. (Modified with permission from Weitz JI: Low molecular weight heparins, *N Engl J Med* 337:688–698, 1997.)

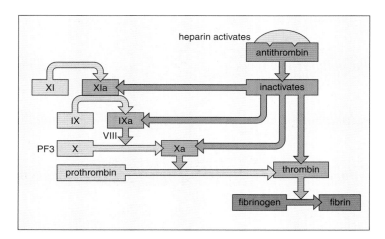

Fig. 26-23. The action of heparin: this activates antithrombin, which then forms complexes with activated serine protease coagulation factors (thrombin, Xa, IXa, and XIa) and so inactivates them. (Modified with permission from Hoffbrand AV, Pettit JE: *Essential hematology,* ed 3, Oxford, 1993, Blackwell Scientific.)

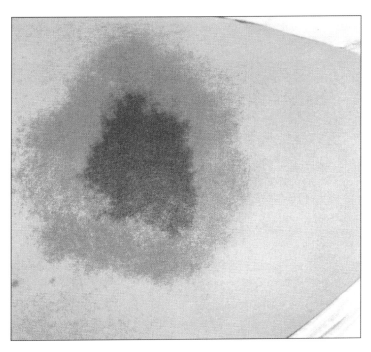

Fig. 26-25. Heparin: skin necrosis. After local subcutaneous injection of unfractionated heparin.

WARFARIN

The traditional oral anticoagulants are derivatives of coumarin and indanedione. Warfarin, a coumarin derivative, is used most widely. These drugs are vitamin K antagonists, and therapy results in reduced activity of coagulation factors II, VII, IX, and X.

The mechanism of action is shown in Fig. 26-26. Therapy is monitored by prothrombin time testing and international normalized

TABLE 26-7. WARFARIN THERAPY: RECOMMENDED RANGES FOR INTERNATIONAL NORMALIZED RATIO FOR DIFFERENT CLINICAL INDICATIONS

Target INR	Clinical state
2.5 (2.0–3.0)	Treatment of DVT, pulmonary embolism, atrial fibrillation, recurrent DVT off warfarin; symptomatic inherited thrombophilia, cardiomyopathy, mural thrombosis, cardioversion
3.0 (2.5–3.5)	Recurrent DVT while on warfarin, mechanical prosthetic heart valves, antiphospholipid syndrome (some cases)

DVT, Deep vein thrombosis; *INR,* international normalized ratio.

ratio (INR) (Table 26-7). The activity of warfarin can be enhanced or inhibited by a wide variety of drugs (Table 26-8). Warfarin resistance may also be caused by mutations in the gene that codes the enzymatically active component in the vitamin K epoxide reductase complex *(VKORC 1)*. This site is likely to be the site of warfarin action. The mutations do not appear to interfere with the vitamin K metabolism. Sensitivity to warfarin may be increased with polymorphisms in cytochrome P450 CYP2C9, which are associated with a low dose requirement. A recommended approach to the management of overdose and bleeding complication is outlined in Table 26-9.

FACTOR Xa INHIBITORS

Fondaparinux, a synthetic analog of the antithrombin-binding pentasaccharide of heparin, is an indirect factor Xa inhibitor. Given subcutaneously with a half-life of 17 hours, it does not require

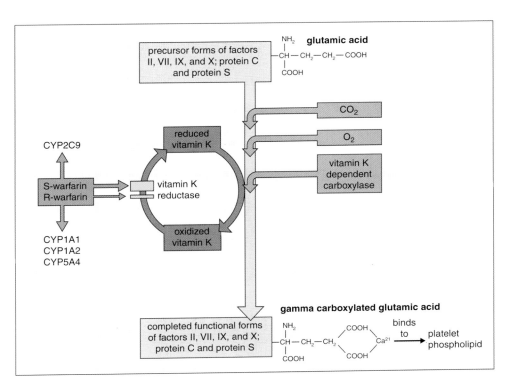

Fig. 26-26. The action of vitamin K in γ-carboxylation of glutamic acid in coagulation factors, which are then able to bind to platelet phospholipid. By inhibiting vitamin K reductase, warfarin interferes with the regeneration of the reduced form of vitamin K required for the carboxylation of coagulation factors. Genetic single-nucleotide polymorphism in the cytochrome P450 complex CYP2C9 may result in

different warfarin dose requirements. Patients with the variants CYP2C9*2 and CYP2C9*3 eliminate warfarin slowly and require lower doses. Single-nucleotide polymorphisms in vitamin K reductase are also associated with increased sensitivity to warfarin.

TABLE 26-8. WARFARIN THERAPY: DRUG INTERFERENCE WITH CONTROL OF THERAPY

Increase warfarin effect

Antibiotics
Cephalosporins
Ciprofloxacin
Clarithromycin
Co-trimoxazole
Erythromycin
Isoniazid
Metronidazole
Penicillins
Quinolones
Roxithromycin
Tetracycline

Antifungals
Fluconazole
Itraconazole
Ketoconazole
Miconazole

Antiinflammatory
Aspirin
Phenylbutazone
Diclofenac
Piroxicam
Other NSAIDs
Paracetamol
Sulfinpyrazone

Cardiac
Amiodarone
Clofibrate
Propranolol
Propafenone
Quinidine
Statins
Verapamil

Central nervous system
Antidepressants
Tricyclics
SSRIs
Valproate

Gastrointestinal
Cimetidine
Cisapride
Omeprazole

Others
Allopurinol
Anabolic Steroids
Danazol
Disulfiram
Flutamide
Fosfamide
Tamoxifen
Thyroxine
Proquanil
Ritonavir

Decrease warfarin effect

Aminoglutethimide
Acetretin
Barbiturates
Carbamazepine
Chlorodiazepoxide
Cholestyramine
Griseofulvin

Oral Contraceptives
Phenytoin
Primidone
Rifampicin
Sucralfate
Vitamin K

NSAIDS, Nonsteroidal antiinflammatory drugs; *SSRIs,* selective serotonin reuptake inhibitors.

TABLE 26-10. BLOOD COAGULATION: ACTIVATION AND INHIBITION: SITES OF ACTION OF NEW ANTICOAGULANTS

Coagulation pathway	Anticoagulants
Initiation — TF/VIIa	**Tissue factor pathway inhibitors –** TFPI, NAPc2, VIIai
Thrombin generation — X, IX	**IXa inhibitors –** IXai, IXa antibody
IXa, VIIIa	**Protein C activators** (protein C, thrombomodulin)
Xa Va II	**Xa inhibitors –** TAP, pentasaccharide analogues fondaparinux, idraparinux, rivaroxaban
Thrombin activity — IIa (thrombin)	**IIa (thrombin) inhibitors –** hirudin, bivalirudin, dabigatran

TAP, tick anticoagulating peptide.

laboratory monitoring. Idraparinux, a chemically modified analog of fondaparinux, has a longer half-life, and as a weekly injection in selected patients it may be more convenient than warfarin or LMWH.

Rivaroxaban taken orally has had excellent results in preventing venous thromboembolism.

DIRECT THROMBIN INHIBITORS

Direct thrombin inhibitors (Table 26-10) are effective against both free thrombin and thrombin bound to fibrin, but they do not inhibit

TABLE 26-9. WARFARIN THERAPY: RECOMMENDATIONS FOR THE MANAGEMENT OF BLEEDING AND EXCESSIVE ANTICOAGULATION

INR 3.0–6.0 No bleeding	Reduce or stop warfarin Restart warfarin when INR <5
INR 6.0–8.0 No bleeding or minor bleeding	Stop warfarin Repeat INR next day Restart in reduced dose when INR <5 If INR fails to shorten or if reversal required within 24–48 hours give 1 mg oral vitamin K
If INR >8.0 No bleeding or minor bleeding	Stop warfarin Give 1–2.5 mg oral vitamin K Repeat INR next day; give repeat dose of vitamin K if necessary Restart warfarin in reduced dosage when INR <5
Major bleeding	Stop warfarin Give vitamin K 5 mg intravenously slowly Admit to hospital Give prothrombin complex concentrate or fresh frozen plasma

INR, International normalized ratio.

thrombin generation. Hirudin was originally extracted from the salivary glands of the medicinal leech *Hirudo medicinalis*. It is more effective than heparin in the prevention of venous thrombosis in high-risk patients and has been recommended for use in heparin-induced thrombocytopenia. Bivalirudin has been used as an alternative to heparin in patients having percutaneous coronary interventions, and given alone it suppresses adverse ischemic events to a similar extent as heparin plus glycoprotein IIb/IIIa inhibitors and is associated with a lower risk of hemorrhage.

Dabigatran etexilate (Pradaxa) is a once daily, orally active direct thrombin inhibitor, approved in the UK for the prevention of DVT in orthopedic patients and is undergoing trials for the treatment of DVT.

FIBRINOLYTIC AGENTS

Fibrinolytic agents act by enhancing conversion of plasminogen to plasmin, which degrades fibrin by proteolytic cleavage (Fig. 26-27). They are able to lyse fresh thrombi and are widely used in clinical practice. Systemic intravenous therapy is of proven benefit for patients with acute myocardial infarction, major pulmonary emboli, or iliofemoral DVT. Local therapy via an indwelling catheter is used in acute peripheral arterial or venous thrombosis.

Streptokinase, a peptide produced by hemolytic streptococci, forms a complex with plasminogen that converts other plasminogen molecules to plasmin. Urokinase is a tissue plasminogen activator initially extracted from urine. Second-generation thrombolytic agents include tissue plasminogen activator (tPA), which is synthesized using recombinant DNA technology. Recombinant tPA (alteplase) is more fibrin specific with less systemic activation of fibrinolysis and bleeding than streptokinase. It is superior to streptokinase and has a lower short-term mortality rate. Other newer agents include single-chain, urokinase-type plasminogen activator and acylated plasminogen streptokinase activator complex. Laboratory tests for controlling and monitoring short-term thrombolytic therapy are unnecessary. The possibility of dangerous hemorrhage or other clinical complications may exclude the use of thrombolytic therapy (Table 26-11).

TABLE 26-11.   THROMBOLYTIC THERAPY: CONTRAINDICATIONS TO THERAPY

Absolute contraindications

Active gastrointestinal bleeding
Aortic dissection
Head injury or cerebrovascular accident in the past 2 months
Neurosurgery in the past 2 months
Intracranial aneurysm or neoplasm
Proliferative diabetic retinopathy

Relative contraindications

Traumatic cardiopulmonary resuscitation
Major surgery in the past 10 days
Past history of gastrointestinal bleeding
Recent obstetric delivery
Prior arterial puncture
Prior organ biopsy
Serious trauma
Severe arterial hypertension (systolic pressure >200 mm Hg, diastolic pressure >110 mm Hg)
Bleeding diathesis

POSTTHROMBOTIC SYNDROME

Postthrombotic or postphlebitic syndrome is the development of chronic venous insufficiency after deep vein thrombosis. Injury to the venous system produces symptoms that include edema, pain, changes in skin pigmentation, and venous ulcers. Trophic skin changes may include any of the following: hyperpigmentation, lipodermatosclerosis, asteatosis (acquired ichthyosis), atrophy blanche, and venous ulceration (Figs. 26-28 to 26-30). In a minority of patients, extensive proximal venous thrombosis is complicated by thrombosis in collateral veins, and this may be associated with phlegmasia. Many patients with this serious complication have widespread cancer. In the milder

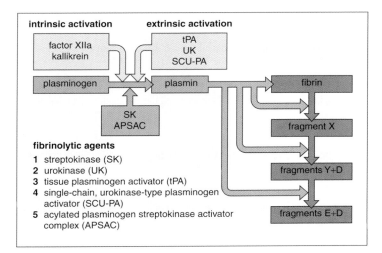

Fig. 26-27. The fibrinolytic system and fibrinolytic agents. (Modified with permission from Hoffbrand AV, Pettit JE: *Essential hematology*, ed 3, Oxford, 1993, Blackwell Scientific.)

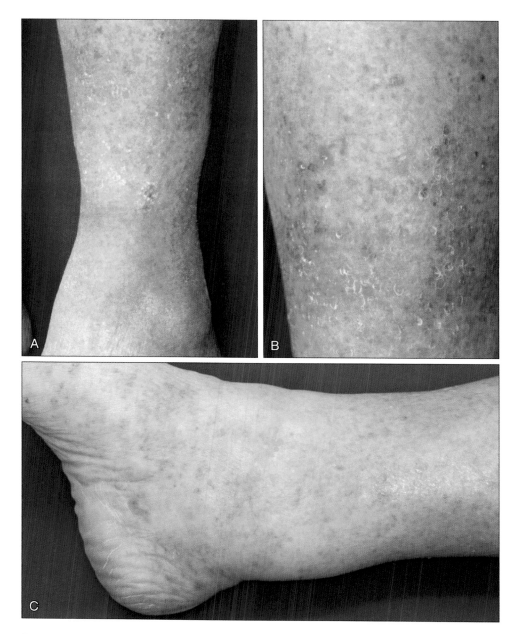

Fig. 26-28. Postthrombotic syndrome: skin changes in chronic venous insufficiency. **A,** Lower left leg pigmentation, lipodermatosclerosis, and a small venous ulcer. **B,** A closer view of the same leg showing central atrophy blanche and lateral changes of asteatosis (acquired ichthyosis). **C,** Lower leg and ankle edema in a different patient. (All images courtesy of Dr. Kenneth Macdonald.)

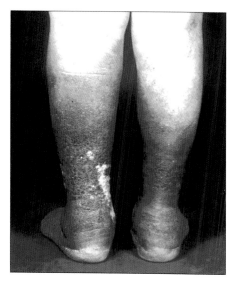

Fig. 26-29. Postthrombotic syndrome: both lower legs show marked pigmentation and lipodermatosclerosis. (Courtesy of Professor George Hamilton.)

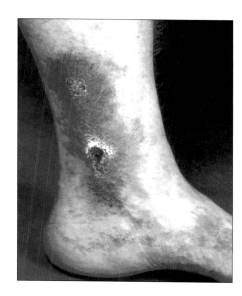

Fig. 26-30. Postthrombotic syndrome: a healing venous ulcer with surrounding pigmentation. (Courtesy of Professor George Hamilton.)

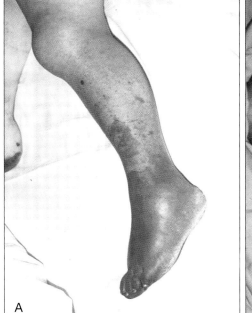
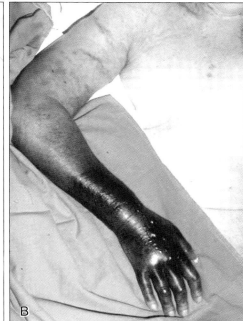

Fig. 26-31. Postthrombotic syndrome: phlegmasia cerulea dolens. **A,** Grossly swollen left leg with marked cyanosis and early ischemic changes in the foot. **B,** Swollen right arm with marked cyanosis and early venous gangrene of the hand. (Courtesy of Professor George Hamilton.)

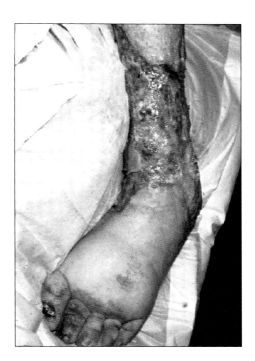

Fig. 26-32. Postthrombotic syndrome: Marjolin's ulcer. Squamous cell carcinoma at the margins of a very extensive and neglected venous ulcer. (Courtesy of Professor George Hamilton.)

form of phlegmasia (alba dolens) there is severe edema, pain, and blanching (alba) without cyanosis. In fulminant or progressive disease associated with ischemia (phlegmasia cerulea dolens), there is marked cyanosis in addition to massive edema and, in many patients, venous gangrene (Fig. 26-31). Involvement of the arm occurs in less than 5% of patients. Long-standing untreated venous ulceration may be complicated by the development of squamous cell carcinoma (Fig. 26-32).

SECONDARY ANEMIA AND BONE MARROW IN NONHEMATOPOIETIC DISORDERS

ANEMIA OF CHRONIC DISORDERS

The anemia of chronic disorders, sometimes referred to as secondary anemia, is found in patients with infections, inflammation, and malignancy (Table 27-1). Less well recognized is its association with some patients with severe heart disease, diabetes, severe trauma, and acute and chronic immune activation. The blood count usually shows a moderate normocytic, normochromic anemia, although occasionally hemoglobin levels may be less than 8.0 g/dL.

A number of factors may contribute to the pathogenesis of this anemia (Fig. 27-1). The dominant problem is reduced red cell production. Hemoglobin production is restricted by reduced release of iron from macrophages with low serum iron levels. Increased hepcidin levels in patients with infections, inflammation, and malignancy have a dominant role in this disturbance of iron metabolism. Erythropoiesis is unable to respond to the anemia despite moderate increases in erythropoietin levels. It has been suggested that there may be increased apoptosis of erythroblasts. An inadequate erythropoietin production in response to the anemia has been suggested as a minor contributing factor. Cytokine and growth factor release (e.g., interleukin 1, interleukin 6, tumor necrosis factor) by the primary condition may initiate activation of other factors (e.g., interferons β and α), which have been shown to replicate a similar anemia in animals. A minor factor in the pathogenesis of anemia may be some reduction in red cell survival.

The blood film shows mild red cell changes, including anisocytosis and poikilocytosis. There may be obvious rouleaux formation (Fig. 27-2). The reticulocyte count is inappropriately low. The extent of elevations in erythrocyte sedimentation rate (ESR), C-reactive protein, and fibrinogen are determined by the underlying illness. In most patients, the serum iron and transferrin or total iron-binding capacity are low with a normal iron saturation.

A minority show low saturation similar to iron deficiency. The serum ferritin level is usually normal or elevated, but this may be inaccurate as an indicator of iron stores because of its release by inflammatory and necrotic tissue. Serum transferrin receptor levels are not increased.

The bone marrow may show minor changes in erythropoiesis. There may be clusters of erythroblasts in close proximity to macrophages (Fig. 27-3). Iron staining usually shows normal or increased storage of iron with reduced or absent siderotic granulation in erythroblasts (Fig. 27-4).

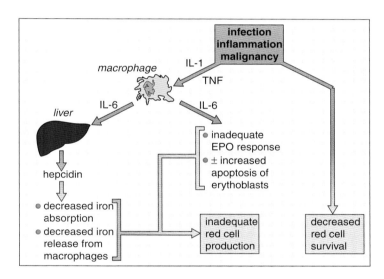

Fig. 27-1. Factors involved in the pathogenesis of anemia of chronic disorders.

TABLE 27-1.	CONDITIONS ASSOCIATED WITH ANEMIA OF CHRONIC DISORDERS

Chronic inflammatory diseases

Infectious
For example, pulmonary abscess, tuberculosis, osteomyelitis, pneumonia, bacterial endocarditis

Noninfectious
For example, rheumatoid arthritis, systemic lupus erythematosus and other connective tissue diseases, sarcoid, Crohn's disease, cirrhosis

Malignant disease

For example, carcinoma, lymphoma, sarcoma, myeloma

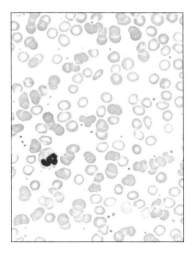

Fig. 27-2. Anemia of chronic disorders: blood film showing mild red cell anisocytosis, poikilocytosis, and rouleaux formation.

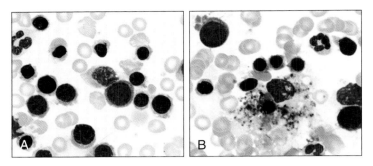

Fig. 27-3. Anemia of chronic disorders: bone marrow aspirate. **A,** Normoblastic erythroblasts showing minor irregularity. **B,** Erythroblasts in close association with a macrophage.

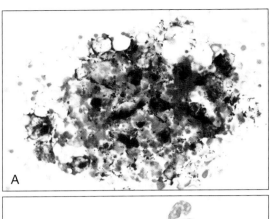

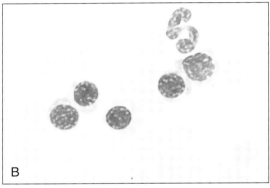

Fig. 27-4. Secondary anemia: bone marrow aspirate showing fragments containing adequate iron in the reticuloendothelial cells **(A)** and no siderotic granules in the developing erythroblasts **(B).** (Perls' stain.)

MALIGNANT DISEASES (OTHER THAN LEUKEMIAS, LYMPHOMAS, AND HISTIOCYTIC/MYELOPROLIFERATIVE DISORDERS)

Anemia may result from multiple factors. The anemia of chronic disorders, blood loss, iron deficiency, bone marrow failure from extensive marrow replacement by metastatic disease, folate deficiency, hemolysis, and marrow suppression from chemotherapy or radiotherapy may be involved in different malignancies (Table 27-2).

TABLE 27-2. HEMATOLOGIC ABNORMALITIES IN MALIGNANT DISEASE

Hematologic abnormalities	Tumor or treatment associated
Pancytopenia	
Marrow hypoplasia	Chemotherapy, radiotherapy
Myelodysplasia	Metastases in marrow
Leukoerythroblastic	Folate deficiency
Megaloblastic	B_{12} deficiency (carcinoma of stomach)
Red cells	
Anemia of chronic disorders	Most forms
Iron-deficiency anemia	Especially gastrointestinal, uterine
Pure red-cell aplasia	Thymoma
Immune hemolytic anemia	Lymphoma, ovary, other tumors
Microangiopathic hemolytic anemia	Mucin-secreting carcinoma
Polycythemia	Kidney, liver, cerebellum, uterus
White cells	
Neutrophil leukocytosis	Most forms
Leukemoid reaction	Disseminated tumors, those with necrosis
Eosinophilia	Hodgkin's disease, others
Monocytosis	Various tumors
Platelets and coagulation	
Thrombocytosis	Gastrointestinal tumors with bleeding, others
Disseminated intravascular coagulation	Mucin-secreting carcinoma, prostate
Activation of fibrinolysis	Prostate
Acquired inhibitors of coagulation	Most forms
Paraprotein interfering with platelet function	Lymphomas, myeloma
Tumor cell procoagulants – tissue factor and cancer procoagulant (direct activation of factor X)	Especially ovarian, pancreas, brain, colon

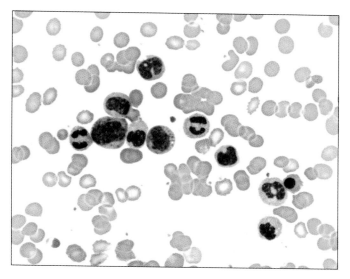

Fig. 27-5. Malignant disease: blood film in a patient with carcinoma of the breast and metastatic marrow involvement showing leukoerythroblastic features.

Blood film leukoerythroblastic change (Fig. 27-5) is found when there is extensive metastatic involvement of marrow. Leukemoid changes may occur if there is associated inflammation or tumor necrosis.

Microangiopathic hemolysis occurs with mucin-secreting adenocarcinoma, for example, some tumors of the stomach, lung, or breast (Fig. 27-6). Autoimmune hemolytic anemia occurs in some malignant lymphomas and rarely in other tumors. Primary red cell aplasia has been found in association with thymomas and lymphoma, and myelodysplastic syndrome may follow chemotherapy or radiotherapy. Some cases of carcinoma of the stomach may occur in association with pernicious anemia.

Secondary polycythemia (see Chapter 15) is seen in occasional renal, hepatic, cerebellar, and uterine tumors.

Malignancy may be associated either with thrombocytosis or thrombocytopenia. Disseminated intravascular coagulation occurs with mucin-secreting adenocarcinoma. There may be activation of fibrinolysis in some carcinomas of the prostate.

Venous thromboembolism is most common in tumors of the ovary, brain, pancreas, and colon and may also follow surgical treatment of any cancer.

The bone marrow is involved most commonly by metastatic deposits from carcinomas of the breast (Fig. 27-7), prostate (Figs. 27-8 and 27-9), lung (Fig. 27-10), kidney (Fig. 27-11), and thyroid.

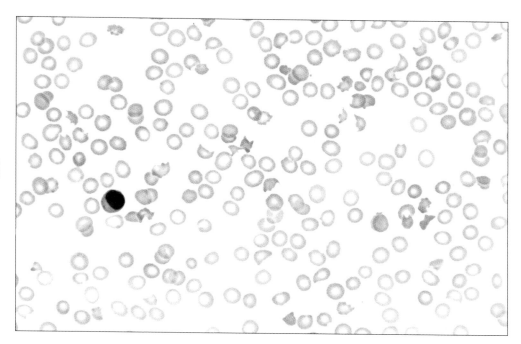

Fig. 27-6. Carcinoma of the stomach: blood film showing red cell fragmentation and thrombocytopenia.

Fig. 27-7. Metastatic carcinoma of the breast. **A,** Marrow aspirate cell trail showing a nest of neoplastic epithelial cells with features of a large undifferentiated carcinoma. **B,** The trephine biopsy also shows sheets and clumps of similar neoplastic epithelial cells. **C,** Immunohistologic staining in the same biopsy showing positivity for estrogen receptor (ER).

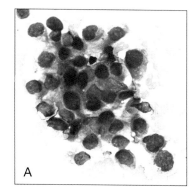

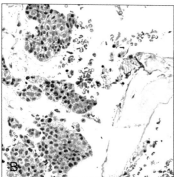

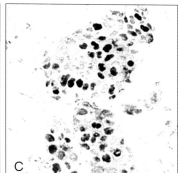

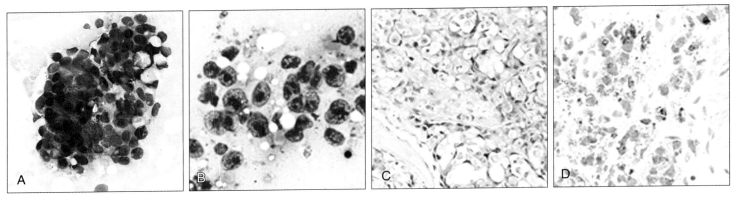

Fig. 27-8. Metastatic carcinoma of the prostate. **A,** Marrow aspirate showing a sheet of neoplastic cells. **B,** A trephine biopsy "roll" in the same patient shows nuclear detail, including prominent nucleoli. **C,** The trephine sections from the same patient show almost complete replacement of hematopoietic cells by sheets of pleomorphic cells from a poorly differentiated adenocarcinoma. **D,** Immunohistologic staining for prostate-specific antigen (PSA) shows strong cytoplasmic positivity in the tumor cells.

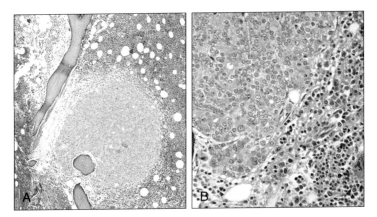

Fig. 27-9. Metastatic carcinoma. **A,** A prominent paratrabecular deposit of neoplastic epithelial cells; the patient had chronic lymphocytic leukemia and a primary carcinoma of the prostate. **B,** Higher power shows a clear separation of malignant epithelial tissue from hematopoietic tissue that contains increased numbers of lymphocytes.

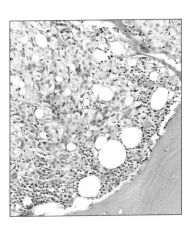

Fig. 27-11. Metastatic carcinoma: sheets of pleomorphic neoplastic epithelial cells (primary carcinoma of kidney).

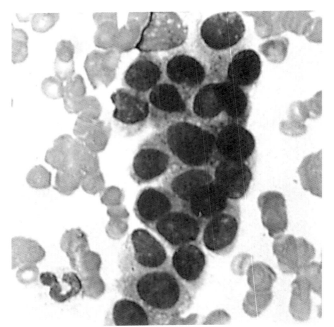

Fig. 27-10. Metastatic carcinoma: of the lung. The marrow aspirate shows a loose collection of pleomorphic neoplastic cells.

Metastatic involvement by carcinomas of the stomach (Fig. 27-12), colon (Fig. 27-13), and pancreas occur less frequently, but virtually any malignant tumor may involve the marrow (Figs. 27-14 and 27-15). Skeletal lesions are predominantly osteolytic, appearing as radiolucent areas in radiographic examination (Fig. 27-16). Extensive osteoclastic resorption of bone is often found in trephine biopsies (Fig. 27-17). Most tumors provoke some healing and sometimes new bone deposition; osteoblastic activity is most pronounced in metastatic spread from carcinoma of the prostate (Fig. 27-18) and breast (Fig. 27-19).

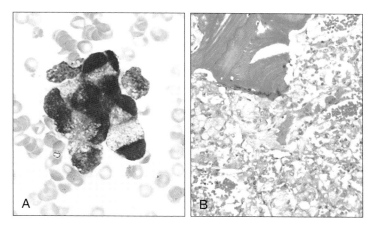

Fig. 27-12. Metastatic carcinoma. **A,** A clump of distended and vacuolated neoplastic epithelial cells in a patient with microangiopathic hemolytic anemia and laboratory evidence of disseminated intravascular coagulation. **B,** Sheets and acini of mucin-secreting adenocarcinoma in the same patient as described in **A,** who had a primary tumor of the stomach.

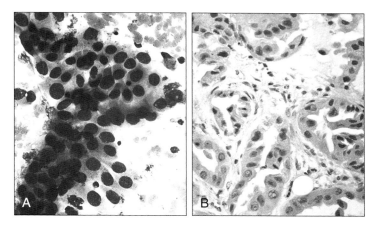

Fig. 27-13. Metastatic carcinoma: **(A)** a sheet of neoplastic columnar cells in bone marrow; **(B)** replacement of normal hemopoietic tissue by acini of neoplastic columnar cells in the same patient, who had a primary carcinoma of the ascending colon.

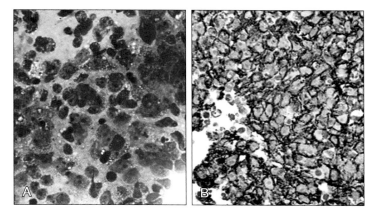

Fig. 27-14. Metastatic carcinoma: marrow aspirate from a patient with a primary nasopharyngeal carcinoma. **A,** The cell trails contained sheets of neoplastic epithelial cells. **B,** Immunohistologic staining shows strong positivity for anti low molecular weight cytokeratin CAM 5.2.

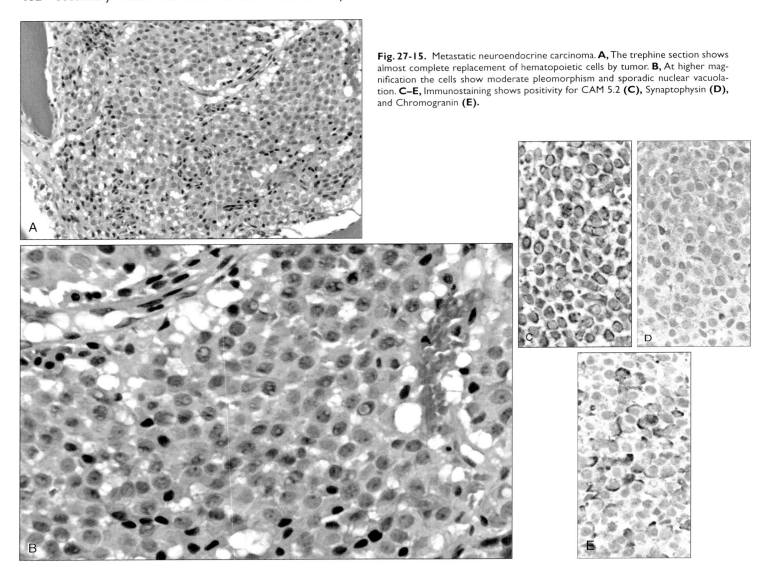

Fig. 27-15. Metastatic neuroendocrine carcinoma. **A,** The trephine section shows almost complete replacement of hematopoietic cells by tumor. **B,** At higher magnification the cells show moderate pleomorphism and sporadic nuclear vacuolation. **C–E,** Immunostaining shows positivity for CAM 5.2 **(C),** Synaptophysin **(D),** and Chromogranin **(E).**

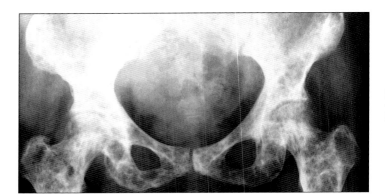

Fig. 27-16. Metastatic carcinoma: radiograph of the pelvis of a 58-year-old man with carcinoma of the lung. Metastatic deposits of tumor have produced widespread lytic lesions, most marked in the lower pelvis and upper parts of the femurs.

Fig. 27-17. Metastatic carcinoma: metastatic deposits from a carcinoma of the kidney. Sheets of neoplastic epithelial cell surrounding residual trabecular bone with osteoclasts adjacent to the scalloped edges.

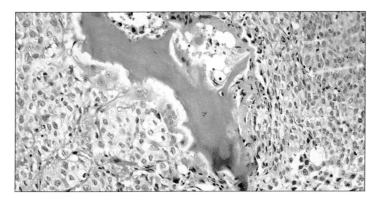

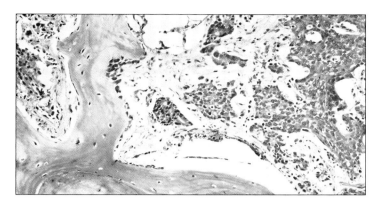

Fig. 27-18. Metastatic carcinoma: There is thickening of medullary trabecular bone, and osteoblasts are prominent along the right-hand margin of the vertical trabecula. The intertrabecular space contains nests of malignant epithelial cells supported by an abundant fibrous stroma. The patient had carcinoma of the prostate.

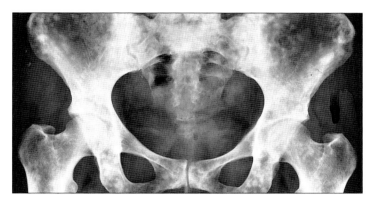

Fig. 27-19. Metastatic carcinoma: radiography of the pelvis of a 45-year-old woman with carcinoma of the breast. The widespread foci of increased bone density are the result of osteoblastic activity surrounding metastases.

Occasionally, fragments of epidermis are carried into the marrow cavity by the trephine biopsy (Fig. 27-20), but the well-differentiated nature of such fragments allows easy distinction from metastatic carcinoma.

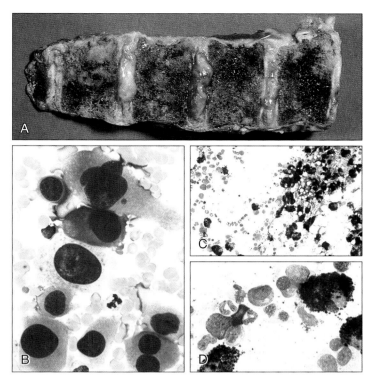

Fig. 27-21. Metastatic malignant melanoma. **A,** Postmortem section of spine showing multiple black deposits. **B,** Large malignant melanoma cells of variable size with primitive chromatin patterns and nucleoli. **C** and **D,** Lower- and higher-power views show no malignant cells, but numerous melanin-filled macrophages are evident. The patient had a malignant melanoma on the skin of the back. (*A,* Courtesy of Dr. R. Britt.)

Metastatic spread of malignant melanoma frequently involves the bone marrow (Fig. 27-21). Occasionally melanin is found in blood monocytes (Fig. 27-22). Bone marrow examination may detect marrow involvement by other tumors, including metastatic neuroblastoma (Fig. 27-23), medulloblastoma (Fig. 27-24), and Kaposi sarcoma (Fig. 27-25). Metastatic rhabdomyosarcoma (Fig. 27-26) may be confused with other blastic tumors, but immunopositivity with anti-desmin (intermediate filaments) is able to confirm a mesodermal origin.

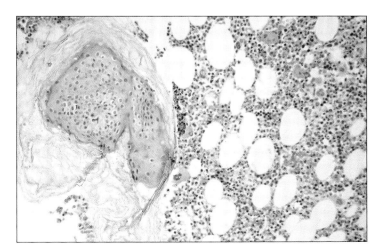

Fig. 27-20. Artifact on trephine biopsy: A small fragment of well-differentiated keratinized squamous epithelium has been carried into the bone marrow cavity. Normal hematopoietic tissue is on the right.

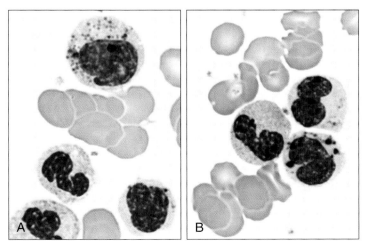

Fig. 27-22. Malignant melanoma: blood film showing monocytes with inclusions of phagocytosed melanin.

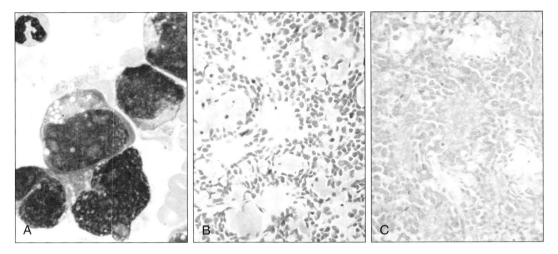

Fig. 27-23. Metastatic neuroblastoma. **A,** Bone marrow from a 3-year-old boy with neuroblastoma in the right thorax shows malignant "neuroblasts," somewhat larger and more pleomorphic than hematopoietic blast cells and with fine chromatin patterns and prominent nucleoli. **B,** Rosettes of neuroblastoma cells, some pyriform or fibrillar, with neurofibrils within amorphous extracellular material. **C,** Staining for neuron-specific enolase, using an immunoperoxidase–avidin biotin complex technique, demonstrates the antigen within the cells and in the neurofibrillary extracellular material. (*B* and *C*, Courtesy of Dr. P. O. G. Wilson.)

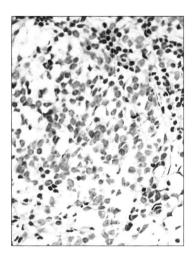

Fig. 27-24. Metastatic medulloblastoma: extensive replacement of hematopoietic tissue by small primitive cells with round nuclei, open chromatin, and scanty cytoplasm.

Although the majority of primary bone tumors do not spread to parts of the skeleton distant from their origin, bone marrow examination may reveal evidence of dissemination in Ewing's tumor of bone (Fig. 27-27).

Blood and bone marrow involvement by malignant lymphoma and histiocytic proliferations are discussed in Chapters 16 and 19 to 21.

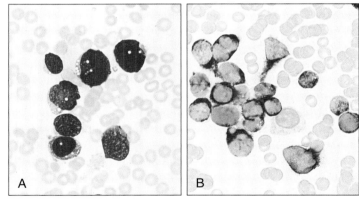

Fig. 27-26. Metastatic rhabdomyosarcoma: May-Grünwald/Giemsa stain **(A);** anti-desmin antibody **(B)** (AP-AAP technique). (*A* and *B,* Courtesy of Professor D. Y. Mason.)

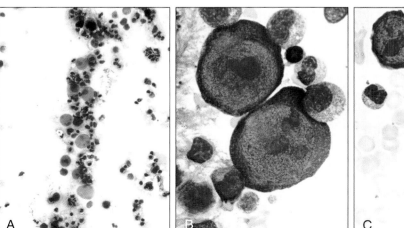

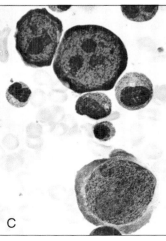

Fig. 27-25. Kaposi sarcoma: marrow aspirate. **A,** Low-power view of a cell trail showing numerous large pleomorphic cells. **B** and **C,** High-power images showing basophilic cytoplasm and nuclear detail, including large prominent nucleoli.

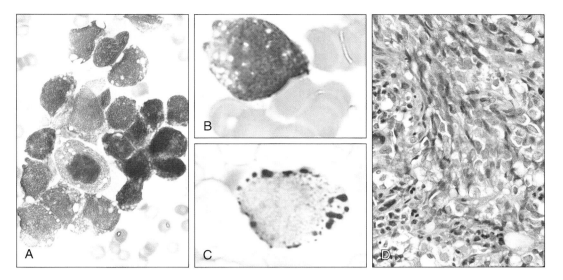

Fig. 27-27. Metastatic Ewing's sarcoma. **A,** Bone marrow aspirate showing vacuolated pleomorphic cells, including a cell in mitosis. **B,** At higher magnification a tumor cell shows a fine chromatin pattern and vacuolated basophilic cytoplasm. **C,** Periodic acid-Schiff base (PAS) staining shows coarse blocks of positive material. **D,** A trephine biopsy shows a sheetlike deposit of primitive cells with normal hematopoietic cells below. (*A* and *B*, May-Grünwald/Giemsa; *C*, PAS; *D*, H & E.) (*A* and *D*, Courtesy of Dr. D. M. Swirsky.)

RHEUMATOID ARTHRITIS AND OTHER CONNECTIVE TISSUE DISEASES

In rheumatoid arthritis, an anemia of chronic disorders is usually proportional to the severity of disease. Gastrointestinal hemorrhage related to therapy with aspirin, corticosteroids, and nonsteroidal anti-inflammatory drugs may cause iron deficiency. Gold therapy may be followed by marrow hypoplasia.

Arthritis with associated neutropenia and splenomegaly is found in Felty's syndrome (Fig, 27-28).

In systemic lupus erythematosus, the anemia of chronic disorders is complicated by neutropenia and lymphopenia. In severe cases a marked pancytopenia occurs. Some patients develop an autoimmune hemolytic anemia (Fig. 27-29). There is an autoimmune thrombocytopenia in 5% of cases. Occasional patients have problems related to thrombosis and recurrent miscarriage related to the presence of the "lupus anticoagulant" and other antiphospholipid antibodies (see Chapter 26). The bone marrow stromal tissue in severe disease may show degenerative changes (Fig. 27-30).

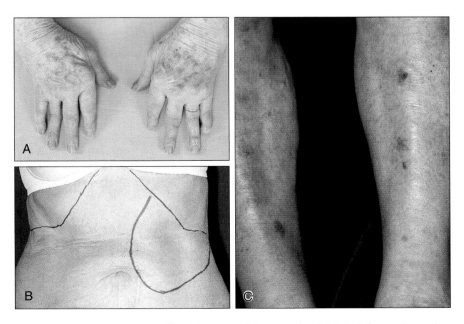

Fig. 27-28. Felty's syndrome. **A,** The deformities of rheumatoid arthritis include prominent ulnar styloids, ulnar deviation of the hands, swan-neck deformities (best seen in the right fourth finger and left fourth and fifth fingers), and wasting of the intrinsic muscles. **B,** Splenic enlargement. **C,** Skin ulceration on the anterior surface of the leg.

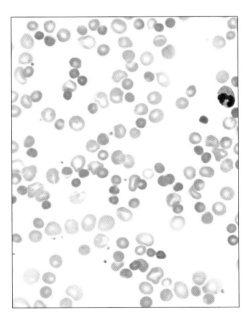

Fig. 27-29. Systemic lupus erythematosus: blood film in autoimmune hemolytic anemia showing prominent red cell spherocytosis and polychromasia.

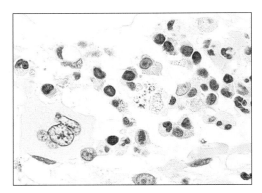

Fig. 27-30. Systemic lupus erythematosus: trephine biopsy showing stromal damage, small irregular fat cells, and a centrally placed macrophage containing iron pigment and ingested nuclei. (Courtesy of Dr. D. Swirsky.)

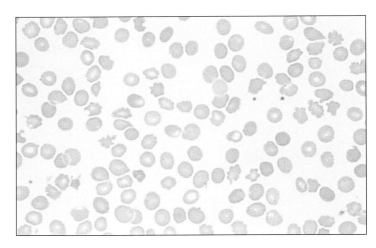

Fig. 27-31. Renal failure: peripheral blood film showing coarse acanthocytes and "burr" cells.

The anemia of chronic disorders is found in other collagen vascular disorders. Patients with polyarthralgia rheumatica and temporal arteritis have marked elevation of ESR, marked red cell rouleaux in blood films, and polyclonal increases in immunoglobulins.

RENAL FAILURE

The hematologic abnormalities found in patients with renal failure are listed in Table 27-3. Normochromic anemia is present in most patients with chronic renal failure. Generally, there is a 2.0 g/dL fall in hemoglobin level for every 10 mmol/L rise in blood urea. There is impaired red cell production as a result of defective erythropoietin secretion. Variable shortening of red cell life span occurs, and in severe uremia the red cells show abnormalities including spicules (spurs) and "burr" cells (Fig. 27-31). Increased red cell 2,3-diphosphoglycerate (2,3-DPG) levels in response to the anemia and hyperphosphatemia

result in decreased oxygen affinity and a shift of the hemoglobin oxygen dissociation curve to the right, which is augmented by uremic acidosis. The patient's symptoms are therefore relatively mild for the degree of anemia. Other factors that may complicate the anemia of chronic renal failure include the anemia of chronic disorders, iron deficiency from blood loss during dialysis or caused by bleeding because of defective platelet function, and folate deficiency in some chronic dialysis patients. Aluminum excess in patients on chronic dialysis also inhibits erythropoiesis. Patients with polycystic kidneys usually have retained erythropoietin production and may have less severe anemia for the degree of renal failure.

The hemolytic-uremic syndrome and thrombotic thrombocytopenic purpura are discussed on p. 440.

A bleeding tendency with purpura, gastrointestinal bleeding, or uterine bleeding occurs in 30% to 50% of patients with chronic renal failure and is marked in patients with acute renal failure. The bleeding is out of proportion to the degree of thrombocytopenia and has been associated with abnormal platelet or vascular function, which can be reversed by dialysis.

In chronic renal failure there is resistance to the action of vitamin D and a compensatory parathyroid hyperplasia. Characteristic changes are found in bone architecture on trephine biopsy (Fig. 27-32). In mild disease the lesions are predominantly osteomalacic. Microscopically, the trabeculae are increased in thickness and in number, and the osteoid seams have defective mineralization, similar to the changes seen in vitamin D deficiency. In severe disease, evidence of osteitis fibrosa is also present (Fig. 27-33).

TABLE 27-3.   HEMATOLOGIC ABNORMALITIES IN RENAL DISEASE

Anemia

Reduced erythropoietin production
Aluminium excess in dialysis patients
Anemia of chronic disorders
Iron deficiency
  blood loss (e.g., dialysis, venesection, defective platelet function)
Folate deficiency
  chronic hemodialysis without replacement therapy

Abnormal platelet function
Thrombocytopenia
Immune complex-mediated (e.g., systemic lupus erythematosus, polyarteritis nodosa) Some cases of acute nephritis and following allograft Hemolytic-uremic sydrome and thrombotic thrombocytopenic purpura
Thrombosis
Some cases of the nephrotic syndrome
Polycythemia
In renal allograft recipients Rarely in renal cell carcinoma, cysts, arterial disease

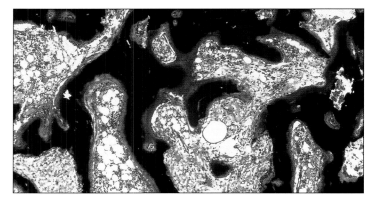

Fig. 27-32. Osteomalacia: thickened trabeculae with prominent layers of uncalcified osteoid on their outer borders. (Von Kossa stain.) (Courtesy of Bullough PG, Vigorita VJ: *Atlas of orthopedic pathology,* New York, 1984, Gower Medical Publishing.)

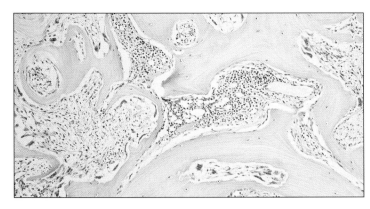

Fig. 27-33. Renal osteodystrophy and osteitis fibrosa cystica: extensive resorption of bone trabeculae with fibrous replacement. Osteoclasts lie adjacent to areas of active resorption.

LIVER DISEASE

The hematologic abnormalities in liver disease are listed in Table 27-4. Chronic liver disease is associated with anemia that is mildly macrocytic and often accompanied by target cells, mainly as a result of increased cholesterol in the membrane (Fig. 27-34). Contributing factors to the anemia may include blood loss (e.g., bleeding varices) with iron deficiency, dietary folate deficiency, and direct suppression of hematopoiesis by alcohol. Alcohol may have an inhibiting effect on folate metabolism and is occasionally associated with sideroblastic changes. Hemolytic anemia may occur in patients with alcohol intoxication (Zieve's syndrome) and in Wilson's disease (see Fig. 8-64), and autoimmune hemolytic anemia is found in some patients with chronic immune hepatitis. Viral hepatitis (usually non A, non B, non C) is associated with aplastic anemia.

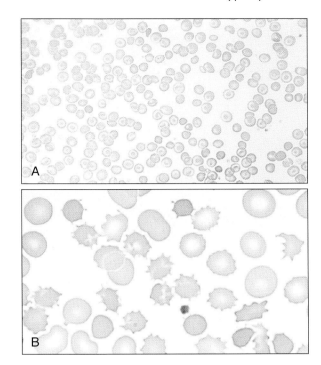

Fig. 27-34. Liver disease: peripheral blood films showing marked target cell formation **(A)** and, at higher magnification, marked red cell acanthocytosis **(B)**.

Bleeding may result from deficiencies of vitamin K–dependent factors (II, VII, IX, and X) and, in severe disease, of factor V and fibrinogen. Thrombocytopenia may occur from hypersplenism or from immune complex–mediated platelet destruction. Dysfibrinogenemia with abnormal fibrin polymerization may occur as a result of excess sialic acid in the fibrinogen molecules. These hemostatic defects may contribute to major blood loss from bleeding varices caused by portal hypertension.

HYPOTHYROIDISM

A moderate anemia is usual and may be caused by lack of thyroxine. T_3 and T_4 potentiate the action of erythropoietin. The blood film may show mild macrocytosis and acanthocytosis (Fig. 27-35). There is also a reduced oxygen need and thus reduced erythropoietin secretion. Autoimmune thyroid disease, especially myxedema or Hashimoto's disease, is associated with pernicious anemia. Iron deficiency may also be present, particularly in women with menorrhagia.

TABLE 27-4.	HEMATOLOGIC ABNORMALITIES IN LIVER DISEASE

Liver failure ± obstructive jaundice ± portal hypertension

Anemia

Usually mildly macrocytic, often with target cells; may be associated with:
  Blood loss and iron deficiency
  Alcohol (± ring sideroblastic change)
  Folate deficiency
  Hemolysis (e.g., Zieve's syndrome, Wilson's disease, autoimmune, hypersplenism from portal hypertension)

Bleeding tendency

Deficiency of vitamin K–dependent factors; also of factor V and fibrinogen
Thrombocytopenia in hypersplenism, immune, platelet function defects
Functional abnormalities of fibrinogen
Increased fibrinolysis
Portal hypertension – hemorrhage from varices

Viral hepatitis

Aplastic anemia

Tumors

Polycythemia
Neutrophil leukocytosis and leukemoid reactions

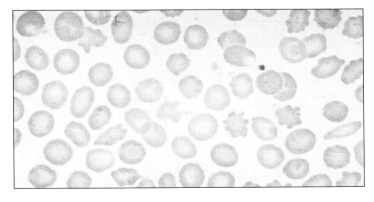

Fig. 27-35. Hypothyroidism: peripheral blood film showing mild macrocytosis, poikilocytosis, and irregular acanthocytosis.

TABLE 27-5.   HEMATOLOGIC ABNORMALITIES IN INFECTIONS

Hematologic abnormality	Infection associated
Anemia	
Anemia of chronic disorders	Chronic infections, especially tuberculosis
Aplastic anemia	Viral hepatitis
Transient red-cell aplasia	Human parvovirus
Marrow fibrosis	Tuberculosis
Immune hemolytic anemia	Infectious mononucleosis, *Mycoplasma pneumoniae*
Direct red-cell damage or	Bacterial septicemia (associated disseminated intravascular coagulation)
microangiopathic	*Clostridium perfringens*, malaria, bartonellosis
	Viruses – hemolytic-uremic syndrome and thrombotic thrombocytopenic purpura
Hypersplenism	Chronic malaria, tropical splenomegaly syndrome, leishmaniasis, schistosomasis
White cell changes	
Neutrophil leukocytosis	Acute bacterial infections
Leukemoid reactions	Severe bacterial infections, particularly in infants
	Tuberculosis
Eosinophilia	Parasitic diseases (e.g., hookworm, filariasis, schistosomiasis)
	Recovery from acute infections
Monocytosis	Chronic bacterial infections – tuberculosis, brucellosis, bacterial endocarditis, typhoid
Neutropenia	Viral infections – human immunodeficiency virus, hepatitis, influenza
	Fulminant bacterial infections (e.g., typhoid, miliary tuberculosis)
Lymphocytosis	Infectious mononucleosis, toxoplasmosis, cytomegalovirus, rubella, viral hepatitis
	pertussis, tuberculosis, brucellosis
Lymphopenia	Human immunodeficiency virus infection
	Legionella pneumophila
Thrombocytopenia	
Megakaryocytic depression,	Acute viral infections, particularly in children (e.g., measles, varicella, rubella,
immune-complex mediated, and	malaria, severe bacterial infection)
direct interaction with platelets	
Prothrombotic state	**All with prolonged inflammation**

INFECTIONS

BACTERIAL INFECTIONS

Blood and bone marrow abnormalities occur in many infections (Table 27-5). In prolonged bacterial infections, mild anemia is common. Severe hemolytic anemia, sometimes associated with disseminated intravascular coagulation, may occur with bacterial septicemia, particularly those associated with meningococcal and gram-negative

organisms. *Clostridium perfringens* organisms produce an α toxin, a lecithinase that produces marked spherocytosis (see Fig. 8-59). In children the hemolytic-uremic syndrome may be associated with infection by *Escherichia coli* with verotoxin 0157 (Fig. 27-36) or with other organisms, for example, *Shigella.* Hemolysis in Oroya fever is caused by direct red cell infection by *Bartonella* organisms (see Fig. 28-24). *Mycoplasma pneumoniae* infections are associated with "cold"-type autoimmune hemolytic anemia.

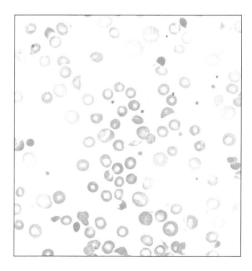

Fig. 27-36. Hemolytic-uremic syndrome: blood film in a child with *E. coli* septicemia. The red cells show marked fragmentation, polychromasia, and anisocytosis.

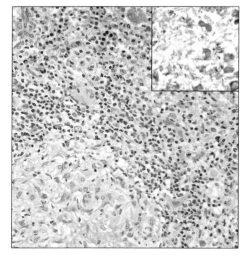

Fig. 27-37. Tuberculosis: a small granuloma surrounded by hyperplastic hematopoietic tissue. The *inset* shows small numbers of acid-fast bacilli. (*Inset,* Ziehl-Neelsen stain.)

Anemia of chronic disorders is found in chronic bacterial infections. In tuberculosis, marrow replacement by granulomatous infiltration and fibrosis (Fig. 27-37) associated with miliary disease may cause leukoerythroblastic change in blood and increase the severity of the anemia.

Bacterial infections are the most common causes of neutrophil leukocytosis, and severe infections may be associated with a leukemoid reaction.

If left untreated, tuberculosis involving bone marrow becomes extensive, particularly in the anterior aspects of the vertebral bodies and in the metaphyseal regions of long bones producing cystic areas of osteomyelitis that erode the endplates and may involve nearby joint spaces. In tuberculous spondylitis (Pott's disease), there is wedging and eventual collapse of the anterior aspects of the vertebral bodies (Fig. 27-38).

In Whipple's disease (infection with *Tropheryma whippelii*), marrow examination may show granulomatous inflammation or other changes (Fig. 27-39).

VIRAL INFECTIONS

Infectious mononucleosis (Epstein–Barr virus [EBV] infection) and human immunodeficiency virus (HIV) infection are associated with a wide range of hematologic changes, and both of these conditions are described and illustrated in Chapter 11.

Acute viral infections are often associated with mild anemia. An immune hemolytic anemia with anti-i autoantibody occurs in infectious mononucleosis, and other viral infections, as well as syphilis, have been associated with paroxysmal cold hemoglobinuria. Viruses have been associated with the hemolytic uremic syndrome, thrombotic thrombocytopenic purpura, and the hemophagocytic syndrome. Aplastic anemia may follow infection with hepatitis A but is more frequently seen in non-A, non-B, non-C hepatitis. Transient red cell aplasia is associated with parvovirus infection and may cause severe anemia in patients who already have a hemolytic anemia (e.g., hereditary spherocytosis or sickle cell disease).

Many viral infections, including rubella and cytomegalovirus (CMV) infection, may be associated with a reactive lymphocytosis with variable numbers of atypical lymphocytes in the blood film. Transient neutropenia is frequently present. CMV transmission by white cells may cause a posttransfusion infectious mononucleosis–like syndrome. In bone marrow transplant recipients or other immunosuppressed patients, CMV infections may cause pancytopenia. CMV infections in infants are associated with massive splenomegaly and hepatomegaly.

Acute and transient immune or nonimmune thrombocytopenia may follow viral infection, particularly in children.

Toxoplasmosis

Toxoplasmosis in adults and children is associated with lymphadenopathy (Fig. 11-20) and large numbers of atypical lymphocytes in the blood (Fig. 27-40). Newborn infants with congenital disease may be hydropic and have gross hepatomegaly, splenomegaly, leukoerythroblastic anemia, and thrombocytopenia. Their condition may be mistaken as hydrops fetalis.

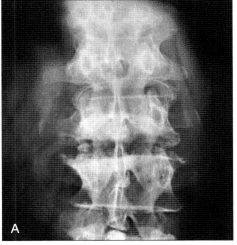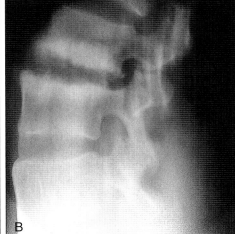

Fig. 27-38. Tuberculosis: radiographs of the lumbar spine seen in anteroposterior view **(A)** and a lateral tomogram **(B).** Inflammatory changes are seen around the disc between the second and third lumbar vertebrae, with sclerosis of the adjacent vertebral endplates. (*A* and *B,* Courtesy of Dr. R. Dick.)

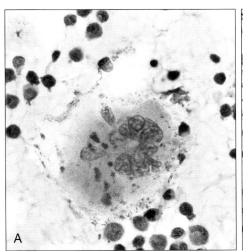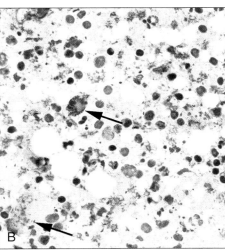

Fig. 27-39. Whipple's disease. **A,** Bone marrow aspirate showing a hypersegmented megakaryocyte with strongly periodic acid-Schiff base (PAS)–positive staining cytoplasmic inclusions. **B,** Mesenteric lymph node section, diastase-resistant PAS stain. *Left arrow,* Diastase-resistant PAS-positive granular material and bacilliform structures in the extracellular space. *Right arrow,* Granular and rod-shaped inclusions in macrophages. (Courtesy of Dr. Roland Walter.)

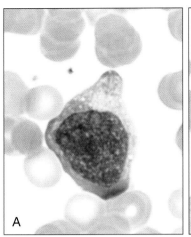 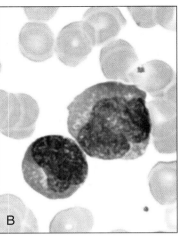 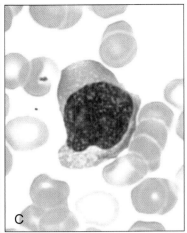

Fig. 27-40. Toxoplasmosis: blood film showing atypical lymphocytes.

PARASITIC INFECTIONS DIAGNOSED IN BLOOD

Parasitic involvement of blood is discussed separately and in more detail in Chapter 28, which includes descriptions of malaria and other protozoan parasites responsible for trypanosomiasis, babesiosis, and toxoplasmosis; the microfilaria of roundworm infections, filariasis and loaiasis; bacterial infection in bartonellosis; and the spirochetes responsible for borreliosis, or sleeping sickness.

Kala-azar (Visceral Leishmaniasis)

Kala-azar is distributed widely throughout tropical and warm regions of the world. The causal organism, *Leishmania donovani,* is transmitted by the bite of sandflies of the genus *Phlebotomus.* Nonflagellated amastigote forms of the organism are distributed widely through macrophages in the bone marrow, spleen, and liver. Diagnosis is made by examining bone marrow (Fig. 27-41), splenic aspirates, or biopsy specimens. Clinical features include fever, lassitude, weight loss, splenomegaly, hepatomegaly, anemia, neutropenia, and polyclonal increases in immunoglobulin.

MARROW INVOLVEMENT IN OTHER INFECTIONS

Bone marrow examination has little part to play in the diagnosis and management of osteomyelitis, although occasionally initial evidence of a disseminated fungal infection may be uncovered (Fig. 27-42).

The bone marrow and spleen may be involved in cases of disseminated histoplasmosis. The *Histoplasma capsulatum* organisms may be seen inside macrophages either in marrow aspirates or trephine biopsies(Fig. 27-43).

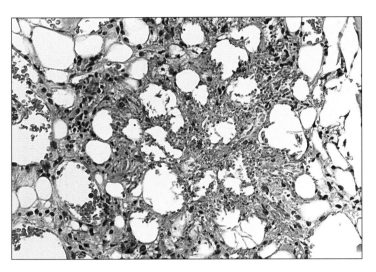

Fig. 27-42. Disseminated aspergillosis: biopsy taken after bone marrow transplantation showing hyphae of *Aspergillus* in an area of necrosis.

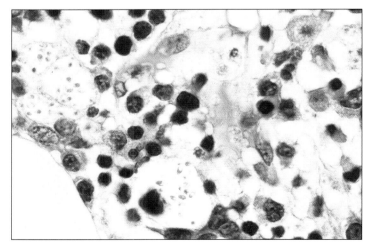

Fig. 27-43. Histoplasmosis: trephine biopsy. The encapsulated organisms are seen clearly inside the macrophages.

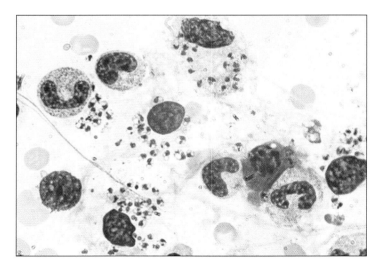

Fig. 27-41. Kala-azar (visceral leishmaniasis): bone marrow showing macrophages that contain Leishman–Donovan bodies. Also seen are neutrophil metamyelocytes and a plasma cell.

GRANULOMATOUS INFLAMMATION

Granulomatous inflammation of bone marrow is found in a wide variety of disorders (Table 27-6).

TABLE 27-6. CONDITIONS ASSOCIATED WITH BONE MARROW GRANULOMATA

Infections

Tuberculosis, atypical mycobacterial infection, disseminated bacillus Calmette–Guerin (BCG), leprosy, brucellosis, syphilis, typhoid fever, legionnaire's disease, Whipple's disease, leishmaniasis, toxoplasmosis, histoplasmosis, cryptococcosis, blastomycosis, coccidioidomycosis, herpes viral infection, and others

Sarcoidosis

Malignancy

Hodgkin's disease, non-Hodgkin's lymphoma, mycosis fungoides, multiple myeloma, acute lymphoblastic leukemia

Foreign material

Anthracosis, silicosis, berylliosis, talc

Drug hypersensitivity

For example, chlorpropamide, phenyl butazone, phenytoin, sulphasalazine, allopurinol

AMYLOIDOSIS

Amyloidosis is caused by extravascular deposition of insoluble abnormal fibrils derived from aggregation of misfolded, normally soluble protein (Fig. 27-50). The fibrillary structure is visible on electron microscopy, and following Congo red staining amyloid shows a distinct apple-green birefringence under polarized microscopy. Many different proteins may form amyloid fibrils, causing different and distinct clinical entities (Table 27-7).

Amyloid fibrils associate with other nonfibrillar components, including serum amyloid P (SAP) and glycosaminoglycans, forming stable deposits that disrupt the structure and function of involved organs and tissues. In systemic amyloidosis there are widespread deposits in viscera, blood vessel walls, and connective tissue. In local amyloidosis, the amyloid is restricted to an organ or tissue. In acquired amyloidosis, preexisting conditions produce an amyloidogenic protein or are associated with production of large amounts of potentially amyloidogenic normal protein. In hereditary amyloidosis, mutant genes encode variant amyloidogenic proteins.

Systemic amyloid precursor monoclonal immunoglobin light chain (AL) primary amyloidosis (see also Chapter 22), is due to an otherwise benign low-grade monoclonal gammopathy. AL amyloidosis may also complicate multiple myeloma (see Chapter 22) or other clonal B-cell proliferative disorders. The fibrils are formed from the

SARCOIDOSIS

This granulomatous disorder of unknown etiology most frequently affects the middle-aged. It is characterized by widespread epithelioid granulomas, depression of delayed hypersensitivity, and lymphoproliferation. Multisystem involvement is characteristic; intrathoracic disease affects 90% of cases, ocular and skin involvement each occur in about 20% of cases, and erythema nodosum occurs in one third of cases. In different series the reticuloendothelial system has been involved in up to 40% of patients. Evidence of disease may be found during bone marrow examination (Fig. 27-44) or at splenectomy (Fig. 27-45).

OTHER GRANULOMAS

Evidence of other granulomatous disease may be found during bone marrow examination (Figs. 27-46 to 27-49). Investigations may reveal a diagnosis, but in many cases no cause is found.

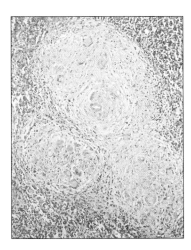

Fig. 27-45. Sarcoidosis: section of spleen showing granulomatous collections of epithelioid cells, including prominent multinuclear forms and peripheral lymphoid cells.

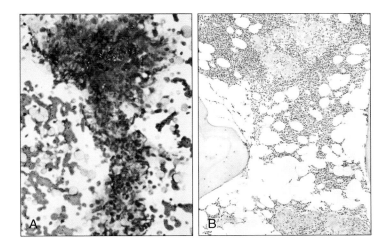

Fig. 27-44. Sarcoidosis. **A,** A sheet of epithelioid histiocytic cells, scattered lymphocytes, and myeloid cells. **B,** Two small granulomas comprising epithelioid cells and lymphocytes.

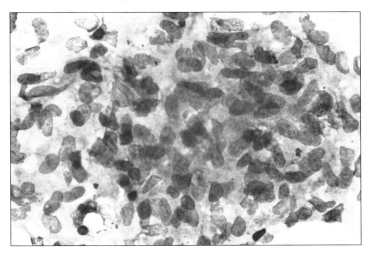

Fig. 27-46. Nonspecific marrow granuloma: This small collection of epithelioid cells was found in a bone marrow cell trail that showed no other abnormality. No specific diagnosis was made.

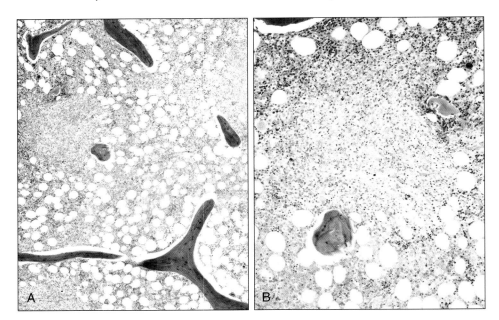

Fig. 27-47. Malignant lymphoma: trephine biopsy in a patient with a diffuse large B-cell lymphoma in cervical lymph nodes. There was no evidence of marrow involvement by malignant lymphoma, but numerous areas of granulomatous inflammation are seen. **A,** Low power. **B,** High-power Giemsa stain.

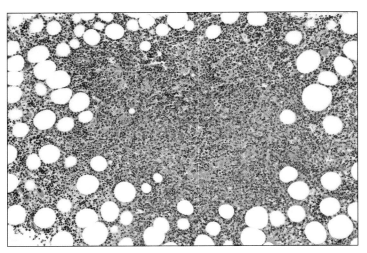

Fig. 27-48. Marrow granuloma: trephine biopsy in a patient with refractory anemia and concurrent allopurinol hypersensitivity. The intertrabecular space contains a large, loosely formed granuloma of lymphocytes and histiocytes.

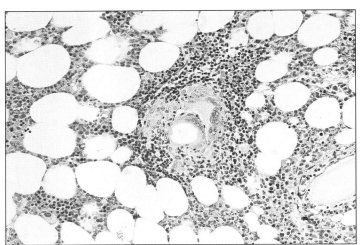

Fig. 27-49. Foreign body granuloma: an isolated granuloma with a central large vacuole that contains a refractile body of uncertain origin surrounded by giant cells.

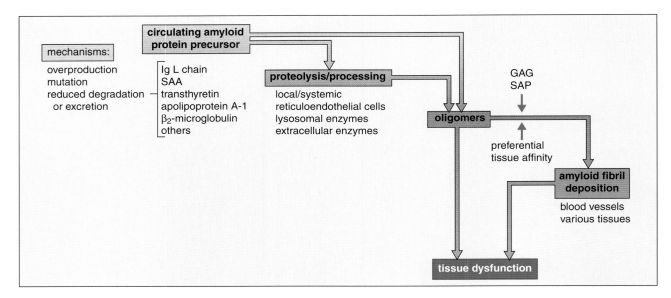

Fig. 27-50. Amyloidosis: The general mechanisms involved in amyloid formation. The amyloidogenic protein can be synthesized in excess and persist in serum in high concentration, as for the acute-phase protein serum amyloid A (SAA) or monoclonal light chains, or can reach high serum concentrations because of reduced clearance, such as β_2-microglobulin in chronic dialysis, or can be mutated as in hereditary amyloidosis. Certain proteins with intrinsic amyloidogenic properties, such as transthyretin, may cause amyloidosis late in life, as in senile systemic amyloidosis. Some of these proteins undergo a proteolytic remodeling that facilitates polymerization. The early protein aggregates may exert a direct cytotoxic effect. The concurrence of tissue components and common constituents, for example, glycoaminoglycans (GAGs) and serum amyloid P (SAP) component, favors deposition of amyloid fibrils. (From Merlini G, Stone MJ: *Blood* 108:2520–2530, 2006.)

TABLE 27-7.   CLASSIFICATION OF AMYLOIDOSIS

Type	Fibril precursor protein	Clinical syndrome
AA	Serum amyloid A protein	Systemic amyloidosis associated with acquired or hereditary chronic inflammatory diseases; formerly known as secondary or reactive amyloidosis
AL	Monoclonal immunoglobulin light chains	Systemic amyloidosis associated with myeloma, monoclonal gammopathy, occult B cell dyscrasia; formerly known as primary amyloidosis
ATTR	Normal plasma transthyretin	Senile systemic amyloidosis with predominant cardiac involvement
ATTR	Genetic variants of transthyretin (e.g., ATTR Met30, Ala60, Ile122)	Familial amyloid polyneuropathy (FAP), with systemic amyloidosis and often prominent amyloid cardiomyopathy
$A\beta_2M$	β_2-Microglobulin	Dialysis-related amyloidosis (DRA) associated with renal failure and long-term dialysis; predominantly musculoskeletal symptoms
$A\beta$	β-Protein precursor (and rare genetic variants)	Cerebrovascular and intracerebral plaque amyloid in Alzheimer's disease; occasional familial cases
AApoAI	Genetic variants of apolipoprotein AI (e.g., AApoAI, Arg26, Arg60)	Autosomal dominant systemic amyloidosis; predominantly nonneuropathic with prominent visceral involvement, especially neuropathy; minor wild-type ApoAI amyloid deposits may occur in the aorta
AFib	Genetic variants of fibrinogen α chain (e.g., AFib Val526)	Autosomal dominant systemic amyloidosis; nonneuropathic usually with prominent nephropathy
ALys	Genetic variants of lysozyme (e.g., ALys His67)	Autosomal dominant systemic amyloidosis; nonneuropathic with prominent renal and gastrointestinal involvement
ACys	Genetic variant of cystatin C (Gln68)	Hereditary cerebral hemorrhage with cerebral and systemic amyloidosis
AGel	Genetic variants of gelsolin (e.g., Asn187)	Autosomal dominant systemic amyloidosis; predominant cranial nerve involvement with lattice corneal dystrophy
AIAPP	Islet amyloid polypeptide	Amyloid in islets of Langerhans in type II diabetes mellitus and insulinoma

From Goodman HJB, Hawkins PN: *Postgraduate haematology,* ed 5, Oxford 2005, Blackwell Publishing.

N-terminal variable domain of immunoglobulin light chains. Deposits may affect almost any part of the body except the brain. Frequent presenting features include proteinuria, peripheral or autonomic neuropathy, symptoms from cardiac involvement, splenomegaly, and hepatomegaly. Macroglossia (Fig. 27-51) is present in about 10% of patients but is almost pathognomonic of AL disease. Amyloid deposition in tendon sheaths may cause a carpal tunnel syndrome (Fig. 27-52). Bone marrow trephine biopsy may reveal the first evidence of amyloidosis (Fig. 27-53, *A-D*).

Reactive systemic amyloid precursor amyloid A protein (AA) amyloidosis is a complication of chronic infectious or inflammatory disease, for example, rheumatoid arthritis, Still's disease, Crohn's disease, familial Mediterranean fever, and bronchiectasis, in which there is a sustained acute-phase response with high levels of serum amyloid A protein. This protein is an apoprotein made in the liver and regulated by proinflammatory cytokines. The plasma concentration may rise 1000-fold during an acute-phase response. Patients may have nephropathy and proteinuria. Liver, gastrointestinal, and splenic involvement occur with advanced disease. Cardiac and neural involvement are rare. Bone marrow involvement may be shown by trephine biopsy (Fig. 27-53, *E-G*). When the disease is suspected, diagnosis may be confirmed by fine needle biopsy of abdominal fat (Fig. 27-54, *A* and *B*), renal biopsy (Fig. 27-54, *C-E*), or rectal biopsy.

The extent of systemic amyloid disease can be assessed by radiolabeled SAP component scintigraphy and progress monitored by measuring serum light-chains (Fig. 27-55).

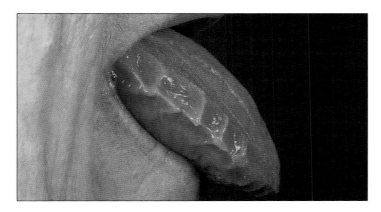

Fig. 27-51. Systemic AL amyloidosis: tongue enlarged, with a waxy, smooth appearance.

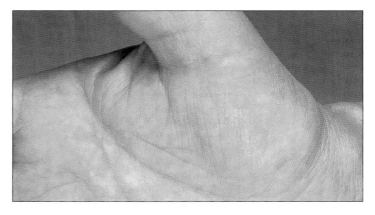

Fig. 27-52. Systemic AL amyloidosis: flattening of thenar eminence caused by carpal tunnel syndrome. Same case as shown in Fig. 27-51.

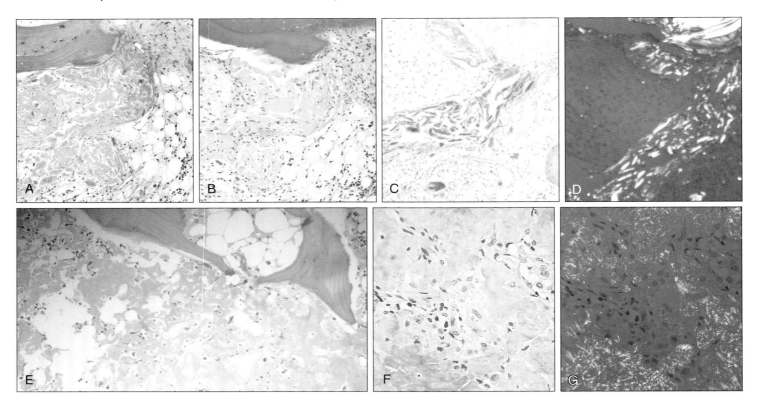

Fig. 27-53. Amyloidosis: trephine biopsies. Systemic AL amyloidosis. Giemsa **(A)** and H&E **(B)** stains show replacement of hematopoietic tissue by loose collections of foamy histiocytes and an amorphous material that is salmon pink in the Congo red stain **(C)** with characteristic yellow green birefringence with polarized light **(D)**. Systemic reactive AA amyloidosis in a patient with bronchiectasis shows extensive replacement of hematopoietic tissue by pale acidophilic material in H&E **(E)** and salmon pink staining with Congo red **(F)** with characteristic yellow green birefringence with polarized light **(G)**.

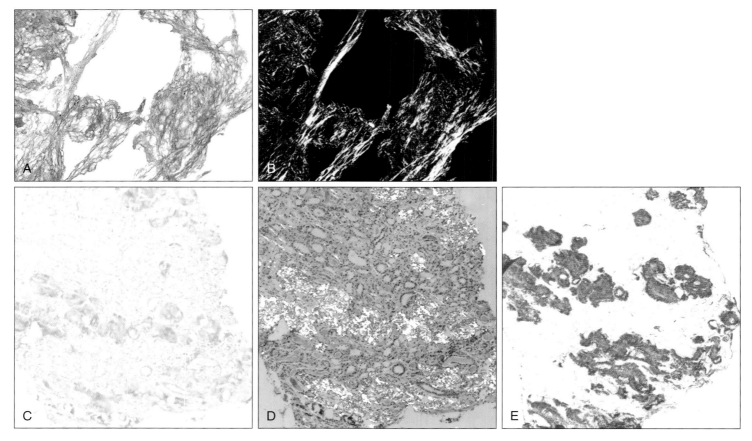

Fig. 27-54. Amyloidosis: fine needle aspirate of abdominal fat stained with Congo red. **A,** strong positivity with light microscopy. **B,** Birefringence under polarized light. Renal biopsy in a patient with a 15-year history of adult-onset Still's disease. **C,** Congo red staining shows pink amyloid deposits. **D,** Under polarized light the deposits show a characteristic apple-green birefringence. **E,** Immunohistologic staining using a monoclonal antiserum amyloid A protein antibody shows intense positivity confirming that the amyloid deposits are of AA type. (*A* and *B,* Courtesy of Professor Giampaolo Merlini; *C-E* Courtesy of Professor Philip Hawkins.)

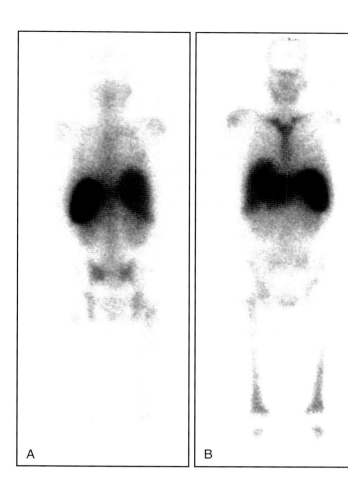

A   B

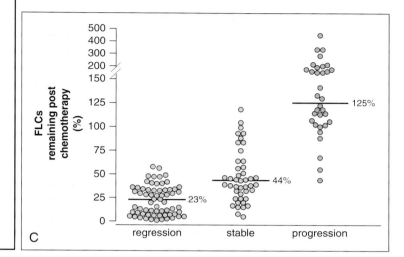

Fig. 27-55. Systemic AL amyloidosis: serum amyloid P component scintigraphy. Posterior **(A)** and anterior **(B)** whole-body scans obtained 24 hours after injection of ^{123}I-labeled serum amyloid P (SAP) component in a 62-year-old woman with systemic AL amyloidosis. The tracer has localized to amyloid deposits in the liver, spleen, and kidneys and throughout the bone marrow. **C,** FLCs in 127 patients with AL amyloidosis before and 12 months after commencing chemotherapy. The mean percentages of remaining serum free light chains (FLCs) in each group are indicated (Kruskal-Wallis test: $P < 0.0001$). (A and B, Courtesy of Professor P. N. Hawkins and Professor M. B. Pepys. C, Courtesy of Bradwell AG: *Serum free light chain analysis,* ed 4, Birmingham, UK, 2005, Binding Site.)

OSTEOPETROSIS (ALBERS–SCHÖNBERG OR MARBLE BONE DISEASE)

Osteopetrosis is a heterogeneous group of inherited disorders in which there is defective bone resorption by osteoclasts. This failure of bone resorption and remodeling leads to an increase in density of all bones. Three mutations responsible for osteopetrosis are shown in Fig. 27-56. The most common, detected in over 50% of patients, causes a defect in the osteoclast vacuolar H^+-ATPase proton pump. Less common mutations result in defects in the osteoclast-specific chloride channel or carbonic anhydrase II dysfunction.

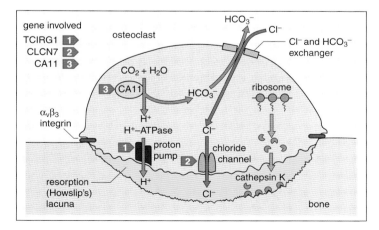

Fig. 27-56. Osteopetrosis: osteoclast mutations and malfunction. To achieve acidification of the resorption lacunae and demineralization, carbonic anhydrase II (CAD II) generates a proton and bicarbonate from carbon dioxide and water. This proton is passed across the ruffled border membrane through the action of a vacuolar H^+ ATPase "proton pump." A chloride channel coupled to the pump facilitates balancing the ions across the membrane. Excess bicarbonate is removed from the cell by passive exchange with chloride. The organic matrix of bone is removed by cathepsin K and other enzymes. The sites of malfunction caused by the mutations are indicated. (Modified from Tolar J et al: *N Engl J Med* 351: 2839–2849, 2004.)

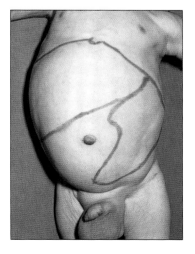

Fig. 27-57. Osteopetrosis: massive hepatosplenomegaly in a 14-month-old infant. Bilateral inguinal hernias are present because of raised intraabdominal pressure.

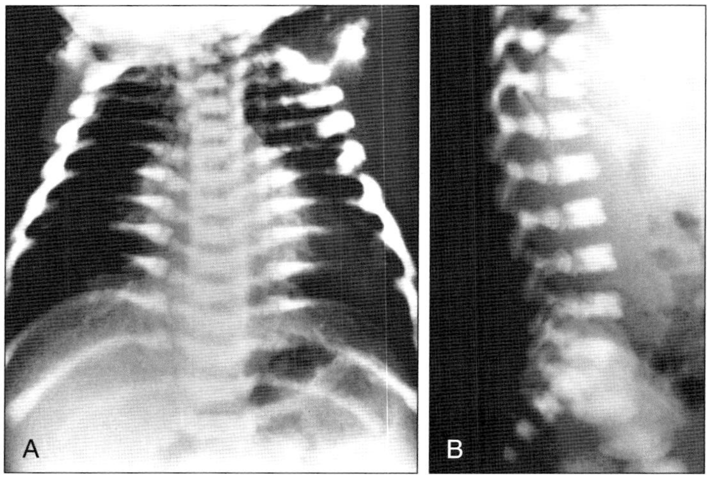

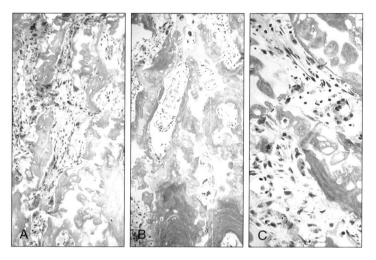

Fig. 27-58. Osteopetrosis: radiographs of the chest **(A)** and the lower spine **(B)** of an infant with a gross generalized increase in bone density. The changes are most marked at the upper and lower margins of the vertebral bodies. The vertebrae also show the characteristic "bone-in-bone" appearance.

Fig. 27-59. Osteopetrosis. **A,** Compacted intramedullary osseous tissue and relatively little hematopoietic tissue; cores of cartilaginous matrix are bordered by areas of primitive bone. **B** and **C,** Persistence of cartilage, lack of bone modeling, and primitive osseous tissue at the edges of and within the cartilage. (*B* and *C,* Picro-Mallory stain.)

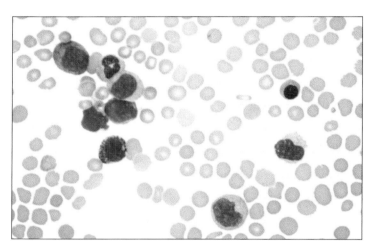

Fig. 27-61. Osteopetrosis: leukoerythroblastic changes. The red cells show anisocytosis and poikilocytosis; the nucleated cells include a myeloblast, a promyelocyte, a myelocyte, and an erythroblast.

Severe forms of the disease manifest in infancy with anemia and hepatosplenomegaly (Fig. 27-57). These children have little or no bone marrow; hematopoiesis is chiefly extramedullary, and blood transfusions are required to sustain life. The typical radiographic appearances are shown in Fig. 27-58; characteristic microscopic abnormalities are found in trephine bone biopsies (Figs. 27-59 and 27-60), and leukoerythroblastic changes are seen in the blood (Fig. 27-61). Failure to resorb bone results in optic atrophy, deafness, and hydrocephalus. Milder cases may manifest later in childhood or in adult life with retarded growth, anemia, and splenomegaly (Figs. 27-62 and 27-63).

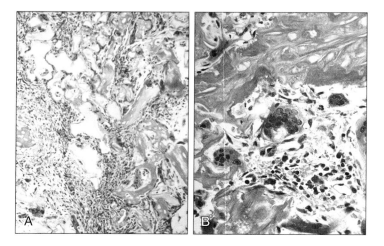

Fig. 27-60. Osteopetrosis: biopsy (same case as shown in Fig. 27-59) **(A)** showing large numbers of osteoclasts, better seen at high power **(B).** There is little evidence of bone resorption, and no trabeculae or hematopoietic marrow spaces are seen. (*A* and *B,* Picro-Mallory stain.)

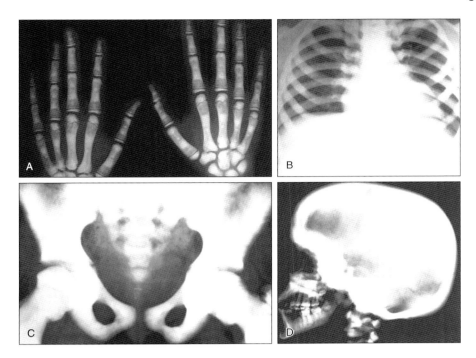

Fig. 27-62. Osteopetrosis: radiographs of the hands **(A)**, the chest **(B)**, the pelvis **(C)**, and the skull **(D)** of a 14-year-old girl with retarded growth, leukoerythroblastic anemia, and massive splenomegaly. The bones are dense with coarse trabeculation and lack the usual corticomedullary demarcation. The mandible appears normal.

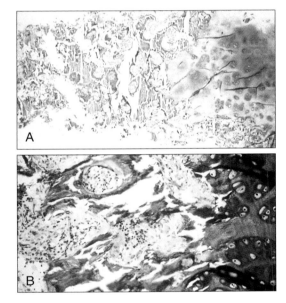

The bony trabeculae may have a striking mosaic appearance created by the pattern of cement lines. In areas of extensive repair the bone may be osteomalacic with wide osteoid seams. If extremely rapid absorption has occurred, areas of fibrosis and intensive osteoclastic activity may resemble the microscopic appearances of osteitis fibrosa.

Fig. 27-63. Osteopetrosis: biopsy of the posterior iliac crest (same case as shown in Fig. 27-62), seen at low **(A)** and high power **(B)**, showing persistence of cartilage in the cortex and medulla and architecturally disordered marrow with islands of hematopoietic tissue surrounded by sheets of primitive osteochondroid material. (*A* and *B*, Courtesy of Dr. J. E. McLaughlin.)

PAGET'S DISEASE OF BONE (OSTEITIS DEFORMANS)

In Paget's disease of bone, which is of unknown etiology, rapid bone formation and resorption occurs in the involved regions of the skeleton. The lesions are essentially local and asymmetric in the early stages and frequently involve the weight-bearing bones, especially the sacrum and pelvis. Unsuspected disease may be found during trephine bone marrow biopsy examination (Figs. 27-64 and 27-65). The plasma calcium and phosphorus levels are usually normal, whereas the alkaline phosphatase level is invariably high.

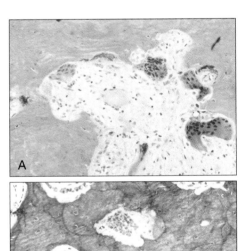

Fig. 27-64. Paget's disease of bone. **A,** Autopsy section shows increased osteoclastic and osteoblastic activity, with scalloping of the bone surface *(green)* adjacent to the osteoclasts. **B,** In the biopsy of more advanced disease, the disturbed bone (undecalcified) architecture is obvious. Irregular cement lines separate the uneven bone sections, and osteoblasts and osteoclasts are prominent. (*A,* Goldner's stain.) (*A* and *B,* Courtesy of Bullough PG, Vigorita VJ: *Atlas of orthopedic pathology,* New York, 1984, Gower Medical Publishing.)

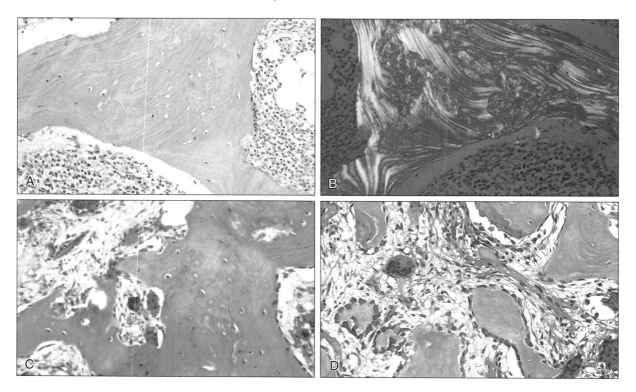

Fig. 27-65. Paget's disease of bone: thickened and irregular trabecular bone **(A)**, seen under polarized light **(B)**; intense bone resorption by osteoclasts **(C)**; bone apposition by osteoblasts during the active phase of the disease **(D)**. The normal intratrabecular hematopoietic tissue has been extensively replaced by vascular loose connective tissues.

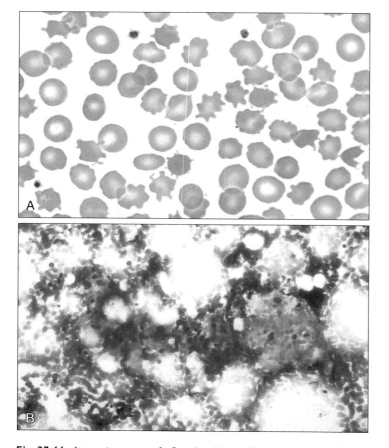

Fig. 27-66. Anorexia nervosa. **A,** Peripheral blood film showing red cell acanthocytosis. **B,** Bone marrow showing extracellular homogeneous pink- and purple-staining material that replaces fat spaces and is composed of acid mucopolysaccharide.

ANOREXIA NERVOSA

These patients suffer from severe deficiency of carbohydrates, fats, and calories, but little protein deficiency. The peripheral blood may reveal mild anemia and thrombocytopenia with acanthocytes; the marrow is hypocellular, with fat cells replaced by acid mucopolysaccharides appearing as pink-staining extracellular material (Fig. 27-66). Similar appearances may occur in other causes of malnutrition, such as carcinomata (Fig. 27-67).

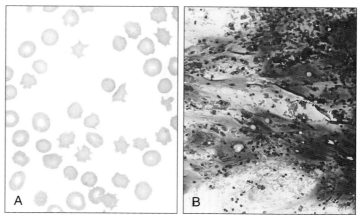

Fig. 27-67. Cachexia caused by carcinomatosis: peripheral blood film **(A)** and bone marrow showing similar appearances to those in Fig. 27-66 **(B)**. (*A* and *B*, Courtesy of Dr. D. Simpson.)

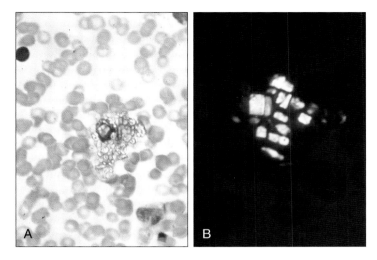

Fig. 27-68. Cystinosis: bone marrow containing histiocytic cells **(A),** which under polarized light **(B)** show the characteristic birefringence of cystine crystals.

CYSTINOSIS

In this recessively inherited disease, cystine crystals are deposited in the reticuloendothelial and corneal tissues. In its more severe form (cystinosis with Fanconi syndrome or the de Toni–Fanconi–Lignac syndrome), progressive renal degeneration is fatal during early childhood. Children with this syndrome usually have anorexia, thirst, polyuria, failure to thrive, rickets, or photophobia. Laboratory tests reveal glycosuria, proteinuria, low serum bicarbonate, hypokalemia, or hypophosphatemia. The diagnosis is established by the demonstration of cystine crystals in macrophages in bone marrow aspirates (Fig. 27-68).

PRIMARY OXALURIA

In this fatal autosomal recessive metabolic disorder, there is widespread deposition of calcium oxalate crystals in the kidneys and elsewhere in the body, including the liver, spleen, and bone marrow (Fig. 27-69). A number of different enzyme deficiencies have been implicated as causal factors.

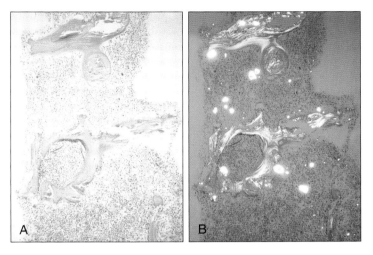

Fig. 27-69. Primary oxaluria: normal **(A)** and polarizing **(B)** microscopy showing birefringent calcium oxalate monohydrate crystals (and normal birefringent cortical bone). The patient, a 3-month-old boy, had renal failure. (*A* and *B,* Courtesy of Dr. S. Milkins.)

PARASITIC DISORDERS

MALARIA

The protozoal disease malaria has a distribution that is essentially worldwide in tropical and warm temperate regions. Mosquito-borne infection is caused by four species of the genus *Plasmodium: P. vivax* (benign tertian), *P. falciparum* (malignant tertian), *P. malariae* (quartan), and *P. ovale* (ovale tertian). Infections caused by *P. vivax* and *P. falciparum* are the most common, and the latter is much more likely to be life threatening.

The malarial life cycle (Fig. 28-1) begins in the female mosquito after ingestion of human blood that contains the sexual forms (gametocytes) of the causal organisms. The resultant conjugate develops into infective forms (sporozoites) within the mosquito, which are transmitted to humans when the insects feed.

The sporozoites pass through the blood to the parenchymal cells of the liver, where they multiply and divide, producing merozoites in

this preerythrocytic phase. When the liver cell ruptures, the parasites enter the red cells.

In the red cells, the parasites pass from early trophozoite, or ring forms, to actively ameboid forms with malarial pigment (hemozoin), which then undergo chromatin division to form merozoites. The mature parasite is called a meront (schizont). The red cell ruptures, releasing merozoites into the plasma, which may enter other red cells and repeat the cycle or form male and female sexual forms (gametocytes).

The four types of malaria organisms may be distinguished by their characteristic appearances within red cells (Table 28-1). In *P. vivax* infection (Fig. 28-2), the red cells are large (because they are young) and Schüffner's dots (degraded red cell microtubules) are present; the ring forms and meronts of the parasites are large, with up to 24 merozoites per meront.

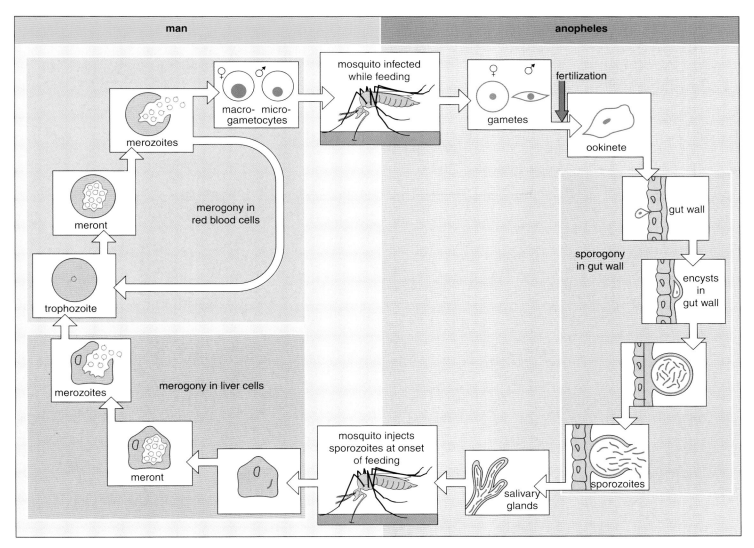

Fig. 28-1. Life cycle of a malarial parasite.

TABLE 28-1.   IDENTIFICATION OF THE DIFFERENT FORMS OF MALARIA IN THE PERIPHERAL BLOOD

	Plasmodium falciparum	*Plasmodium malariae*	*Plasmodium vivax*	*Plasmodium ovale*
Red blood cells (RBCs)				
Enlargement	None	None	Yes	Yes; oval shape; fimbriated edge
Inclusions (not always present)	Maurer's clefts	Ziemann's dots (rare)	Schüffner's dots (coarse red granules)	Red granules similar to Schüffner's dots
Ring form				
Size	Less than one third of RBC	Greater than one third of RBC	Greater than one third of RBC	Greater than one third of RBC
Multiple parasites in RBC	Common; often at margins	Rare	Rare	Rare
Shape	Delicate; often double chromatin dot	Tends to be compact; inverted chromatin dot	Rough; single chromatin dot	Rough; single chromatin dot common
Ameboid forms	Absent	Common; often as band across RBC	Common	Common
Meront (schizont)				
Frequency	Very rarely seen	Common; dense, central, yellow/black hemozoin pigment	Common; with hemozoin pigment	Common
Configuration	Random	Daisy head	Random	Daisy head
Merozoite number	8–24	8–12	12–24	8–12
Gametocyte	Crescent forms; centrally placed chromatin	Small and round; eccentrically placed chromatin; occupies one half to two thirds of RBC	Large and round; eccentrically placed chromatin; fills RBC	Small and round; eccentrically placed chromatin; occupies one half to two thirds of RBC

Infections with two types of malarial parasite are common.

In *P. falciparum* infections (Fig. 28-3), usually a heavy parasitemia with small ring forms occurs, often with double chromatin dots; multiple ring forms may be found, some on the margins within individual red cells, and the red cells may contain blue-staining Maurer's clefts. The gametocytes have a characteristic crescent shape, and meronts are rarely seen.

As in *P. falciparum* infections, with *P. malariae* (Fig. 28-4) the red cells are not enlarged and do not contain pigment; the ring form tends to have an inverted chromatin dot. Occasionally, dustlike stippling (Ziemann's dots) is seen. The ameboid trophozoites often show band forms, and the merozoites may show a "daisy-head" distribution.

P. ovale (Fig. 28-5) infections are distinguished by the parasitized red cells being enlarged and oval shaped, but with fimbriated edges. The red cells show red granules similar to Schüffner's dots, and the meronts have a daisy-head distribution.

Immunochromatography methods (Fig. 28-6) are able to identify *P. falciparum* and distinguish this infection from other malarial species. These techniques use two antibodies, one specific to the histidine protein-rich protein II of *P. falciparum* and the other specific for an antigen common to all four malarial species.

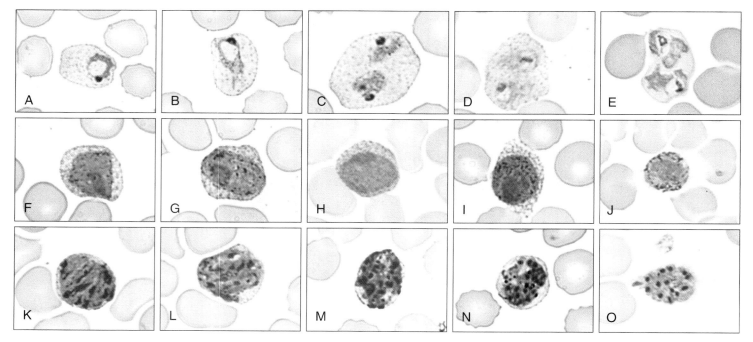

Fig. 28-2. Malaria: peripheral blood films showing various stages of *P. vivax*. **A,** Early trophozoite or ring form. **B** and **C,** Young ameboid trophozoites with Schüffner's dots. **D** and **E,** Developing trophozoites after asexual binary fission. **F–H,** Female gametocytes with localized eccentric chromatin. **I** and **J,** Male gametocytes with more diffuse chromatin. **K–O,** Early and later meronts with hemozoin pigment densities and many merozoites randomly distributed.

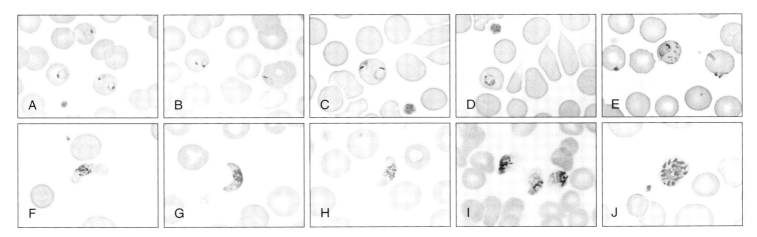

Fig. 28-3. Malaria: peripheral blood films showing various stages of *P. falciparum*. **A–D,** Small ring forms. **E,** Small ring form showing Maurer's clefts, denatured red cell microtubules. **F–H,** Crescentic gametocytes with centrally placed chromatin. **I,** Rarely seen rounded "pink flag" gametocytes. **J,** Rarely seen meront with randomly distributed merozoites. (*E,* Courtesy of Dr. S. Knowles.)

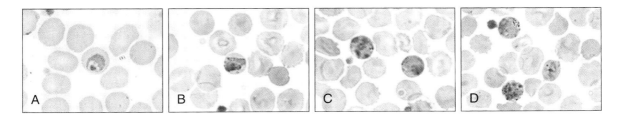

Fig. 28-4. Malaria: peripheral blood films showing various stages of *P. malariae*. **A.** Ring form with inverted chromatin dot. **B,** Band-form ameboid trophozoite. **C,** Developing trophozoite and female gametocyte. **D,** From *top left* clockwise: male gametocyte, ring form, and developing meront with daisy-head merozoite distribution. (*A* and *B,* Courtesy of Dr. S. Knowles and J. Griffiths.)

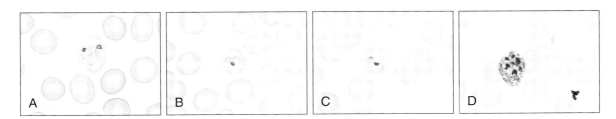

Fig. 28-5. Malaria: peripheral blood films showing various stages of *P. ovale*. **A–C,** Ring forms in enlarged red cells with fimbriated margins and faint red granules. **D,** Meront with daisy-head merozoite distribution.

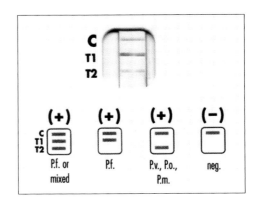

Fig. 28-6. Immunochromatography screening test (Binax Inc.). The result is consistent with *P. falciparum* infection.

EFFECTS OF MALARIA ON VARIOUS ORGANS

Malaria may affect the structure and function of various organs. The most serious complication is cerebral malaria, which may prove fatal. Parasites in cerebral capillaries (Figs. 28-7 and 28-8) may lead to hemorrhage (Figs. 28-9 and 28-10). The placenta may be infested with parasites, but they do not usually cross from the maternal to the fetal circulation (Fig. 28-11).

Anemia is frequent, partly because parasitized red cells are prematurely destroyed and phagocytosed (Fig. 28-12). It may also arise from hypersplenism because frequently there is splenic enlargement, caused by the phagocytosis of infected red cells in splenic macrophages (Fig. 28-13).

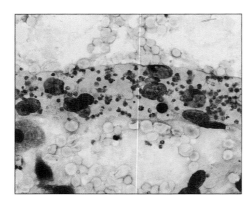

Fig. 28-7. Cerebral malaria: cerebral capillary. This high-power view shows abundant parasites within red cells. (Squash preparation of white matter stained with Giemsa.) (Courtesy of Professor S. Lucas.)

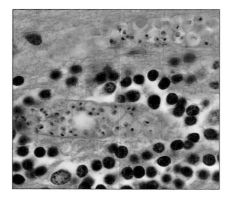

Fig. 28-8. Cerebral malaria: cerebral capillary. In this histologic preparation, two capillaries are seen with parasitized red cells adherent to the endothelium (sequestration). (Courtesy of Professor S. Lucas.)

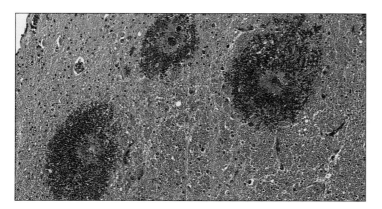

Fig. 28-9. Cerebral malaria: hemorrhage. Low-power view of brain white matter with three ring hemorrhages caused by obstructed vessels. (Courtesy of Professor S. Lucas.)

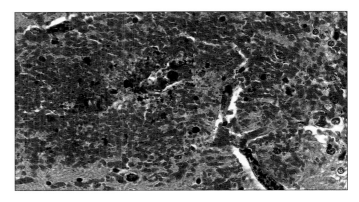

Fig. 28-10. Cerebral malaria: hemorrhage from vessel rupture by *P. falciparum* malaria. The intense pigmentation within the blood vessel indicates the heavy parasitemia at this site. (Courtesy of Professor S. Lucas.)

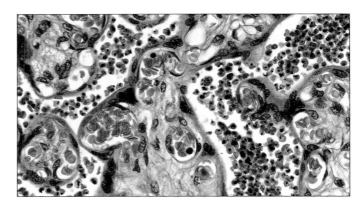

Fig. 28-11. Placental malaria: placental villi and maternal sinus. Nearly all of the red blood cells in the maternal sinus contain parasites, pigment, or both. Note that the fetal vessels in the villi are not infected. (Courtesy of Professor S. Lucas.)

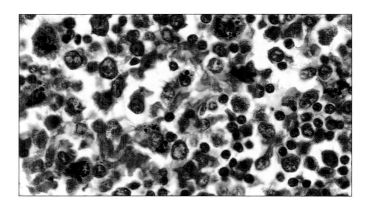

Fig. 28-12. Pediatric malaria: hypercellular bone marrow. Macrophages that contain brown-colored hemozoin malaria pigment are plentiful. Parasites inside red blood cells are not seen in this field. (Courtesy of Professor S. Lucas.)

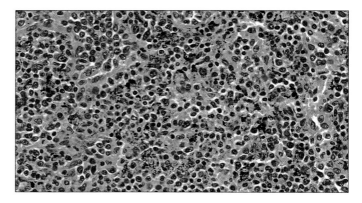

Fig. 28-13. Spleen: red pulp showing abundant macrophages that contain brown-colored hemozoin malaria pigment. (Courtesy of Professor S. Lucas.)

TABLE 28-2.   MALARIA DIAGNOSIS: COMPARISON
               OF METHODS

	Limits of detection (parasites/ml)
Thin film	200
Thick film	10
Quantitative buffy coat	20*
Histidine-rich protein II antigen detection†	50
DNA hybridization	40
Polymerase chain reaction	<5

*The quantitative buffy coat method is as sensitive as thick film for
P. falciparum but less so for other species.
†Histidine-rich protein II antigen is in the red cell membrane and is secreted
by red cells infected by *P. falciparum*.

Courtesy of Dr. W. Erber.

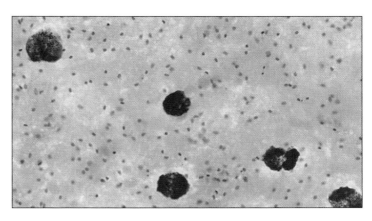

Fig. 28-15. Malaria diagnosis: thick film of *P. falciparum* (heavy infection). Chromatin dots of *P. falciparum* are easily seen in this thick film. (Giemsa stain.) (Courtesy of Dr. W. Erber.)

COMPARATIVE METHODS FOR MALARIA DIAGNOSIS

In Table 28-2 the sensitivities of the different methods for malaria diagnosis are compared. Thick films may improve sensitivity. Red cell lysis is carried out at pH 6.8 in phosphate buffers for 10 minutes.

Thick films are made and stained with Giemsa at pH 7.2 for 30 minutes. Fig. 28-14 shows positive films for *P. vivax* and Fig. 28-15 shows a film with a heavy parasite load in *P. falciparum* infection.

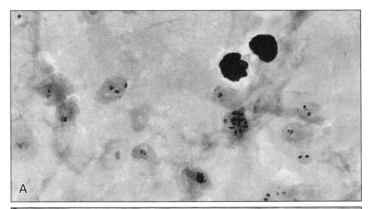
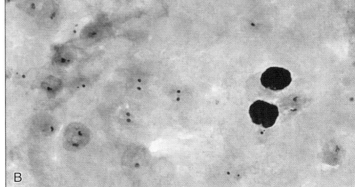
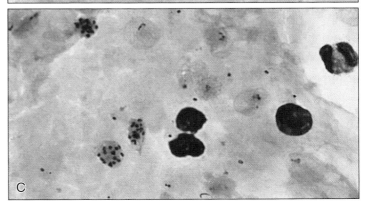

Fig. 28-14. Malaria diagnosis: thick films. **A,** *P. vivax* trophozoites and schizonts. **B,** *P. vivax* trophozoites. **C,** *P. vivax* trophozoites and schizonts. (Giemsa stain.) (A–C, Courtesy of Dr. W. Erber.)

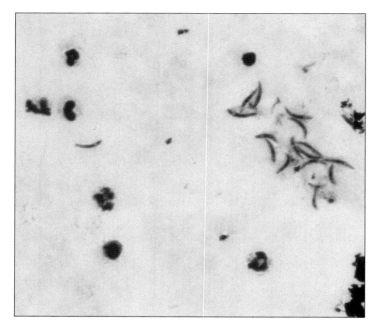

Fig. 28-16. Acute toxoplasmosis: thick peripheral blood film showing trophozoite forms of *T. gondii* from a ruptured monocyte.

TOXOPLASMOSIS

Toxoplasmosis, a common infection, is caused by the protozoan *Toxoplasma gondii*. Most human infections are acquired from cats. Affected patients may be symptomless or suffer a brief febrile illness with lymphadenopathy and fatigue. Severe infection, most commonly seen in the fetus (congenital toxoplasmosis) or in patients with immunodeficiency, is associated with extensive damage to the brain, eyes, muscle, heart, and lungs. Diagnosis is usually confirmed by positive serology, although a lymph node biopsy may be needed (see Fig. 11-XX). Rarely, the trophozoite forms are present in blood monocytes (Fig. 28-16).

BABESIOSIS

Babesiosis is a tick-borne disease caused by protozoan parasites of the genus *Babesia*. Although the disease affects a number of animal species, it is only occasionally transmitted to humans. In most patients the illness is mild and characterized by fever, malaise, myalgia, mild hepatosplenomegaly, and hemolytic anemia. Occasionally, patients who have had previous splenectomy have developed a more fulminating infection with massive intravascular hemolysis, which has sometimes proved fatal.

The majority of human infections are caused by *B. microti*, a species that usually infects rodents. Several cases in splenectomized patients result from *B. bovis*, a species associated with red water fever in cattle. Diagnosis is made by finding the trophozoites, which resemble small ring forms of *P. falciparum*, in the red cells (Fig. 28-17).

TRYPANOSOMIASIS

The East African and West African variants of trypanosomiasis are caused by *Trypanosoma brucei* and *T. brucei gambiense*, respectively. Both are transmitted by tsetse flies of the genus Glossina. The dominant clinical problems are related to involvement of the central nervous system. In the acute phase of the disease, organisms are found in the blood (Fig. 28-18).

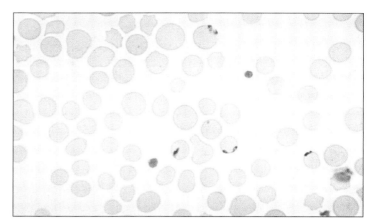

Fig. 28-17. Babesiosis: peripheral blood film showing red cell infestation with the typical small coccoid and dumbbell-shaped *Babesia* organisms. (Courtesy of P. J. Humphries.)

American trypanosomiasis, or Chagas' disease, occurs widely in Mexico and in many countries in Central and South America. The causative organism, *T. cruzi*, is transmitted by a triatomid bug. During the acute febrile stage of the illness, flagellated parasites may be found in the blood (Fig. 28-19). In the chronic stage, which is associated with myocarditis, megacolon, or megaesophagus, nests of amastigote forms are found within the tissues.

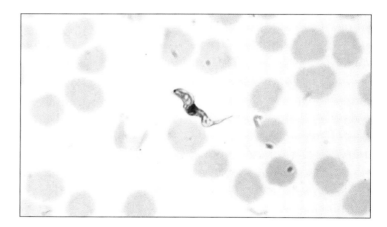

Fig. 28-18. African trypanosomiasis: peripheral blood film showing *T. brucei*.

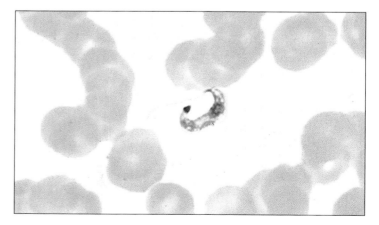

Fig. 28-19. Chagas' disease: peripheral blood film showing the flagellate form of *T. cruzi*. (Courtesy of J. Williams.)

BANCROFTIAN FILARIASIS

Bancroftian filariasis is a widespread disease that occurs throughout the tropical and subtropical regions of the world and is caused by *Wuchereria bancrofti*. A similar condition is caused by infection with the related *Brugia malayi*.

Both organisms are transmitted by infected mosquitoes. Larvae pass into the lymphatic vessels and lymph nodes, where they mature into adult worms (Fig. 28-20). The fertilized females release microfilariae via the lymphatic vessels into the bloodstream.

Many patients are asymptomatic, but others develop a febrile illness with headaches, muscle pains, and lymphadenitis. Chronic inflammatory changes in the infected lymphoid system may lead to lymphatic obstruction and elephantiasis of the scrotum or lower extremities. Diagnosis is usually made by demonstrating microfilariae in the blood (Figs. 28-21 and 28-22). Microfilaremia is usually greatest at night.

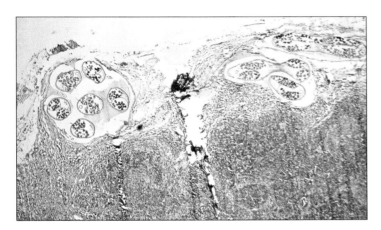

Fig. 28-20. Bancroftian filariasis: section of lymph node showing adult forms of *W. bancrofti* in the peripheral sinus area.

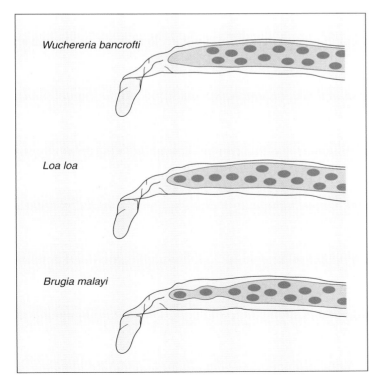

Fig. 28-21. Posterior ends of sheathed microfilariae found in blood. In *W. bancrofti* the nuclei do not extend to the tip of the tail; in *L. loa* there is a continuous line of nuclei to the end of the tail; in *Br. malayi* the nuclei are not continuous, with two isolated nuclei at the tip of the tail.

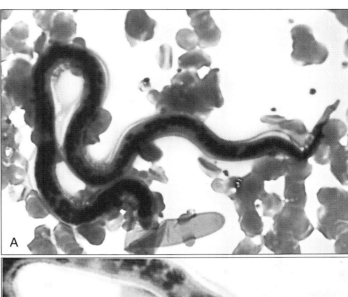

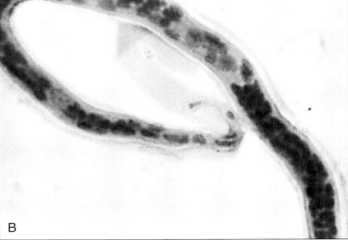

Fig. 28-22. Filariasis: thick preparations of peripheral blood showing the center and tail portions of the microfilariae of *W. bancrofti* **(A)** and *Br. malayi* **(B).** (*B*, Courtesy of Dr. A. E. Bianco.)

LOIASIS

Infection with *Loa loa* occurs in Central and West Africa. The adult worm causes subcutaneous swellings, but occasionally its passage through the subconjunctival tissues produces local pain and acute conjunctivitis. Microfilariae are found in the blood (Fig. 28-23), and infestation is via tabanid flies.

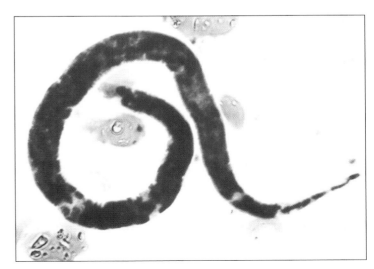

Fig. 28-23. Loiasis: peripheral blood film with sheathed microfilaria of *L. loa.*

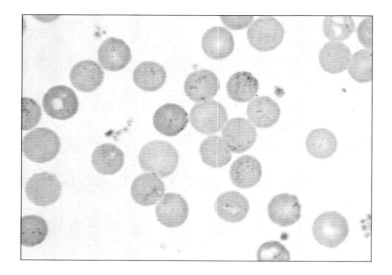

Fig. 28-24. Bartonellosis: peripheral blood film showing rod-shaped coccobacilli of *Ba. bacilliformis* in the red cells in Oroya fever. (Courtesy of H. Furze.)

BARTONELLOSIS

Bartonella bacilliformis causes a severe febrile hemolytic anemia. The disease occurs in inhabitants of the Andes Mountains in Peru, Colombia, and Ecuador. The characteristic rod-shaped coccobacilli are found in red cells (Fig. 28-24). The infection is also known as Oroya fever and Carrión's disease and is transmitted by *Phlebotomus* sandflies.

RELAPSING FEVER

Various spirochetes of the genus *Borrelia* cause relapsing fever. Louse-borne relapsing fever is a human disease caused only by *Bo. recurrentis,* but tick-borne relapsing fever is a zoonosis caused by a number of different species. It is during the febrile period of the disease that the organisms are present in the blood (Fig. 28-25). With the production of antibodies, the *Borrelia* spirochetes disappear and the patient becomes afebrile. Relapses occur after 7 to 10 days, with the production of new antigenic variants of the organisms. In louse-borne relapsing fever, a single relapse is usual, whereas in the tick-borne forms of the disease, multiple relapses may occur.

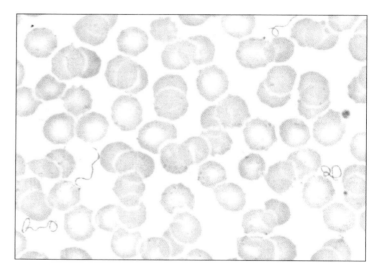

Fig. 28-25. Relapsing fever. Peripheral blood film showing the coiled spirochetes *Bo. recurrentis.*

BLOOD TRANSFUSION

Blood transfusion involves transfusion of whole blood or a blood component (red cells, platelets, fresh frozen plasma, cryoprecipitate, or white cells) from an individual (the donor) into the recipient. In the case of red cells, autologous (self) transfusion is also carried out. The major clinical need is for red cells, for which compatibility between donor red cell antigens and the antibodies in the recipient's plasma must be ensured.

RED CELL ANTIGENS

Over 400 red cell antigens have been identified and the best characterized are listed in Table 29-1. They are inherited in a simple mendelian fashion and are stable. Subjects who lack any antigen are likely to make antibodies to that antigen if they are exposed to it. The clinically important red cell blood group systems are detailed in Table 29-2.

TABLE 29-1. RED CELL ANTIGENS: THOSE BEST CHARACTERIZED ARE ASSIGNED TO RECOGNIZED BLOOD GROUP SYSTEMS. OTHER ANTIGENS INCLUDE Sd^a, VEL, At^a BG (HLA ON RED CELLS)

ABO	'Lewis'	I	P	Rh		MNS		Lutheran	Kell
A	Le^a	I	P$_1$	D	CE	M	m^v	Lu^a	K
A$_2$	Le^b	i	P	C	D^w	N	FAR	Lu^b	$\bar{\text{k}}$
A$_3$		I^T	p^k	E		Hu	'N'	Lu^3	Kp^a
A$_x$			Luke	$\bar{\text{c}}$	Rh26	S	S^D	Lu^4	Kp^b
A$_m$			$\bar{\text{p}}$	e	cE	$\bar{\text{s}}$	Mit	Lu^5	
B				$\bar{\text{f}}$	hr^H	He	Dantu	Lu^6	Ku
B$_3$				C$\bar{\text{e}}$	Rh29	Mi^a	HOP	Lu^7	Js^a
B$_m$				C^w	Go^a	U	Nob	Lu^8	Js^b
B$_w$				C^x	hr^b	M^c	ENKT	Lu^9	K^w
H				V	Rh32	V^w	DANE	Lu^{11}	KL
O				E^w	Rh33	Mg	TSEN	Lu^{12}	Ul^a
				G	Rh34	Vr	Or	Lu^{13}	K11
					Rh35		MINY	Lu^{14}	K12
					Be^a	Mur	MUT	Lu^{16}	K13
					Rh37	M^e	SAT	Lu^{17}	K14
					Rh38	Mt^a	ERIK	Au^a	K16
				Hr$_o$	Rh39	St^a	OS^a	Au^b	WK^a
				Hr	Rh40	Ri^a	ENEP	Lu20	K18
				hr^S	Rh41	Cl^a	ENEH	probably	K19
				VS	Rh42	Ny^a	HAG		K20
				C^G	Rh43		ENAV		K21
					Rh44	Hut	MARS		K22
					Rh45	Hil			K23
					Rh46				K24
					Rh47				K25
					Rh48				K26
					Rh49				K27
					Rh50				KX
					Rh51				
					Rh52				
					Rh53				

Continued

TABLE 29-1. RED CELL ANTIGENS: THOSE BEST CHARACTERIZED ARE ASSIGNED TO RECOGNIZED BLOOD GROUP SYSTEMS. OTHER ANTIGENS INCLUDE Sd^a, VEL, At^a BG (HLA ON RED CELLS)—cont'd

Lw	Duffy	Kidd	Xg^a	Diego	Cartwright	Scianna	Dombrock	Colton	Chido/Rogers
Lw^a	Fy^a	JK^a	Xg^a	Di^a	Yt^a	Sc1	Do^a	Co^a	Ch
Lw^b	Fy^b	JK^b		Di3-21	Yt^b	Sc2	Do^b	Co^b	Rg
Lw^{ab}	Fy^x	JK^3				Sc3	Do^3	Co^3	
	Fy^3					Rd	Do^4		
	Fy^4						Do^5		
	Fy^5								
	Fy^6								

Courtesy of G. Hazlehurst.

TABLE 29-2. RED CELL ANTIBODIES: THOSE THAT CAUSE HEMOLYTIC REACTIONS AND HEMOLYTIC DISEASE OF THE NEWBORN

Blood group system	Frequency of antibodies	Hemolytic transfusion reactions	Hemolytic disease of the new-born
ABO	Very common	Yes (common)	Yes
Rh	Common	Yes (common)	Yes
Kell	Occasional	Yes (occasional)	May
Duffy	Occasional	Yes (occasional)	May
Kidd	Occasional	Yes (occasional)	May
Lutheran	Rare	Rare	No
Lewis	Common	Rare	No
P	Rare	Rare	No
MNSs	Rare	Rare	Rare
Ii	Rare	Unlikely	No

RED CELL ANTIBODIES

There are two types of red cell antibodies: natural and immune. Natural antibodies are a normal occurrence in plasma in the absence of transfusion or pregnancy. Immune antibodies develop in response to exposure to the antigen by transfusion or by exposure to red cells that cross the placenta during pregnancy. Natural antibodies, usually immunoglobulin M (IgM), react best in the cold and include anti-A and anti-B. Immune antibodies, usually immunoglobulin G (IgG), react best at 37° C and include Rhesus (Rh) antibody anti-D. Ig antibodies, but not IgM, cross the placenta.

ABO SYSTEM

The structure of the A, B, and H antigens is shown in Fig. 29-1. The relative incidence in the U.K. population is shown in Table 29-3. The A, B, and H antigens occur in most body cells, including leukocytes and platelets, and in so-called secretors (80% of the population); they also occur in body fluids such as saliva, tears, semen, and sweat.

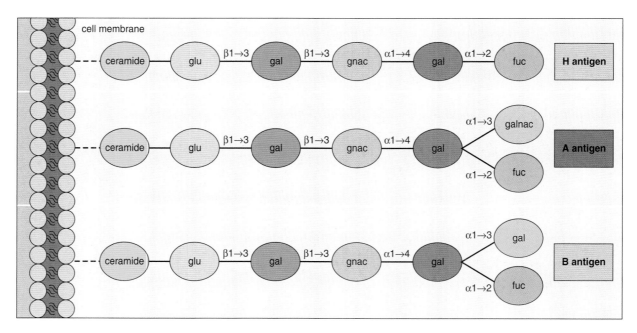

Fig. 29-1. Structure of the ABO blood group antigens: each consists of a chain of sugars, in a or b conformation, linked through different carbon atoms (numbered 1 to 4). The H antigen of the O blood group has a terminal fucose (fuc). The A antigen has an additional *N*-acetylgalactosamine (galnac), whereas the B antigen has an additional galactose (gal). (*glu*, Glucose; *gnac*, *N*-acetylglucosamine.)

TABLE 29-3. ABO BLOOD GROUPS: INCIDENCE IN THE U.K. POPULATION

	Blood group			
	O	**A**	**B**	**AB**
Antigens on red (and other) cells	None	A	B	A+B
Antibody in serum	Anti-AB	Anti-B	Anti-A	None
Approximate percentage in UK population	47	42	8	3

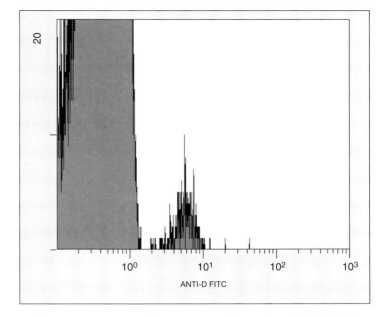

Fig. 29-2. Determination by flow cytometry of the number of RhD fetal cells in the maternal circulation using a fluorescence-labeled antibody to RhD, the mother being Rhdd. (Courtesy of Dr. W. Erber.)

RH SYSTEM

The Rh system is more complex than the ABO system. There are three closely linked loci with alternative antigens, Cc, D or no D (termed "d," for which there is no antigen), and Ee (Table 29-4). They are immune antibodies, and before the introduction of prophylaxis with Rh anti-D after delivery or miscarriage, anti-D was the dominant cause of hemolytic disease of the newborn. The number of fetal cells entering the maternal circulation at delivery or miscarriage can be determined by the Kleihauer technique (Fig 9-106) or by flow cytometry using a fluorescent-labeled antibody to RhD (Fig. 29-2) or by DNA techniques.

BLOOD GROUPING AND CROSS-MATCHING

Blood grouping and cross-matching is carried out by a tile (Fig. 29-3), microplate (Fig. 29-4), E gel microtube (Fig. 29-5), or IgM agglutination (Fig. 29-6, *A*) technique. The patient's cells are mixed with known antisera and the patient's serum is mixed with cells of known A, B, or O type (see Figs. 29-3 and 29-4). An indirect antiglobulin test (IAT) may be used to detect irregular red cell antibodies in the patient's serum (Fig. 29-6, *B*). This technique can also be used to detect antibodies in the serum of the recipient that react against the donor red cells. For patients with antibodies, the selection of red cell units should be based on antigen specificity and clinical significance (Table 29-5).

RED CELL COMPONENTS

SAG-M (saline-adenine-glucose-mannitol) blood may be provided as buffy coat–depleted red cells (Fig. 29-7) or as a multisatellite red cell pack (Fig. 29-8).

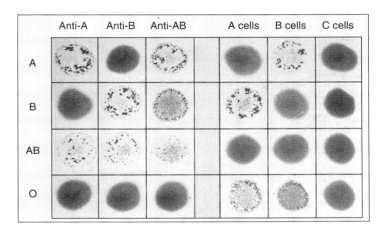

Fig. 29-3. ABO blood group testing: reactions observed. Agglutination denotes reactivity. The three left-hand columns denote patient cells (A, B, AB, or O) mixed with anti-A, anti-B, or anti-AB. The three right-hand columns denote plasma from the patients, mixed with A, B, or O cells.

TABLE 29-4. THE RH SYSTEM: GENOTYPES

CDE nomenclature	Short symbol	Caucasian frequency (%)	RhD status
cde/cde	rr	15	Negative
CDe/cde	R1r	32	Positive
CDe/CDe	R1R1	17	Positive
cDE/cde	R2r	13	Positive
CDe/cDE	R1R2	14	Positive
cDE/cDE	R2R2	4	Positive
Other genotypes		5	Positive (almost all)

Modified from Hoffbrand AV, Pettit JE: *Essential haematology,* ed 5, Oxford, 2006, Blackwell.

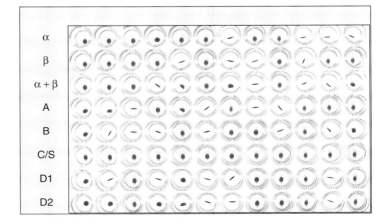

Fig. 29-4. ABO grouping: standard layout for 96-well microplate blood grouping (12 patients grouped on one plate). Symbols along the vertical side are as follows: α, anti-A; β, anti-B; α+β, anti-A+B; A, B, known A or B cells; C/S, patient cells and serum; D1, D2, two sources of anti-D. Sharp agglutination ("comma-like") shows a positive reaction, and no agglutination shows a negative reaction. (Courtesy of G. Hazlehurst.)

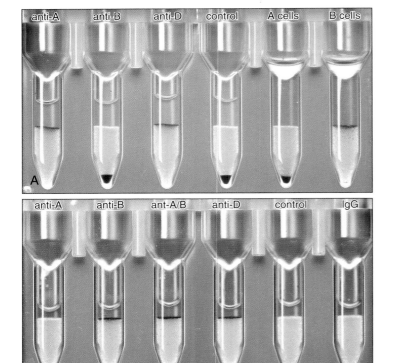

Fig. 29-5. Blood grouping using microcolumn (gel) system. **A,** A Rh(D) positive. The three left hand tubes contain patient cells, the two right hand, patient plasma. Control = patient cells and plasma. **B,** The patient is B Rh(D) positive, with an additional direct antiglobulin test using anti IgG, which is negative. (Courtesy of G. Hazlehurst.)

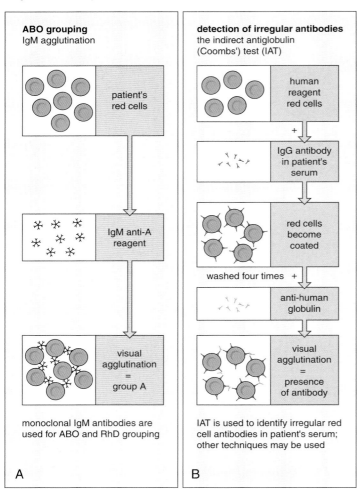

Fig. 29-6. ABO grouping. **A,** IgM agglutination. Monoclonal IgM antibodies are used for ABO and RhD grouping. **B,** The indirect antiglobulin (Coombs') test (IAT). The IAT is used to identify irregular red cell antibodies in the patient's serum. (A, B, Courtesy of Professor M. Contreras and North London Blood Transfusion Centre.)

TABLE 29-5. RED CELL UNITS: SELECTION BASED ON ANTIGEN SPECIFICITY AND CLINICAL SIGNIFICANCE

Specificity	Clinical significance	Selection of units and compatibility testing
Rh antibodies (reactive in IAT)	Yes	Antigen negative
Kell antibodies	Yes	Antigen negative
Duffy antibodies	Yes	Antigen negative
Kidd antibodies	Yes	Antigen negative
Anti-S, -s	Yes	Antigen negative
Anti-A$_1$, -P$_1$, -N	Rarely	IAT cross-match compatible at 37°C
Anti-M	Rarely	IAT cross-match compatible at 37°C
Anti-M IAT reactive at 37°C	Sometimes	Antigen negative
Anti-Le^a, anti-Le^{a+b}	Rarely	IAT cross-match compatible at 37°C
Anti-Le^b	No	Not clinically significant and can be ignored
High-titer low-avidity antibodies	Unlikely	Seek advice from blood center
Antibodies against high-frequency antigens	Depends on specificity	Seek advice from blood center

Courtesy of British Committee for Standardization in Haematology, 1996.

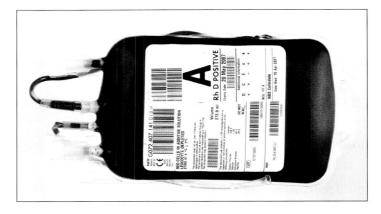

Fig. 29-7. Leukocyte-depleted red cells: the average volume of this product, which contains CPDA-1 as the anticoagulant, is 280 ml. SAG-M additive solution (100 ml) is added to give a final hematocrit of 50% to 70%. The storage temperature of these red cells is 4° ± 2° C and the shelf life is 35 days. Depletion in the white cell content of red cell products to less than 5×10^6/unit reduces the incidence of reactions caused by human leukocyte antigen (HLA) alloimmunization and of transfusion of CMV or prions. (Courtesy of G. Hazlehurst.)

CLINICAL BLOOD TRANSFUSION

A schedule of the normal quantities of blood ordered by type of surgical procedure is set at hospital level (Fig. 29-9). In some patients, especially those with sickle cell anemia, exchange transfusion is needed, which can be carried out using a cell separator (Fig. 29-10) or manually in infants. A transfusion management guideline for major hemorrhage is given in the *Handbook of Transfusion Medicine,* fourth edition, edited by D. B. L. McClelland (Blood Services, 2007).

COMPLICATIONS OF BLOOD TRANSFUSION

Complications of blood transfusions include hemolytic reactions, immediate or delayed (Fig. 29-11), as a result of red cell incompatibilities, and allergic or pyrogenic reactions to white cells, platelets, or proteins. A number of other nonimmune reactions may occur acutely (e.g.,

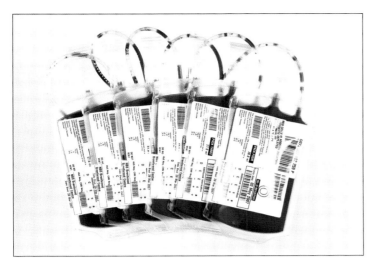

Fig. 29-8. Small volume neonatal transfusions: it is usually supplied as group O RhD-negative blood, which should be stored at 4° C for up to 35 days. It may be anti-CMV antibody negative, HbS negative, and have up to seven attached satellite bags. This enables a single unit of blood to be dedicated to an individual infant so that donor exposure is limited. Dosage is 10 to 20 ml/kg. (Courtesy of G. Hazlehurst.)

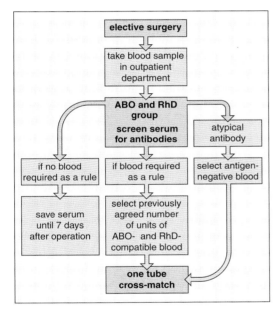

Fig. 29-9. Surgical blood ordering policy.

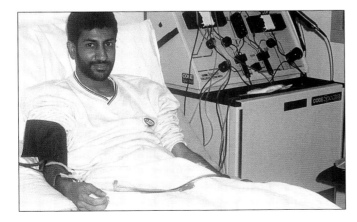

Fig. 29-10. Exchange transfusion: use of a cell separator to exchange red cells in a patient with sickle cell anemia. For neonatal exchange transfusion, use plasma-reduced blood in CPDA1 less than 5 days old, irradiated and CMV negative. A single volume (80 to 100 ml/kg) is used for anemia, and double volume (160 to 200 ml/kg) is used for hyperbilirubinemia.

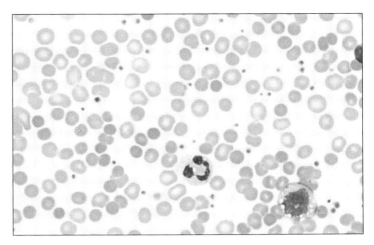

Fig. 29-11. Blood transfusion: delayed transfusion reaction. Peripheral blood film showing microspherocytes and polychromasia. (Courtesy of Dr. W. Erber.)

circulatory overload, air embolism, thrombophlebitis), as may complications of massive transfusion (e.g., clotting abnormalities, citrate toxicity, hyperkalemia) (Table 29-6). Massive transfusion is defined as replacement of one blood volume in 24 hours or of 50% blood volume in 3 hours or a rate of loss of 150 ml per minute in adults.

INFECTIONS

Immediate shock may occur after transfusion if the blood is infected, and a number of different infectious diseases may be transmitted. These may be bacterial, parasitic (Table 29-7), viral, or prions (Table 29-8).

TABLE 29-6.	BLOOD TRANSFUSION: COMPLICATIONS
Immunologic	

Sensitization to red cell antigens
  hemolytic transfusion reactions
  immediate (e.g., ABO)
  delayed (e.g., Rh)	

Reactions as a result of white cell and platelet antibodies
  febrile
  post-transfusion purpura	

Reactions as a result of plasma protein antibodies
  urticaria
  anaphylaxis (e.g., IgA-deficient recipient)	

Transfusion-related acute lung injury (TRALI)	
Graft versus host disease (if host severely immunocompromised)	
Non-immunologic	
Transmission of disease	
Reactions as a result of bacterial pyrogens and bacteria	
Circulation overload	
Thrombophlebitis	
Air embolism	
Transfusion hemosiderosis	
Complications of massive transfusion	
Coagulation abnormalities	
Citrate toxicity	
Hyperkalemia	

TABLE 29-7.   BLOOD TRANSFUSION: TRANSMISSIBLE BACTERIA AND PARASITES

Bacteria

Occasional bacterial contaminants (e.g., *Staphylococcus* spp, *Klebsiella*, *Pseudomonas*, *Salmonella*, *Sarcina*, *Micrococcus*)

Treponema pallidum (syphilis)

Yersinia enterocolitica

Brucellosis (donors giving a history are not accepted in the UK)

Borrelia burgdorferi (Lyme disease)

Parasites

Plasmodium spp. (malaria)

Trypanosoma cruzi (Chagas disease)
    endemic in Latin America, this parasite is present in 75% of seropositive subjects; up to 22% of donors in Latin America may be seropositive

Toxoplasma gondii
    Only a risk in granulocytes transfused to immunosuppressed seronegative recipients

Babesia microti (Nantucket fever)
    Potential risk in certain areas of North America

Leishmania spp

TABLE 29-8.   BLOOD TRANSFUSION: TRANSMISSIBLE VIRUSES; PRIONS ARE ALSO POTENTIALLY TRANSMISSIBLE

Plasma-borne viruses

Hepatitis B

Hepatitis A (rarely)

Hepatitis C

Parvovirus B19

HIV-1 and HIV-2

West Nile virus

Cell-associated viruses

Cytomegalovirus (CMV)

Epstein–Barr (EB) virus (more than 95% of adults are immune)

HTLV-1 (causes human T-cell leukemia and tropical spastic paraparesis)

HTLV-11 (clinical relevance not clear, may be more common than HTLV-1 in Western developed countries)

Prions

Transmissible by blood transfusion from asymptomatic donors

TABLE 29-9.   BLOOD DONATIONS: MANDATORY TESTING FOR INFECTIOUS AGENTS IN ENGLAND

Hepatitis B	Surface antigen
Anti-HCV	(On pools of 48 samples)
Anti-HIV-1, anti-HIV-2	HIV-1 antigen
Anti-HTLV	(On pools of 48 samples)
Anti-*Treponema pallidum*	
Anti-*Plasmodium falciparum*	
Anti-Chagas disease	

Prion Disease

Four definite cases of Creutzfeldt-Jacob disease (CJD) have been caused by blood transfusion. The donors have been traced and recipients informed and undergo surveillance. Also if patients with CJD have received blood, the donors are traced. It is clear that the disease can be transmitted by infectious agents (e.g., in pituitary-derived growth hormone and gonadotrophins). The cause of the disease is transmission of an abnormal form of a naturally occurring protein, prion (PrP). In prion disease, it is considered that a natural protein (PrP) is converted into an abnormal form (PrP scrapie or PrPSc). This has the ability to convert the normal protein, which has a multiple helical structure, into the abnormal variant in which much of the backbone is straightened out. The abnormal PrP may arise by a random change in a normal protein, which probably accounts for sporadic CJD. In familial CJD, a point mutation occurs in the DNA coding for the protein. Thus there is the potential for transmission of

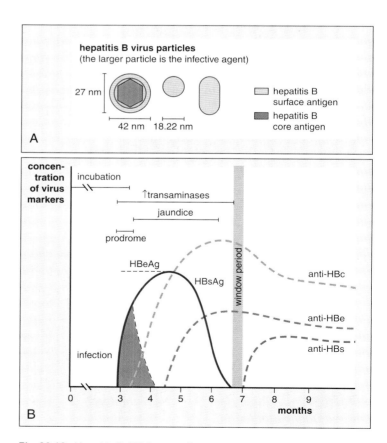

Fig. 29-12. Hepatitis B: **(A)** hepatitis B virus particles (the larger particle is the infective agent); **(B)** typical course of an acute infection with hepatitis B virus (HBV). (HbeAg, hepatitis Be antigen; HbsAg, hepatitis B surface antigen; HBc, hepatitis B core antigen.) (*A, B,* Courtesy of Professor M. Contreras and the NHS Blood Transfusion Service.)

Viruses

Viral infections are the most common, so blood donations are tested for these infectious agents (Table 29-9). Hepatitis B (Fig. 29-12, *A*) was frequently transmitted. A typical course of an acute infection is illustrated in Fig. 29-12, *B*. The sequelae may be cirrhosis and, in a minority of cases, hepatocellular carcinoma. A similar outcome may occur after hepatitis C infection (see Fig. 9-39). The risk that a donation is positive for human immunodeficiency virus (HIV) is now estimated to be 1 in 4.5 million, the risk that a donation is positive for hepatitis B is 1 in 450,000, and the risk that a donation is positive for hepatitis C is 1 in 20 million.

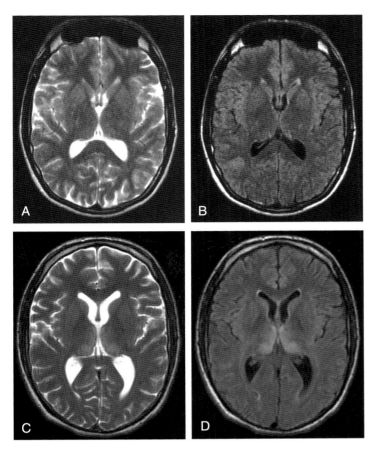

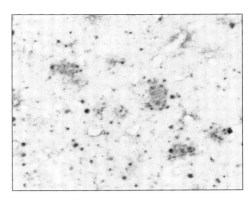

Fig. 29-15. New variant Creutzfeldt-Jacob disease (nvCJD): immunocytochemistry for PrP in the occipital cortex in nvCJD shows strong staining of individual plaques, with diffuse PrP deposits around neurons and blood vessels (KG9 monoclonal antibody). (Courtesy of Dr. J. W. Ironside.)

Fig. 29-13. New variant Creutzfeldt-Jacob (nvCJD) disease: magnetic resonance imaging (MRI) appearances late in the clinical course. **A, B,** Normal appearances on T_2 and FLAIR. **C, D,** Abnormal increased T_2 and FLAIR: high signal within the posteromedial thalamus 18 months later. (Wroe SJ, Pal S, Siddique D et al: Clinical presentation and pre-mortem diagnosis of variant Creutzfeldt-Jakob disease associated with blood transfusion: a case report, *Lancet* 368: 2061-2067, 2006. Courtesy of Proffesor John Collinge.)

the disease to recipients of the blood, if it is present in the blood of asymptomatic individuals. New variant CJD (nvCJD) is caused by the same prion as bovine spongiform encephalitis (BSE; Figs 29-13 to 29-17). Non-U.K. plasma is now used for fractionation. Potential blood donors who have themselves received blood or blood product transfusion are excluded as donors.

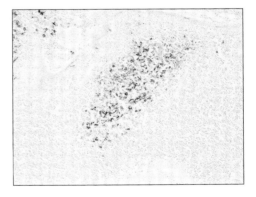

Fig. 29-16. New variant Creutzfeldt-Jacob disease (nvCJD): the tonsil in a 27-year-old woman with nvCJD shows positive staining for PrP within the germinal center in follicular dendritic cells (KG9 monoclonal antibody). (Courtesy of Dr. J. W. Ironside.)

IRON OVERLOAD

Iron overload may become a major clinical problem in multitransfused anemic patients. In such cases, iron chelation therapy is required (see Chapter 9).

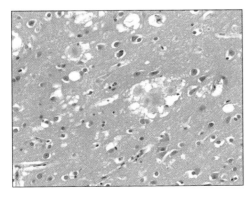

Fig. 29-14. New variant Creutzfeldt-Jacob disease (nvCJD): frontal cortex from a 22-year-old man with nvCJD showing the characteristic florid plaques (center), which are composed of aggregates of the prion protein. (Courtesy of Dr. J. W. Ironside.)

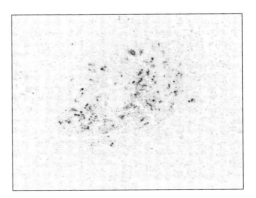

Fig. 29-17. New variant Creutzfeldt-Jacob disease (nvCJD): follicular dendritic cells in the spleen surrounding a small arteriole show strong positive staining for PrP in a 32-year-old woman with nvCJD (3F4 monoclonal antibody). (Courtesy of Dr. J. W. Ironside.)

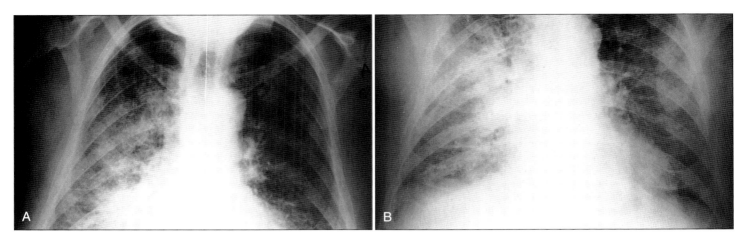

Fig. 29-18. Transfusion-related acute lung injury: chest radiographs **(A)** 3 hours and **(B)** 48 hours after onset of dyspnea in a 55-year-old man receiving chemotherapy for acute myeloid leukemia. The patient had received 1 unit of platelets 12 hours before the onset of symptoms, then 4 units of blood and a further unit of platelets 30 minutes before the onset. The patient was treated with high-dose corticosteroids and made a full recovery, with chest radiographs clear 7 days after onset of symptoms. (*A, B,* Courtesy of Dr. A. Virchis.)

TRANSFUSION-RELATED ACUTE LUNG INJURY

Transfusion-related acute lung injury (TRALI) is an acute respiratory distress syndrome, resembling adult respiratory distress syndrome, that occurs within 6 hours (rarely, 1 to 2 days). It is characterized by dyspnea and hypoxia, with transient pulmonary infiltrates on chest radiographs (Fig. 29-18). Oxygen support is needed and mechanical ventilation is needed in more than 50% of patients. It is rare, occurring in about 1 in 5000 transfusions, and patients usually (greater than 90%) recover. The etiology is unclear; it may result from a combination of different mechanisms, including reaction of the recipient's neutrophils with human leukocyte antigen (HLA) or neutrophil antibodies in donor plasma, which leads to increased permeability in the pulmonary circulation, or from cell membrane–derived lipids in the donor plasma priming the recipient's neutrophils. The donors are often multiparous women and, once identified as the cause of a reaction, should be removed from the donor panel. All U.K. fresh frozen plasma (FFP) is now prepared from male donors.

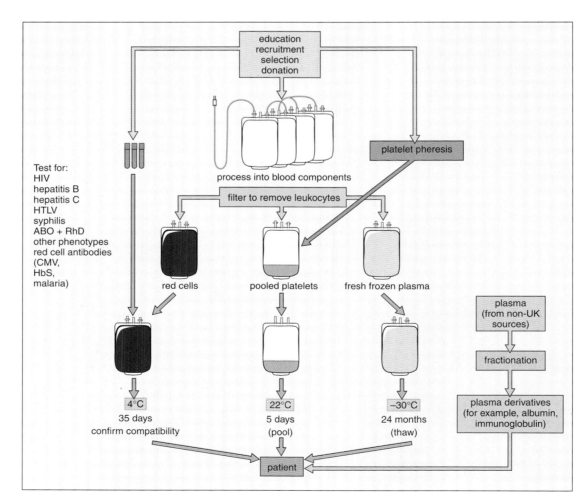

Fig. 29-19. Production of blood components and plasma derivatives: preparation. (Adapted from McClelland DBL, editor: *Handbook of transfusion medicine,* ed 4, 2007, United Kingdom Blood Services.)

GRAFT-VERSUS-HOST DISEASE

Transfusion of viable lymphocytes to a heavily immunosuppressed host may result in "grafting" of the lymphocytes, which may proliferate in the host and cause a disease similar to graft-versus-host disease (GVHD) in stem cell transplant recipients. Transfusion GVHD is rare, is likely to be associated with marrow aplasia and pancytopenia, and is usually fatal. It is diagnosed by finding lymphocytes in the blood of the recipient that are of the HLA type of the donor, and it is prevented by irradiation of all blood products before transfusion into immunosuppressed patients.

OTHER BLOOD COMPONENTS

The preparation of blood components from whole blood is illustrated in Fig. 29-19.

PLATELET CONCENTRATES

Platelet concentrates may be prepared from whole blood donors (Fig. 29-20) or from a single donor apheresis (see Fig. 19-21). They are required for patients with severe thrombocytopenia as a result of bone marrow failure (e.g., caused by acute leukemia, myelodysplasia, aplastic anemia, chemotherapy, or radiotherapy). The usual adult therapeutic dose (ATD) is 2.5 to 3.0 × 10^{11}/L platelets. They are used prophylactically because the platelet count is extremely low, less than 5 × 10^9/L, or likely to fall that low, or is 10 to 20 × 10^9/L and associated with infection; or before minor surgery (e.g., liver biopsy, insertion of indwelling catheter), or in patients with less severe degrees of thrombocytopenia (and established hemorrhage) to raise the platelet count to greater than 50 × 10^9/L.

Patients with platelet functional defects require platelet support at higher platelet counts. Platelets express only HLA Class I antigens, whereas leukocytes express both HLA Class I and Class II antigens. Both are required to stimulate the reticuloendothelial system to make HLA antibodies. These antibodies may cause refractoriness to mixed-platelet pools. If this occurs, HLA-compatible platelets may be needed, from a special tissue-typed panel of donors.

LEUKOCYTES

Leukocytes are not often used because of the difficulties in obtaining sufficient quantities, their short life span in vivo, the lack of data on a beneficial effect, and the danger of transmission of disease (e.g., cytomegalovirus [CMV]). Buffy coat preparations or cells harvested by leukapheresis from patients with chronic myeloid leukemia may have a restricted place in therapy, particularly in severely neutropenic patients with local infections.

FRESH FROZEN PLASMA

Fresh frozen plasma (FFP; Fig. 29-22) is provided in doses of 240 to 300 ml and in pediatric doses of 50 ml. It is used to replace clotting factors, for example, in patients after massive transfusion or

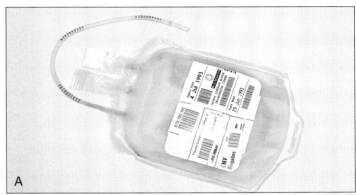

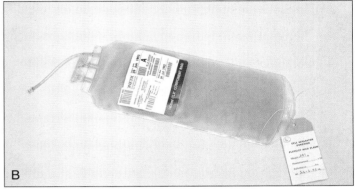

Fig. 29-21. Platelet concentrates **(A)** from a single donor. These platelet concentrates are derived from a single blood donation and are approximately 50 ml in volume. The concentrate is derived from CPDA-1 plasma and contains platelets >55×10^9 and leukocytes <0.05×10^9 per unit. Platelets should be maintained at 22° C, and they have a shelf life of 5 days. **(B)** Platelet concentrates can also be made by apheresis from a single donor. These platelet concentrates are approximately 215 ml in volume and contain about 290 × 10^9 platelets and 0.3×10^6 white cells per pack. In addition, they may be HLA-matched or cross-matched to be compatible with recipient serum in cases of refractory patients. (Courtesy of G. Hazlehurst.)

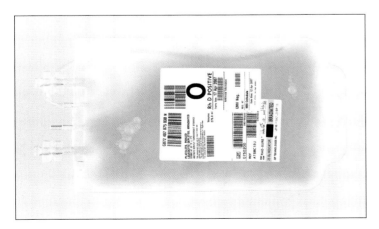

Fig. 29-20. Platelet pool: this may be derived from four to six donors depending on the place of manufacture. When produced by the buffy coat method a pool of platelets contains more than 250 × 10^9/L platelets per pool.

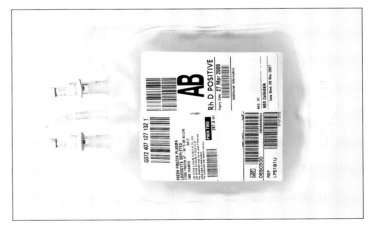

Fig. 29-22. Fresh frozen plasma (FFP): this is provided in 240 to 300 ml volumes including adult and pediatric doses. It can be supplied from volunteer plasmapheresis donors or recovered from routine blood donations. Illustrated here is a 240 ml FFP pack anticoagulated with CPDA-1. It should be stored at −30° C, and will then keep for up to 2 years. It should not be used as a plasma expander. Its use should be monitored with tests of coagulation when administered to correct a documented coagulation abnormality. (Courtesy of G. Hazlehurst.)

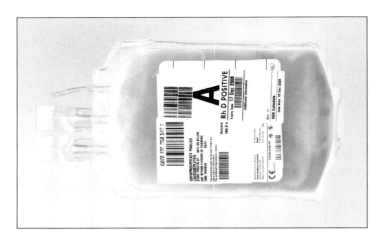

Fig. 29-23. Batched cryoprecipitate: individual cryoprecipitates from different donors may be batched together in groups of six to represent an adult dose. Each unit contains approximately 20 ml and is derived from CPDA-1 plasma. It contains fibrinogen greater than 140 mg per unit and factor VIII greater than 70 IU per unit. It should be stored at −30° C and has a shelf life of 1 year. In general, group A donors have higher levels of factor VIII than group O donors. (Courtesy of G. Hazlehurst.)

cardiopulmonary bypass, in liver disease, or for plasma exchange in thrombotic thrombocytopenic purpura (see p. 440). The dose is 15 to 20 ml/kg body weight, monitored by coagulation factor assays. Prothrombin complex concentrates are now preferred over FFP to reverse a warfarin effect in a bleeding patient.

Cryoprecipitate (Fig. 29-23) is obtained by thawing FFP at 4° C, and is widely used as a replacement for fibrinogen if no concentrate is available.

PLASMA DERIVATIVES

Human albumin solution (4.5%) is used mainly to treat shock. Human albumin solution (20%) is used for patients with severe hypoalbuminemia (e.g., with liver disease or nephrotic syndrome).

Clotting factor concentrates (e.g., factor VIII or factor IX) and immunoglobulin concentrates can also be made from human plasma (Fig. 29-22). Other concentrates include fibrinogen and prothrombin complex concentrated (which contain zymogen or activated IX, VII, and to a lesser extend X, XI, and thrombin) with or without factor X.

INDEX

Page numbers followed by t indicate tables.

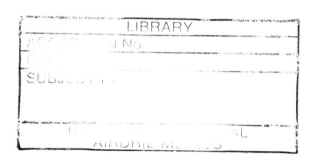
LIBRARY